Knee Ligament Rehabilitation

Todd S. Ellenbecker, MS, PT, SCS, CSCS
Clinic Director
Physiotherapy Associates[SM]
Scottsdale Sports Clinic
Scottsdale, Arizona

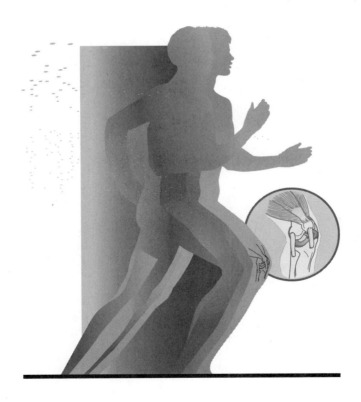

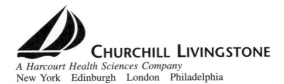
CHURCHILL LIVINGSTONE
A Harcourt Health Sciences Company
New York   Edinburgh   London   Philadelphia

CHURCHILL LIVINGSTONE
A Harcourt Health Sciences Company

The Curtis Center
Independence Square West
Philadelphia, Pennsylvania 19106

Library of Congress Cataloging-in-Publication Data

Knee ligament rehabilitation/[edited by] Todd S. Ellenbecker.

p.; cm.

ISBN 0–443–07534–4

1. Knee—Wounds and injuries—Patients—Rehabilitation.   2. Ligaments—
   Wounds and injuries—Patients—Rehabilitation.   3. Knee—Surgery —
   Patients — Rehabilitation.   I. Ellenbecker, Todd S.
   [DNLM: 1. Knee Injuries—rehabilitation.   2. Ligaments, Articular—
   injuries.   3. Ligaments, Articular—surgery.   4. Reconstructive Surgical
   Procedures—rehabilitation.   WE 870 K6741 2000]

RD561.K576 2000

617.5′82044—dc21   99–089460

Acquisitions Editor: Andrew Allen
Project Manager: Mary Anne Folcher
Production Manager: Peter Faber
Illustration Specialist: Francis Moriarty
Book Designer: Steven Stave

KNEE LIGAMENT REHABILITATION   ISBN 0–443–07534–4

Printed in the United States of America.

Last digit is the print number: 9   8   7   6   5   4   3   2   1

To my wife, Gail, whom I love dearly and thank for her constant support and love
To my grandmother, Hattie Meyer, who taught me the value of hard work, dedication, and devotion

Contributors

James R. Andrews, MD
Clinical Professor of Orthopaedic
   Surgery, Department of
   Orthopaedics, University of
   Alabama School of Medicine,
   University of Alabama at
   Birmingham; Orthopaedic Surgeon,
   Alabama Sports Medicine and
   Orthopaedic Center; Medical
   Director, American Sports Medicine
   Institute, Birmingham, Alabama;
   Medical Director, Tampa Bay Devil
   Rays Baseball Team, Tampa Bay,
   Florida
   *Assessment and Treatment of Medial
   Capsular Injuries*

Sue D. Barber-Westin, BS
Director, Clinical Studies, Cincinnati
   Sports Medicine Research and
   Education Foundation, Deaconess
   Hospital, Cincinnati, Ohio
   *Autogeneic and Allogeneic Anterior
   Cruciate Ligament Rehabilitation;
   Posterior Cruciate Ligament and
   Posterolateral Reconstruction*

Brian L. Becker, PT
Covington, Kentucky
   *Nonoperative Posterior Cruciate Ligament
   Rehabilitation*

John A. Bergfeld, MD
Medical Director, Cleveland Clinic
   Hospital; Team Physician, NFL
   Cleveland Browns, NBA Cleveland
   Cavaliers, and Cleveland Public
   Schools, Cleveland, Ohio
   *Posterolateral Instability; Posterior
   Cruciate Ligament Reconstruction and
   Rehabilitation*

Turner Blackburn, MEd, PT, ATC
Director, Tulane Institute of Sports
   Medicine, New Orleans, Louisiana
   *Proprioception and Balance Training and
   Testing Following Injury*

Richard R. Boeckmann, PT
Clinical Coordinator, Scottsdale Health
   Care, Grainey Ranch, Scottsdale,
   Arizona
   Biomechanics

Lori Thein Brody, MS, PT, SCS, ATC
Sports Specialty Track Chair, Rocky
   Mountain University of Physical
   Therapy, Provo, Utah; Senior Clinical
   Specialist, University of Wisconsin
   Sports Medicine Spine Center,
   Madison, Wisconsin
   *Anterior Cruciate Ligament Injury in the
   Female Athlete; Aquatic Therapy*

Gary J. Calabrese, PT
Director, Cleveland Clinic Sports
   Health and Orthopaedic
   Rehabilitation, Cleveland Clinic
   Hospital; Consulting Physical
   Therapist, NFL Cleveland Browns,
   NBA Cleveland Cavaliers, Cleveland,
   Ohio
   *Posterolateral Instability; Posterior
   Cruciate Ligament Reconstruction and
   Rehabilitation*

Patrick W. Cawley, OPA, RT, CRA
Vista, California
   Bracing: Science or Psychology?

Donald A. Chu, PhD, PT, ATC, CSCS
Professor and Director, Physical
   Therapist Assistant Program,
   Ohlone College, Newark Campus,
   Newark; Center Manager, NovaCare,
   Castro Valley, California
   Plyometrics in Rehabilitation

William G. Clancy, Jr, MD
Clinical Professor of Orthopaedic
  Surgery, Department of
  Orthopaedics, University of
  Alabama School of Medicine,
  University of Alabama at
  Birmingham; Orthopaedic Surgeon,
  Alabama Sports Medicine and
  Orthopaedic Center, Birmingham,
  Alabama
  *Assessment and Treatment of Medial
  Capsular Injuries*

Michael Clark, MS, PT, CSCS
Director, Sports Performance
  Physiotherapy Associates; Director
  of Sports Science, The Athletic
  Institute, Tempe, Arizona
  *Open and Closed Kinetic Chain
  Rehabilitation; Core Stabilization Training*

Nathaniel T. Cohen
New York, New York
  Effects of Instability on Articular Cartilage

H. Royer Collins, MD
Institute of Bone and Joint Disorders,
  Phoenix, Arizona
  *Synthetic Ligaments in Anterior Cruciate
  Ligament Reconstruction*

Douglas J. Cordier, MS, PT, ATC, CSCS
Physical Therapist, Outpatient Center,
  Baptist Hospital, Miami, Florida
  Plyometrics in Rehabilitation

P. Dean Cummings, MD
Medical Director, The Athletic
  Institute, Seneca, Pennsylvania
  Core Stabilization Training

J.F. James Davidson, MD
Chairman, Department of Surgery,
  Maryvale Samaritan Medical Center,
  Phoenix, Arizona
  *Synthetic Ligaments in Anterior Cruciate
  Ligament Reconstruction*

George J. Davies, MEd, PT, SCS, ATC, CSCS
Professor, Graduate Physical Therapy
  Program, University of Wisconsin-
  LaCrosse, LaCrosse; Director,
  Clinical and Research Services,
  Gundersen Lutheran Sports
  Medicine, Onalaska, Wisconsin
  *Open and Closed Kinetic Chain
  Rehabilitation; Functional Progression of
  Exercise During Rehabilitation*

Mark DeCarlo, MHA, PT, SCS, ATC
Chief Operating Officer, Methodist
  Sports Medicine Center,
  Indianapolis, Indiana
  Anterior Cruciate Ligament

Robert Donatelli, PhD, PT, OCS
Orthopaedic Track Chairman, DPT
  Program, Rocky Mountain
  University; National Director, Sports
  Rehabilitation Physiotherapy
  Association, Rocky Mountain
  University, Provo, Utah
  Foot Mechanics and Knee Pathology

Todd S. Ellenbecker, MS, PT, SCS, CSCS
Clinic Director, Physiotherapy
  Associates^SM, Scottsdale Sports
  Clinic, Scottsdale, Arizona
  *Biomechanics; Clinical Examination;
  Isokinetics in Rehabilitation*

Gregory M. Fox, MD
Clinical Assistant Professor,
  Department of Orthopaedics,
  Indiana University School of
  Medicine; Orthopaedic Surgeon,
  Bloomington Bone and Joint Clinic,
  Bloomington, Indiana
  *Assessment and Treatment of Medial
  Capsular Injuries*

William Garrett, Jr, MD, PhD
Professor and Chairman, Orthopaedic
  Surgery; Vice-Chairman of Staff,
  University of North Carolina School
  of Medicine, Chapel Hill, North
  Carolina
  Neuromuscular Concepts

Bruce Greenfield, MMSc, PT, OCS
Instructor, Physical Therapy, Emory
  University, Atlanta, Georgia
  Foot Mechanics and Knee Pathology

**Ola Grimsby, PT, MOMT, MNSMT, FAA,
OMPT**
Ola Grimsby Institute, San Diego,
  California
  *Manual Therapy Approach to Knee
  Ligament Rehabilitation*

Timothy P. Heckmann, PT, ATC
Administrator, HealthSouth Sports
  Medicine and Rehabilitation Center,
  Cincinnati, Ohio
*Autogeneic and Allogeneic Anterior
Cruciate Ligament Rehabilitation;
Posterior Cruciate Ligament and
Posterolateral Reconstruction*

Bryan C. Heiderscheit, MS, PT, CSCS
Teaching Assistant, Physical
  Therapist, University Health Center,
  University of Massachusetts–
  Amherst, Amherst, Massachusetts
*Open and Closed Kinetic Chain
Rehabilitation; Optimizing Treatment of
Joint Contracture Following
Reconstruction*

Ron M. Johnson, PT, MPT, ATC, LAT, CSCS
HealthSouth Sports Medicine,
  Houston, Texas
Instrumented Examination

David Joseph, MD
New York, New York
Effects of Instability on Articular Cartilage

W. Ben Kibler, MD
Medical Director, Lexington Sports
  Medicine Center, Lexington,
  Kentucky
Kinetic Chain Concept

Thomas Klootwyk, MD
Orthopaedic Surgeon, Methodist
  Sports Medicine Center,
  Indianapolis, Indiana
Anterior Cruciate Ligament

Janice Kuperstein, PT, MSEd, Del-CHA
Assistant Professor, Physical Therapy,
  College of Allied Health, University
  of Kentucky, Lexington, Kentucky
Neuromuscular Concepts

Terry Malone, EdD, PT, ATC
Professor and Director of Physical
  Therapy, College of Allied Health,
  University of Kentucky, Lexington,
  Kentucky
Neuromuscular Concepts

Robert E. Mangine, MEd, PT, ATC
Covington, Kentucky
*Nonoperative Posterior Cruciate Ligament
Rehabilitation*

Jenny McConnell, BApp Sci (Phty)
Director, McConnell Institute, Neutral
  Bay, NSW, Australia
*Patellofemoral Joint Complications and
Considerations*

Van C. Mow, PhD
Professor of Mechanical Engineering,
  Orthopaedic Engineering; Director,
  Orthopaedic Research Laboratory,
  Columbia University, New York, New
  York
Effects of Instability on Articular Cartilage

Michael J. Mullin, ATC, PTA
Coordinator of Rehab Services, The
  Stone Clinic, Orthopaedic Surgery,
  Sports Medicine and Rehabilitation,
  San Francisco, California
*New Techniques for Cartilage Repair and
Replacement*

Arthur J. Nitz, PhD, PT, OCS, ECS
Professor, Physical Therapy, College of
  Allied Health, University of
  Kentucky, Lexington, Kentucky
Neuromuscular Concepts

Frank R. Noyes, MD
Clinical Professor, Department of
  Orthopaedic Surgery, University of
  Cincinnati Medical Center; Director,
  Cincinnati Sportsmedicine and
  Orthopaedic Center; Director,
  Cincinnati Sportsmedicine Research
  and Education Foundation,
  Cincinnati, Ohio
*Autogeneic and Allogeneic Anterior
Cruciate Ligament Rehabilitation;
Posterior Cruciate Ligament and
Posterolateral Reconstruction*

Kathy Oneacre, MA, ATC
Research Coordinator, Physical
  Therapy, Methodist Sports Medicine
  Center, Indianapolis, Indiana
Anterior Cruciate Ligament

Russell M. Paine, PT
Associate Clinical Professor, Texas
  Woman's University; Rehabilitation
  Consultant, Houston Rockets and
  NASA, Houston, Texas
Instrumented Examination

Brian Power, PT, MOMT
Physical Therapist, Atlanta, Georgia
Manual Therapy Approach to Knee Ligament Rehabilitation

Michael S. Roh, MD
New York, New York
Effects of Instability on Articular Cartilage

David A. Schulz, PT, CSCS
Physical Therapist, Physiotherapy Associates, Mesa, Arizona
Anatomy

K. Donald Shelbourne, MD
Associate Professor, Indiana University School of Medicine; Orthopaedic Surgeon, Methodist Sports Medicine Center, Indianapolis, Indiana
Anterior Cruciate Ligament Reconstruction: Evolution of Rehabilitation

Kevin R. Stone, MD
Orthopaedic Surgeon, The Stone Clinic; Chairman, The Stone Foundation for Sports Medicine and Arthritis Research, San Francisco, California
New Techniques for Cartilage Repair and Replacement

Jill M. Thein, MPT, ATC
Faculty Associate, University of Wisconsin–Madison, Madison, Wisconsin
Aquatic Therapy

Rocci V. Trumper, MD
Orthopaedic Center of the Rockies, Fort Collins, Colorado
Anterior Cruciate Ligament Reconstruction: Evolution of Rehabilitation

Michael Voight, DPT, OCS, SCS, ATC
Associate Professor, School of Physical Therapy, Belmont University, Nashville, Tennessee
Proprioception and Balance Training and Testing Following Injury

Kevin E. Wilk, PT
Adjunct Associate Professor, Programs in Physical Therapy, Marquette University, Milwaukee, Wisconsin; National Director, Research and Clinical Education, HealthSouth Rehabilitation; Associate Clinical Director, HealthSouth Sports Medicine and Rehabilitation Center, Birmingham, Alabama; Rehabilitation Consultant, Tampa Bay Devil Rays Baseball Team, Tampa Bay, Florida
Assessment and Treatment of Medial Capsular Injuries

Debra A. Zillmer, MD, PT
Adjunct Clinical Professor, University of Wisconsin–LaCrosse, LaCrosse, Wisconsin; Medical Director, Athletic Training Program, Winona State University, Winona, Minnesota; Orthopaedic Surgeon, Gundersen Lutheran Sports Medicine, LaCrosse, Wisconsin
Functional Progression of Exercise During Rehabilitation

Preface

As a young student in physical therapy school in the mid 1980s, I was given a small, information-rich book called *Rehabilitation of the Surgical Knee*. In this paperback book were the current state-of-the-art guidelines for knee rehabilitation written by leaders in the field of orthopedic and sports physical therapy. Issues regarding immobilization and range-of-motion restriction and protection, as well as isokinetic strengthening and exercise progression, were discussed by therapists such as George Davies, Terry Malone, and Bob Mangine. It is a text that I have to this day. It provided me with an invaluable resource as I began treating patients with knee ligament injuries, both non-operative and postoperative.

This revised edition of *Knee Ligament Rehabilitation* is released in the new millennium with exactly the same purpose as that paperback text that I read as a student: to provide current state-of-the-art information for specialists of rehabilitation of the knee with a ligament injury. Much has clearly changed since the first edition of this text was expertly edited by Robert Engle.

To address and update the changes in surgical and rehabilitative concepts, this edition contains specific chapters on collateral and cruciate ligament reconstruction and rehabilitation. Two chapters deal with evaluation and treatment of injury to the posterolateral structures of the knee. Updates in biomechanical research and instrumented evaluation methods are included. The changes in current rehabilitation focus are reflected in the inclusion of chapters on open and closed chain rehabilitation, functional progression, core stabilization, and kinetic link concepts. New areas in rehabilitation, such as that of the female athlete as well as aquatic therapy, are also included in this revision of *Knee Ligament Rehabilitation*.

The continuing challenges in rehabilitation of the patient with knee ligament injury are addressed with chapters that detail patellofemoral complications, range-of-motion limitation, and effects of ligamentous instability on articular cartilage. It is hoped that this text will provide a detailed, research-oriented reference for the clinician to assist in the rehabilitation of the patient with knee ligament injury.

TODD S. ELLENBECKER, MS, PT, SCS, CSCS

Acknowledgments

My career has been guided by several individuals who deserve special mention. I must thank and acknowledge George Davies, Janet Sobel, and Gary Derscheid for their tremendous gifts of mentorship, something that I am completely thankful for and can never repay. I would also like to thank David Feiring and Paul Roetert for their professional guidance and research assistance, and to CE for always being there.

I would also like to thank the team of contributors that has been assembled. They devoted their time and talent to producing the chapters that contain current state-of-the-art information in their areas of expertise. The willingness of these clinicians, researchers, and contributors to write these chapters reflects their commitment to our profession and the advancement of knee ligament rehabilitation.

I would like to also thank Michael Wooden for giving me this and other opportunities, and Carol Bader, Marie Pelcin, Peter Faber, and Andrew Allen of Harcourt Health Sciences for their hard work in producing this text.

Contents

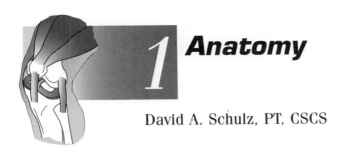

1 Anatomy

David A. Schulz, PT, CSCS

*T*he knee joint, or tibiofemoral joint, is the largest joint in the body. It is ginglymoid, or modified hinged, in nature, providing a large degree of range of motion.[1] The knee joint itself is able to move in six degrees of freedom: three translations (anterior-posterior, medial-lateral, and proximal-distal), and three rotations (internal-external, varus-valgus, and flexion-extension).[2] There is little inherent knee stability because the joint is located at the ends of two long lever arms, the femur and tibia; therefore, the joint greatly depends on muscular and ligamentous structures for stability and strength.[3] Secondary to this lack of osseous stability, soft tissue structures are required to withstand vast external forces, often resulting in tissue overload and injury. Consequently, knee injuries are common in the medical realm.[4] To adequately diagnose and treat knee injuries, a comprehensive understanding of general anatomy is essential.

In this chapter, the osseous and cartilagenous components of the knee are discussed as well as the dynamic and static soft tissue stabilizers of the joint.

OSSEOUS STRUCTURE

The knee joint consists of three bones: the proximal tibia, the distal femur, and the patella (Fig. 1–1). The tibiofemoral joint is the articulation between the distal femur and the proximal tibia. The weight-bearing surfaces on the femur are convex and asymmetric medial and lateral condyles are found on the distal end of the femur (Fig. 1–2). They blend anteriorly to create a shallow

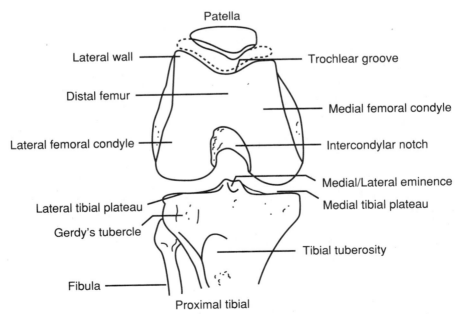

Figure 1–1. Osseous structure of the tibiofemoral joint. (From Engle R: Knee Ligament Rehabilitation. New York, Churchill Livingstone, 1991, p. 2.)

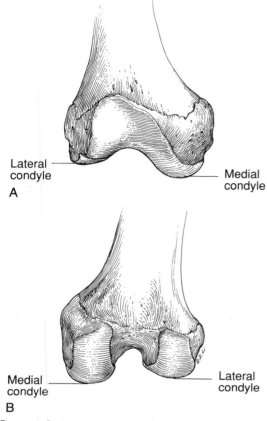

Lateral condyle

A

Medial condyle

Medial condyle

B

Lateral condyle

Figure 1–2. Anterior (A) and posterior (B) aspects of the distal femur. (From Tria AJ Jr, Klein KS: An Illustrated Guide to the knee. New York, Churchill Livingstone, 1992, p. 16.)

concave trochlear groove, in which the patella is positioned in an articulating fashion. Posteriorly, the condyles are separated by the intercondylar notch. The femoral condyles are convex in both the frontal and sagittal planes.[4-6] The articulating surface of the medial condyle is longer than the contact surface of the lateral condyle. The height of the lateral condyle's wall is greater along the trochlear groove, thereby aiding in prevention of lateral subluxation of the patella. Corresponding to the articulating surfaces of the femur are two concave and asymmetric plateaus on the proximal tibia (Fig. 1–3). The lateral and medial tibial plateaus are separated by two spines called the lateral and medial eminences or tubercles. Incongruencies and asymmetries exist between the medial and lateral tibial plateaus. First, the contact surface of the medial tibial plateau is 50 percent larger that that of the

lateral plateau (Fig. 1–4). Second, the lateral plateau is concave in the frontal plane and convex in the sagittal plane.[4, 7] It is this incongruency that permits several separate motions to occur at the tibiofemoral joint. Motion at the knee may be characterized as a combination of rolling, sliding, and spinning.

The patellofemoral joint is the articulation between the patella and the femur. The patella is characterized as a triangular sesamoid bone. Anteriorly, the patella is minimally convex in all directions. Distally, it is V-shaped and encompassed by the infrapatellar tendon. The lateral border of the patella is thinner than the medial border. Both borders nonetheless secure attachments of the synovium, joint capsule, and quadriceps expansion.[4] The femoral sulcus angle is normally considered to be 137 degrees (Fig. 1–5). The sulcus itself articulates with the patellar facets throughout the range of motion of the knee. The retropatellar surface is composed of seven facets, four on the medial side and three on the lateral aspect (Fig. 1–6). The medial facets are generally more convex and smaller than the lateral counterparts, which are not only larger but also more concave. The medial "odd facet" is nonarticulating except during full knee flexion, at which time there is minimal contact with the medial femoral condyle. As the knee proceeds from full extension into flexion, the distal patellar surface comes into contact with the femoral sulcus. The area of contact on the patella moves proximally and onto the medial and lateral facets as flexion advances. The zone of contact on the lateral and medial aspects of the femur moves distally from anterior to posterior as flexion proceeds.[8] In addition to improving the efficiency of the quadriceps during the final 30 degrees of extension, the patella also serves as a guide for the quadriceps tendon, diminishes friction of the quadriceps mechanism, controls knee capsular tension, and acts as a shield for femoral condyle cartilage.[3] Optimal tracking of the patella is essential for normal biomechanics. Tracking of the patellofemoral joint is deemed normal if the apex of the patella is centered in the femoral trochlear groove through all degrees of flexion.[9]

MENISCI

The menisci are asymmetric, wedge-shaped crescentic plates of fibrocartilage lo-

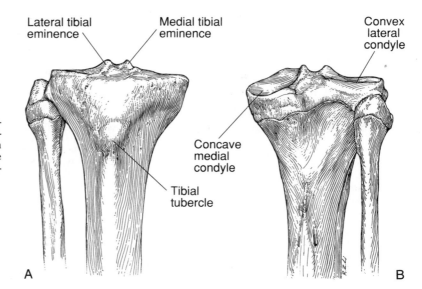

Figure 1–3. Anterior *(A)* and posterior *(B)* aspects of the proximal tibia. (From Tria AJ Jr, Klein KS: An Illustrated Guide to the knee. New York, Churchill Livingstone, 1992, p. 17.)

cated on the articular surface of the tibia. They are often referred to as the semilunar cartilages because of their shape (Fig. 1–7). Both menisci possess two fibrous horns: posterior and anterior. The outer portion of the meniscus is convex and the medial border is concave. The superior surface is concave, thereby deepening the tibial surface on which the femoral condyles roll, slide, and spin. The inferior surface of the meniscus is flat. In addition to deepening the articular surface of the tibia, the menisci serve as shock absorbers, transmitting approximately half the axial loads across the joint.[10–12] Research evidence indicates that removal of the meniscus via the surgical approach can lead to destructive degenerative articular changes as well as joint space narrowing, flattening of the femoral condyles,

and development of osteophytes.[13–15] Furthermore, the menisci are essential for joint stability, lubrication, and proprioception.[16]

The medial meniscus is C-shaped and is broader posteriorly than anteriorly. The posterior horn attaches to the posterior intercondylar area of the tibia, roughly 3 to 5 mm anterior to the anterior border of the posterior cruciate ligament. The anterior horn of the medial mensicus is made up of two separate segments. One segment extends anteriorly and inferiorly, attaching to the anterior intercondylar area of the tibia (approximately 5 to 8 mm anterior to the insertion site of the anterior cruciate ligament) (see Fig. 1–7). The second segment,

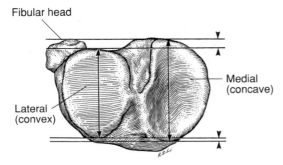

Figure 1–4. Contact surfaces of the medial and lateral tibial plateaus. (From Tria AJ Jr, Klein KS: An Illustrated Guide to the knee. New York, Churchill Livingstone, 1992, p. 17.)

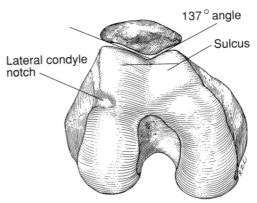

Figure 1–5. The femoral sulcus, illustrating an angle of 137 degrees. (From Tria AJ Jr, Klein KS: An Illustrated Guide to the knee. New York, Churchill Livingstone, 1992, p. 18.)

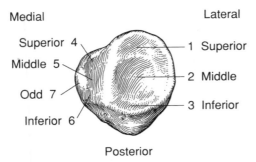

Medial Lateral

Superior 4 — 1 Superior

Middle 5 — 2 Middle

Odd 7 —

— 3 Inferior

Inferior 6

Posterior

Figure 1-6. Patellar facets. (From Tria AJ Jr, Klein KS: An Illustrated Guide to the knee. New York, Churchill Livingstone, 1992, p. 18.)

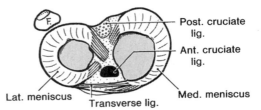

— Post. cruciate lig.

— Ant. cruciate lig.

Lat. meniscus Med. meniscus

Transverse lig.

Figure 1-8. Transverse ligament uniting the anterior horns of the medial and lateral menisci. (From Moore KL: Clinically Oriented Anatomy, 2nd ed. Baltimore, Williams & Wilkins, 1985, p. 537.)

situated more posteriorly, gives rise to the transverse ligament.[17] The transverse ligament unites the anterior horns of both menisci (Fig. 1-8). The external margins of the medial meniscus are attached to the tibial condyles via capsular fibers known as the coronary ligaments. Deep fibers of the medial or tibial collateral ligament and joint capsule additionally secure the periphery of the medial third of the medial meniscus.[18]

The lateral meniscus is larger than its medial counterpart and is much more circular.

It is consistent in width throughout. The posterior horn of the lateral meniscus is secured posterior to the intercondylar eminence of the tibia, just anterior to the central attachment of the posterior horn of the medial meniscus. The anterior horn is affixed to the tibia anterior to the intercondylar eminence, approximately 3 to 4 mm posterior and lateral to the site of the anterior cruciate ligament attachment to the tibia (see Fig. 1-7). The meniscofemoral ligaments stabilize the posterior horn of the lateral meniscus. Humphry's ligament extends from the posterolateral aspect of the meniscus anteri-

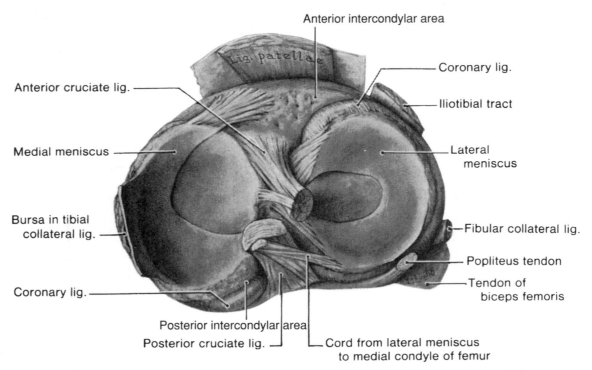

Anterior intercondylar area

Coronary lig.

Anterior cruciate lig. —

Iliotibial tract

Medial meniscus —

Lateral meniscus

Bursa in tibial collateral lig. —

Fibular collateral lig.

Popliteus tendon

Tendon of biceps femoris

Coronary lig. —

Posterior intercondylar area

Posterior cruciate lig. — Cord from lateral meniscus to medial condyle of femur

Figure 1-7. Attachment sites of the medial and lateral menisci. Additionally note tibial attachments of the cruciate and coronary ligaments. (From Moore KL: Clinically Oriented Anatomy, 2nd ed. Baltimore, Williams & Wilkins, 1985, p. 537.)

orly into the medial femoral condyle, passing anterior to the posterior cruciate ligament. Wrisberg's ligament also extends from the posterolateral meniscus to the medial femoral condyle. The latter, however, passes posterior to the posterior cruciate ligament. Both are intimately related to the posterior cruciate ligament. It is thought that either one of these two ligaments may be present in up to 70 percent of individuals.[8, 17, 19] The coronary ligaments bind the peripheral margin of the lateral meniscus, except posterolaterally where the popliteus tendon crosses obliquely, laterally, and upward.[17] Since the lateral meniscus does not attach to the fibular (lateral) collateral ligament and is interrupted by the presence of the popliteus tendon, it has greater mobility than does the medial meniscus. This increased mobility decreases the incidence of damage to the lateral meniscus during torsion injuries.[20–23] The medial and lateral menisci receive vascularization from the medial and lateral geniculate arteries. Branches of the geniculate arteries form a perimensical capillary plexus within the knee joint capsular tissues and synovium. It is by this freely branching network of capillaries that the border of the meniscus is supplied through its direct attachment to the joint capsule. Studies have illustrated that vascular penetration may be 10 to 30 percent of the width of the medial meniscus and 10 to 25 percent of the width of the lateral meniscus.[4, 24, 25]

PRIMARY LIGAMENTS

Anterior Cruciate Ligament

The anterior cruciate ligament (ACL) arises from the posterior aspect of the medial surface of the lateral femoral condyle. It then travels anteriorly, medially, and distally to insert onto the tibial plateau anterior and lateral to the anterior tibial spine. The tibial attachment of the ACL is generally stronger and wider than the femoral attachment, as the ligament has a tendency to "fan out" as it proceeds distally (see Fig. 1–7). At the same time, the ACL laterally twists approximately 5 mm distal to the femoral attachment. This twist is more pronounced with knee flexion.[26–28] The ACL is attached to the femoral and tibial surfaces as an aggregation of individual fascicles rather than as a dis-

tinct single cord. The ACL may be divided into separate bands: the anteromedial and the posterolateral. The anteromedial band, coursing from the posterior medial surface of the lateral femoral condyle to the anteromedial aspect of the tibial attachment, is taut in flexion and lax in extension. The posterolateral bundle or band, consisting of the remaining fascicles off the posterolateral aspect of the tibial attachment and medial surface of the lateral femoral condyle, is thought to represent the largest portion of the ACL. The posterolateral band is tight in extension and lax in flexion.[29–31] The orientation of the anteromedial and posterolateral bands furnishes a general idea of the dynamics of the ACL but in many respects may be an oversimplification. Between the two bands there is a continuum or intermediate region that allows a portion of the ACL to remain tight throughout the range of motion of the knee. In addition, in the cruciate ligaments, each fiber has a unique point of origin and insertion. These fibers are not always parallel and are often of unequal length. The significance of this type of structure is that different groups of fascicles may function together throughout the joint range of motion.[32] The primary function of the ACL is to prevent anterior translation of the tibia on the femur. It furthermore checks external rotation of the tibia in flexion and assists in controlling the normal rolling and gliding movement of the knee.[3]

Posterior Cruciate Ligament

The posterior cruciate ligament (PCL) arises from the posterior aspect of the tibial intercondylar region and travels anteromedially behind the ACL to the lateral surface of the medial femoral condyle (see Fig. 1–7).[18] The cruciate ligaments are intra-articular but extrasynovial. The synovium, resembling a mesentery, lines the entire capsule but is cast back from the posterior capsule covering the cruciate ligaments. This overlying synovial membrane ordinarily does not allow joint fluid to enter the extrasynovial space of the cruciate ligaments. As a result, fluid accumulations in the extrasynovial space as seen on magnetic resonance images are likely to come from direct cruciate ligament injury.[33] The posterior aspect of the PCL merges with the posterior capsule and periosteum. The fascicular PCL, like the ACL, is made up of two separate bundles: anterolateral and posteromedial. The anterolateral bundle is taut in flexion and the posteromedial component is taut in extension. It has been found that the anterolateral component has a notably greater linear stiffness and ultimate load than the posteromedial component and meniscofemoral ligaments (ligaments of Humphry and Wrisberg).[34-36] The PCL is considered the strongest ligament in the knee. Its primary function is to prevent posterior translation of the tibia on the femur. The PCL additionally serves to prevent hyperextension at the knee, maintain rotary stability, and act as the knee's central axis of rotation.[3]

Medial (Tibial) Collateral Ligament

The medial collateral ligament originates at the adductor tubercle on the medial femoral condyle and advances distally to insert into the medial tibial diaphysis approximately 3 to 4 inches below the joint line inferior to the insertion of the pes anserinus (Fig. 1–9). It consists of two separate layers: superficial and deep. Both layers originate at the adductor tubercle. As they pass distally, the deep layer diverges, inserting into the medial meniscus. This attachment serves to stabilize and secure the medial semilunar cartilage. From the inferior aspect of the medial meniscus, the deep layer continues and proceeds again distally until it

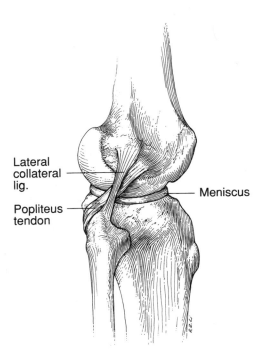

Figure 1–10. Lateral collateral ligament, passing over the popliteus tendon. (From Tria AJ Jr, Klein KS: An Illustrated Guide to the knee. New York, Churchill Livingstone, 1992, p. 19.)

merges with the superficial layer, where both insert onto the medial side of the tibia. The medial collateral ligament and associated capsular structures are strong stabilizers of the medial aspect of the knee, protecting against valgus stresses and tibial external rotation stresses, most notably when the knee is flexed.[8, 37]

Lateral (Fibular) Collateral Ligament

The lateral collateral ligament, round and pencil-like, is much shorter and smaller than the medial collateral ligament. It originates from the lateral femoral condyle, passes distally and posteriorly over the popliteus tendon and inserts onto the lateral proximal fibular head (Fig. 1–10). This separates the lateral meniscus from the lateral collateral ligament and gives the meniscus the previously discussed increased freedom of movement. The lateral collateral ligament additionally serves to split the tendon of the distal biceps femoris as it inserts into the head of the fibula. The tendon of the biceps femoris is easily palpable and serves as a

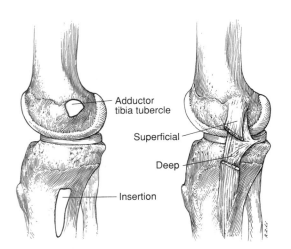

Figure 1–9. The medial collateral ligament. (From Tria AJ Jr, Klein KS: An Illustrated Guide to the knee. New York, Churchill Livingstone, 1992, p. 19.)

guide to the insertion of the distal end of the fibular collateral ligament. The lateral collateral ligament protects against varus stresses at the knee. Injury to this ligament is rare secondary to its great strength and the rarity of lateral joint line stresses or medial knee blows during competitive and noncompetitive activities.[18]

CAPSULAR AND SUPPORTING STRUCTURES

Medial Aspect of the Knee

According to Warren and Marshall,[38] the medial aspect of the knee may be subdivided into three separate layers consisting of the superficial layer (I), the intermediate or middle layer (II), and the deep layer (III), commonly referred to as the true joint capsule (Fig. 1–11).

The superficial layer I is encompassed by the crural fascia that envelops the sartorius muscle. Layer I unites anteriorly with layer II to attach to the medial patellar retinaculum and, in turn, the patella. This layer is further reinforced by fascial fibers of the vastus medialis. Posteriorly, layer I overlies the heads of the gastrocnemius and the popliteal fossa. The semitendinosus and gracilis tendons are located beneath layer I proximally, but merge with this layer proximal to the pes anserinus.

Layer II consists of the superficial portion of the medial collateral ligament (superficial medial ligament). This ligament unites with layer III posteriorly to surround the posterior medial condyle. The superficial medial ligament is separated from the deep medial ligament (layer III) by fat and intervening bursal tissue.[39, 40] At the anterior border of the superficial medial ligament, layer II is divided in a vertical plane. Fibers traveling anterior to this cut-off point join layer I and

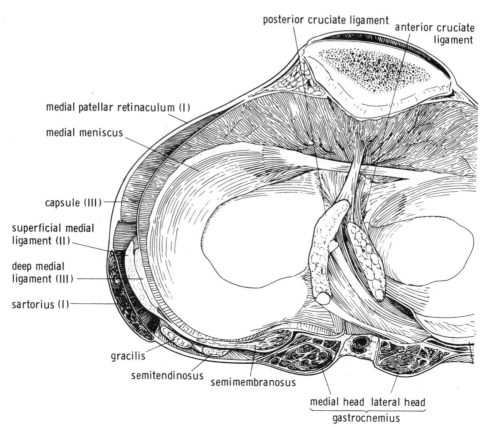

Figure 1–11. Anatomy of the medial compartment. (From Tria AJ Jr, Klein KS: An Illustrated Guide to the knee. New York, Churchill Livingstone, 1992, p. 212.)

the fibers of the vastus medialis to create the patellar retinaculum.

Layer III is considered the true capsule of the knee. This layer is securely attached to the medial meniscus. The deep medial ligament (middle capsular ligament or deep portion of the tibial collateral ligament), as noted earlier, is found in this layer. Posteriorly, layer III joins with layer II to form the posteromedial capsule. The semimembranosus muscle, inserting into the posteromedial aspect of the tibia behind the tibial collateral ligament, reinforces the posteromedial capsule. The semimembranosus insertion has five reflections: one insertion into the rim of the medial meniscus; one into the medial tibial metaphysis beneath the superficial medial collateral ligament insertion; one across the posterior knee, intensifying the oblique popliteal ligament; one into the fascia covering the popliteus; and one into the posteromedial tibia. The pouch of the posteromedial capsule, formed by layers II and III and the semimembranosus, surrounds the posterior medial femoral condyle and gives it rotational support. Anteriorly, layer III is separate from the retinacular fibers. Superiorly, this layer is secured firmly to the medial femoral condyle.

Lateral Aspect of the Knee

Seebacher et al.[41] have divided the lateral aspect of the knee likewise into three distinct layers: the superficial layer (I), the intermediate layer (II), and the capsule layer (III) (Fig. 1–12).

The superficial layer I of the lateral aspect of the knee is created anteriorly by the iliotibial tract expansion and posteriorly by the expansion of the biceps femoris muscle. Layer I extends from the prepatellar bursa to the popliteal fossa. It blends with layer II anteriorly to create a thick, well-defined band.

Layer II encompasses the lateral collateral ligament. The lateral collateral ligament, running from the lateral femoral condyle to the fibular head, is covered by the superficial lamina of layer III. The patellar retinaculum of the quadriceps forms layer II anteriorly, while the patellofemoral ligaments form this layer posteriorly.

Layer III, the deepest layer, forms the lateral joint capsule. Posterior to the overlying iliotibial tract, layer III separates, forming two laminae. The superficial lamina comprises the lateral collateral ligament and the lateral inferior genicular vessels. The lateral

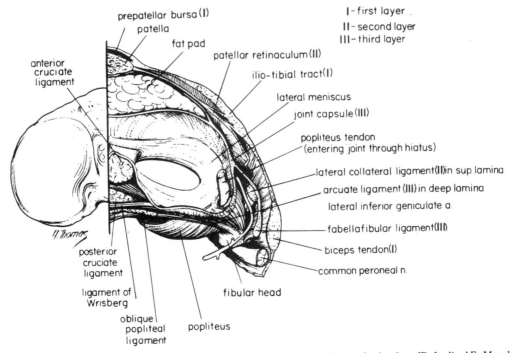

Figure 1–12. The three layers of the lateral compartments of the knee. (From Seebacher JR, Inglis AE, Marshall JL, et al: The structure of the posterolateral aspect of the Knee. J Bone Joint Surg 64A:536–541, 1982.)

collateral ligament, although enveloped by this portion of layer III, is nonetheless considered an entity of layer II. The superficial lamina ends at the fabellofibular ligament posteriorly. The fabellofibular ligament takes its origin on the fibular head, inserts into the fabella (the sesamoid bone located in the lateral head of the gastrocnemius muscle), and then extends into the posterior capsule. The lateral aspect of the lateral meniscus is covered by the deeper lamina. After forming a passage or hiatus for the popliteus tendon, the deep lamina terminates posteriorly at the arcuate ligament. The arcuate ligament itself originates from the fibular head, ascends superomedially, and merges into the posterior capsule. The presence of the fabella varies from individual to individual. If present, the fabellofibular ligament is deemed the major posterolateral ligament. If the fabella is lacking, the acruate liament is considered the primary structure.

Posterior Aspect of the Knee

The posterior aspect of the knee consists of Winslow's ligament (oblique popliteal ligament), the afore-mentioned posterolateral and posteromedial capsular structures, the popliteus muscle, and the deep capsule. The oblique popliteal ligament extends from the inferomedial aspect of the posterior knee at the site of the semimembranosus insertion on the tibia and travels superolaterally, inserting into the capsule behind the lateral femoral condyle.[8] The popliteus will be further discussed later in this chapter.

MISCELLANEOUS STRUCTURES

Bursae

Bursae are closed, fluid-filled sacs lined with synovium. Synovium is the tissue or membrane most commonly found in joints that produces lubricating fluid called synovial fluid. The primary function of bursae is to diminish the friction between adjoining structures, for example between bone and overlying muscle tissue. Bursae are prevalent throughout the knee and are susceptible to anomaly, including infection, neoplasm, trauma, rheumatic affliction, and metabolic

abnormality. Anteriorly, bursae are found between the lower patella and skin (subcutaneous or prepatellar bursa), between the tibia and patellar ligament (deep infrapatellar bursa), between the patellar ligament and skin (subcutaneous or superficial infrapatellar bursa), and between the femur and quadriceps femoris (suprapatellar bursa). Laterally, bursae are present between the lateral head of the gastrocnemius and joint capsule, between the lateral collateral ligament and the biceps femoris tendon, between the lateral collateral ligament and the popliteus, and between the popliteus and the lateral femoral condyle. Medially, bursae are found between the medial collateral ligament and the pes anserinus (anserine bursa), between the tendon of the semimembranosus and the medial tibial condyle and the gastrocremius medial head, and variably below the medial collateral ligament between the capsule, femur, medial meniscus, tibia, and tendon of the semimembranosus (Figs. 1–13 and 1–14). The presence of bursae posteriorly is variable.[42, 43]

Infrapatellar Fat Pads

The infrapatellar fat pad is situated deep to the patellar tendon anterior to the femoral condyles. The infrapatellar fat pad is highly vascular, as it is lined posteriorly by

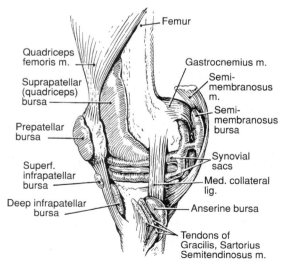

Figure 1–13. The bursae about the knee (medial aspect). (From O'Donaghue DH: Treatment of Injuries to Athletes, 4th ed. Philadelphia, W.B. Saunders, 1984, p. 466.)

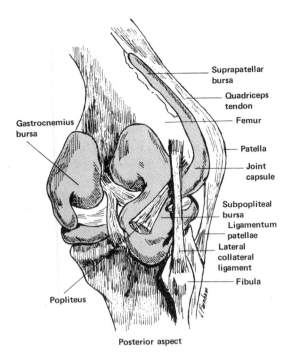

Figure 1–14. A drawing of the posterolateral aspect of the knee complex, showing the knee joint capsule and bursae. (From Norkin C, Levangie P: Joint Structure & Function: A Comprehensive Analysis. Philadelphia, F.A. Davis, 1983, p. 300.)

synovium. The middle genicular artery, a branch of the popliteal artery, penetrates the knee joint capsule and supplies the synovium and infrapatellar fat pad. The fat pad acts to disperse synovial fluid over the joint surface of the femur before contact with the tibia during knee flexion and extension.[4, 18, 44]

Plica

Plica is a crescent-shaped fold of synovium attaching laterally in the vicinity of the vastus lateralis tendon insertion into the patella. Medially, it traverses from the medial femoral condyle to the medial infrapatellar fat pad. Superiorly, it attaches to the deep surface of the quadriceps tendon. Plica arises from an incomplete fusion of the synovial cavity of the knee during the embryonic stage of life.[4]

MUSCULOTENDINOUS STRUCTURES

Knee Extensors

The four extensors of the knee, consisting of the rectus femoris, vastus intermedius, vastus lateralis, and vastus medialis, are collectively known as the quadriceps femoris (Fig. 1–15). The patellar ligament (also known as the ligamentum patellae, patellar tendon, and infrapatellar tendon) is the extension of the quadriceps muscle complex from the inferior pole of the patella to the tibial tubercle on the proximal anterior tibia.

The rectus femoris, originating on the anterior inferior iliac spine and upper margin of the acetabulum and inserting onto the tibial tubercle via the patellar ligament, is the only muscle in the quadriceps complex that crosses both the hip and knee joints. It acts to extend the knee and assists in hip flexion. The vastus intermedius arises from the anterior and lateral femoral shaft. The vastus lateralis and vastus medialis originate from the linea aspera on the posterior femur and, along with the vastus intermedius, insert also onto the tibial tubercle via the patellar ligament. The primary function of these three is to extend the knee. Occasionally blended with the vastus intermedius is a small muscle called the articularis genus (Fig. 1–16). It originates from the inferoanterior aspect of the femur and inserts into the synovial capsule of the knee joint and the suprapatellar bursa. The articularis genus acts to pull the synovial capsule superiorly during knee extension. Sweeping, fibrous expansions on the lateral and medial sides of the patella, made up of extensions of the vastus lateralis and vastus medialis, cross over the knee joint and insert onto the tibia. These expansions, known as the lateral and medial retinacula, function to assist the quadriceps muscle complex in extending the knee. The medial retinaculum, along with the vastus medialis, serves a very important role in patellar stabilization and prevention of lateral subluxation or dislocation of the patella. The quadriceps femoris group is innervated by the femoral nerve (L2,3,4).[7, 18, 42, 45]

The vastus medialis segment of the quadriceps muscle group consists of two parts separated by fascia: the vastus medialis longus and the vastus medialis obliquus. Muscle fibers in the former are large and oriented vertically, whereas, those in the latter are smaller and positioned more horizontally.[7] The angulation of these fibers is crucial for proper patellar stabilization. The vastus medialis obliquus (VMO) ordinarily has a fiber angulation of 65 degrees on the quadriceps tendon and medial border of the

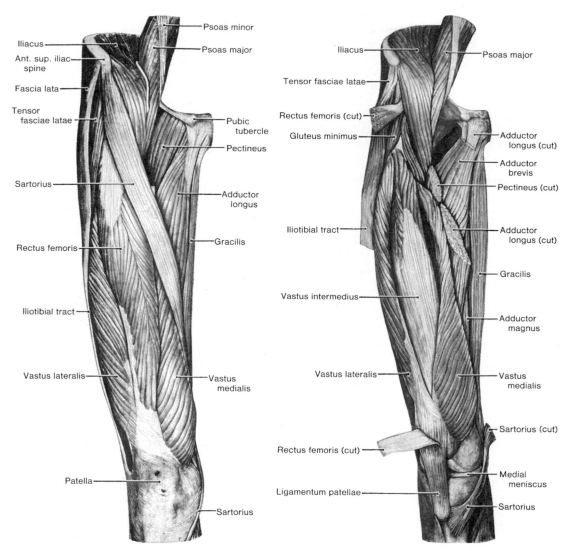

Iliacus
Psoas minor
Psoas major
Ant. sup. iliac spine
Fascia lata
Tensor fasciae latae
Pubic tubercle
Pectineus
Sartorius
Adductor longus
Rectus femoris
Gracilis
Iliotibial tract
Vastus lateralis
Vastus medialis
Patella
Sartorius

Iliacus
Psoas major
Tensor fasciae latae
Rectus femoris (cut)
Gluteus minimus
Adductor longus (cut)
Adductor brevis
Pectineus (cut)
Iliotibial tract
Adductor longus (cut)
Gracilis
Vastus intermedius
Adductor magnus
Vastus lateralis
Vastus medialis
Sartorius (cut)
Rectus femoris (cut)
Medial meniscus
Ligamentum patellae
Sartorius

Figure 1–15. The quadriceps femoris muscle complex. (From Moore KL: Clinically Oriented Anatomy, 2nd ed. Baltimore, Williams & Wilkins, 1985, p. 422.)

Figure 1–16. The articularis genus, lying directly below and blended with the vastus intermedius. (From Moore KL: Clinically Oriented Anatomy, 2nd. ed. Baltimore, Williams & Wilkins, 1985, p. 422.)

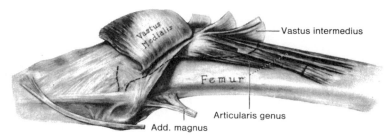

Vastus Medialis
Vastus intermedius
Femur
Articularis genus
Add. magnus

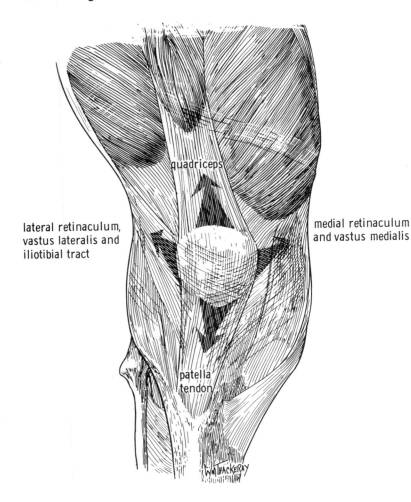

lateral retinaculum,
vastus lateralis and
iliotibial tract

medial retinaculum
and vastus medialis

quadriceps

patella
tendon

Figure 1–17. Static and dynamic patellar stabilizers. (From Engle R: Knee Ligament Rehabilitation, New York, Churchill Livingstone, 1991, p. 6.)

patella. An angle less than 65 degrees would not provide adequate stabilization of the patella during an explosive contraction of the remaining quadriceps complex.[5] The vastus lateralis is considered the largest of the four quadriceps muscles and may in some individuals (eg, those with insufficient VMO strength, poor VMO fiber orientation, shallow femoral sulcus) overpower the VMO, pulling the patella laterally when moving into full extension (Fig. 1–17).[4, 42, 46]

Knee Flexors

The primary flexors of the knee consist of three large femoral muscles collectively known as the hamstrings: the biceps femoris, semitendinosis, and semimembranosus (Fig. 1–18). The hamstrings cross both the knee and hip joints and therefore act not only as knee flexors but also as hip extensors.

The biceps femoris is positioned along the posterolateral aspect of the thigh. It has two proximal attachments. The long head attachment orginates from the distal portion of the sacrotuberous ligament and the posterior aspect of the ischial tuberosity of the pelvis. The short head does not cross the hip joint. It originates from the femur at the lateral lip of the linea aspera, the proximal two-thirds of the supracondylar line, and the lateral intramuscular septum. Both the long head and the short head form the muscle belly and travel distally. The primary part of the tendon splits around the fibular collateral ligament and inserts onto the lateral aspect of the fibular head. The remainder of the distal biceps femoris tendon divides into three laminae: the intermediate lamina blends with the fibular collateral ligament while the remaining two advance superficial

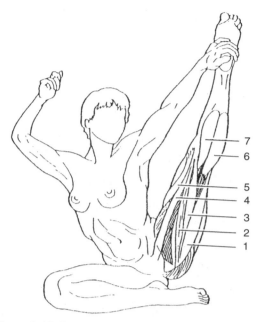

Figure 1–18. Posterior lower extremity musculature: biceps femoris (1), semitendinosus (2), semimembranosus (3), gracilis (4), sartorius (5), gastrocnemius (6 and 7). Note that the semitendinosus, gracilis, and sartorius make up the pes anserinus. (From Kapandji IA: The Physiology of the Joints, Vol. 2. New York, Churchill Livingstone, 1970.)

and deep to the ligament, attaching to the lateral condyle of the tibia.[18, 43, 47, 48]

The medial hamstrings consist of the semitendinosus and semimembranosus muscles. The semitendinosus originates from the upper portion of the ischial tuberosity via a shared tendon with the long head of the biceps femoris. It travels distally, becoming a slender cord-like tendon approximately two-thirds of the way down the posteromedial thigh. It passes over the tibial collateral ligament and inserts into the medial surface of the tibia and deep fascia of the lower leg posterior to the attachment of the sartorius and distal to the attachment of the gracilis. Collectively, the semitendinosus, sartorius, and gracilis are known as the pes anserinus. The semimembranosus derives its name from the flattened, long, and thick appearance of its proximal tendon. By way of this tendon, the semimembranosus originates from the ischial tuberosity proximal and medial to the biceps femoris and semitendinosis. The semimembranosus inserts distally via five fibrous expansions: (1) posterior aspect of the medial tibial condyle via a tubercle termed the tuberculum tendinis;

(2) medial margin of the tibia, immediately posterior to the tibial collateral ligament; (3) over the popliteus by way of a thin fibrous expansion to fascia; (4) inferior lip and adjacent portion of the groove on the posterior aspect of the medial tibial condyle, deep to the tibial collateral ligament; and (5) femoral intercondylar line and lateral femoral condyle via a secure expansion, forming a substantial portion of the oblique popliteal ligament. The hamstrings are innervated by the sciatic nerve (L5, S1, and S2) through the tibial and common peroneal divisions.[18, 43, 48]

Gastrocnemius

The gastrocnemius (see Fig. 1–18) derives its name from the Greek word *gastro*, which means "belly." It is therefore the "belly" of the calf. The gastrocnemius originates via two heads. The larger medial head originates from a depression at the superoposterior aspect of the medial condyle of the femur behind the adductor tubercle and from a minimally raised area on the popliteal surface of the femur above the medial condyle. The lateral head emanates from the lateral surface of the lateral condyle and from the lower aspect of the supracondylar line. Both heads additionally originate from the knee joint capsule. The fleshy component of both heads extends distally to approximately midcalf. At midcalf, the muscle fibers begin to insert into an expansive aponeurosis. Prior to this point, both muscular heads remained separate. The aponeurosis progressively contracts and accepts the soleus tendon. The soleus is a flat broad muscle deep to the gastrocnemius shaped somewhat like a fish. The aponeurosis and soleus tendon, in turn, form the tendo calcaneus or Achilles tendon, which attaches directly to the calcaneus. The two heads of the gastrocnemius along with the soleus form a tripartite muscle mass called the triceps surae. The gastroc-soleus complex is the primary plantar flexor of the foot. The gastrocnemius moreover acts as a flexor of the knee. The gastrocnemius is innervated by the tibial nerve (S1 and S2).[43, 35]

Popliteus

The popliteus (see Fig. 1–10) is a thin triangular muscle originating from the lateral aspect of the lateral condyle of the femur, inferior to the attachment of the lateral collateral ligament, as well as from the posterior portion of the lateral meniscus and posterolateral knee joint capsule. It then travels inferomedially, inserting along the posterior tibial surface, superior to the soleal line.[18] The popliteus acts as an internal rotator of the tibia and further functions to unlock the fully extended knee during the beginning phases of flexion.[49] It has furthermore been shown to retract the lateral meniscus during knee flexion[50] and function as a strong stabilizer of the lateral knee compartment via tendinous reinforcement of the lateral meniscus and posterolateral capsule.[4, 51] Popliteus nerve supply comes from the tibial nerve (L4, L5, and S1).[18]

Iliotibial Tract

The iliotibial tract (ITT) is characterized as an extremely strong lateral band of fascia originating from the iliac crest with tendinous reinforcements from the tensor fasciae latae and gluteus maximus muscles. The ITT inserts onto the lateral femoral condyle, lateral knee capsule, proximal tibia at Gerdy's tubercle, and fibula.[4, 18, 52] The ITT performs several complex tasks. It serves as an extensor when the knee is in 0 to 30 degrees of flexion. When the knee is flexed in excess of 40 degrees, the ITT functions as a knee flexor. Between 30 and 40 degrees, the ITT plays a neutral role.[53] The ITT also plays an integral part in static lateral stability of the knee.[54]

SUMMARY

It is apparent that the knee is an intricate joint, relying on optimal balance between dynamic and static soft tissue stabilizers and osseous and cartilagenous components. Given the complex nature of this joint and its propensity for injury, a sound understanding of its anatomic components is crucial. It was the goal of this chapter to provide this information so as to establish a solid base for the rehabilitation of the injured knee.

References

1. Hoppenfeld S: Physical Examination of the Spine and Extremities. Norwalk, CT, Appleton-Century-Crofts, 1976.
2. Yoshitsugu T, Xerogeanes JW, Livesay GA, et al.: Biomechanical function of the human anterior cruciate ligament. Arthroscopy 10:140, 1994.
3. Magee DJ: Orthopedic Physical Assessment. Philadelphia, W.B. Saunders 1987.
4. Gill DM, Corbacio EJ, Lauchle LE: Anatomy of the knee. In Engle RP (ed): Knee Ligament Rehabilitation. New York, Churchill Livingstone, 1991, p. 1.
5. Hughston JC: Subluxation of the patella. J Bone Joint Surg 50A:1003, 1968.
6. Kennedy JC, Fowler PJ: Medial and anterior instability of the knees: An anatomic and clinical study using stress machines. J Bone Joint Surg 53A:1257, 1971.
7. Norkin CC, Levangie PK: Joint Structure and Function: A Comprehensive Analysis. Philadelphia, F.A. Davis, 1990.
8. Tria AJ: Ligaments of the Knee. New York, Churchill Livingstone, 1995.
9. Hayes CW: MRI of the patellofemoral joint. Semin Ultrasound CT MRI 15:383, 1994.
10. Turek SL: Orthopaedics: Principles and Their Application, 4th ed. Philadelphia, J.B. Lippincott, 1984.
11. Seedhom BB, Dowson D, Wright V: The function of the menisci: A preliminary study. J Bone Joint Surg 56B:381, 1974.
12. Shrive N: The weight-bearing role of the menisci of the knee. J Bone Joint Surg 56B:381, 1974.
13. Fairbank TJ: Knee joint changes after meniscectomy. J Bone Joint Surg Br 30:664, 1976.
14. Allen PR, Denham RA, Swan AV: Late degenerative changes after meniscectomy: Factors affecting the knee after operation. J Bone Joint Surg Br 66:666, 1984.
15. Johnson RJ, Kettlekamp DB, Clark W, Leaverton P: Factors affecting late results after meniscectomy. J Bone Joint Surg 56:719, 1974.
16. Johnson DL, Swenson TM, Livesay GA et al: Insertion-site anatomy of the human menisci: Gross, arthroscopic, and topographical anatomy as a basis for meniscal transplantation. Arthroscopy 11:386, 1995.
17. Firooznia H, Golimbu C, Rafii M: MR imaging of the menisci: Fundamentals of anatomy and pathology. MRI Clin of North Am 2:325, 1994.
18. Moore KL: Clinically Oriented Anatomy, 2nd ed. Baltimore, Williams & Wilkins, 1985.
19. VanDommelen BA, Fowler PJ: Anatomy of the posterior cruciate ligament: A review. Am J Sports Med 17:24, 1989.
20. Fritz JM, Irrgang JJ, Harner CD: Rehabilitation following allograft meniscal transplantation: A review of the literature and case study. J Ortho Sports Phys Ther 24:98, 1996.
21. Kapandji IA: The Physiology of the Joints, Vol 2, 2nd ed. New York, Churchill Livingstone, 1970.
22. Last RJ: The popliteus muscle and the lateral meniscus: With a note on the attachment of the medial meniscus. J Bone Joint Surg Br 32:93, 1950.
23. Thompson WO, Fu FH: The meniscus in the cruciate-deficient knee. Clin Sports Med 12:771, 1993.
24. Arnoczky SP: Anatomy of the anterior cruciate ligament. Clin Orthop 172:19, 1983.

25. Arnoczky SP, Warren RF: Microvasculature of the human meniscus. Am J Sports Med 10:90, 1982.
26. Arnoczky SP, Warren RF: Anatomy of the cruciate ligaments. In Feagin JA Jr (ed): The Crucial Ligaments, 2nd ed. New York, Churchill Livingstone, 1994, p. 271.
27. Schutte MJ, Dabezies EJ, Zimny ML, Happel LT: Neural anatomy of the human anterior cruciate ligament. J Bone Joint Surg 69:243, 1987.
28. Samuelson TS, Drez D, Maletis GB: Anterior cruciate ligament graft rotation: Reproduction of normal graft rotation. Am J Sports Med 24:67, 1996.
29. Smith BA, Livesay GA, Woo SL-Y: Biology and biomechanics of the anterior cruciate ligament. Clin Sports Med 12:637, 1993.
30. Fuss FK: Anatomy of the cruciate ligaments and their function in extension and flexion of the human knee joint. Am J Anat 184:165, 1989.
31. Clark JM, Sidles JA: The interrelation of fiber bundles in the anterior cruciate ligament. J Orthop Res 8:180, 1988.
32. Dodds JA, Arnoczky SP: Anatomy of the anterior cruciate ligament: A blueprint for repair and reconstruction. Arthroscopy 10:132, 1994.
33. Lee SH, Petersilge CA, Trudell DJ, et al.: Extrasynovial spaces of the cruciate ligaments: Anatomy, MR imaging, and diagnostic Implications. AJR Am J Roentgenol 166:1433, 1996.
34. Harner CD, Xerogeanes JW, Livesay GA, et al.: The human posterior cruciate ligament complex: An interdisciplinary study. Am J Sports Med 23:736, 1995.
35. Girgis FG, Marshall JL, Al Monajem ARS: The cruciate ligaments of the knee joint: Anatomical, functional, and experimental analysis. Clin Orthop 106:216, 1975.
36. Van Dommelen BA, Fowler PJ: Anatomy of the posterior cruciate ligament. Am J Sports Med 17:24, 1989.
37. Hunter L, Funk FJ: Rehabilitation of Injured Knees. St. Louis, CV Mosby, 1984.
38. Warren LF, Marshall L: The supporting structures and layers on the medial side of the knee: An anatomical analysis. J Bone Joint Surg 61A:56, 1979.
39. Lee JK, Yao L: Tibial collateral ligament bursa: MR imaging. Radiology 178:855, 1991.
40. Ruiz, ME, Erickson SJ: Medial and lateral supporting structures of the knee: Normal MR imaging anatomy and pathologic findings. MRI Clin North Am 2:381, 1994.
41. Seebacher JR, Inglis AE, Marshall JL, et al.: The structure of the posterolateral aspect of the knee. J Bone Joint Surg 64A:536, 1982.
42. American Academy of Orthopaedic Surgeons: Athletic Training and Sports Medicine, 2nd ed. Rosemont, IL, American Academy of Orthopaedic Surgeons, 1991.
43. Soames RW: Skeletal system. In Williams PL (ed): Gray's Anatomy, 38th ed. New York, Churchill Livingstone, 1995, p. 425.
44. Jackson WO, Drez D, Jr: The Anterior Cruciate Deficient Knee. St. Louis, CV Mosby, 1987.
45. Sieg KW, Adams SP: Illustrated Essentials of Musculoskeletal Anatomy. Gainesville, FL, Megabooks, 1994.
46. Zakaria D, Harburn KL, Kramer JF: Preferential activation of the vastus medialis oblique, vastus lateralis, and hip adductor muscles during isometric exercises in females. J Orthop Sports Phys Ther 26:23, 1997.
47. Terry GC, LaPrade RF: The biceps femoris muscle complex at the knee: Its anatomy and injury patterns associated with acute anterolateral-anteromedial rotatory instability. Am J Sports Med 24:2, 1996.
48. Worrell TW, Perrin DH: Hamstring muscle injury: The influence of strength, flexibility, warm-up, and fatigue. J Orthop Sports Phys Ther 16:12, 1992.
49. Basmajian JV, Lovejoy JF: Function of the popliteus muscle in man. J Bone Joint Surg 53B:557, 1971.
50. Jones CDS, Keene GCR, Christie AD: The popliteus as a retractor of the lateral meniscus of the knee. Arthroscopy 11:270, 1995.
51. Muller W: The Knee: Form, Function, and Ligamentous Reconstruction. New York, Springer-Verlag, 1982.
52. Matsumoto H, Seedhom B: Tension characteristics of the iliotibial tract and role of its superficial layer. Clin Orthop 313:253, 1995.
53. Muller W: Kinematics of the cruciate ligaments. In Feagin JA Jr (ed): The Crucial Ligaments, 2nd ed. New York, Churchill Livingstone, 1994, p. 295.
54. Insall JN: Disorders of the patella. In Insall JN (ed): Surgery of the Knee. New York, Churchill Livingstone, 1984, p. 191.
55. Tria AJ Jr, Klein KS: An Illustrated Guide to the Knee. New York, Churchill Livingstone, 1992.
56. O'Donoghue DH: Treatment of Injuries to Athletes 4th ed. Philadelphia, W.B. Saunders, 1984.

2 Biomechanics

Richard R. Boeckmann, PT, and
Todd S. Ellenbecker, MS, PT, SCS, CSCS

*A*n understanding of the biomechanics of the human knee forms the basis for the design and progression of rehabilitation programs for the patient with knee ligament injury. Knowledge of the biomechanical principles of the tibiofemoral joint and surrounding ligamentous structures is of vital importance both to the clinical evaluation and treatment and to better understanding of the demands placed on the surgically reconstructed knee.

TIBIOFEMORAL JOINT

The tibiofemoral joint is the most complex joint in the human body. It is made up proximally by the medial and lateral femoral condyles, which are the distal articulating surfaces of the femur. These surfaces are biconvex, asymmetrical, and separated posteriorly by the deep intercondylar notch. Anteriorly, the condylar surfaces merge to form the trochlear groove. The condyles do not follow the shape of a circle, but their radius decreases from anterior to posterior, with the medial condyle presenting with a more gradual change in radii.[1] The lateral condyle is narrower, but its circumferential length is larger than that of the medial condyle.[2, 3]

The proximal articulating surface of the tibia is made up of two asymmetrical condyles. The medial tibial condyle is larger and oval, with a biconcave joint surface. This allows for a more congruent fit for the medial femoral condyle. The smaller lateral tibial condyle is concave mediolaterally and convex anteroposteriorly.[1, 3] The result of this is reduced congruency and increased mobility in the lateral joint articulation.[3, 4]

Menisci

Resting on top of the tibial plateaus are the asymmetric, wedge-shaped mensci. The medial meniscus is semicircular in shape and securely attached peripherally to the joint capsule and to the tibial condyle by the coronary ligaments.[5] It also has an attachment to the deep fibers of the medial collateral ligament, which is considered to limit the amount of posterior meniscal translation available with knee flexion.[6] There is a dynamic attachment from the semimembranosis, which sends a tendinous slip to attach to the posterior horn of the medial meniscus. This will assist in the posterior movement of the medial meniscus during flexion.[1, 3]

The lateral meniscus is more oval and also is attached peripherally to the joint capsule and to the lateral tibial plateau via the coronary ligaments. What is different is the absence of an attachment to the lateral collateral ligament. This allows for more anteroposterior mobility of the lateral meniscus relative to the medial. This was supported by Thompson et al.[7] through the use of three-dimensional magnetic resonance imaging of the unloaded knee with a flexion-extension arc. The medial meniscus was found to translate posteriorly 5.1 mm, as compared with 11.2 mm of posterior movement in the lateral meniscus.[7] There is an additional ligamentous attachment to the posterior horn of the lateral meniscus by the meniscofemoral ligaments. These ligaments, known as the ligament of Wrisberg and the ligament of Humphery, run from the posterior horn of the lateral meniscus obliquely medially and superiorly to the lateral aspect of the femur.[8–10] They run fairly close to the posterior cruciate ligament, although they are believed to function to improve congruency between the lateral meniscus and the lateral femoral condyle by pulling the anterior horn forward.[10] The popliteus has an attachment to the posterior horn of the lateral meniscus and assists in gliding the meniscus posteriorly with knee flexion.[3, 11]

The menisci serve important functions, including absorption and even distribution of stress to the articular cartilage through increasing joint congruency[12, 13] and dispersing of joint lubrication and nutrients to the cartilage.[7, 13] There has been ongoing debate as to the role of the menisci in joint stability. The research data demonstrate that the menisci do not play any role in the primary stability of the anterior cruciate ligament (ACL)–intact knee.[7] However, research does indicate that the meniscus plays a considerable role in assisting with knee stability in the ACL-deficient knee.[14, 15] The more stable posterior horn of the medial meniscus is thought to act as a wedge, limiting the amount of anterior translation of the tibia in the ACL-deficient knee.[7]

Knee Joint Kinetics and Kinematics

Six degrees of freedom (DOFs) are available in the tibiofemoral joint: three translational movements described as anteroposterior, mediolateral and proximodistal (distraction-compression), and three rotational movements described as flexion-extension, internal-external rotation, and varus-valgus (Fig. 2–1).[16, 17] The availability of these multiple movements allows for the complex functioning of this system, whether it be maximal stability (terminal extension) or various amounts of mobility, depending on the degree of tibiofemoral flexion present. Calculation of the instant center of rotation of the tibiofemoral joint is very complex and has been accomplished by several authors.[18, 19] These authors conclude that the tibiofemoral joint does not function as a true hinge joint because of the movement of the instant center of joint rotation. The instant center of rotation for the saggital plane motion of flexion-extension changes during the range of motion, with the joint centers falling within a circle with a diameter of 2.3 cm with axes piercing the lateral femoral condyle.[19] The vertical axis of the knee passes via the medial femoral condyle because of the normal orientation of the femur and tibia.[20]

KNEE JOINT RANGE OF MOTION

The saggital plane range of motion available in a normal knee varies from 5 to 10 degrees hyperextension to 135 to 160 degrees flexion.[3, 13, 21] Limitation of further flexion is secondary to soft tissue approximation of the posterior calf with the thigh. Further extension is restricted by tightening of the capsular and ligamentous structures, primarily the posterior capsule and the collateral and cruciate ligaments. The available range of motion in rotation, which occurs in a transverse plane, is dependent on the flexion-extension position of the knee. At 90 degrees of flexion, rotation of 70 to 80 degrees is possible, with external rotation (0–40 degrees) being greater than internal rotation (0–30 degrees).[3, 11, 22] The amount of rotation available progressively increases from no rotation at terminal extension to 70 or 80 degrees of rotation at 90 degrees flexion, and then decreases again as further flexion occurs.[23]

Ranges of motion of the tibiofemoral joint have been calculated during activities of daily living and recreational activities and give clinicians insight into the biomechanical demands and movement patterns patients require following knee ligament reconstruction or injury. Table 2–1 outlines tibiofemoral joint ranges of motion and corresponding activities for the human knee.

TIBIOFEMORAL ARTHROKINEMATICS

The basic arthrokinematics of the femur and tibia are a combination of rolling and

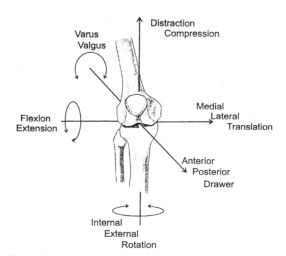

Figure 2–1. The six degrees of freedom of the human knee joint. (From Stowers S: Biomechanical terminology applied to the knee joint. Sports Med Arthroscop Rev 4(4):310, 1996.)

Table 2–1. Tibiofemoral Joint Ranges of Motion Required for Activities of Daily Living and Recreational Activities

Activity	Tibiofemoral Joint Range of Motion, degrees
Walking	0–67
Slow walking	0–6*
Fast walking	12–18*
Stair climbing	0–83
Sitting down	0–93
Tying a shoe	0–106
Lifting an object	0–117
Descending stairs	0–90
Running	18–30*

Modified from Frankel VH, Nordin M: Basic Biomechanics of the Skeletal System. Philadelphia, Lea & Febiger, 1980.

*Data from Perry J, Norwood L, House K: Knee posture and biceps and semimembranosis muscle action in running and cutting. (An EMG study). Trans Orthop Res Soc 2:258, 1977.

gliding.[3, 4, 24] This can be described as the femur moving on tibia or tibia moving on femur; the former description is used here. Flexion and extension involves an intermix of femoral condyle rolling and gliding on the tibial plateau. During flexion, the femoral condyles roll posteriorly while they glide anteriorly on the tibial plateau. The opposite occurs with extension, in which case the femoral condyles roll anteriorly and glide posteriorly. The ratio of the amount of roll to glide varies throughout all degrees of flexion and is described by Müller[24] as approximately 1:2 in early flexion and 1:4 by the end of flexion. Kapandji[3] describes this ratio as pure rolling of the femoral condyles during early flexion; 10 to 15 degrees for the medial femoral condyle and 20 degrees for the lateral femoral condyle, at which time gliding begins to accompany the rolling. The gliding will progressively increase as further flexion occurs, until there is pure gliding of the condyles without rolling at the end of flexion.

The absence of either the roll or glide component does not allow for normal functioning of the knee. The circumference of the femoral condyles is twice the length of the tibial plateau.[3] In the absence of gliding, the femoral condyles would roll off the posterior lip of the tibial plateau after a certain degree of flexion (Fig. 2–2A).[3, 5] In the absence of the rolling with only the gliding component, the contact points between the femur and tibia would remain the same. Here, flexion would be limited, as the posterior femur would abut the posterior lip of the tibial plateau (Fig. 2–2B). In the normally functioning knee, this combination of roll and glide during flexion creates a posterior movement of the tibiofemoral contact point[3, 24] to the degree that dislocation is avoided, yet further range of motion is achieved (Fig. 2–2C).

There is also a spin component to knee arthrokinematics, which results in knee rotation in the transverse plane during flexion and extension. During knee flexion from an

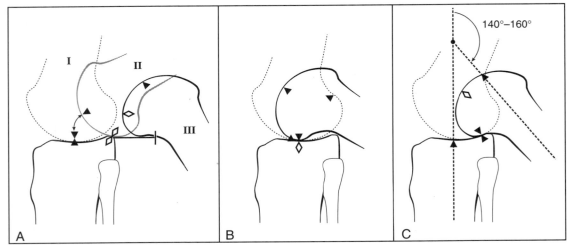

Figure 2–2. Movements of the femoral condyles on the tibial plateau during flexion and extension. *A*, Absence of rolling component with only gliding; *B*, absence of glide component with only rolling; *C*, normal combination of both rolling and gliding. (From Kapandji IA: The Physiology of the Joints. Vol II, Lower Extremity, 5th ed. New York, Churchill Livingstone, 1988, p. 85.)

extended knee position, the lateral tibiofemoral contact point will move a greater distance posteriorly than the medial contact point.[4] This will result in an automatic external rotation of the femur on the tibia or relative internal rotation of the tibia. The greater posterior migration of the lateral tibiofemoral contact point is secondary to (1) the convex-on-convex saggital plane joint surface geometry of the lateral compartment, (2) the increased mobility of the lateral compartment, including the lateral meniscus,[3, 4] and (3) the greater circumferential length of the lateral femoral condyle.[3]

During knee extension from a flexed position, there is greater anterior excursion of the lateral tibiofemoral contact point than medially. This results in a combined movement of knee extension with femoral internal rotation or relative tibial external rotation.[2, 3] The last few degrees of this combined tibial extension and external rotation is referred to as the "screw-home" mechanism.[2, 9, 22] This mechanism, which locks the knee at terminal extension, is a result of the joint orientation just described but is also influenced by the winding and tightening of the cruciate ligaments.[1, 2]

LIGAMENTOUS STRUCTURES

Anterior Cruciate Ligament

The ACL consists of two primary fiber bundles (anteromedial and posterolateral) that traverse from the lateral femoral condyle to the anterior aspect of the tibial plateau. The ACL assists in controlling the six degrees of freedom of knee motion and is one of the most frequently injured knee ligaments.[25] In evaluating the biomechanical properties of human ligaments, scientists typically report both a linear stiffness and ultimate tensile load. Stiffness is the resistance offered to external loads by a specimen or structure as it deforms, and ultimate tensile load is the load and accompanying elongation between the clamped ends of a specimen recorded during tensile testing.[25] Trent et al.[26] tested the ACL with bone blocks of the femur ACL tibial complex (FATC) of cadavers between the ages of 29 and 55 years. A linear stiffness of 141 N/mm and ultimate tensile load of 633 N were reported. In a similar investigation, Noyes and Grood[27] tested the FATC in younger ca-

davers between the ages of 16 and 26 and found stiffness to be 182 N/mm and ultimate tensile loads of 1725 N.

A recent investigation by Rowden et al.[28] compared the biomechanical properties of the human ACL and patellar tendon and semitendonosis autographs in fresh, young (age <42 years) cadavers. They determined the stiffness and ultimate tensile load of the ACL to be 306 N/mm and 2195 N, respectively. Biomechanical testing of the specimens was repeated following either autogenous 10 mm wide bone–patellar tendon–bone graft with interference screws or a quadruple stranded semitendinosis graft with titanium button fixation. Results showed ultimate tensile strengths of 416 N in the patellar tendon group and 612 N in the semitendinosis group (Fig. 2–3). Stiffness did not differ between the two types of autogenous grafts and was 47 N/mm. The authors conclude that current methods of autogenous ACL reconstruction produce grafts that have only 20 to 30 percent of the ultimate tensile strength of the ACL at the time of surgery.

The effect of knee motion on the length and orientation of the human ACL is well documented.[18, 25, 28] Changes in the length of the ACL during extension-flexion, internal-external, and varus-valgus rotations have both surgical and rehabilitative connota-

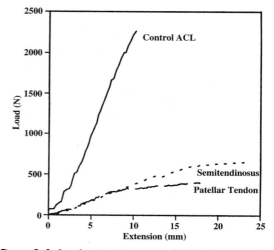

Figure 2–3. Load extension curves for the human anterior cruciate ligament, patellar tendon, and semitendinosus bone-ligament-bone complexes. (From Rowden NJ, Sher D, Rogers GJ, Schindhelm K: Anterior cruciate ligament graft fixation: Initial comparison of patellar tendon and semitendinosus autografts in young fresh cadavers. Am J Sports Med 25(4):472–478, 1997.)

tions and deserve discussion. Because of the broad attachments on the tibia and femur of the ACL, some collagenous bundles experience heightened tension whereas others carry less load based on range of motion and rotational orientation.[18, 25, 28] In general, fibers of the ACL located anteriorly on the femur lengthen with increases in knee flexion, whereas posterior insertions decreased in length during knee flexion.[25, 29–31]

The ability of the ACL to control anterior translation of the tibia relative to the femur throughout the range of motion has been extensively documented.[25–27, 30–32] The ACL and posterior cruciate ligament (PCL) have been described together in their ability to control saggital plane translation by Müller[24] throughout knee extension and flexion using a four-bar linkage system. Some fibers of the cruciate ligaments are nearly isometric through a full range of motion and cross at the instant center of the knee. (Fig. 2–4).[33]

Stresses placed on the human ACL have been studied with simulated active motion and passive motion. More and Markolf[34] measured the force on the ACL to be highest (40 N) at full extension, increasing to 60 N with simulated active quadriceps activity. This force dropped to only 20 N at 20 degrees of knee flexion. With similar direct testing of ACL stresses, Markolf et al.[29] measured greater forces within the ACL with internal tibial rotation when compared with measurements generated throughout knee flexion angles with external tibial rotation. Rotational measurements increased stress on the ACL as the knee was extended, with the greatest stress being imparted with superimposed hyperextension with internal rotation.[29]

Finally, several studies have closely documented stresses in the ACL with quadriceps contraction.[29, 32, 35] Shoemaker et al.[35] studied the effects of quadriceps contraction on anteroposterior tibial translation. Their findings are consistent with others[36, 37] who found peak anterior tibial translation, and hence stress to the ACL, to occur in the last 25 to 30 degrees of knee extension. Shoemaker's study also showed that ACL graft load and anterior tibial translation at 100 degrees of knee flexion decreases with quadriceps contraction, as opposed to increases in graft tension in the ACL near terminal extension.

Posterior Cruciate Ligament

The PCL exhibits a simple parallel fiber orientation that is most evident with the

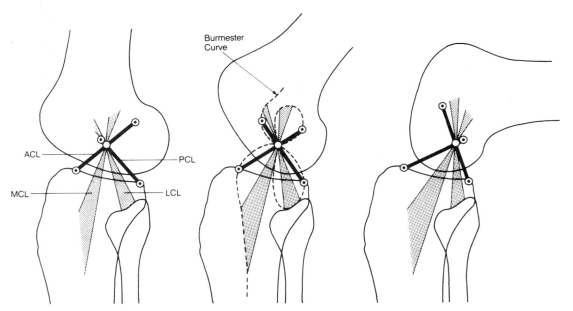

Figure 2–4. Crossed four-bar linkage system mechanism of cruciate ligaments and relationship to Burmester's curve. ACL = anterior cruciate ligament; PCL = posterior cruciate ligament; LCL = lateral collateral ligament; MCL = medial collateral ligament. (From Feagin JA Jr: The Crucial Ligaments: Diagnosis and Treatment of Ligamentous Injuries About the Knee, 2nd ed. New York, Churchill Livingstone, 1994, p. 308.)

knee fully flexed, where the fibers appear to be under full and equal tension.[33] Information regarding the tensile strength of the PCL is quite scarce as compared with that of the human ACL. Kennedy et al.,[38] in 1976, published findings on the tensile strength of the human PCL. Their research showed the strength of the PCL to be twice that of the ACL. Prietto et al.[39] tested PCL in young cadavers and found the stiffness and ultimate tensile load to be 204 N/mm and 1624 N, respectively. Most research studying the PCL identifies two distinct bands: the anterolateral and the posteromedial. The posterior edge of the PCL contacts the roof of the intercondylar notch.[33] The anterolateral band is two to three times stiffer and three to four times more resistant to tensile loads than the posteromedial band in the same knee.[40]

The biomechanical function of the PCL has been studied using selected cutting experiments.[40, 41] The application of a posteriorly directed load to the tibia with the knee flexed 90 degrees in neutral rotation produced a significant increase in the load in the PCL.[41] Application of the same amount of posterior loading with the knee in full extension did not increase the load in the PCL.[41] The lack of significant loading to the PCL with the knee in full extension indicates the ability of the posterior capsular structures to function by absorbing the applied load. Simulation of a quadriceps contraction with tension via the quadriceps tendon increased the force in the PCL with the knee in 80 and 90 degrees of flexion only.[41]

Removal of only the PCL in a cadaveric specimen increases the limit of posterior tibial translation (up to 11.4 mm at 90 degrees of knee flexion) but does not change the limit in varus or valgus angulation or tibial rotation.[42] Transection of the posterolateral extra-articular capsular structures (lateral collateral ligament, arcuate complex, and popliteus tendon) increases the amount of tibial external rotation and varus angulation.[42] These results show that the posterolateral extra-articular structures provide the primary restraint to tibial external rotation, particularly in the range of flexion between 20 and 40 degrees. This information has clinical ramifications, especially for interpretation of information from manual laxity tests in the patient with knee ligament injury.

Hyperextension of the knee has often been cited as the mechanism of injury of the PCL.[41, 42] Wascher et al.[41] compared the stresses in the ACL and PCL during hyperextension force placed on the knee under experimental conditions. They found forces in the PCL to be considerably lower than forces in the ACL during hyperextension of the knee, indicating that damage to the PCL alone is unlikely from a straight hyperextension movement. These researchers also found forces in the ACL to be almost twice those in the PCL during hyperflexion.[41] Therefore, isolated rupture of the PCL is typically incurred with the application of a posteriorly directed force applied to a knee flexed 90 degrees.[41] The application of this posteriorly directed force is significantly negated by internal or external tibial rotation, indicating the important role of the posteromedial and posterolateral capsular secondary constraints.[41]

Collateral Ligaments

The medial and lateral collateral ligaments can be represented by a curve derived mathematically by Burmester and published in a kinematic textbook in 1888[24] (Fig. 2–4). Mechanical testing data are also scarce for the collateral ligaments as compared with the ACL, as mentioned earlier in this chapter. Woo et al.[43] studied the ACL and medial collateral ligament in rabbits and found that the ACL values of ultimate tensile stress were only one-half those of the medial collateral ligament in age-matched experimental subjects. This study indicates significant differences in the mechanical properties of the medial collateral ligament.

The medial collateral ligament's parallel fibered superficial portion was the primary restraint at both 5 and 25 degrees of knee flexion to valgus stress, providing 57 percent at 5 degrees and 78 percent at 25 degrees of knee flexion. The increased responsibility of the medial collateral ligament with increased knee flexion is attributed to the decrease in secondary restraint provided from the posterior medial capsule, which becomes slack with knee flexion.[44] At 5 degrees of knee flexion, the posterior capsule and cruciate ligaments were also important secondary restraints.[44] Lateral joint opening with varus stress was tested in a similar fashion in cadaveric knees, with the lateral collateral ligament providing 54 percent of the total restraint to varus stress at 5 degrees of flexion and 69 percent at 25 degrees of flexion. Again, the contribution of the posterior lateral half of the capsule was minimized with increased knee flexion and required greater control from the lateral collateral ligament for stabilization. In both varus and valgus stress testing conditions with the knee in full extension, the secondary restraints were nearly able to completely block joint opening even after transection of both collateral ligaments.[44]

Shapiro et al.[45] studied what effect sectioning of the medial collateral ligament had on the ACL. They found that sectioning of the medial collateral ligament did not affect the ACL during varus stress; however, with valgus stress, the forces imparted to the ACL increased dramatically, especially with 45 degrees of knee flexion.[45] Increased stress on the ACL was also reported with external tibial rotation, with a variable influence reported for internal tibial rotation.[45] The findings of this study have clinical relevance for the patient with residual medial laxity from a medial collateral ligament sprain. The results of this study demonstrate that a greater load on the ACL is borne with valgus stress and with external tibial rotation in this condition and may subject the individual to further, more serious ligament injury.

SUMMARY

Reviewing the tibiofemoral joint biomechanical features highlights the complex interplay between the joint arthrokinematics that allow specific motions to occur and the capsular and ligamentous structures that attempt to control and limit them. Applied research on the ligamentous structures of the human knee demonstrates the complex function and biomechanical limits of both the existing anatomy and the reconstructive grafts. The application of future research will allow the clinician to better understand the function and demands placed on the knee with activities of daily living as well as sport-specific movement patterns to promote optimal rehabilitation following injury.

References

1. Hertling D, Kessler RM: Management of Common Musculoskeletal Disorders, 2nd ed. Philadelphia, J.B. Lippincott, 1990.
2. Residency Program. Ola Grimsby Institute, Course Notes, 1994.
3. Kapandji IA: The Physiology of the Knee Joints, Vol 2, 5th ed. New York, Churchill Livingstone, 1987.
4. Dye SF: An evolutionary perspective. In Feagin JA Jr (ed): The Crucial Ligaments, 2nd ed. New York, Churchill Livingstone, 1994.
5. Moore KL: Clinically Oriented Anatomy, 2nd ed. Baltimore, Williams & Wilkins, 1985.
6. Palmer I: On the injuries to the ligaments of the knee joint: A clinical study. Acta Chir Scand 53(suppl):282, 1938.
7. Thompson WO, Fu FH: The meniscus in the cruciate deficient knee. Clin Sport Med, 12:771–796, 1993.
8. Brantigan OC, Voshell AF: Ligaments of the knee joint. The relationship of the ligament of Humphery to the ligament of Wrisberg. J Bone Joint Surg 28A:66–67, 1946.
9. Clancy WG Jr, Shelbourne KD, Zoellner GB, et al.: Treatment of knee joint instability secondary to rupture of the posterior cruciate ligament. J Bone Joint Surg, 65A:310–322, 1983.
10. Heller L, Langman J: The menisco-femoral ligaments of the human knee. J Bone Joint Surg 46B:307–313, 1964.
11. Cailliet R: Knee Pain and Disability. Philadelphia, F.A. Davis, 1973.
12. Lanzer WL, Komenda G: Changes in articular cartilage after meniscectomy. Clin Orthop 252:41–48, 1990.
13. Canner GC: Biomechanics and Biomaterials of the knee: Knee ligament rehabilitation. In Engle RP (ed): Knee Ligament Rehabilitation. New York, Churchill Livingstone, 1991, pp 17–24.
14. Levy IM, Torzilli PA, Warren RF: The effect of medial meniscectomy on anterior-posterior motion of the knee. J Bone Joint Surg 64:883–888, 1982.
15. Sullivan D, Levy IM, Sheskier S, et al.: Medial restraints to anterior-posterior motion of the knee. J Bone Joint Surg 66:930–936, 1984.
16. Yoshitsugu T, Xerogeanes JW, Livesay GA, et al.: Biomechanical function of the human anterior cruciate ligament. Arthroscopy 10:140, 1994.
17. Smith, Livesy GA, Fu FH: Biomechanics of the knee. In Tria AJ Jr (ed): Ligaments of the Knee. New York, Churchill Livingstone, 1995, pp 27–44.
18. Soderberg GL: Kinesiology: Application to Pathological Motion. Baltimore, Williams & Wilkins, 1986.
19. Smidt GL: Biomechanical analysis of knee flexion and extension. J Biomech 6:79–92, 1973.
20. Steindler A: Kinesiology of the Human Body under Normal and Pathological Conditions. Ligaments of the Knee. Springfield, IL, Charles C Thomas, 1955.
21. American Academy of Orthopaedic Surgeons: Joint Motion: Method of Measuring and Recording. Rosemont, IL, AAOS, 1994.
22. Frankel VH, Nordin M: Basic Biomechanics of the Skeletal System. Philadelphia, Lea & Febiger, 1980.
23. Norkin C, Levangie P: Joint Structure & Function. Philadelphia, F.A. Davis, 1992.
24. Müller W: Kinematics of the cruciate ligaments. In Feagin JA (ed): The Crucial Ligaments, 2nd ed. New York, Churchill Livingstone, 1994, pp. 289–305.
25. Woo SLY, Livesay GA, Engle C: Biomechanics of the human anterior cruciate ligament. Orthop Rev. July: 835–842, 1992.
26. Trent PS, Walker PS, Wolf P: Ligament length patterns, strength and rotational axes of the knee joint. Clin Orthop 117:263–270, 1976.

27. Noyes FR, Grood ES: The strength of the anterior cruciate ligament in humans and rhesus monkeys: Age-related and species-related changes. J Bone Joint Surg 58A:1074–1082, 1976.
28. Rowden NJ, Sher D, Rogers GJ, Schindhelm K: Anterior cruciate ligament graft fixation: Initial comparison of patellar tendon and semitendonosis autografts in young fresh cadavers. Am J Sports Med 25:4, 472–478, 1997.
29. Markolf KL, Gorek JF, Kabo M, Shapiro MS: Direct measurement of resultant forces in the anterior cruciate ligament. J Bone Joint Surg 72A:557–567, 1990.
30. Butler DL, Martin ET, Kaiser AD, et al.: The effects of flexion and tibial rotation on the 3-D orientations and lengths of human anterior cruciate ligament bundles. Trans Orthop Res Soc 13:59, 1988.
31. Sidles JA, Larson RV, Garbini JL, et al.: Ligament length relationships in the moving knee. J Orthop Res 6:593–610, 1988.
32. Woo SLY, Livesay GA, Engle C: Biomechanics of the human anterior cruciate ligament. Muscle stabilization and ACL reconstruction. Orthop Rev August: 935–941, 1992.
33. O'Brien WR, Friederich NF: Fiber recruitment of the cruciate ligaments. In Feagin JA (ed): The Crucial Ligaments, 2nd ed. New York, Churchill Livingstone, 1994, pp 307–317.
34. More RC, Markolf KL: Measurement of stability for the knee and ligament force after implantation of a synthetic anterior cruciate ligament graft. J Bone Joint Surg 70A:1020–1031, 1988.
35. Shoemaker SC, Adams D, Daniel DM, Woo SL: Quadriceps/anterior cruciate graft interaction: An invitro study of joint kinematics and anterior cruciate ligament graft tension. Clin Orthop Rel Res 294:379–390, 1993.
36. Wilk KE, Andrews JR: The effects of pad placement and angular velocity on tibial displacement during isokinetic exercise. J Orthop Sports Phys Ther 17(1):24–30, 1993.
37. Grood ES, Suntay WJ, Noyes FR, Butler DL: Biomechanics of knee extension exercise. J Bone Joint Surgery 66-A(5):725–734, 1984.
38. Kennedy JC, Hawkins RJ, Willis RB, Danylchuk KD: Tension studies of human knee ligaments, yield point, ultimate failure, and disruption of the cruciate and tibial collateral ligaments. J Bone Joint Surg 58-A:350, 1976.
39. Prietto MP, Bain JR, Stonebrook SN, Settlage RA: Tensile stress of the human posterior cruciate ligament (PCL). Trans Orthop Res Soc 13:195, 1988.
40. Harner CD, Kusayama T, Carlin GJ, et al.: Structural and mechanical properties of the human posterior cruciate and meniscofemoral ligaments. Trans Orthop Res Soc 19:629, 1994.
41. Wascher DC, Markolf KL, Shapiro MS, Finerman GAM: Direct in vitro measurement of forces in the cruciate ligaments. J Bone Joint Surg 75-A(3):377–386, 1993.
42. Grood ES, Stowers SF, Noyes FR: Limits of motion in the human knee. J Bone Joint Surg 70-A(1):88–97, 1988.
43. Woo SLY, Newton PO, MacKenna DA, Lyon RL: A comparative evaluation of the mechanical properties of the rabbit medial collateral ligament and anterior cruciate ligaments. J Biomech 25:377, 1992.
44. Grood ES, Noyes FR, Butler DL, Suntay WJ: Ligamentous and capsular restraints preventing straight and lateral laxity in intact human cadaver knees. J Bone Joint Surg 63-A(8):1257–1269, 1981.
45. Shapiro MS, Markolf KL, Finerman GAM, Mitchell PW: The effect of section of the medial collateral ligament on force generated in the anterior cruciate ligament. J Bone Joint Surg 73-A(2):248–256, 1991.

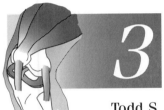

3 *Clinical Examination*

Todd S. Ellenbecker, MS, PT, SCS, CSCS

A comprehensive examination of an individual with a suspected injury to the ligamentous structures of the knee is the initial step in the complete treatment and rehabilitation process. Knowledge of the anatomy and biomechanics of the knee joint is of paramount importance, as is an understanding of the demands of the human knee in daily activities as well as in sports-specific movement patterns. The purpose of this chapter is to summarize salient portions of the examination process for the patient with a suspected acute or chronic knee ligament injury. Although it is beyond the scope of this chapter to provide an exhaustive description of all knee examination procedures, the reader will be directed, where applicable, to sources contained within and beyond this text.

SUBJECTIVE EVALUATION

The subjective evaluation begins with a thorough patient medical history consistent with the initial evaluation of any musculoskeletal injury.[1] Establishment of the presence of an acute or chronic knee injury or pathologic condition is usually obvious, but it is important to delineate. Use of directed questioning to rule out systemic medical conditions as well as referral symptoms must be included. The presence of symptoms typically inconsistent with musculoskeletal syndromes must be documented and should alert the examiner to possible neurologic or systemic complications in the individual. Numbness or loss of sensation and radiating pain from the spine or hip are examples of symptoms that alert the examiner to the presence of additional symptoms beyond the possible knee ligament injury that may be contributory factors.

Mechanism of Injury

Additional questioning specific to the knee joint regarding the mechanism of injury is also important for gaining insight into the possible structures involved. Gleaning from the patient information regarding whether an audible "pop" was felt or heard during the injury may indicate a complete ligament tear, and establishing whether contact with another person or object occurred also assists in providing a better understanding for the examiner. Re-creation of the mechanism of injury whenever possible with emphasis on cutting, foot placements (open or closed chain), and general lower extremity positioning can only add to the diagnostic accuracy.

In addition to the general medical history, establishing the history of other lower extremity injuries is important. Repeated episodes of instability or giving way over a period of months or years may heighten the examiner's suspicion of injury to secondary restraints, meniscus, or patellofemoral complications. A history of injury immediately proximal or distal to the knee joint is also extremely important to note, particularly in reference to the kinetic chain rehabilitation methods employed and biomechanical interfaces between interposing joints in the lower extremity (see Chapter 22).

Location of Symptoms

Identification of the location, and intensity of the pain is always included in the subjective examination. In a study of 90 patients with knee pain, patients and physicians completed pain diagrams blinded to each other's finding.[2] Eighty-five percent of all patient complaint zones were included in the physician's pain diagram following evaluation. These findings indicate that areas of tenderness located on examination of a patients' knee do correspond closely to the areas of patient complaint and facilitate proper diagnosis by directing attention to these specific zones during examination. The use of subjective rating is also recommend.[3, 4] The analogue pain scale using the baseline of "0" (no pain) and "10" (worst pain ever experienced) enables the examiner to place a value on the patient's symptoms and allows for comparison on re-evaluations and treatment sessions.

Finally, in the postoperative patient, it is important to obtain information from the patient regarding the exact surgical procedure performed as well as whether any additional procedures were required to address the meniscus or secondary ligament or capsular support structures. A close relationship with the referring surgeon as well as access to the operative report is recommended. Inclusion of surgical techniques is presented in many chapters of this book to enable clinicians to obtain a greater understanding of current surgical techniques and their subsequent rehabilitation indications and contraindications.

OBJECTIVE PHYSICAL EXAMINATION

Weight-Bearing Posture

In both the acutely and the chronically injured knee, a significant amount of information can be gathered simply by visual observation of weight-bearing stance for an anterior, posterior, and lateral view. General lower extremity alignment factors, including genu varum or valgum, genu recurvatum, and foot and ankle parameters, can be observed (Table 3–1). Additionally, a bilateral comparison of general quadricep and calf girth can be attained, as well as an initial idea of swelling location and extent. Finally, the patient's ability to bear weight on the injured extremity is gauged by stance posture, leg length difference, and trunk posture. For a complete description of the weight-bearing and non-weight-bearing foot examination, the reader is referred to Chapter 23. In addition to the static variables listed, a dynamic gait evaluation when possible can give additional information, such as the identification of a quadriceps avoidance

◯━ Table 3–1. Lower Extremity Postural Factors Observed During Weight-Bearing Stance

Postural Factor	Description/Detail
Genu varum	Feet together, one to two fingerbreadths between knees or more
Genu valgum	Knees together, distance of 9–10 cm considered excessive
Genu recurvatum	Extension beyond neutral (0 degrees)
Tibia varum	Medial bowing of the tibia
Foot pronation	Collapse of medial longitudinal arch
Helbings sign	Medial bowing of Achilles tendon due to rear foot valgus in weight-bearing
Hallux valgus	Valgus angulation of first metatarsophalangeal joint secondary to compensatory pronation
Leg length difference	Pelvic asymmetry of anterosuperior and posterosuperior iliac spine and iliac crest
Patellar position	Squinting patellae: inward-pointing patellae Grasshopper eyes: outward-pointing patellae

gait pattern,[5] or patient apprehension during weight-bearing or turning.

Effusion

Several tests are typically used in addition to visual observation of the knee in stance and in extension or position of most comfort with the patient in a supine position on a plinth.[4, 6] Typical locations for swelling following knee ligament injury are in the suprapatellar pouch, along the medial and lateral joint lines, and posteriorly in the popliteal fossa (Baker's cyst). Two tests described by Hoppenfeld[6] are the milking and ballotable patella tests. The milking test, or sign, tests for the presence of an intra-articular effusion and is performed with the knee in extension on a plinth with the subject in a supine position. One hand brushes or milks the swelling from the distal thigh downward toward the superior pole of the patella, attempting to squeeze or gather the intra-articular fluid from within the suprapatellar pouch. The second hand then gently pokes the medial or lateral side of the knee joint. A positive milking sign is when pressure on one side of the knee produces a wave-like response on the contralateral side of the joint, indicating the presence of fluid in the joint capsule.

With larger amounts of swelling, a ballotable patella sign is often present. This test is performed with the knee in as much extension as is comfortable and possible with the quadriceps relaxed. A downwardly directed force (tap) is applied to the patella with one or two fingers, with a quick release of the pressure on the top of the patella, similar to dribbling a basketball. A ballotable patella is present when a sensation or feeling of a floating patella is felt along with a rebound of the patella due to the presence of fluid in the joint.

Careful measurement and attention to joint effusion are not only important to better understanding of the potential injured structures within the knee but also have rehabilitative ramifications. Stratford[7] and Spencer et al.[8] studied the effects of knee effusion on quadriceps activity. Both found marked decreases in quadricep activity and a reflex shut-down of the quadriceps mechanism with as little as 20 to 30 mL of saline injection into the knee. Inhibition of the quadriceps due to effusion is thought to be mediated by afferent receptor input in the joint capsule triggered by pressure from the knee joint effusion. Attention to the degree of effusion in the acute or chronically injured patient is important both diagnostically and in rehabilitation, when efforts are geared at improving volitional quadricep activation.

Anthropometric Measurements

In addition to visual observation of a patient's swelling and overall quadriceps atrophy or thigh girth, anthropometric measurement of the limb is indicated. Objective quantification of girth using a tape measure is indicated to provide a baseline for both swelling and atrophy of the limb. Although significant differences in measurement protocol exist, typical locations for measurement are at the joint line or mid-patella level as well as over the vastus medialis obliquus and suprapatellar region, at mid-thigh, and over the belly of the gastrocnemius muscle.[3] This author's protocol consists of midpatellar measurement, and measurement 3 and 6 inches proximal and distal to that point. Use

of a Gulick tape measure is also recommended. A Gulick tape measure has a spring-loaded cylinder attached to the end of the tape measure and allows for a more consistent tension applied during anthropometric testing at multiple sites and across multiple occasions.

Palpation

Although it is beyond the scope of this chapter to completely list all palpable structures of the knee, the reader is referred to two references that detail a logical and complete sequence of palpation.[4, 6] It is recommended that the examiner follow a sequence of palpation rather than simply palpating the most indicated or obvious regions. According to Clancy,[9] the most painful areas should be palpated last, not first, upon examining a patient with a knee injury. Elevating the patient's pain level by first touching the most sensitive areas may mask less involved areas and create apprehension by the patient during further testing.

Patellar Testing

Examination of the patellofemoral joint is of key importance in both the nonoperative and postoperative evaluation of the patient with a knee ligament injury. Measurement of the Q-angle is an important indicator of the static and dynamic alignment of the lower extremity and, when coupled with the lateral pull test[10], gives the examiner insight into the degree of lateral deviation and tracking of the patellofemoral joint. The lateral pull test is performed by simply having the patient contract the quadriceps muscle with the knee in full extension. The direction of patellar movement is noted and compared bilaterally. The presence of lateral patellar tracking as opposed to superior or superolateral movement of the patella is noted and indicates the resultant pull of the quadriceps force vector (dynamic) as well as the static position of the patella near full extension (static). Use of the patellofemoral grinding test or Clarke's test gives the examiner insight into the condition of the undersurface of the patellae, as well as the degree of discomfort and inhibition of the quadriceps produced by a quadriceps contraction through the patellofemoral joint.

Of particular importance in the evaluation of the patellofemoral joint in the patient following a traumatic or acute injury is the apprehension test. Attempting to laterally or medially sublux the patella from the trochlear groove and monitoring the reaction of the patient to this maneuver can give the evaluator insight regarding possible patellar instability.

More subtle patellar positioning is also indicated in the overall evaluation of the patellofemoral joint. This is outlined by McConnell in this book and includes the factors of patellar tilt, glide, and rotation (see Chapter 15 for complete description). Careful evaluation of the patellofemoral joint will assist the clinician in both nonoperative and postoperative rehabilitation by identifying individuals who are at risk for patellofemoral complications from the lower extremity resistive training inherent in knee ligament rehabilitation, as well as providing a framework for the clinician in deciding which patients may need altered exercise prescriptions secondary to their patellofemoral joint status or lower extremity alignment.

Range of Motion

Careful documentation of knee range of motion (ROM) is necessary to both establish baseline ROM values and identify patients who need particular emphasis on ROM reattainment following injury or surgery. Considerable variation in knee ROM is reported in the literature.[11] Knee extension values range from 0 degrees to 5 to 10 degrees of genu recurvatum or hyperextension and 135 to 160 degrees flexion in the sagital plane.[12–15] DeCarlo et al.[16] recommend documenting range of motion using three measures: hyperextension, extension, and flexion. Therefore, a patient with 5 degrees of genurecurvatum and 135 degrees of flexion would be documented as 5-0-135. Measurement of passive knee extension, by placing the extremity on a towel roll or bolster, as well as active knee extension is also recommended.[16] Transverse plane motion of the tibiofemoral joint is 20 to 30 degrees of medial rotation and 30 to 40 degrees of lateral rotation with the knee flexed to 90 degrees.[4]

Additionally, passive motion and endfeels are of importance when evaluating the knee joint. Endfeels are described by Cyriax and Cyriax[17] as the feeling transmitted to the examiner's hands at the extreme ends of range of motion. The typical description of endfeels at the tibiofemoral joint for flexion is soft tissue approximation, while the endfeel for extension and medial and lateral rotation of the tibia on the femur is tissue stretch or capsular.[4] Table 3–2 outlines the common classifications of endfeel as outlined by Cyriax and Cyriax.[17]

Use of a standard universal goniometer to measure knee joint ROM has been subjected to critical analysis and study. Results of intratester reliability produced intraclass correlation coefficients of 0.99 for flexion and 0.98 for extension, whereas intertester reliability was reported as 0.90 for flexion and 0.86 for extension.[18] Comparison of goniometric measurements to visual estimates by clinicians ranged between 0.80 and 0.94.[18] These results support the use of goniometric measurements to precisely document ROM in the evaluation of the human knee as opposed to visual estimates.[18, 19]

Stability Testing

GENERAL CONCEPTS

One of the most important evaluations applicable to the patient with instability in the knee is ligamentous stability tests. Although there are many variations in techniques and interpretation, it is imperative that every clinician have a competent arsenal of clinical tests to evaluate the stability and integrity

Table 3–2. Classification and Description of Endfeels

Classification	Description
Bony	Two hard surfaces meeting, bone to bone (elbow extension)
Capsular	Leathery feel, further motion available (tibial rotation)
Soft tissue approximation	Soft tissue contact limits further motion (knee flexion)
Spasm	Muscular spasm limits motion (vibrant twang)
Springy block	Intra-articular block prohibits motion (rebound is felt)
Empty	Movement causes pain, pain limits movement

of, primarily, the collateral and cruciate ligaments.

Several important concepts accompany a successful stability examination for the patient with a suspected knee ligament injury. The first concept involves primary versus secondary constraints. Information regarding the primary and secondary restraints for each test described in this chapter come from laboratory research using selective cutting experimentation.[20] For a specific motion, the structure that provides the greatest limitation to movement or motion is considered the primary restraint.[21] When a primary restraint is disrupted, motion in that plane is limited by the remaining structures that are considered secondary restraints. What is important to note, however, is that disruption of a secondary restraint will not result in pathologic motion if the primary restraint is intact, but sectioning a secondary restraint when the primary restraint is already disrupted or affected will significantly increase the pathologic motion.[21]

While performing stability tests on the tibiofemoral joint, several additional factors must be considered and understood to optimize the interpretation of the movement or translation that is being evaluated. The human knee ligaments are only able to resist tibiofemoral motion along the line of their attachments and cannot limit motion perpendicular to their orientation.[22] Two ligaments are required to limit translation, one for each direction. For the example of anteroposterior translation, the primary restraint for anterior translation is the anterior cruciate ligament, while the primary restraint for posterior translation is the posterior cruciate ligament. Additionally, a single ligament is unable to resist rotation, since a bone is always able to rotate around a single attachment.[22] Therefore, when assessing anteroposterior translation, or tibiofemoral rotation, it is important to understand that several structures are working together to limit movement, not just one isolated structure.

Another important concept that is applied when clinically evaluating the ligamentous structures of the knee is "just taut length."[22] Just taut length is the amount of motion that occurs before a ligament can begin to provide a resisting force. Experienced examiners develop a clinical sense of the normal amount of motion that is typically required before a particular ligament or combination of ligaments can provide a resistive force

that will limit motion. Always examining the contralateral or uninjured extremity is recommended to provide the examiner with a baseline reference prior to examination of the injured extremity.

SPECIFIC CONCEPTS

In addition to always examining the uninjured extremity first, several specific concepts are required for successful examination of ligamentous structures of the knee. Examiners must denote not only the amount of tibiofemoral motion, but also the quality of the motion and endfeel. The stress imparted to the joint must be developed gently using light hand contacts to promote relaxation by the patient. A consistent application of the test by the examiner, with regard to hand placements and patient and extremity positioning, will enhance the reliability and validity of each of the stability tests contained in this text. Individual variation and adaptation of the tests may have to be carried out on occasion because of patient extremity size, examiner hand size, and patient positioning complications caused by other injuries or patient immobility.

Finally, grading of stability examinations for the knee has been discussed and several classification systems have been established to allow for consistent interpretation and communication of results of tibiofemoral stability testing. The classic orthopedic terminology of grade I (0–5 mm), grade II (5–10 mm), and grade III (>10 mm) has been used for many years.[23] Hughston and associates[24] graded instability according to the amount of tibial translation present compared with the contralateral side. Grade I injuries or instability consists of 0 to 5 mm of increased laxity, grade II consists of 5 to 10 mm of increased laxity or translation, grade III has 10 to 15 mm greater translation, and grade IV represents laxity above 15 mm compared with the unaffected side.

STABILITY TESTS FOR THE TIBIOFEMORAL JOINT

Testing the stability of the knee includes tests for both straight (one-plane) and rotational (rotary) instability. The breakdown of testing order for this chapter occurs in the following sequence:

- One-plane medial instability tests
- One-plane lateral instability tests

- One-plane anterior instability tests
- One-plane posterior instability tests
- Anteromedial rotary instability tests
- Anterolateral rotary instability tests
- Posteromedial rotary instability tests
- Posterolateral rotary instability tests

One-Plane Medial Instability Tests

The primary clinical test employed to assess the medial stability of the tibiofemoral joint is the valgus stress test. This test is done in both complete extension and with 20 to 30 degrees of knee flexion. The test is performed with the patient supine, with neutral axial rotation of the femur. The examiner grasps the distal femur by cupping and supporting the proximal segment of the extremity, placing the hand as a block along the lateral joint line (Fig. 3–1A). The opposite hand grasps the medial aspect of the distal tibia to further support the extremity. With the hand on the distal tibia, an axial load is applied to place the tibiofemoral joint in a neutral position.[21] The distal leg is then abducted without axial rotation while the proximal hand stabilizes and blocks the motion, opening the medial joint line as pictured (Fig. 3–1B). The medial joint space

opening as well as the stiffness and endfeel are noted and compared with the contralateral side. Grood et al.[25] have shown that the medial collateral ligament accounts for 57 percent of the restraining force against valgus stress at 5 degrees of knee flexion and 78 percent at 25 degrees knee flexion.[4, 25] Additional structures stabilizing the knee against valgus stress are the following:

- Medial collateral ligament
- Posterior oblique ligament
- Anterior cruciate ligament (ACL)
- Posterior cruciate ligament (PCL)
- Medial middle one-third of joint capsule.

One-Plane Lateral Stability Tests

The primary test to assess lateral stability of the tibiofemoral joint is the varus stress or adduction stress test. This test is performed at both complete extension and 25 to 30 degrees of flexion in a similar manner to the valgus stress test. Hand placements are demonstrated in Figure 3–2 which shows the proximal hand placed on the medial aspect of the knee to block, and the distal hand of the examiner placed along the lateral side of the distal tibia. Separation of the lateral joint space is assessed along with the

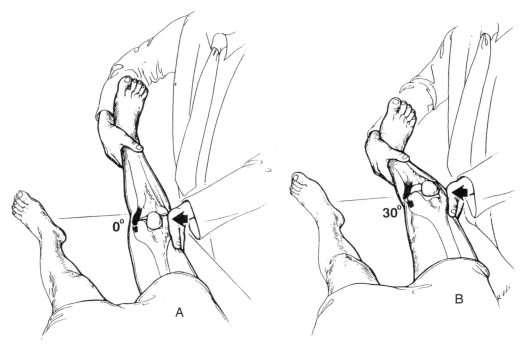

Figure 3–1. The valgus stress test. (From Tria AJ Jr, Klein KS: An Illustrated Guide to the Knee. New York, Churchill Livingstone, 1992, p. 57.)

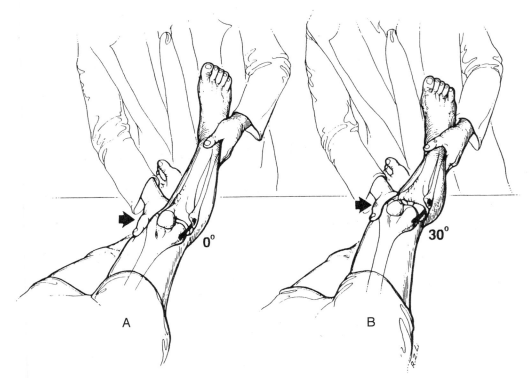

Figure 3–2. The varus stress test. (From Tria AJ Jr, Klein KS: An Illustrated Guide to the Knee. New York, Churchill Livingstone, 1992, p. 58.)

endfeel and compared with the contralateral side. The primary restraint against lateral joint space widening is the lateral or fibular collateral ligament.[25] Additional noncontractile structures assessed with this test are the following:[4, 23]

- Lateral collateral ligament
- Middle one-third of lateral capsule
- Arcuate-popliteus complex
- ACL
- PCL
- Illiotibial band.

One-Plane Anterior Instability Tests

Lachman Test. The Lachman test has been reported to be the best test for assessing the integrity of the posterolateral band of the anterior cruciate ligament (ACL) and is the most practical test for assessing the integrity of the ACL in an acutely injured knee because of the position utilized with testing.[4, 11, 20, 26] The original test for assessing the integrity of the ACL was described by Jones[27] in the first decade of the 20th century.[26] It utilized a fully extended position until modified by Torg et al.[28] who detailed

the test, named it the Lachman test, and recommended this test as the standard for assessment of the ACL.

Performing the Lachman test as recommended by Wroble and Lindenfeld using a stabilized technique is illustrated in Figure 3–3. Owing to complications arising from examiner hand size, patient extremity size, and axial rotation of the testing extremity encountered with the standard Lachman examination,[24] the stabilized method stabilizes the limb using a support or the examiner's thigh to maintain a consistent flexion position, and allows hand placements that can more accurately asses anterior tibial translation.[4, 26] The patient lies supine on the examination table, with the examiner's right knee or a firm 6 inch diameter bolster placed under the left knee of the patient.[4] This places the knee in approximately 20 to 35 degrees of flexion as recommended.[11] The thigh is further stabilized by placing the top hand over the thigh with the fingers extending distally to palpate the medial joint line (see Fig. 3–3). The distal hand then applies an anteriorly directed force to the tibia, while the proximal hand is able to palpate

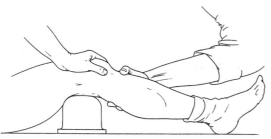

Figure 3–3. The supported Lachman test (From Feagin JA: The Crucial Ligaments: Diagnosis and Treatment of Ligamentous Injuries About the Knee. New York, Churchill Livingstone, 1994, p. 390.)

the motion. Care must be taken to be certain the force is directed straight anterior during the test without induction of axial rotation of the tibia or femur. Additional modifications of this classic test include the prone Lachman test described by Feagin and Cooke.[29] The primary and secondary noncontractile structures tested during the Lachman test are the following:[4]

- ACL, posterolateral bundle
- Posterior oblique ligament
- Arcuate ligament.

Improved diagnostic accuracy was reported by Donaldson et al.[30] using the Lachman test as compared with the anterior

drawer test, with accuracy improving from 70 percent to 100 percent. Further support for the Lachman clinical test comes from research performed by Fleming et al.[31] who compared clinical tests to instrumented tests on autopsy specimens. They found that Lachman and anterior drawer tests were more reliable than either the Genucom or Knee Signature System (KSS) instrumented devices. Additional research was performed comparing magnetic resonance imaging (MRI), arthrometry, and clinical examination in the diagnosis of acute complete tears of the ACL.[32] The Lachman test was found to be 95 percent sensitive and was the single best clinical test for diagnosing complete ACL tears.

Anterior Drawer Test. Another straight plane test to assess anterior stability of the knee is the anterior drawer test. This test involves flexing the knee to 90 degrees and the hip to 45 degrees. The examiner is seated and places the forefoot of the extremity being tested under his or her buttock to stabilize the distal portion of the extremity (Fig. 3–4). The foot should be in neutral rotation. The examiner's hands are placed around the tibia, palpating the hamstring tendons medially and laterally to establish a relaxed state of these muscle-tendon units.

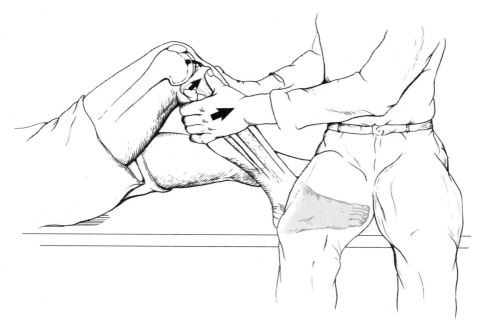

Figure 3–4. The anterior drawer test. (Modified from Tria AJ Jr, Klein KS: An Illustrated Guide to the Knee. New York, Churchill Livingstone, 1992, p. 59.)

Care must be taken to determine whether the tibia is starting from a neutral position, which is imperative for true interpretation of the anterior tibial translation garnered during this test. The thumbs can be used to align the anterior-most part of the tibial plateaus in line with the femoral condyles prior to starting the test. Posterior sagging of the tibial condyles indicates possible injury to the posterior cruciate ligament (see discussion of tests in the next section). Once the neutral position has been established, the examiner draws the tibia forward on the femur, noting both the amount of translation and the endfeel or endpoint. The anterior drawer test examines the integrity of the following noncontractile tissues[4, 23]:

- ACL, anteromedial bundle
- Middle and posterior one-third of medial and lateral capsule
- MCL, deep fibers
- Illiotibial band
- Posterior oblique ligament
- Arcuate complex
- PCL.

Traditionally, the anterior drawer test has shown a lower sensitivity in both chronic and acutely injured ACLs. This has led examiners to utilize the Lachman and pivot shift maneuvers. Several reports have been published highlighting an additional complication to diagnosis of ACL injury.[33] Kong et al.[33] reported on displaced bucket handle tears of the medial meniscus masking ACL deficiency and caution examiners against ruling out ACL injury in the presence of negative results of anterior drawer or Lachman tests if the mechanism of injury and history suggest ACL injury. These clinical tests, when used together or in isolation, provide the clinician with the best available clinical tests for diagnosis of ACL injury.

One-Plane Posterior Instability Tests

Tibial Sag Sign. The traditional tibial sag sign is described with 90 degrees of knee flexion and 45 degrees of hip flexion with the patient lying supine. In this position, the patient's involved tibia will appear to sag posteriorly, creating a concave appearance of the patellar tendon. This posterior sagging is indicative of injury to the PCL and posterior capsular structures (posterior medial oblique ligament and arcuate complex) as well as the ACL. A common variation of the tibial sag sign is Godfrey's test. In Godfrey's test, the patient lies supine and the hips and knees are simultaneously flexed to 90 degrees. Again, a posterior or downward sagging of the tibia and bowing of the patellar tendon indicates injury to the previously mentioned structures.

Posterior Drawer Test. Using identical procedures and positioning as the anterior drawer test, the posterior drawer test examines the competency of, primarily, the PCL (Fig. 3–5). A posterior force is exerted on the tibia in an attempt to sublux it posteriorly beneath the femur. Noncontractile tissues tested during the posterior drawer test are the following:

- PCL
- Middle and posterior one-third of medial and lateral capsule
- MCL, deep fibres
- Illiotibial band
- Posterior oblique ligament
- Arcuate complex
- ACL, anteromedial bundle.

Tests to Determine Rotary Instability

Anteromedial Rotary Instability Test. The anteromedial rotary instability test, also called Slocum's test[34] is performed with 80 to 90 degrees of knee flexion, and 15 degrees of lateral or external tibial rotation. This position tenses the medial capsular structures. The examiner pulls the tibia forward, and a positive result includes increased anterior tibial translation, particularly on the medial side relative to the lateral side of the knee being examined, as well as greater translation relative to the contralateral extremity. A positive result indicates injury to the following structures[4]:

- Medial collateral ligament
- Posterior medial oblique ligament
- Posterior and middle one-third of medial capsule
- ACL.

Anterolateral Rotary Instability Test. One test used to assess anterolateral rotary instability is one portion of Slocum's test.[34] This test, like the test for anteromedial rotary instability, uses an identical patient and examiner position as the anterior drawer test (see Fig. 3–4), except for the use of 30 degrees of internal or medial rotation of the tibia. For a positive anterolateral rotary instability test, movement is primarily located on the lateral side of the knee with an anteriorly directed force of the tibia upon the fe-

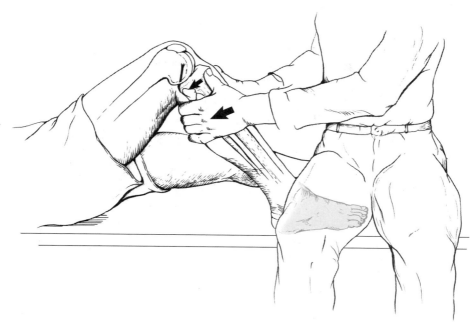

Figure 3–5. The posterior drawer test. (Modified from Tria AJ Jr, Klein KS: An Illustrated Guide to the Knee. New York, Churchill Livingstone, 1992, p. 62.)

mur.[4, 11] A positive anterolateral rotary instability test indicated injury to the following structures:

- ACL
- Lateral collateral ligament
- Arcuate ligament
- Middle and posterior one-third of lateral joint capsule
- PCL
- Illiotibial band.

Pivot Shift Test. The pivot shift test has been described by numerous authors as the Losee test, side-lying test, and flexion-rotation drawer test.[21] The classic pivot shift test has been described as an anterior subluxation and internal axial rotation of the tibia on the femur. The pivot shift test is performed with the patient in a supine position with the hip flexed approximately 30 degrees and in slight (20 degrees) internal rotation.[4, 21] The examiner holds the patient's foot as pictured in Figure 3–6, with one hand, while the other hand is placed with the heel of the hand or thumb over the fibular head and lateral head of the gastrocnemius. The tibia is internally rotated as the knee is extended, causing the tibia to sublux anteriorly and medially indicating involvement of the ACL and the following lateral restraint structures:

- ACL

- Posterolateral capsule
- Arcuate ligament
- Lateral collateral ligament
- Illiotibial band.

Following the passive extension of the knee, a valgus stress is imparted to the knee while maintaining the position of medial tibial rotation. The knee is then passively flexed with a reduction of the anteriorly displaced tibia occurring at approximately 30 to 40 degrees. This relocation or reduction occurs because of the illiotibial band's change of function from an extensor to a flexor at this 30- to 40-degree flexed range of motion (see Fig. 3–6). Factors contributing to or negating a positive pivot shift test are torn meniscus or a tear in the illiotibial band, which would prevent tibial excursion.[4, 21] The relationship between tears of the ACL and the configuration of the lateral tibial plateau and the pivot shift test have been statistically identified with MRI.[35]

Posteromedial Rotary Instability Test. The primary test to assess posteromedial stability in the human knee is the posteromedial drawer sign. Starting position for this test is identical to the posterior drawer test discussed earlier in this chapter, with the exception of the addition of slight internal or medial rotation of the tibia. As the examiner

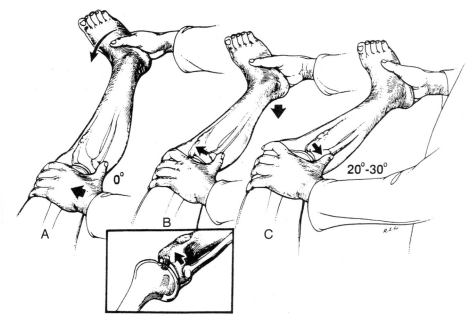

Figure 3–6. The pivot-shift test. (From Tria AJ Jr, Klein KS: An Illustrated Guide to the Knee. New York, Churchill Livingstone, 1992, p. 60.)

pushes the tibia backward, care is taken to determine whether most of the posterior movement occurs on the medial side relative to the lateral side of the joint, as well as relative to the contralateral extremity. The following structures are involved in a positive result to the posteromedial drawer test[4]:

- PCL
- Posterior medial oblique ligament
- Medial collateral ligament
- Posteromedial joint capsule
- ACL.

Posterolateral Rotary Instability Test. Hughston's posterolateral drawer test can be used to test for posterolateral rotary instability.[4, 36] Again, identical patient positioning and hand placements are followed, as compared with the posterior drawer test, with the exception of lateral or external tibial rotation relative to the femur. The presence of increased posterior tibial translation on the lateral side of the knee joint from the posterior pressure exerted by the examiner indicates a positive result. The result will be positive only if the PCL is torn.[4] Additional structures indicated with a posterolateral rotary instability test are as follows:

- PCL
- Arcuate complex
- Lateral collateral ligament
- Posterolateral joint capsule
- ACL.

External Rotation Recurvatum Test. The external rotation recurvatum test is performed with the patient in the supine position with the knees in complete extension. The quadriceps remain relaxed during the test while the examiner grasps the great toe of each extremity simultaneously (Fig. 3–7). As the knees are fully extended passively, the amount of hyperextension or genu recurvatum is noted. Particular attention is given to the hyperextension of the lateral aspect of the joint, which is greater in a positive test, along with external rotation or lateral rotation of the tibial tubercle.

Active Posterolateral Drawer Sign. As opposed to the above-mentioned passive tests for posterolateral rotary instability, this test utilizes an active contraction of the hamstrings, specifically the biceps femoris to create a posterior subluxation of the lateral tibial plateau. The test is typically conducted with the patient in a seated position with the knee comfortably flexed and tibia in lateral rotation.

Reverse Pivot Shift Test. The reverse pivot shift test has been reported as the most reliable test for posterolateral rotary instability.[21, 36] One description of the reverse pivot shift test states that the test commences with the examiner's hand supporting the limb, grasping under the heel of the extremity to be examined in neutral axial

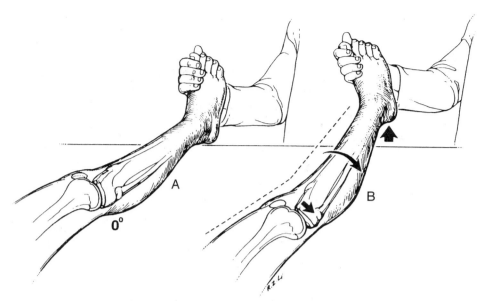

Figure 3-7. The external rotation recurvatum test. (From Tria AJ Jr, Klein KS: An Illustrated Guide to the Knee. New York, Churchill Livingstone, 1992, p. 63.)

rotation with the knee extended.[21] The second hand of the examiner is placed on the lateral side of the calf, applying a valgus stress to the knee while the knee is flexed. In a positive reverse pivot shift, the tibia will rotate externally at about 20 to 30 degrees of knee flexion with the lateral tibial plateau displacing posteriorly and remain in this position during further flexion.[21] Extension of the knee will produce a reduction of the lateral tibial plateau.

Summary. Each ligamentous examination detailed in this chapter must be performed by the examiner using a reliable and consistent application. Standardization of patient positioning and examiner hand placements and forces is necessary to allow proper interpretation of the translation produced. The difficulty in interpretation of these ligamentous examination techniques lies in the subtle discrimination between normal and abnormal movement patterns. An experienced examiner is usually able to detect ACL disruption, even when there is only a 4 mm bilateral difference between the injured and the uninjured extremity. Although the ultimate difference in translation is important, the difference in endpoint stiffness or endfeel enables the experienced examiner to detect pathologic conditions as well.[21] Development of a consistent examination method of at least one technique to assess both straight plane and rotary instability for the tibiofemoral joint is of paramount importance.

Meniscal Tests

The classic clinical tests to rule out meniscal pathology are McMurray's and Apley's tests. Many variations in the technique and interpretation of McMurray's test exist.[37] The simplest description of the test has the patient in the supine position on a plinth with the hip flexed and knee acutely flexed.[37] The knee is brought to 90 degrees of flexion while full internal and then full external rotation of tibia is maintained. A click that reproduces the patient's pain is thought to represent a tear in the meniscus. A notable addition to this basic description of McMurray's test is the use of a varus stress with internal tibial rotation and a valgus stress with lateral or external tibial rotation. Diagnostic accuracy using McMurray's test consistently places the sensitivity at about 26 percent and the specificity at 94 percent.

Apley's test involves a prone position, with 90 degrees of knee flexion. The examiner then stabilizes the thigh with his or her leg and internally and externally rotates the tibia while compressing the tibiofemoral joint. A meniscal injury is suspected if the combination of tibial rotation and compression reproduces the patient's symptoms.[4]

Comparison of clinical meniscal examination techniques with MRI in the diagnosis of meniscal tears was made in 93 competitive athletes.[38] The correct diagnosis of a meniscal tear was made 89 percent of the time with clinical examination alone, and 89 percent of the time with MRI. The results of this study show that the use of clinical examination techniques by an experienced examiner can produce similar degrees of accuracy and sensitivity as those achieved by MRI. Care must be taken, however, to properly interpret the findings of the clinical examination for the meniscus, as the inexperienced examiner can incorrectly assume that crepitance and other types of joint irregularities felt during clinical meniscal tests are meniscal lesions.

Muscular Strength Testing

The use of manual muscle testing (MMT) has become a clinical standard for muscular strength assessment since its initial development in the early 1900s on patients with poliomyelitis. This technique has been found to be reliable between examiners within one grade (MMT is graded from 0, absent, to 5, normal).[39] MMT is an inexpensive and quick assessment technique that ultimately depends on the subjective rating of muscular strength by the examiner. It is nonetheless the primary initial examination method used clinically to quickly discern the strength of the musculature surrounding the knee joint as well as proximal, stabilizing musculature in the patient with a knee ligament injury. MMT of the quadriceps and hamstrings, as well as testing of hip flexion, extension, abduction and adduction, and internal-external rotation, is recommended. Testing proximal muscle groups is recommended because of the frequent presence of proximal muscular weakness found in extremities with distal injury.[40]

In addition to MMT, individuals with higher levels of function may require more advanced methods of muscular strength assessment. The reader is directed to Chapters 4 and 20 outlining details of isokinetic strength testing for patients in this injury population.

Sensation

Evaluation of neurologic deficits in the patient with a knee ligament injury includes assessing both motor and sensory function. Motor function is usually assessed with MMT, as mentioned above, while monitoring of the patient's sensory function is performed via the patient's ability to detect light touch sensation. Sharp or dull, or hot or cold sensation is often tested to establish a pattern or region of sensory loss in the patient, particularly following open surgery when peri-incisional sensory loss is often encountered. Testing the dermatomal regions of L_2–S_1 is often carried out, with particular emphasis being placed around surgical scars. Use of the Semmes-Weinstein monofilaments constitutes a threshold test that allows the examiner to determine at what threshold sensation can be detected by the patient using various sizes of calibrated monofilaments.[41] The use of the Semmes-Weinstein monofilaments allows the examiner to determine a baseline and perform follow-up evaluations to discern improvement.

Functional Testing

Functional testing is an important element in every musculoskeletal examination and can vary in intensity from basic functions such as gait, stair climbing, or crouching ability to more advanced tasks such as hopping, cutting motions and performing sports-specific tests. The primary functional test used and recommended by the International Knee Documentation Committee (IKDC) is the one-leg hop test. The one-leg hop test involves jumping off of and landing upon the same limb, with the results on the involved limb being compared with those on the uninvolved limb.[42] An excellent result on the horizontal one-leg hop test is achievement of a distance greater than 90 percent or more of the uninvolved limb, with 75 to 89 percent being a good result.[42] A fair result is deemed 50 to 74 percent of the distance of the uninvolved limb, whereas less than 50 percent of the distance is considered a poor result. Hu et al.[43] reported acceptable test-retest reliability of the one-leg hop test (ICC range 0.79–0.96) between sessions.

Additional functional testing is outlined in Chapter 21 and includes lower extremity test examples as well as normative data. One additional test used by this author is the hexagon test. This test has been used by the

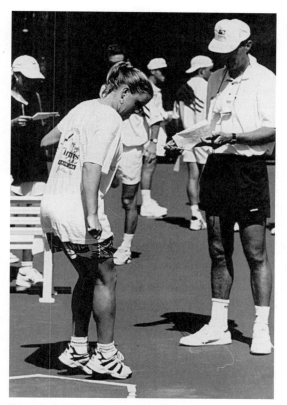

Figure 3–8. The hexagon functional test.

hexagon facing the same forward direction as each of the hexagon lines is crossed. Three complete revolutions are performed and timed with a stopwatch. Normative data for the hexagon test are listed for adults and junior-aged tennis players in Table 3–3.[45]

KNEE RATING OR SCORING SCALES

One final topic to be discussed in this chapter is the use of subjective rating scales. These scales are recommended for use to quantify the patient's perception of his or her own function and pain levels, to serve as a baseline following injury or surgery and during serial evaluations and follow-up. The simplest form of subjective rating scale is the visual analog pain scale. With this scale, the patient is asked to quantify his or her pain with rest or certain activities using the scale from 0, no pain, to 10, worst pain ever experienced. Either a number is given or a single line with endmarkings is given to patients and they are asked to place a mark on the blank line where they feel their symptoms currently place them. A ruler or scaling device is then used to objectively measure the location of their mark along the pain continuum. Subjective rating scales can be very general, such as general health and well-being questionnaires, ranging to very specific, such as rating systems designed only for one type of clinical pathology.

The Lysholm scale[46] is commonly used in patients with knee ligament injuries (Table 3–4). This scale uses subheadings for instability, pain, ambulation independence, and general activities of daily living movement patterns. It is easily administered to patients and can assist in research outcomes for patients with knee ligament injuries.[47] Addi-

United States Tennis Association as a lower extremity agility test because of the use of explosive muscular contractions, presence of multiple changes of direction, and reliance on optimal center of mass control.[44, 45] The hexagon test is laid out using athletic tape on a smooth surface with 24-inch lengths at 120 degree angles arranged in the shape of a hexagon (Fig. 3–8). The test begins with the patient in the hexagon. Upon receiving the command to start, the patient jumps over the line and back into the hexagon. The patient then continues around the

Table 3–3. Hexagon Functional Test Normative Data*

	Excellent	Good	Average	Poor
Female				
Adult	<12:00	12:00–12:10	12:10–12:40	>13:40
Junior	<10:48	10:48–11:70	11:70–12:30	>12:30
Male				
Adult	<11:80	11:80–13:00	13:00–13:50	>13:50
Junior	<11:10	11:10–11:80	11:80–12:70	>12:70

*Data expressed in seconds.
Data from United States Tennis Association, Roetert EP, Ellenbecker TE: Complete Conditioning for Tennis. Champagne, IL, Human Kinetics Publishers, 1998.

●━━ Table 3–4. **Lysholm Knee Scoring Scale**

Limp (5 points)	
None	5
Slight or periodical	3
Severe and constant	0
Support (5 points)	
None	5
Stick or crutch	2
Weight-bearing impossible	0
Locking (15 points)	
No locking and no catching sensations	15
Catching sensation but no locking	10
Locking	
Occasionally	6
Frequently	2
Locked joint on examination	0
Instability (25 points)	
Never giving way	25
Rarely during athletics or other severe exertion	20
Frequently during athletics or other severe exertion (or incapable of participation)	15
Occasionally in daily activities	10
Often in daily activities	5
Every step	0
Pain (25 points)	
None	25
Inconstant and slight during severe exertion	20
Marked during severe exertion	15
Marked on or after walking more than 2 km	10
Marked on or after walking less than 2 km	5
Constant	0
Swelling (10 points)	
None	10
On severe exertion	6
On ordinary exertion	2
Constant	0
Stair-climbing (10 points)	
No problems	10
Slightly impaired	6
One step at a time	2
Impossible	0
Squatting (5 points)	
No problems	5
Slightly impaired	4
Not beyond 90 degrees	2
Impossible	0

struction and reported no significant differences in the Lysholm scale between groups. Many types of scales are available for the lower extremity and specifically the knee joint with a ligament injury. It is recommended that each clinician and or clinic review the literature and consider using a rating scale or group of rating scales on a consistent basis. Use of tests with established validation and test-retest reliability is of paramount importance. Self-reported questionnaire data have recently been studied and found to be reliable in patients with musculoskeletal injury.[49]

SUMMARY

The primary elements most integral in a comprehensive evaluation of the patient with knee ligament injury are summarized in this chapter. Although it is beyond the scope of this chapter to completely discuss every test in total detail, where applicable, additional resources contained within this text have been referenced. It is important that every examiner have a structured and standardized method for testing the integrity of the noncontractile stabilizing structures of the knee, and that every examiner is able to interpret these findings in both normal and pathologically extreme conditions.

tional scales used are included in this text, such as the Cincinnati Knee Rating System (Chapter 9, Appendix 9–B) and the Modified Noyes Questionnaire (Chapter 8, Appendix 8–A). These scales increase the amount of measurable and quantifiable information regarding patient outcomes and assist in the rehabilitation and treatment of patients with knee ligament injury.

Subjective rating or scoring scales are also used in research when comparing rehabilitation or surgical methods.[48] Bynum et al.[48] compared open-chain to closed-chain rehabilitation protocols following ACL recon-

References

1. Gould JA, Davies GJ: Orthopaedic and sports rehabilitation concepts. In Gould JA, Davies GJ (eds): Orthopaedic and Sports Physical Therapy. St. Louis, Mosby, 1985.
2. Post WR, Fulkerson J: Knee pain diagrams: Correlation with physical examination findings in patients with anterior knee pain. Arthroscopy 10(6):618–623, 1994.
3. Timm KE: The knee. In Richardson JK, Iglarsh ZA (eds): Clinical Orthopaedic Physical Therapy. Philadelphia, W.B. Saunders, 1994.
4. Magee DJ: Orthopedic Physical Assessment, 3rd ed. Philadelphia, W.B. Saunders, 1997.
5. Brownstein B: Movement skills in sports. In Brownstein B, Bronner S (eds): Functional Movement in Orthopaedic and Sports Physical Therapy. New York, Churchill Livingstone, 1997.
6. Hoppenfeld S: Physical Examination of the Spine and Extremities. London, Prentice-Hall Inc., 1976.
7. Stratford P: Electromyography of the quadriceps femoris muscles in subjects with normal knees and acutely effused knees. Phys Ther 62(3):279–283, 1981.
8. Spencer JD, Hayes KC, Alexander IJ: Knee joint effusion and quadriceps reflex inhibition in man. Arch Phys Med Rehabil 65:171–177, 1984.

9. Clancy WG: Acute Injuries in the Knee: Evaluation and Treatment. 11th Annual Injuries in Baseball Course. Birmingham, AL, 1993.
10. Kolowich PA, Paulos LP, Rosenburg TD, Farnsworth S: Lateral release of the patella: Indications and contraindications. Am J Sports Med 18:359–362, 1990.
11. Engle RP: Examination of the knee. In Engle RP (ed): Knee Ligament Rehabilitation. New York, Churchill Livingston, 1991.
12. Kapandji IA: The Physiology of the Joints, Vol 2, 5th ed. New York, Churchill Livingstone, 1987.
13. American Academy of Orthopaedic Surgeons: Joint Motion: Method of Measuring and Recording. Chicago, AAOS, 1965.
14. DeCarlo MS, Sell K: Normative data for range of motion and single leg hop in high school athletes. J Sport Rehab 6:246, 1997.
15. DeCarlo MS, Sell K: The effects of the number and frequency of physical therapy treatments on selected outcomes of treatment in patients with ACL reconstruction. J Orthop Sports Phys Ther 26:332–339, 1997.
16. DeCarlo, Shelbourne KD, McCarroll JR, Rettig AC: Traditional versus accelerated rehabilitation following ACL reconstruction: A one year follow-up. J Orthop Sports Phys Ther 15(6):309–316, 1992.
17. Cyriax JH, Cyriax PJ: Illustrated manual of orthopaedic medicine. London, Butterworths, 1983.
18. Watkins MA, Riddle DL, Lamb RL, Personius WJ: Reliability of goniometric measurements and visual estimates of knee range of motion obtained in a clinical setting. Phys Ther 71(2):90–97, 1991.
19. Gajdosik RL, Bohannon RW: Clinical measurement of range of motion. Review of goniometry emphasizing reliability and validity. Phys Ther 67(12):1867–1872, 1987.
20. Woo SLY, Livesay GA, Engle C: Biomechanics of the human anterior cruciate ligament: ACL structure and role in knee motion. Orthop Rev July:835–842, 1992.
21. Daniel DM, Stone ML: Diagnosis of knee ligament injury: Tests and measurement of knee motion limits. In Feagin JA (ed): The Crucial Ligaments, 2nd ed. New York, Churchill Livingstone, 1994.
22. Grood ES, Noyes FR: Diagnosis of knee ligament injuries: Biomechanical precepts. In Feagin JA (ed): The Crucial Ligaments, 2nd ed. New York, Churchill Livingstone, 1994.
23. Wallace LA, Mangine RE, Malone T: The knee. In Gould JA, Davies GJ (eds): Orthopaedic and Sports Physical Therapy. St. Louis, Mosby 1985.
24. Hughston JC, Andrews JR, Cross MJ, Noschi A: A classification of knee ligament instabilities: Part I. The medial compartment and cruciate ligaments. J Bone Joint Surg 58A:159, 1976.
25. Grood ES, Noyes FR, Butler DL, Suntay WJ: Ligamentous and capsular restraints preventing medial and lateral laxity in intact human cadaver knees. J Bone Joint Surg 63-A(8):1257–1269, 1981.
26. Wroble RR, Lindenfeld TN: The stabilized Lachman test. Clin Orthop Rel Res 237:209–212, 1988.
27. Jones R: On certain derangements of the knee. Clin J 28:51, 1906.
28. Torg JS, Conrad W, Kalen V: Clinical diagnosis of anterior cruciate ligament instability in the athlete. Am J Sports Med 4:84, 1976.
29. Feagin JA, Cooke TDV: Prone examination for anterior cruciate ligament insufficiency. J Bone Joint Surg 71-B(5):863, 1989.
30. Donaldson WF, Warren RF, Wickiewicz T: A comparison of acute anterior cruciate ligament examinations. Am J Sports Med 13:5, 1985.
31. Fleming BC, Johnson RJ, Shapiro E, et al.: Clinical versus instrumented knee testing on autopsy specimens. Clin Orthop Rel Res 282:196–207, 1992.
32. Liu SH, Osti L, Henry M, Bocchi L: The diagnosis for acute complete tears of the anterior cruciate ligament. J Bone Joint Surg 77-B(4):586–588, 1995.
33. Kong KC, Hamlet MR, Peckham T, Mowbray MAS: Displaced bucket handle tears of the medial meniscus masking anterior cruciate ligament deficiency. Arch Orthop Trauma Surg 114:51–52, 1994.
34. Slocum DB, Larson RL: Rotary instability of the knee. J Bone Joint Surg 50-A:211, 1968.
35. Kujala UM, Nelimarkka O, Koskinen SK: Relationship between the pivot shift and the configuration of the lateral tibial plateau. Arch Orthop Trauma Surg 111:228–229, 1992.
36. Cooper DE: Tests for posterolateral instability of the knee in normal subjects: Results of examination under anesthesia. J Bone Joint Surg 73-A(1):30–36, 1991.
37. Stratford PW, Binkley J: A review of the McMurray test: Definition, interpretation, and clinical usefulness. J Orthop Sports Phys Ther. 22(3):116–120, 1995.
38. Muellner T, Weinstabl R, Schabus R, Vecsei V, Kainberger F: The diagnosis of mensical tears in athletes: A comparison of clinical and magnetic resonance imaging investigations. Am J Sports Med 25(1):7–12, 1997.
39. Aitkens S, Lord J, Bernauer E, Fowler WM, Lieberman JS, Berck P: Relationship of manual muscle testing to objective strength measurements. Muscle Nerve 12:173–177, 1989.
40. Nicholas JA, Strizak AM, Veras G: A study of thigh muscle weakness in different pathological states of the lower extremity. Am J Sports Med 4:241, 1976.
41. Wadsworth C: The wrist and hand. In Malone TR, McPoil T, Nitz AJ (eds): Orthopaedic and Sports Physical Therapy, 3rd ed. St. Louis, Mosby, 1997.
42. Wallace LA, Mangine RE, Mangine TR: The knee. In Malone TR, McPoil T, Nitz AJ (eds): Orthopaedic and Sports Physical Therapy, 3rd ed. St. Louis, Mosby, 1997.
43. Hu HS, Whitney SL, Irrgang J, Ianosky I: Test-retest reliability of the one-legged vertical jump test and the one legged standing hop test (abstract). J Orthop Sports Phys Ther 15(1):51, 1992.
44. Roetert EP, Garrett GE, Brown SW, Camaione DN: Performance profiles of nationally ranked junior tennis players. J Appl Sports Sci Res 6(4):225–231, 1992.
45. United States Tennis Association, Roetert, EP, Ellenbecker TE: Complete Conditioning for Tennis. Champaign, IL: Human Kinetics Publishers, 1998.
46. Tegner Y, Lysholm J: Rating systems in the evaluation of knee ligament injuries. Clin Orthop Rel Res 198:43–49, 1985.
47. Jenkins W, Bronner S, Mangine R: Functional evaluation and treatment of the lower extremity. In Brownstein B, Bronner S (eds): Functional Movement in Orthopaedic and Sports Physical Therapy. New York, Churchill Livingstone, 1997.
48. Bynum EB, Barrack RL, Alexander AH: Open versus closed chain kinetic exercises after anterior cruciate ligament reconstruction. A prospective randomized study. Am J Sports Med 23:401–406, 1995.
49. Roddey TS, Oslon SL, Gartsman GM, Hanten WP: Reliability of self-report sections of four shoulder scales in shoulder patients (abstract). Phys Ther 78(5):S28, 1998.

4 Instrumented Examination

Russell M. Paine, PT,
and Ron M. Johnson, PT, MPT, ATC, LAT, CSCS

*C*urrently, measuring outcomes is at the forefront of the changing health-care environment. As we progress toward measures of functional outcomes, techniques and tools for recording data continue to be developed. To document these outcome measures, commercially available instrumented testing devices have been used to objectively quantify various biomechanical and kinematic characteristics of the knee.

To date, knee ligament arthrometers have been the predominantly used devices in instrumented testing. These arthrometers attempt to objectively measure in millimeters the various diagnostic knee examination tests, the results of which were previously quantified by a grading system. The development of isokinetic testing dynamometers has made it possible to objectively quantify knee muscular characteristics and predict possible functional limitations of the knee in ligamentous disorders. Finally, a new instrumented device called the Functional Active System for Testing and Exercise (FASTEX) has been introduced that offers the capability of quantifiably measuring functional lower extremity tests.

The purpose of this chapter is to provide an overview of instrumented testing and provide specific clinical techniques that may be useful in obtaining reproducible and accurate results during an instrumented testing examination. The less inherent margin for error a device has, the greater its reliability will be. As is true with any instrument that has been proven to be reliable, its reliability is totally dependent on the expertise of the examiner.

BIOMECHANICS OF THE KNEE

For successful use of knee-testing devices, the individual performing the testing must have a working knowledge of the arthrokinematics of the knee. With the aid of bioengineers, the language of knee motion has become more specific. Using engineering terms, motion of the knee can be described as three rotations and three translations about three different axes, *x*, *y*, and *z*. The interactions of these three movements make up the six degrees of freedom of the knee. Combinations of these translations and rotations provide coupled motions that are often described as "rolling and gliding" of the femur on the tibia.

The knee is a modified hinged joint, with flexion and extension being its primary motions. Flexion and extension occur about the *y* axis (mediolateral). The translations that occur along the *y* axis are medial and lateral. Rotations about the *x* axis (anteroposterior) are abduction and adduction. Translations about the *x* axis are anterior and posterior. Rotations along the *z* axis (proximodistal) are internal-external and translations are penetration and distraction. The diagram in Figure 4–1 illustrates these movements.

An example of coupled motion that occurs during knee arthrometer testing may be described when performing an anterior drawer test. As the tibia is pulled anteriorly on the fixed femur, it translates anteriorly and rotates internally.[1] It is the belief of some that constraining this normally occurring motion during an examination would lead to erroneous readings.[2–7] When performing an anterior drawer test, constraining internal rotation of the tibia on the femur may decrease anterior translation readings. To impose or increase internal rotation of the tibia on the femur would increase anterior translation. This is why it is of utmost importance to apply loads in line with the particular axis that is being tested (Fig. 4–2).

Testing position has definite effects on laxity measurements. Anterior tibial displace-

40

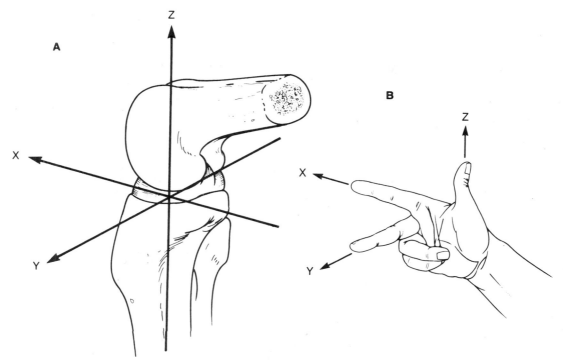

Figure 4–1. *A*, The knee with conventional three-axis system superimposed. *B*, This sketch of the hand shows a simple way to use the right-hand rule. The index finger is pointed along the *x* axis, the long finger along the *y* axis, and the thumb along the *z* axis. (From Jackson DW, Drez D Jr: The Anterior Cruciate Deficient Knee: New Concepts in Ligament Repair. St. Louis, CV Mosby, 1987.)

ment has been reported to be less at 90 degrees of flexion than at 30 degrees. When the anterior cruciate ligament (ACL) has been injured, there is a greater increase in pathologic laxity at 30 degrees than at 90 degrees.[8–13] Thus, to maximally demonstrate pathologic laxity for ACL tears, the proper test position is between 25 and 30 degrees of knee flexion.

Active testing is a new area of interest. Because of the orientation of the patellar tendon's pull on the tibia, there will be anterior displacement of the tibia with quadriceps contraction when the knee is positioned between 25 and 30 degrees (Fig. 4–3).[14] This active anterior translation is increased in the ACL-deficient knee. As the knee is flexed to approximately 70 degrees,

Figure 4–2. Examiner must apply load perpendicular to axis of rotation (*arrow*). Care must also be taken not to impose rotation during testing procedure.

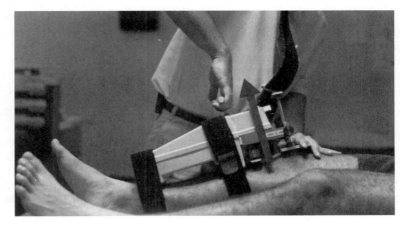

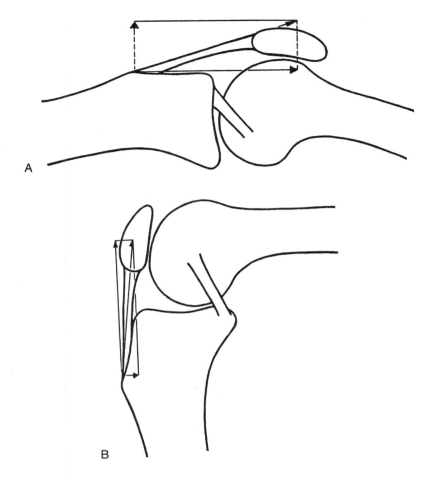

Figure 4–3. *A*, With the normal knee positioned between 25 and 30 degrees, active quadriceps contraction results in anterior tibial translation. This is due to the anterior orientation of the patellar tendon. *B*, With the normal knee positioned at 90 degrees, the patellar tendon orientation becomes posterior, resulting in posterior translation. (From Daniel DM, Stone ML, Barnett P, et al.: The Active Drawer Test. Pamphlet presented at the Annual Meeting of the American Academy of Othopaedic Surgeons, Anaheim, CA, 1983.)

there is a point in the normal knee where the resultant vector of the patellar tendon causes neither anterior nor posterior displacement of the tibia. Active quadriceps contraction in this position results in no translation of the tibia. Daniel et al.[14] have defined this position as the neutral quadriceps active position. As knee flexion approaches 90 degrees, the vector orientation changes, so that there is actually a posterior resultant force acting on the tibia during active quadriceps contraction. In the normal knee, this causes a slight posterior displacement of the tibia on the femur (see Fig. 4–3). In the posterior cruciate ligament (PCL)–deficient knee, the tibia will be in a posterior sag position at 90 degrees. In the PCL-deficient knee, active quadriceps contraction with the knee positioned at 90 degrees will cause an anterior displacement of the tibia (Fig. 4–4). According to Daniel et al.,[14] an arthrometer reading of anterior displacement at 90 degrees is a positive sign for a PCL tear.

Definitions of Biomechanical Terminology

Ultimate tensile strength (breaking point) is the point at which all components of a material fail. For the ACL, the ultimate tensile strength is approximately 1700 N.[15]

Plastic deformation occurs when an object does not return to its original resting state when a load is removed. Thus, there has been failure of some of the components of the material.

Elastic deformation is defined as a return to original length of a material after removal of a load.

Elastic hysteresis is the lack of coincidence of curves on a stress-strain curve. The area bounded by the two curves (hysteresis loop) is equal to the energy dissipated within the elastic material. The loop is commonly observed when testing with instrumented devices that allow display of force versus displacement graphs (Fig. 4–5).

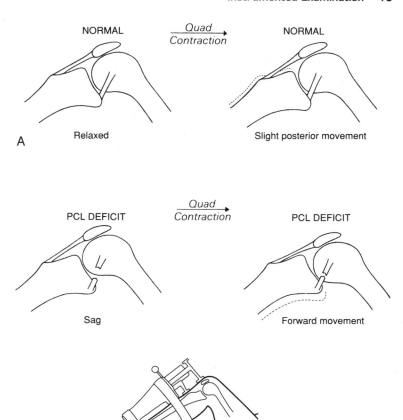

NORMAL ⟶ *Quad Contraction* NORMAL

Relaxed — Slight posterior movement

PCL DEFICIT ⟶ *Quad Contraction* PCL DEFICIT

Sag — Forward movement

Figure 4–4. *A,* In the normal knee, active quadriceps contraction with the knee positioned at 90 degrees results in 0 to 2 mm of posterior translation. *B,* In the posterior cruciate ligament–deficient knee, a posterior tibial sag is present. Active quadriceps contraction brings the tibia anterior. An instrumented testing device can be used to detect the anterior translation. (From Daniel DM, Stone ML, Barnett P, et al.: The Active Drawer Test. Pamphlet presented at the Annual Meeting of the American Academy of Othopaedic Surgeons, Anaheim, CA, 1983.)

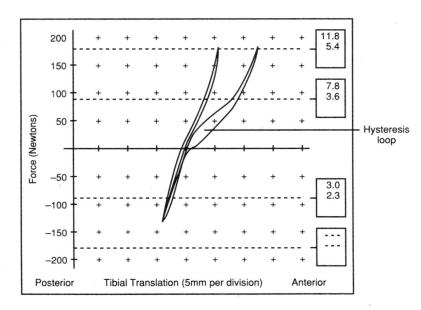

Force (Newtons) vs. Tibial Translation (5mm per division), Posterior — Anterior

Hysteresis loop

Figure 4–5. Typical hysteresis loop seen on graphic representation when using computerized instrumented testing devices. Curve shown is taken from force versus displacement graph of CA-4000 device (manufactured by Orthopedic Systems, Inc. Hayward, CA).

Stiffness is the amount of force required to deform a ligament a given distance (ratio of the change in force divided by the change in length). The normal stiffness for the ACL is 175 N/mm.[15]

Compliance is the distance in millimeters a ligament deforms when a predetermined force is applied (ratio of the change in length divided by the change in force). For the normal ACL, this is 0.006 mm/N.[15] The compliance figure can be calculated with any of the various devices and is the amount of increase in displacement between two displacement loads (eg, change in length between 15- and 20-lb forces). The compliance figure may be the most important postoperative information retrieved because it tests the actual elasticity of the ligament or graft.

KNEE LIGAMENT ARTHROMETERS

History

Instrumented testing using knee ligament arthrometers began in 1971 when Kennedy and Fowler[16] measured knee laxity with a clinical stress machine and serial radiographs. Kennedy's testing device required the patient to sit in a machine while anterior displacement loads were applied at 90 degrees of flexion. The recorded radiographs were compared, and side-to-side displacements were measured. Torzilli et al.[17] and Jacobsen[18] observed that while Kennedy did measure anterior and varus-valgus laxity, he did not take into consideration tibial rotation. The next major study was in 1978 when Markolf et al.[8] used a modified dental chair with potentiometers that measured anteroposterior (AP) translation and constantly measured the amount of applied tibial force. However, it was not until 1983 that Daniel et al.[5] introduced a commercially available device to measure anterior and posterior laxity called the KT-1000. Since 1983, several instrumented ligament arthrometers have been marketed. Oliver and Raab[19] introduced the Genucom knee analysis system, which was designed to measure all six degrees of freedom of the knee. Although the Genucom device is no longer produced, it continues to be used within clinical and testing facilities. The CA-4000 (formerly called the Knee Signature System) is another device similar to the Genucom. This ligament arthrometer was designed to quantify four degrees of freedom and was introduced in 1986.[20] The KLT (Knee Laxity Tester) is a device similar to the KT-1000 and was initially marketed in 1985.[21]

Clinical Uses

As instrumented testing gains greater acceptance through studies documenting reproducibility and reliability, more frequent clinical usage has been observed. Initial skepticism from some clinicians has been overcome as they see the beneficial effects of clinical use of the instrumented testing devices.

One of the primary uses of knee ligament arthrometers is that of verification of suspected ACL and PCL tears. The data retrieved are not meant to replace the hands of the physician but to act as a finely tuned gauge to document more accurately the severity of the suspected pathologic laxity. Decisions regarding treatment options may hinge on accurate assessment by instrumented testing.

As noted earlier, the goal of knee ligament arthrometer testing is to objectively quantify in millimeters the ligamentous laxity found during common knee evaluation tests. To date, the predominant test using instrumented devices that have been reported in the literature is the Lachman test performed between 25 and 30 degrees of knee flexion. It is the general agreement that greater than 3 mm difference between the injured and noninjured knee is indicative of an ACL tear.[3, 22] Daniel et al.[23] reported that 96 percent of the subjects in their study (N=144) with an ACL disruption confirmed by arthroscopy had an injured minus normal anterior displacement difference of more than 3 mm. The authors further reported on anterior laxity measurements as they relate to "copers" and "noncopers." These data revealed that of the individuals who had side-to-side anterior laxity differences greater than 3 mm (KT unstable) and elected to forego surgical measures (copers), 44 percent were able to return to an active sports level. Of those patients who were determined to be KT unstable and elected to undergo surgical reconstruction (noncopers), 49 percent were able to resume pre-injury activity levels. The ability to relate numerical values to patient function is an exciting and practical benefit of instrumented testing.

Daniel et al.[5] and Markolf et al.[9] have also reported on the compliance index found in individuals with documented ACL disruption. The anterior compliance index was calculated as the difference in anterior displacement found between 67 N (15 lb) and 89 N (20 lb) of force. Daniel et al. found that 85 percent of the subjects (N=89) with ACL disruption had a compliance index greater than 0.5 mm. In two studies,[5, 22] they concluded that a compliance index of 1.5 mm or greater was considered positive for an ACL tear. Daniel et al.[22] later reported that the compliance index is a helpful test in establishing pathologic laxity in individuals who have marginal side-to-side anterior displacement differences, especially in acutely injured patients.

Markolf et al.,[8] Wroble et al.,[24, 25] and Reiderman et al.[26] prefer the use of total AP translations (anterior plus posterior measurements) rather than reporting separate anterior and posterior measurements. Wroble et al. and Reiderman et al. believe that reporting total AP translation eliminates the need to identify the neutral position of the knee, thus eliminating this as a potential source of error. Other investigators have noted that by adding the posterior and anterior readings, one may be introducing a source of error rather than reducing potential source of error. Thus, as numerous investigators have reported,[3, 5, 12, 14, 19, 21–23, 27] we prefer to use separate anterior and posterior measurements in our clinical testing.

DeMaio et al.[28, 29] and Mangine[30] have recommended the frequent use of instrumented testing during postoperative rehabilitation of the patient with a reconstructed ACL. This program enlists weekly testing to document the compliance and stability of the healing graft. DeMaio et al.[29] have noted that an increase in the difference of the ACL-reconstructed and noninvolved knee of 2 mm or more at 89 N (20 lb) of testing force during the initial 5 weeks after surgery warrants a more conservative rehabilitation program. This may allow for greater scarring to occur in the posterior capsule to help shield the healing graft. After 6 weeks, a critical value of 3 mm or more side-to-side difference is accepted as representing possible impending graft failure. Additionally, it is suggested that beginning at the eighth postoperative week, testing may be performed at 134 N (30 lb) of force. At that time, if confirmed increases greater than 3 mm displacement become evident, a more conservative treatment approach should be implemented. Conversely, a more aggressive program may be followed if the measurements show that the involved knee has lower anterior displacement values than the normal knee.

Although anterior laxity measurements are more commonly reported relative to side-to-side differences, some investigators believe that day-to-day changes in individual knee measurements should be considered when evaluating for possible pathologic changes.[25, 26, 31–33] To monitor for changes in anterior laxity as a rehabilitation program is progressed, previous measurements must be compared to current readings. Because of inherent variability found in ligament arthrometers, the tester must know what magnitude of change in displacement specific for that arthrometer is considered significantly greater than what is expected by chance alone. The following differences are required in anterior laxity measurements between subsequent tests to assume that a true change has occurred (α = .05): KT-2000, 2.0 mm; CA-4000, 4.2 mm; and Genucom, 5.9 mm.[33] In our clinic, we agree with Wroble et al.[25] as they state that reporting side-to-side differences on subsequent testing days is more useful because of the fact that changes may be secondary to patient relaxation from altered anxiety levels, dietary intakes, or affective levels. By using right-left differences, these changes and possible sources of error are eliminated.

Knee ligament arthrometers also offer research applications that are very exciting to knee ligament rehabilitation. The CA-4000 has been utilized to document anterior tibial translation during both weight-bearing and non-weight-bearing and open and closed chain exercises.[34] The KT-1000 has also been used to measure anterior tibial displacement in open and closed kinetic chain exercises.[35]

TESTING TECHNIQUES TO IMPROVE ACCURACY: KT-1000

The following techniques are specific to the KT-1000 (and KT-2000) but may also be applied to the other testing devices.

Patient Position

Initial set-up of the patient is vital in obtaining accurate and reproducible results. The patient should be supine with his or her head resting on one pillow. It is helpful to ask patients to rest their hands on their chest. The thigh support should be positioned so that the support rests just above the superior poles of the patella, so as not to reduce measurements by blocking the tibia. The thigh support should place the knee in approximately 25 degrees of flexion. The foot rest is then positioned so that support is given just below the lateral malleoli (Fig. 4–6). This position helps to ensure initial limb symmetry but should not limit tibial rotation when testing forces are applied. Daniel et al.[5] reported a 30 percent decrease in tibial translation when the rotation was constrained. Markolf et al.[9] showed that anteroposterior laxity was greatest at approximately 15 degrees of tibial external rotation. Similarly, Fiebert et al.[7] demonstrated statistically less translation when the tibia was positioned in internal rotation. If excessive external rotation of the tibia on the femur is present, a circumferential thigh strap may be used to decrease rotation.

Arthrometer Positioning

Proper position of the arthrometer is of utmost importance for accurate results. The arthrometer is positioned along the crest of the tibia, aligning the V-shaped undersurface of the device to the tibial crest. The most proximal portion of the patellar sensor pad is positioned to be even with the inferior pole of the patella. Caution should be used so that the patellar sensor pad is not resting on the patellar tendon. This technique will position the arthrometer properly and is more reproducible and simpler than aligning the instrument by using the joint line arrow located on the side of the arthrometer. Kowalk et al.[36] demonstrated the importance in positioning as they reported larger anterior displacement measurements with the device positioned 1 cm proximal to the joint line and smaller measurements when positioned 1 cm distal to the joint line. After aligning the device properly, the upper strap is then tightened firmly and the arthrometer is positioned so that it lies in the same plane as the tibial crest. It is helpful to then release the skin under the proximal strap to restore the normal conformity of the calf. The lower strap is then tightened around the distal lower leg.

Patient Testing

Most ligament arthrometers enable anterior displacement measurements to be recorded for forces up to 30 lb. To test for ACL tears, the examiner first applies two to three posterior pushes to set the tibia in a starting position and to establish a zero recording on the arthrometer dial. The 20-lb posterior

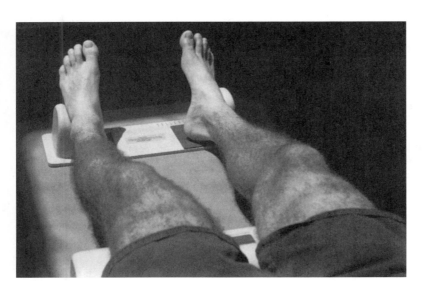

Figure 4–6. Proper patient positioning showing no constraint to rotation.

value is then recorded. The tibia is then pulled anteriorly and readings are taken at 15, 20, and 30 lb of force. Care must be taken not to impose or restrict tibial rotation during testing. As noted earlier, a conscious effort must be made to pull the arthrometer in a plane perpendicular to the shaft of the tibia (see Fig. 4–2). Kowalk et al.[36] demonstrated decreased reliability of translation measurements when forces were applied away from the vertical position. Even patellar pressure must also be maintained to obtain accurate results. The examiner should change hand positions when testing right and left knees (right hand pulls on right knee, left hand pulls on left knee).

An anterior manual maximum force is then applied to the calf. This anterior force should be applied with the hand positioned just below the head of the fibula (Fig. 4–7). Using the fingertips, a maximum force is directed by the examiner until there is no further anterior displacement shown by the device. This test applies anterior forces that attempt to replicate the Lachman test. Daniel et al.[23] and other investigative groups[37, 38] concluded that the manual maximum test revealed the greatest side-to-side anterior displacement difference and was the most sensitive test of an ACL disruption. To perform this test properly, it is important not to impose tibial rotation. This test is also most useful when testing a large individual who requires more than 30 lb of force to demonstrate pathologic laxity.

When testing for a suspected PCL tear, the quadriceps active test is used as described by Daniel et al.[14] to demonstrate posterior tibial subluxation. Before the involved knee is tested, the quadriceps neutral angle must be determined in the patient's normal knee. This will give the examiner a reference position from which anterior and posterior laxity may be distinguished. The patient is positioned supine with the normal knee flexed approximately 70 degrees. The thigh should be supported by the tester to ensure sufficient muscle relaxation. The patient is then asked to perform a quadriceps active test by gently contracting the quadriceps while the tester observes the resultant tibial motion with the arthrometer. The angle of knee flexion is adjusted until there is no resultant movement of the tibia. In the study performed by Daniel et al.,[14] the quadriceps neutral angle ranged from 60 to 90 degrees, with the mean being 71 degrees. The arthrometer is then repositioned properly on the injured knee. With the involved knee positioned in the quadriceps neutral angle found in the normal knee, the amount of tibial translation is recorded for the quadriceps active test and for anterior and posterior translation with applied 20 lb of testing force.

As discussed earlier, if the PCL is ruptured, the tibia will sag posteriorly and the patellar ligament will then be directed anteriorly. When the quadriceps contracts in the PCL-deficient knee, the tibia will shift anteriorly and reveal the PCL pathology. The

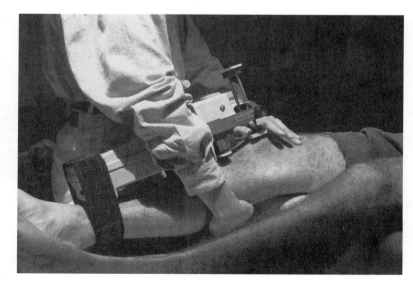

Figure 4–7. Manual maximum displacement test. Care is taken to load knee below head of fibula. A maximum displacement is applied to the calf until there is no further increase in translation (endpoint is reached). This test is most diagnostic for ACL tears.

amount of forward displacement of the tibia seen indicates the magnitude of posterior tibial subluxation.

When assessing anterior and posterior laxity of the knee, the tester must compensate for the posterior sag seen in the PCL-disrupted knee. This is accomplished by calculating the corrected posterior and anterior translations.[14] Corrected posterior translation is determined by adding the resultant posterior translation seen from the 20-lb posterior force and the amount of displacement found in the quadriceps active test. Corrected anterior translation is calculated by subtracting the quadriceps active contraction displacement from the amount of anterior translation produced from the 20-lb anterior force (Fig. 4–8).

Markolf et al.[9] and other investigators[4, 14, 27] have reported that lack of quadriceps relaxation may account for 25 to 50 percent reduction in anterior translation. This is the most common source of lowered anterior translation values. An excellent technique for determining quadriceps relaxation is to palpate the patellar tendon just prior to testing (Fig. 4–9). If there is stiffness in the tendon, the patient should be reminded to attempt to relax the quadriceps muscle. Techniques to aid in relaxation include oscil-

lating the lower leg, massaging the thigh, and contract-relax proprioceptive neuromuscular facilitation techniques. Testing done with quadriceps tension will result in lowered and inaccurate anterior translation values.

Visual observation of the displacement needle becomes more accurate by slowing the rate of pull on the force handle. Three reproducible pulls should be made. The latest version of the device, the KT-2000, obviates the need for visual observation of the displacement needle.

Several investigators have also discussed the effects of exercise on knee laxity measurements.[39–42] Increases in tibial translation were demonstrated in subjects after bouts of exercise. It was concluded that viscoelastic changes in the knee's passive restraint system allowed for this increase. Wojtys et al.[39] specifically illustrated that increases in anterior tibial translation are due in part to muscle fatigue of the quadriceps and hamstring musculature. Therefore, it is suggested that when monitoring knee laxity during a rehabilitation program, ligament arthrometer testing should be performed before exercise to ensure consistent measurements.

These techniques may be applied to the other devices as well. Errors encountered

INJURED KNEE

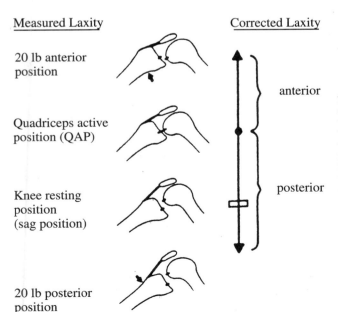

Measured Laxity

20 lb anterior position

Quadriceps active position (QAP)

Knee resting position (sag position)

20 lb posterior position

Corrected Laxity

anterior

posterior

Figure 4–8. In the posterior cruciate ligament–disrupted knee, corrected anterior tibial translation is the distance from the resting position to the superior *arrowhead*. The corrected posterior translation is the displacement given from the resting position to the inferior *arrowhead*. (From Daniel D, et al: Use of the quadriceps active test to diagnose posterior cruciate-ligament disruption and measure posterior laxity of the knee. J Bone Joint Surg 70A:386, 1988.)

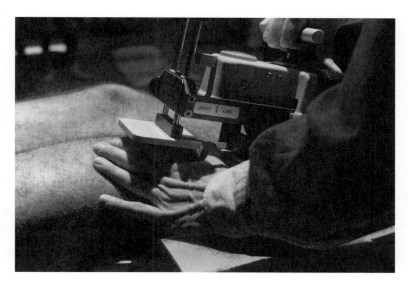

Figure 4–9. Palpation of the patellar tendon with the thumb allows quick and accurate assessment of quadriceps relaxation. Testing must not proceed if tension is detected in the quadriceps mechanism.

when performing instrumented ligament testing are not only due to the arthrometer itself, but also are due to the interaction between the tester, subject, and testing device. Clinical application of any instrumented arthrometer requires special attention to detail to control and limit potential sources of error.

RELIABILITY

As is true with much of the equipment that is introduced into the marketplace today, there is a great need for documentation of the perceived results that manufacturers claim. Although each of the arthrometers that are outlined here has been advocated as producing accurate and reproducible results, there are noted differences in accuracy and laxity measurements documented by these devices. Appendix 4–A outlines the various features and advantages/disadvantages of each arthrometer. The following is a review of literature for the various ligament arthrometers.

KT-1000, KT-2000 (MEDmetric Corp., San Diego, CA)

Daniel et al.[5] reported that measurements of 338 normal subjects with the KT-2000 demonstrated a side-to-side difference of no more than 2 mm with a 20-lb test. Similarly, Daniel and Stone reported a side-to-side dif-

ference of less than 3 mm with the 20-lb test, quadriceps active test, and manual maximum displacement test in 98 percent of the normal subjects tested with the KT-1000 (N= 120).[43] In separate studies, Daniel et al.[22, 23] revealed that 90 and 96 percent of patients with greater than 3 mm of side-to-side difference were shown to have ACL tears. They have also tested normal knees in cadaveric specimens to verify the reproducibility of the KT-1000.[5] They showed that there was no more than 1 mm difference in measurements of specimens after three repeated tests. Daniel and Stone also tested 10 normal subjects and found that total anterior translation varied by 1 mm or less (personal communication). Involved minus noninvolved differences were also less than 1.0 mm. Intertester reliability was addressed in another study by Daniel and Stone in which two examiners tested 34 high school football players (personal communication). All testing was performed on the same day. There was only a 0.9 ± 0.8 mm difference between the two examiners for the right-left difference.

Several other investigators have found the KT arthrometer to be both a valid and a reliable instrument.[5–7, 25, 31, 33, 36, 37, 44–48] Conversely, Fiebert et al.[7] reported poor intertester reliability with anterior tibial translation measurements. Forster et al.[49] showed substantial intertester and intratester variation in both absolute and side-to-side differences in recorded values obtained from the KT-1000. It should be noted in the study done by Fiebert et al. that the examiners only performed 1 week of trials with the KT arthrometer before testing. Likewise, two of the four examiners in that research group had little experience with testing. Therefore, the low intertester reliability could be due to the lack of experience with the KT arthrometer. Hanten and Pace[6] have recommended using the testing device for at least 1 month prior to collecting data.

In our literature search, we found only one study that determined the reliability of anterior and posterior translation measurements in subjects after PCL rupture while describing the use of the quadriceps neutral angle in the methodology.[50] Only moderate reliability was found with intratester and intertester recordings. The authors recommended that examiners use caution when diagnosing injury and documenting changes in laxity in knees with PCL tears or reconstruction.

Wroble et al.[25] found no significant difference between trials (within installation) or between installations (within day) for all parameters recorded for the KT-1000. However, a significant difference was found between days for individual right and left knee measurements at 89 and 134 N force levels. Most importantly, no significant difference was found between days for the right-to-left differences. The authors concluded that the side-to-side differences should be reported rather than individual knee measurements.

Genucom (Faro Medical Technologies, Inc., Lake Mary, FL)

The Genucom knee analysis system was designed to simultaneously measure applied forces and resulting displacements in the six degrees of freedom found in the knee. This testing device uses a multidimensional electrogoniometer, dynamometer, and computer-assisted analysis system.

Oliver and Raab[19] tested the reliability of the Genucom in cadaver specimens and reported data of less than 2.2 mm in AP translation at 90 N with the knee positioned in 90 degrees of flexion. Emery et al.[11] and Highgenboten et al.[45] also addressed reliability by test-retest protocols. Emery et al. found good intratester reliability for AP and varus-valgus tests and poor intertester reliability for the same measures. Highgenboten et al. provided high reliability findings for anterior

and posterior laxity readings in their analysis of 40 knees for three trials.

Oliver and Coughlin[51] stated that 95 percent of patients with a demonstrable result on a Lachman test also had a positive Genucom AP test result at 30 degrees of flexion. They further stated that they found good correlation between the Genucom and the total clinical evaluation of the knee.

In contrast, several investigators found problems with the Genucom's reliability. Wroble et al.[24] demonstrated significant day-to-day differences in individual subjects. Significant differences were also found between the two examiners. Anderson and Lipscomb[44] found that only 70 percent of clinically detectable acute ACL tears had a positive Genucom 30 degree test result. Several other authors have concluded that there is poor reproducibility of measurements with the Genucom knee analysis system and indicate its limited usefulness within the clinical setting.[31, 33, 42, 52, 53]

CA-4000 (Orthopedic Systems, Inc., Hayward, CA)

The CA-4000 arthrometer, formerly called the Knee Signature System, consists of an extraskeletal metal tubular system that is secured in place on the subject's knee using Velcro straps. A potentiometer fixed over the tibial tuberosity and a moveable arm positioned over the center of the patella measures AP tibial translation. The device also measures the knee joint angle via an electrogoniometer along the lateral joint line of the knee. The major advantage of the CA-4000 is its ability to provide objective measures during knee motion.

Riderman et al.[26] found no significant difference between trials (within installation) or between installations (within day) for all but two of the parameters (posterior translation at 20 and 40 lb in left knees) recorded for the CA-4000. Likewise, Queale et al.[33] found good reliability between trials and between installations using the CA-4000. Like the KT-1000, Riderman et al.[26] noted a significant difference between days for individual right and left knee measurements. However, when paired right-to-left differences were examined, no significant differences were found for between-day measurements. Thus, reporting of side-to-side differences is recommended to eliminate this potential error source. Steiner et al.[31] also found good reliability of the CA-4000 and reported a diagnostic correctness of 90 percent when identifying normal subjects and ACL-deficient patients.

KLT (Stryker Corp., Kalamazoo, MI)

The Knee Laxity Tester (KLT) consists of a patient-positioning seat, a force applicator, and a measuring instrument. With the use of the KLT, the subject is seated in a reclined position with the leg held in a leg support apparatus with thigh and ankle straps. Passive AP drawer forces are then applied. Boniface et al.[54] found correlated differences between mean anterior displacements of 8.1 mm in the knees of patients with known ACL disruptions, compared with a mean of 2.5 mm of displacement in the uninjured knees. Highgenboten et al.[45] revealed that no significant differences were found between trial or test sessions using the KLT on normal subjects. Similarly, Stiener et al.[31] and Anderson et al.[37] found the KLT to be reliable and diagnostically accurate in detecting ACL disruptions in more than 85 percent of their subjects.

Others

The Dyonics Dynamic Cruciate Tester (DCT, Dyonics, Andover, MA) is another computerized arthrometer that measures AP laxity, much like the KT-1000 and KLT. Passive drawer tests are performed at 67 N and 89 N of force with the patient in a reclined position. Using the DCT, Anderson et al.[37] reported good reliability and a diagnostic accuracy of 86 percent when the manual maximum test was applied to patients with an ACL deficiency.

In 1978, Markolf et al.[8] introduced the University of California, Los Angeles, instrumented clinical knee-testing apparatus (UCLA). While the subject is reclined and the thigh and patella are stabilized, the ankle is strapped to an adjustable foot rest that allows the knee to be flexed at various angles. The examiner is then able to manipulate the tibia while the testing device records AP tibial force versus displacement

and varus-valgus moment versus angulation. Kochan et al.[55] tested 35 patients with documented ACL deficiency using the UCLA device. When compared with the uninjured knee, the injured knee demonstrated significantly increased AP laxity. Markolf and Amstutz[56] later defined a 95 percent confidence interval for anterior laxity and side-to-side differences in the normal population when tested with the UCLA device. They reported that 95 percent of the normal knees have an anterior laxity less than 7.5 mm and side-to-side anterior laxity difference of less than 2 mm.

The literature reveals that several other knee ligament arthrometers have been constructed. Although evidence is given that these devices can measure uniplanar and multiplanar laxity, they are often too cumbersome and are not well suited for clinical use.[2, 4, 27, 57]

Interdevice Comparison

It is obviously important that these knee ligament arthrometers should provide accurate, reliable, and objective measurements of knee laxity to be of value in the understanding of knee injuries. Furthermore, an understanding of the relationships among laxity measurements between various instrumented devices is also needed when reviewing and applying various investigations involving laxity measurements.

In a comparison of the KT-1000, KLT, and Genucom with ACL-deficient patients, Anderson and Lipscomb[44] found similar values for the KT-1000 and KLT. These measurements were significantly different than the Genucom recordings, however.

Queale et al.[33] and Highgenboten et al.[45] reported significantly larger mean laxity values using the Genucom when compared with the KT-2000 and KT-1000, respectively. Highgenboten et al.,[45] also noted that the KT-1000 produced significantly higher anterior laxity measurements than the KLT.

In contrast, Anderson et al.[37] did not find a significant difference in laxity measurements between the Genucom and the KT-1000. Their investigations did reveal significant differences between these two devices and the others compared in their study—the KLT, KSS, and DCT (Dynamic Cruciate Tester). Similarly, the measurements recorded with the DCT and KSS were not significantly different from each other, but each was significantly less than the other devices. The highest correlation between testing instruments has been given for the KT-2000 and KSS.[33, 58]

Although literature advocates each knee ligament arthrometer as being accurate and reproducible in objectively determining knee laxity, there are differences in the accuracy and laxity reading between these devices. It is assumed that the differences seen in measurements are due to the variability in design and measurement techniques of the devices. Therefore, it has been concluded that laxity measurements cannot be generalized from one device to another.[41, 45]

Examination Under Anesthesia

The Lachman test, pivot shift, and drawer signs are all useful clinical tools when evaluating the chronically injured knee. However, the acutely injured knee may exhibit pain, effusion, and protective muscle spasm, which will render the examination unreliable. In such cases, examination under anesthesia may be used to supplement the clinical evaluation to increase diagnostic accuracy.

Several authors have performed stability examinations of the knee in ACL-deficient patients in both conscious and anesthetized states.[4, 22, 59–63] Donaldson et al.[59] and Anderson and Lipscomb[60] found significant increases in the diagnostic accuracy of the pivot shift, Lachman test, and anterior drawer sign when these tests were performed with the patient under anesthesia. Jonsson et al.[62] examined 45 patients with acute ACL injuries and determined 39 to have positive Lachman test results and 15 to have positive anterior drawer signs. Under anesthesia, these tests produced 44 positive Lachman and anterior drawer results. Similarly, Daniel et al.[22] found increased accuracy of arthrometer laxity tests when applied under anesthesia.

Drez and Paine (unpublished data) used the KT-1000 to document and compare anterior tibial translation values in patients in a conscious clinical examination and under anesthesia. Comparing conscious and unconscious values, they found in 36 patients with ACL injuries a mean increase in side-to-

side differences from 7.3 to 7.5 mm with 30 lb of force and from 7.7 to 8.6 mm with a manual maximum test. These displacement changes were determined to be statistically nonsignificant, indicating that a clinical arthrometer test can be accurate when properly performed. Malcolm et al.[63] and Dahlstedt and Dalen[61] performed comparable studies to those by Drez and Paine and found similar increases in anterior translation under anesthesia. However, these investigators did not report whether these values were of significant value. Highgenboten et al.[64] demonstrated significantly higher anterior translation values in their subjects under anesthesia. Edixhoven et al.[4] tested patients before and after spinal anesthesia. They found no significant differences between anesthetized and unanesthetized states. Coaching the patients on relaxation techniques played an important role in results of these studies.

ISOKINETIC DYNAMOMETERS

History

The concept of mechanically controlled isokinetic exercise and testing was first developed in the late 1960s by James Perrine and was later introduced in the scientific literature by Hislop and Perrine[65] and Thistle et al.[66] In actuality, the concept of isokinetic resistance has been used by clinicians for many years through the use of manually resisted exercises. However, with the introduction of the Cybex dynamometer, rehabilitation specialists were given the opportunity to objectively measure muscular performance through a range of motion for the first time. The introduction of computer software has allowed further enhancement of data analysis and has since greatly expanded the interpretations and applications of isokinetic devices.

As initially stated by Hislop and Perrine,[65] the unique factor in the concept of isokinetic testing and exercise is the control of speed of the muscular performance. Through isokinetic evaluation and exercise, the limb is kept at a constant, predetermined angular velocity through the dynamometer's application of accommodating resistance. That is, an individual using an isokinetic device is able to apply as much force and angular movement as he or she can generate up to a predetermined velocity. When the limb being tested meets the preset angular velocity, the dynamometer produces an equal counterforce to ensure that a constant angular rate is maintained. Thus, increased muscular output results in increased resistance rather than increased acceleration, as is the case with gravity-loaded (isotonic) resistive exercises.

Isokinetic testing and exercise offer several advantages over other modalities. The major advantage is that the tested muscle group can be loaded to its maximum capability throughout its entire range of motion, thereby allowing a more efficient and effective form of exercise. For example, at the beginning and end ranges of motion for a joint, when the muscle is at a physiologic and mechanical disadvantage, the dynamometer will offer less resistance to the limb to maintain its preset velocity. Conversely, the dynamometer will give more resistance at the midrange of joint motion when the muscle has its greatest mechanical advantage. Isokinetic methods are inherently safer because the dynamometer will accommodate for changes due to muscular fatigue and pain experienced by the user throughout the motion. Isokinetic dynamometer testing methods also allow the clinician to have significant control of existing variables and therefore ensures a more objective and reliable outcome.

Since the conception of isokinetic dynamometry, several commercially available dynamometers have been introduced, with subsequent advanced models being marketed. The most common isokinetic dynamometers used by clinicians and referenced in the literature are the Cybex, Kin-Com, Biodex, and Lido models. Although each of these systems has its own individual features, all have the same fundamental components. Appendix 4–B offers a brief description and specifications of each of the above-mentioned isokinetic dynamometers.

Corresponding with the advent of isokinetic testing and exercise, thousands of abstracts and articles have appeared in the scientific literature over the past 25 years. It is the purpose of this section to introduce relevant biomechanical issues and cover measurement and testing aspects of isokinetic dynamometers. The validity and reliability of these methods will also be discussed.

STANDARDIZED ISOKINETIC EVALUATION

The purpose of the isokinetic evaluation is to provide an objective and accurate record of dynamic muscular performance.[67] Before testing, it is imperative that a standard clinical examination is performed to establish possible contraindications for testing and determine general patient responses. Davies[68] has listed the following relative contraindications to testing: pain, limited range of motion, effusion or synovitis, joint instability, or subacute strain. A more severe presentation of any of these factors would present as absolute contraindications.

Several different testing protocols are available through the various isokinetic devices: concentric, eccentric, concentric/concentric, concentric/eccentric, eccentric/concentric, and endurance testing. Regardless of the isokinetic system used or type of test conducted, the hallmark of any isokinetic assessment is the application of a consistent, standardized, and reproducible testing format. To obtain reliable and valid results, the following guidelines and parameters must be established for each testing situation.

System Calibration

Calibration is an essential condition for reliability measures. Calibration is the process by which measured quantities are compared with a known standard and, if necessary, are corrected.[69] Accurate calibration is the ultimate responsibility of the operator and should be performed according to the guidelines of the specific manufacturer. For research and legal purposes, it is recommended that calibration be instituted before each subject testing and data collection.

System Stabilization

The computerized isokinetic system should be adequately stabilized for each data collection period. Proper attachments for included joints, computer interfaces, and additional components should be stabilized as necessary. The tester must document the application of nonstandard components to ensure proper replication on subsequent testing days.

Patient Education

Each patient should be adequately informed about the purpose and necessity of the test he or she is performing. The patient's duties should be outlined with clear and basic instructions throughout the testing protocol. The verbal instructions and testing procedures must be consistent to ensure adequate test reproducibility. The patient should also know how the results of the isokinetic evaluation will be used for his or her benefit during the rehabilitation program.

Patient Position

The patient may be placed in one of three positions for testing: seated, supine, or prone. When placing the patient in the seated position, the tester must consider that the angle of recline has significant effects on the testing outcome.[66, 70] Bohannon et al.[70] found that the angle of incline in sitting (95 degrees versus 150 degrees of thigh-trunk angle) did not significantly affect the strength of the quadriceps but did demonstrate significantly higher hamstring scores with the subject in the upright position. Similarly, Yang and Lieska[71] demonstrated significantly greater knee flexion peak torques with subjects sitting in a more upright position while finding no significant differences in extension torque between different inclinations (hip angles 5, 80, and 110 degrees). When comparing seated versus supine positions Davies and Ellenbecker[72] reported greater peak torque values when seated for the knee flexors and extensors. Apparently, when reviewing previous studies, changing the hip angle in sitting has a greater effect on hamstring torque than on quadriceps torque.

When comparing the supine and prone testing positions, Kramer et al.[73] and Siewart et al.[74] concluded that the moments generated by the hamstrings in the prone position were significantly higher than the supine position. Although no studies were found that compared the hamstring torques in the prone and sitting positions, it does seem that the prone position is particularly suitable for hamstring testing. However, the upright sitting position is probably the optimal position when testing both the knee extensors and flexors, at least in terms of testing efficiency and time.

Patient Stabilization

Most isokinetic dynamometers provide patient stabilization by using pelvic and femoral strapping. However, Hart et al.[75] proved that adding thoracic stabilization improved quadriceps peak torque significantly. Magnusson et al.[76] studied the effect of four stabilization techniques on flexion and extension strength in sitting. Hands and back stabilization were compared to back stabilization, hand stabilization, and no stabilization. They concluded that maximal torque output was observed when the trunk was strapped to the seat and the hands were allowed to grasp the chair. Because different methods of trunk stabilization can significantly affect testing results, it is important that standardized methods are followed for each testing situation.

Alignment

Aligning the anatomical axis of the joint being tested with the input axis of the dynamometer is critical for the reliability of the test data. When testing the knee in the usual sitting position, assuming there is proper stabilization of the distal thigh, a convenient alignment axis extends through the lateral femoral condyle. Proper alignment will not only allow for the collection of more reliable data, but will also ensure the patient's safety and will allow for the maintenance of a more consistent lever arm length.[77]

Position of the Resistance Pad

The resistance pad is normally placed at a level immediately proximal to the medial malleolus. When using this placement, the tester should ensure that the subject is able to maximally dorsiflex his or her ankle and that the strap around the pad is not too tight.

A number of investigators have found that alterations in the placement of the resistance pad result in significant differences in the torque outputs generated by the knee musculature.[77–82] As the resistance pad is placed nearer to the knee joint, the torque outputs for the flexors and extensors become successively smaller. If pad placement is altered by more than 2 inches, or by 25 percent of the lower leg length, peak torque for the flexors and extensors will be altered.[75, 79] Furthermore, Epler and Nawoczenski[78] found significant decreases in peak torque and total work of the quadriceps when a Johnson anti-shear device was employed for Cybex testing. Therefore, it is critical that the researcher is consistent in the testing situation with choice of pad placement and shin adapter.

When testing patients with ACL disorders, the examiner must control the anterior directed force of the rotatory component of the contracting quadriceps. Wilk and Andrews[79] determined that the greatest magnitude of tibia displacement occurs when the knee is extended between 30 and 0 degrees of flexion during isokinetic exercise. Because of the resultant stresses placed on the ACL during open chain knee extension, some have advocated the use of an anti-shear device when performing isokinetic knee extension.[82–84] Johnson[81] concluded that the anti-shear device should be applied when isokinetically testing patients with known or suspected knee ligamentous laxity to significantly limit the resultant anterior tibial translation. Other investigators have suggested using a 20- to 30-degree block of terminal knee extension to avoid the deleterious effects of open chain terminal knee extension.[85–87] Furthermore, Wilk and Andrews[79] and Nisell et al.[88] reported significantly lower anterior directed shear forces during isokinetic knee extension when a single, more proximally placed resistance pad is used. In conclusion, if the tester is concerned about the stress applied to the ACL or ACL graft, the tester should either apply an anti-shear device or place the resistance pad more proximately or limit terminal knee extension.

Warm-Ups

Before actual testing procedures are initiated, it is important that the individual being tested has performed an adequate warm-up to prepare his or her muscles for the testing at hand. In most cases, bicycle ergometry and relevant stretches are sufficient. Because isokinetic movements are unique to most patients being tested, it is recommended that the individual perform three to five submaximal and two to three maximal repetitions at each test speed. This allows the individual to become acclimated to the speed of movement at each preset testing velocity. If the patient appears unsure of the speed or movement, more repetitions can be performed. It is important that the patient perform warm-up repetitions at maximal effort to allow positive transfer to testing conditions.

Gravity Compensation

Proper gravity compensation is another variable that must be standardized prior to testing, to increase testing reliability. When the patient is performing isokinetic knee extension (in sitting), the extensors must overcome the weight of the leg and the resistance provided by the dynamometer. Likewise, the knee flexors are assisted by the limb and dynamometer weights. Thus, if gravity is not compensated for, the strength of the extensors will be underestimated and that of the flexors overestimated. When performing tests in the prone position, the knee flexor strengths will be underestimated if gravitational effects are not accounted for. Several investigators did conclude that significant differences result when tests are gravity compensated verses those that are not.[83, 84, 88–90]

Visual Feedback

Isokinetic muscular performance can be influenced by immediate visual feedback. Isokinetic performance with and without simultaneous feedback was initially investigated by Figoni and Morris.[91] These authors explored the effects of visual feedback on knee extensor and flexor peak torque and fatigue during slow and fast reciprocal testing speeds. Figoni and Morris reported higher peak torque and fatigue values during the slow test speed (15 degrees per second) but not at the fast test speed (300 degrees per second). They suggested that the fatigue (strength decrement) values were higher because of greater strength levels at the beginning of the slow speed fatigue test. The selectivity of effects at test speeds was explained by the longer available period to process the visual information in the slow test. Hald and Bottjen[92] and Baltzopoulos et al.[93] found similar speed-dependent improvements with visual feedback on isokinetic testing. These studies do suggest that testing outcomes can be altered when visual feedback is introduced. It is therefore important to standardize this input across testing sequences to allow for increased reliability of measures.

Verbal Feedback

Consistent verbal commands and encouragement are also important to the testing protocol. Wilk et al.[94] empirically stated that loud aggressive commands often lead to increased torque values, as well as earlier onset of fatigue during testing. It is recommended that verbal encouragement during testing be moderate and consistent in intensity to ensure standardized reporting of results.

Angular Velocities

The knee musculature has been tested using an extensive range of angular velocities. Wilk et al.[94] classified the current angular velocities for isokinetic dynamometers (Table 4–1). Various functional and sporting activities have been estimated as having angular velocities ranging from 700 to 2000 degrees per second. For instance, the angular velocity about the knee has been estimated as occurring at 233 degrees per second during walking and at 1200 degrees per second while running. If the goal of rehabili-

tation is to return the individual to functional activity, it would appear that patients need to be tested and trained at high speeds.

A reasonable and comfortable range for test velocities that has been recommended is between 60 and 300 degrees per second.[62, 63] Other than for high-level athletes, testing at higher velocities is not advised.

The use of very low testing velocities is contraindicated in ligamentous and painful patellofemoral disorders. Wilk and Andrews[79] demonstrated significant anterior translation forces in ACL-deficient knees at 60 degrees per second and therefore advised clinicians to test at speeds of 180 degrees per second or greater.

Angular Velocity Test Order

Davies and Ellenbecker[95] have recommended ordering isokinetic testing speeds from slower to faster velocities. Because it is easier for the patient to achieve and maintain the preset angular velocity at slower speeds, he or she can better adapt to the movement pattern. If there is question as to the patient's ability to perform slow speed testing because of pain, the testing can be initiated at faster angular velocities and then progressed to slower speeds.

Rest Intervals

Another controlled variable during isokinetic testing is the rest interval between testing sets. Ariki et al.[96] recommend a rest time of 90 seconds between testing bouts to aid in the reduction of lactic acid accumulation in the muscles. Further rest should be granted or testing should be terminated if the patient obviously requires additional time to recover.

Test Repetitions

Repetitions performed during testing should also be a standardized testing parameter. Davies[97] indicated that 10 repetitions were sufficient to produce optimal peak torque and power testing values. For tests of muscular endurance, Davies and Ellen-

Table 4–1. Isokinetic Angular Velocity Classification

Speed (degrees/sec)	Classification
15–60	Slow
60–180	Intermediate
180–300	Fast
300–450	Functional

becker[95] suggested using at least 20 to 30 repetitions.

DATA COLLECTION AND INTERPRETATION

Through computer interface, frequently collected data from isokinetic testing were found to include peak torque (general and angle-specific), bilateral peak torque comparisons, peak torque-to-body weight ratios, force decay rate, unilateral peak torque comparisons between agonist and antagonist muscle groups, work, power, and endurance/fatigue. With proper understanding and interpretation of these values, the identification of joint and muscular pathologies and the development of rehabilitation programs can be enhanced.

Torque Parameters

Torque is a force that acts about an axis of rotation and is a function of force times the perpendicular distance from the axis of rotation. Peak torque (PT) represents the highest point on the patient's extension-flexion curve. Mean peak torque can also be calculated and is given as the average of the peak torque readings throughout a series of repetitions. Wilk[98] states that mean peak torque is actually a better estimate of function than peak torque because it considers repetition of movement.

Time rate to torque development (TRTD) measures the time it takes an individual to reach his or her highest torque development. In most cases, PT is seen in the initial third of the upward slope of the torque curve.[98] A delayed PT development may demonstrate decreased accelerative ability, which should be considered when evaluating return to function capabilities.

Torque values displayed at given angles of motion may also provide the clinician with important information about the patient's functional abilities. The quadriceps's torque development at 30 degrees of flexion gives insight as to the patient's ability to provide stabilization at this critical angle during loading response of gait and during various stance activities.[99] Torque may also be noted at the predetermined duration of 0.2 seconds from the start of the torque curve,

which coincides with the time it takes the quadriceps to generate enough force to support the body weight after heelstrike during gait.[99] Wilk et al.[100] noted that the knee should be able achieve 80 to 90 percent of its peak torque by 0.2 seconds of the torque curve.

Bilateral Peak Torque Comparisons

Precise bilateral comparison is one of the major distinguishing facets and advantages of isokinetic testing. It is generally accepted that a difference of 10 percent or less of the opposite side is considered normal; 20 percent is considered minimal; 30 percent is considered moderate; and greater than 30 percent is considered severe.[101, 102]

It should be noted, however, that any deficit in the contralateral limb will render this method of evaluation inaccurate. Therefore, the tester must be cautious before applying such values to patient performance.

Ratio of Peak Torque to Body Weight

Comparing peak torque to total body weight (versus lean body mass) is another technique used to assess patient strength characteristics. Wilk[98] reported the following normative values when analyzing the peak torque to body weight ratios of the patient population (Table 4–2). Davies[95] offered similar percentages as well as applying these values to older populations by suggesting there is a 10 percent decrease in this muscular performance value per decade after 30 years of age.

Table 4–2. **Normative Values for Ratios of Peak Torque to Body Weight**

Speed (degrees/sec)	Males (%)	Females (%)
60	110–115	85–95
180	65–75	55–65
300	45–55	35–45
450	35–40	25–30

From Wilk KE: Isokinetic testing: Goals, standards and knee test interpretation. Isokinetic Source Book. Biodex System 2 Manual, 1992.

Force Decay Rate

The force decay rate (FDR) is defined as the downslope of the torque curve from the point of peak torque.[99] A normal torque should present with a either a straight or a convex slope. A concave slope indicates that the individual is unable to generate sufficient force as terminal extension approaches. Wilk[98] demonstrated this concavity, occurring between 20 and 30 degrees, in ACL-deficient patients and concluded that the FDR may be used in the assessment of knee pathologies (Fig. 4–10). In more severely involved knees, the quadriceps strength appears on the torque curve as a dip at approximately 30 to 45 degrees as the pivot-shift phenomenon occurs.

Unilateral Muscle Ratio

The ratio of the hamstring and quadriceps peak torque is another parameter of isokinetic test data analysis that evaluates the integrity of the knee. Giove et al.[103] first implied that increased strength of the hamstring musculature will enhance dynamic control of the ACL-deficient knee. In separate studies, Walla et al.[104] and Wojtys and Huston[105] noted positive relationships between increased hamstring reflex activity and anterior tibial translation when ACL-deficient knees were exposed to extensor loads. Several other studies have been published that offer calculations for the hamstring-to-quadriceps ratio.[101–106, 108–110] It has been well documented in these studies that this ratio is velocity-dependent, with the ratio approaching and exceeding 1 with increasing speed. Table 4–3 provides the pub-

Table 4–3. Normative Hamstring/ Quadriceps Ratio Data

Speed (degrees/sec)	Normal (%)	ACL (%)
60	60–69	70–79
180	70–79	80–89
240	80–85	90–95
300	85–95	95–105

ACL = anterior cruciate ligament.

lished normative values for unilateral hamstring to quadriceps ratio. As noted, for the ACL-deficient knee, the ratios are often 10 percent higher; in the PCL-deficient knee, they are frequently 10 percent lower.

Although the importance of obtaining a higher hamstring-to-quadriceps ratio has been implicated, correlations with significantly improved outcomes have not been found. Walla et al.[104] were unable to report a significant relationship between increased isokinetic hamstring strength and functional ability. Likewise, Murray et al.[107] stated that no correlation was found between the presence of strength deficits and the need for surgery in ACL-deficient knees. Kannus et al.[111] and Seto et al.[115] offered that the hamstring-to-quadriceps ratio and its relationship to ACL deficiency is more accurately paralleled to weakness of the involved quadriceps, rather than strength of the hamstrings. The use of this parameter for clinical inference, therefore, may not be essential.

Work

Total work is defined as force multiplied by distance throughout the entire range of motion.[99] Work values allow the clinician to

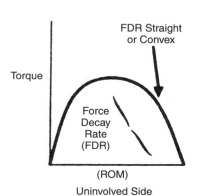

Figure 4–10. The normal FDR pattern (*left*) demonstrates a straight or convex downslope. A concave downslope (*right*) indicates difficulty maintaining force and may suggest knee pathology. (From Wilk KE: Isokinetic testing: Goals, standards, and knee test interpretation. Isokinetic Source Book. Biodex System 2 Manual, 1992.)

evaluate the patient's ability to maintain sufficient force for a number of repetitions. Work is represented as the "area under the curve" along the *x*-axis. Because work is dependent on ROM, standardized testing is vital to obtain valid comparisons between limbs or results between testing days.

Power

Power is calculated by dividing the work performed by the time it takes to perform the work.[99] This value can be used to help identify the patient's actual work rate intensity. Furthermore, the average power can reveal the individual's most efficient exercise velocity.[99]

Fatigue and Endurance

Isokinetic and endurance testing involves evaluating a series of repetitive contractions performed at a predetermined angular velocity. Various methods of quantifying endurance has been found in the literature. Burdett and Van Swearingen[112] defined the use of a fatigue index in which the decline in peak torque after 50 repetitions is expressed as a percent of the highest of the first three contractions. The BIODEX manufacturers define work fatigue as the percentage difference between the work in the first third of the testing set to the work in the last third.[99] The number of contractions performed during an endurance test is most often dependent upon the patient's functional level. Davies[68] suggests 20 repetitions for the average person, 30 repetitions for the recreational athlete, and 40 repetitions for high-performance athletes. Lumex, Inc.,[113] the manufacturers of Cybex equipment, report that fatigue can be measured by counting the number of repetitions performed until the peak torque falls below 50 percent of the initial peak torque. Montgomery et al.,[114] displayed good reliability values for endurance testing when evaluating the number of contractions performed in 45 seconds at 180 degrees per second.

CORRELATION OF ISOKINETIC TESTING WITH FUNCTIONAL PERFORMANCE

Because the ultimate goal for any rehabilitation program is to return the patient to his or her previous functional ability, the clinician is faced with the often difficult task of evaluating the muscular performance required for such functional tasks. Ideally, the most valid form of assessment would be to simulate the muscular contractions and movement patterns reflective of the desired function. Because isokinetic testing is commonly performed in the evaluation of muscular strength in sports and orthopedic clinical settings, it is important to investigate the correlation between isokinetic knee testing and functional testing.

Various functional tests have been derived and are described in the literature. These tests have been developed to better assess an individual's ability to return to a higher functional level. These performance tests include various sprinting, agility runs, hopping, and stair-climbing techniques.[101, 115–124]

An extensive review of the literature reveals conflicting results when various authors investigated the correlation between isolated isokinetic knee testing and functional testing. The discrepancies in results may be derived from differences in subject populations, testing methods, equipment, and pathologic conditions.

Anderson et al.[116] examined varsity-level athletes (N=39) and compared isokinetic concentric and eccentric peak torque with athletic performance tests. Although statistical trends were found between eccentric muscular forces and agility-running and between concentric forces and 40-yard dash, no statistically significant relationships existed. Similarly, although Noyes et al.[101] found a statistical trend toward isokinetic limb function and hop-testing in their study, no statistical relationship was reported. Delitto et al.[117] found no significant correlation between isokinetic testing of the knee and single leg hopping for distance when testing 30 ACL-reconstructed knees. Likewise, Swarup et al.[118] did not find a correlation between isokinetic concentric peak torque and work and the one-legged hop test. Barber et al.,[119] Tegner et al.,[120] Lephart et al.,[121] Greenberger and Paterno,[122] and Tibone et al.[123] all concluded that low correlations were evident between isokinetic testing and various functional tests.

In contrast, several authors have concluded that positive correlation between isokinetics and functional testing do exist. Although Barber et al.[119] stated that no correlation existed between the results of isokinetic knee tests and four functional tests, the authors did find a significant relationship with quadriceps deficit scores at 60 degrees per second and abnormal scores in ACL-deficient patients with the one-legged hop for distance. Wilk et al.[124] documented a positive relationship between quadriceps peak torque at 180 and 300 degrees per second and three hop tests. Paine and Bowman (unpublished data) found in their study a high correlation between quadriceps isokinetic data at 300 degrees per second and the single leg hop for distance. Similarly, Barber et al.,[125] found a significant relationship between quadriceps scores at 60 degrees per second and single leg hop tests. Sachs et al.[126] reported that patients with strength deficits at 60 degrees per second had poorer scores on the one-legged hop for distance test.

Although statistical trends are evident with isokinetic testing and functional activities, isokinetic testing alone is an insufficient criterion for returning patients to play or to functional activities. However, many authors do believe that the combination of isokinetic and functional testing, along with a thorough clinical examination, works to support a more functional environment and thorough evaluation process.

RELIABILITY OF ISOKINETIC DYNAMOMETERS

A sample of some of the reliability studies for the various isokinetic dynamometers is given in Table 4–4. The reader is referred to the References for specific articles regarding information on the various test parameters used for the different dynamometer investigations.[127-147]

FASTEX

For reasons given previously, clinicians should realize that isokinetic and arthrom-

eter measurements will not complete a total assessment of an individual's functional capacity. Therefore, such measurements used exclusively as criteria to determine return to activity are inadequate. Although isokinetic and arthrometer readings should be addressed during rehabilitation, the clinician should also incorporate objective testing under simulated activity conditions to more effectively evaluate the functional status of the patient.

The FASTEX (Cybex, Lumex Inc., Ronkonkoma, NY) is an instrumented device that provides a means to quantify and train functional movement skills (Fig. 4–11). The FASTEX consists of an arrangement of eight to 20 sensitive force platforms interfaced with computer software that provides the clinician with a means to measure functional closed chain movement capabilities. The force platforms contain peizoelectric film sensors that detect impact forces from the foot of the subject and translate the data into quantitative parameters.[148] The FASTEX system configurations are given in Appendix 4–C.

The FASTEX testing and training protocols include simple single- or double-leg balance tests, standard hops tests, plyometric movements, and agility tests. The FASTEX is able to measure static balance from the detection

Table 4–4. Reference Numbers for Dynamometer Reliability Studies

Dynamometer	References
Cybex	72, 121–130
Biodex	103, 109, 119, 122, 123, 131
Kin-Com	132–136
Lido	124, 137–139
Merac	140, 141

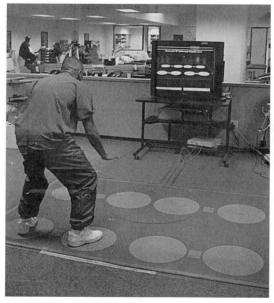

Figure 4–11. FASTEX (Functional Activity System for Testing and Exercise). (Courtesy of CYBEX, Lumex, 1994.)

of the force and frequency of oscillations incurred from the subject's weight-bearing limb. Dynamic movement skills are challenged by the computer through visual cues that direct the subject through a series of movements much like an interactive video game.[148] Hopping and jumping skills are tested and trained similarly. Therefore, the clinician is able to test the subject's ability to stabilize his or her knee during functional movements through such factors as recognition of joint position sense, muscle coordination, and the ability to stabilize the joint as movement occurs.

STANDARDIZED TESTING PROCEDURES

Because the FASTEX is a relatively new testing and training device, there are currently no published data regarding the various testing parameters and their effects on testing values and outcomes. However, it can be inferred that testing must be standardized for such factors as system calibration and set-up, proper patient education, sufficient warm-up, consistent visual and verbal feedback, standard rest periods, proper testing order, and consistent shoe type and clothing worn. Without replication of such parameters between testing sessions, reliable and comparable testing results will not be achieved.

RELIABILITY

Paine et al.[149] have presented the only known reliability study for the FASTEX system. In their study, the test-retest reliability of three functional tests were investigated in 29 healthy, active subjects. The one-legged stand test, single-leg hop-down test, and lateral slide test were all found to exhibit high reliability, with ICC values of .89, .87, and .95, respectively. Obviously, additional research is warranted to determine the reliability and validity of the testing protocols advocated by the FASTEX system.

In a related study, Paine and Bowman (unpublished data) investigated the relationship between the three FASTEX functional tests just described, isokinetic testing, and the single-leg hop for distance. Moderately high correlations were found between the quadriceps isokinetic data at 180 and 300 degrees per second and the FASTEX lateral sliding test, indicating that a relationship does exist between isokinetic strength and

functional agility testing in their study. Low correlations were found between all other test parameters. Although further research is needed to validate FASTEX testing, the implications of testing and training functional movement deficits are promising.

FUTURE OF INSTRUMENTED TESTING

Paine et al.[150] have outlined various products that are now available that claim to measure a wide range of proprioceptive and movement skills. However, these authors have outlined four basic questions that remain in regards to the use of such devices: (1) What measure is needed?, (2) How are the data interpreted?, (3) Is the test meaningful?, and (4) Is the test reproducible?

As these testing devices gain greater acceptance, and as improvements are made to increase the accuracy of the devices, there will be a greater demand for utilization of objective information obtained from an instrumented knee testing examination. Currently, research efforts that report postoperative results of ACL-reconstructed procedures routinely include instrumented knee testing results. Finally, with the introduction of relatively new instrumented devices that offer the capability of quantifiably measuring functional lower extremity tests, further advances can be made in the evaluation of functional abilities and outcomes.

SUMMARY

In closing, there are five guidelines for the clinician to follow when performing instrumented testing of the knee:

Correlate the results to the clinical examination.

Use pre-established criteria for the interpretations.

Be sure all tests are standardized to ensure valid and reproducible results.

Remember that each test has its own value and is only one piece of the clinical picture.

Reliability and validity of testing devices should be a prerequisite for clinical use.

References

1. Torzilli PA, Greenberg RL, Insall J: An *in vivo* biomechanical evaluation of anterior-posterior motion of the knee. J Bone Joint Surg 63A:960, 1981.

2. Sullivan D, Levy M, Sheskier S, et al: Medial restraints to anterior-posterior motion of the knee. J Bone Joint Surg 66A:930, 1984.

3. Sherman OH, Markolf KL, Ferkel RD: Measurements of anterior laxity in normal and anterior cruciate knees with two instrumented test devices. Clin Orthop 215:156, 1987.

4. Edixhoven P, Huskes R, de Graaf R, et al.: Accuracy and reproducibility of instrumented knee-drawer tests. J Orthop Res 5:378, 1988.

5. Daniel DM, Malcom LL, Losse G, et al.: Instrumented measurement of anterior laxity of the knee. J Bone Joint Surg 67A:720, 1985.

6. Hanten WP, Pace MB: Reliability of measuring anterior laxity of the knee joint using a knee ligament arthrometer. Phys Ther 57:357, 1987.

7. Fiebert I, Gresley J, Hoffman S: Comparative measurements of anterior tibial translation using the KT-1000 knee arthrometer with the leg in neutral, internal rotation, and external rotation. J Orthop Sports Phys Ther 19:331, 1994.

8. Markolf KL, Graff-Radford A, Amstutz HC: In vivo knee stability. J Bone Joint Surg 60A:664, 1978.

9. Markolf KL, Kochan A, Amstutz HC: Measurement of knee stiffness and laxity in patients with documented absence of the anterior cruciate ligament. J Bone Joint Surg 66A:242, 1984.

10. Nielson S, Kromann-Anderson C, Rasmussen O, et al.: Instability of cadaver knees after transection of capsule and ligaments. Acta Orthop Scand 55:30, 1984.

11. Emery M, Moffroid M, Boerman J, et al.: Reliability of force/displacement measures in a clinical device designed to measure ligamentous laxity at the knee. J Orthop Sports Phys Ther 10:441, 1989.

12. Granberry WM, Noble PC, Woods W: Evaluation of the electrogoniometric instrument for measurement of laxity of the knee. J Bone Joint Surg 72A:1316, 1990.

13. Daniel D, Lawler L, Malcolm L, et al.: The quadriceps-ACL interaction. Orthop Trans 6:199,1982.

14. Daniel DM, Stone ML, Barnett P, et al: Use of the quadriceps active test to diagnose posterior cruciate-ligament disruption and measure posterior laxity of the knee. J Bone Joint Surg 70A:386, 1988.

15. Noyes FR, Grood ES: The strength of the anterior cruciate ligament in humans and rhesus monkeys. J Bone Joint Surg 58A:1074, 1976.

16. Kennedy JC, Fowler PJ: Medial and anterior instability of the knee. An anatomical and clinical study using stress machines. J Bone Joint Surg 53A:1257, 1971.

17. Torzilli PA, Greenberg RL, Hood RW, et al.: Measurement of anterior-posterior motion of the knee in injured patients using a biomechanical stress technique. J Bone Joint Surg 66A:1438, 1984.

18. Jacobsen K: Stress radiographical measurement of the anteriorposterior, medial and lateral stability of the knee joint. Acta Orthop Scand 47:335, 1976.

19. Oliver JH, Raab S: A new device for in vivo knee stability measurement: The Genucom knee analysis system. Company Memorandum #84-1. FAR Orthopaedics, Montreal, 1984.

20. Neuschwander D, Drez D, Paine R, Young J: Comparison of anterior laxity measurements in anterior cruciate deficient knees with two instrumented testing devices. Orthopedics 13(3):299, 1990.

21. Boniface RJ, Fu FH, Ilkhanipour K: Objective anterior cruciate ligament testing. Orthopedics 9:391, 1986.

22. Daniel DM, Stone ML, Sachs R, et al.: Instrumented measurement of anterior knee laxity in patients with acute anterior cruciate ligament disruption. Am J Sports Med 13:401, 1985.

23. Daniel DM, Stone ML, Dobson BE: Fate of the ACL-injured patient. Am J Sports Med 22:632, 1994.

24. Wroble RR, Grood ES, Noyes FR, et al: Reproducibility of Genucom knee analysis system testing. Am J Sports Med 18:387, 1990.

25. Wroble RR, Van Ginkel LA, Grood ES, et al: Repeatability of the KT-1000 arthrometer in a normal population. Am J Sports Med 18:396, 1990.

26. Reiderman R, Wroble RR, Grood ES, et al: Reproducibility of the Knee Signature System. Am J Sports Med 19:660, 1991.

27. Shino K, Inoue M, Horibe S, et al: Measurement of anterior instability of the knee: A new apparatus for clinical testing. J Bone Joint Surg 69B: 608, 1987.

28. DeMaio M, Noyes FR, Mangine RE: Principles for aggressive rehabilitation after reconstruction of the anterior cruciate ligament. Orthopedics 15: 1992.

29. DeMaio M, Mangine RE, Noyes FR, et al.: Advanced muscle training after ACL reconstruction: Weeks 6 to 52. Orthopedics 15:757, 1992.

30. Mangine RE, Noyes RE, DeMaio M: Minimal protection program: Advanced weight bearing and range of motion after ACL reconstruction—weeks 1 to 5. Orthopedics 15:504, 1992.

31. Steiner ME, Brown C, Zarins B, et al.: Measurement of anterior-posterior displacement of the knee. A comparison of the results with instrumented devices and with clinical examination. Bone Joint Surg 72A:1307, 1990.

32. Myrer JW, Schulthies SS, Fellingham GW: Relative and absolute reliability of the KT-2000 arthrometer for injured knees. Am J Sports Med 24:104, 1996.

33. Queale WS, Snyder-Mackler L, Handling KA: Instrumented examination of knee laxity in patients with anterior cruciate deficiency: A comparison of the KT-1000, Knee Signature System, and Genucom. J Orthop Sports Phys Ther 19:345, 1994.

34. Yack HJ, Riley LM, Whieldon TR: Anterior tibial translation during progressive loading of the ACL-deficient knee during weight-bearing and non-weight-bearing isometric exercise. J Orthop Sports Phys Ther 20:247, 1994.

35. Jenkins WL, Munns SW, Jayaraman G, et al: A measurement of anterior tibial displacement in the closed and open kinetic chain. J Orthop Sports Phys Ther 25:49, 1997.

36. Kowalk DL, Wojtys EM, Disher J, et al: Quantitative analysis of the measuring capabilities of the KT-1000 knee ligament arthrometer. Am J Sports Med 21:744, 1993.

37. Anderson AF, Snyder RB, Federspiel CF, et al: Instrumented evaluation of knee laxity: A comparison of five arthrometers. Am J Sports Med 20:135, 1992.

38. Torzilli PA, Panariello RA, Forbes A, et al: Measurement reproducibility of two commercial knee test devices. J Orthop Res 9:730, 1991.

39. Wojtys EM, Huston LJ: Neuromuscular performance in normal and anterior cruciate ligament-deficient lower extremities. Am J Sports Med 22:89, 1994.

40. Grana WA, Muse G: The effect of exercise on laxity in the anterior cruciate deficient knee. Am J Sports Med 16:586, 1988.

41. Skinner HB, Wyatt MP, Stone ML, et al.: Exercise-related knee joint laxity. Am J Sports Med 14:30, 1986.

42. Steiner ME, Grane WA, Chillag K, et al.: The effect of exercise on anterior-posterior knee laxity. Am J Sports Med 14:24, 1986.

43. Daniel DM, Stone ML: KT-1000 anterior-posterior displacement measurements. In Daniel DM, Akeson WH, O'Connor JJ (eds): Knee Ligaments: Structure, Function, Injury, and Repair. New York, Raven Press, 1990.

44. Anderson AF, Lipscomb AB: Preoperative instrumented testing of anterior and posterior knee laxity. Am J Sports Med 17:387, 1989.

45. Highgenboten CL, Jackson A, Meske NB: Genucom, KT-1000, and Stryker knee laxity measuring device comparison. Am J Sports Med 17:743, 1989.

46. Staubli H, Jakob RP: Anterior knee motion analysis. Am J Sports Med 19:172, 1991.

47. Meneta T, Ezurw Y, Sekiya, et al: Anterior knee laxity and loss of extension after anterior cruciate ligament injury. Am J Sports Med 24:603, 1996.

48. Highgenboten CL, Jackson AW, Jansson KA, et al.: KT-1000 arthrometer: Conscious and unconscious test results using 15, 20, and 30 pounds of force. Am J Sports Med 20:450, 1992.

49. Forster IW, Warren-Smith CD, Tew M: Is the KT-1000 knee ligament arthrometer reliable? J Bone Joint Surg 71B:843, 1989.

50. Huber FE, Irrgang JJ, Harner C, et al.: Intratester and intertester reliability of the KT-1000 arthrometer in the assessment of posterior laxity of the knee. Am J Sports Med 25:479, 1997.

51. Oliver JH, Coughlin LP: Objective knee evaluation using the Genucom knee analysis system. Am J Sports Med 15:571, 1987.

52. McQuade KJ, Sidles JA, Larson RV: Reliability of the Genucom knee analysis system. Clin Orthop Rel Res 245:216, 1989.

53. Seymour RJ, Webster D, Kahn J, et al: An evaluation of anterior and posterior tibial displacements as measured by the Genucom knee analysis system. Physiother Can 46:196, 1994.

54. Boniface JR, Fu FH, Ilkhanipour K: Objective anterior cruciate testing. Orthopedics 9:391, 1986.

55. Kochan A, Markolf KL, More RC: Anterior-posterior stiffness and laxity of the knee after major ligament reconstruction. J Bone Joint Surg 66A:1460, 1984.

56. Markolf KL, Amstutz HC: The clinical relevance of instrumented testing for ACL insufficiency. Experience with the UCLA clinical knee testing apparatus. Clin Orthop Rel Res 223:198, 1897.

57. Shoemaker SC, Markolf KL: In vivo rotatory knee stability. J Bone Joint Surg 64A:208, 1982.

58. Sommerlath KG, Gillquist J: Mechanical stability tests. Am J Sports Med 17:708, 1989.

59. Donaldson WF, Warren RF, Wickiewicz T: A comparison of acute anterior cruciate examinations: Initial versus examination under anesthesia. Am J Sports Med 13:5, 1985.

60. Anderson AF, Lipscomb AB: Preoperative instrumented testing of anterior and posterior knee laxity. Am J Sports Med 17:387, 1989.

61. Dahlstedt LJ, Dalen N: Knee laxity in cruciate ligament injury. Value of examination under anesthesia. Acta Orthop Scand 60:181, 1989.

62. Jonsson T, Althoff B, Peterson L, et al.: Clinical diagnosis of ruptures of the anterior cruciate ligament: A comparative study of the Lachman test and the anterior drawer sign. Am J Sports Med 10:100, 1982.

63. Malcolm LL, Daniel DM, Stone ML, et al.: The measurement of anterior knee laxity after ACL reconstructive surgery. Clin Orthop 186:35, 1985.

64. Highgenboten CL, Jackson AW, Jansson KA, et al.: KT-1000 arthrometer: Conscious and unconscious test results using 15, 20, and 30 pounds of force. Am J Sports Med 20:450, 1992.

65. Hislop HJ, Perrine JJ: The isokinetic concept of exercise. Phys Ther 47:114, 1967.

66. Thistle HG, Hislop HJ, Moffroid JM, et al.: Isokinetic contraction: A new concept of exercise. Arch Phys Med 48:279, 1967.

67. Malone TR: Concentric isokinetics. Ortho Phys Ther Clin North Am 1:283, 1992.

68. Davies GJ: Isokinetic approach to the knee. In Mangine RE (ed): Physical Therapy of the Knee. New York, Churchill Livingstone, 1988.

69. Dvir Z: Isokinetics: Muscle Testing, Interpretation and Clinical Applications. New York, Churchill Livingstone, 1995.

70. Bohannon RW, Gajdosik RL, LeVeau BF: Isokinetic knee flexion and extension torque in the upright sitting and semireclined sitting positions. Phys Ther 66:1083, 1986.

71. Yang LS, Lieska NG: The effect of hip position on peak torques in isokinetic knee flexion and extension. Isokin Exer Sci 1:181, 1991.

72. Davies GJ, Ellenbecker TS: Eccentric isokinetics. Ortho Phys Ther Clin North Am 1:297, 1992.

73. Kramer JF, Hill K, Jones IC, et al.: Effect of dynamometer application arm length on concentric and eccentric torques during isokinetic knee extension. Physiother Can 41:100, 1989.

74. Siewert MW, Ariki PW, Davies GJ, et al.: Isokinetic torque changes based on lever arm pad placement. Phys Ther 65:715, 1985.

75. Hart DL, Stobbe TJ, Till CW: Effect of trunk stabilization on quadriceps femoris muscle torque. Phys Ther 64:375, 1984.

76. Magnusson P, Geismar R, McHugh M, Gleim G, et al.: The effect of trunk stabilization on knee extension/flexion torque production. J Orthop Sports Phys Ther 15:51, 1992.

77. Taylor RL, Casey JJ: Quadriceps torque production on the Cybex II dynamometer as related to changes in lever arm length. J Ortho Sports Phys Ther 8:148, 1986.

78. Epler ME, Nawoczenski DA: Comparison of the Cybex II standard shin adapter versus the Johnson anti-shear accessory. Phys Ther 65:R-135, 1985.

79. Wilk KE, Andrews JR: The effects of pad placement and angular velocity on tibial displacement during isokinetic exercise. J Orthop Sports Phys Ther 17:24, 1993.

80. Johnson RJ, Wilk KE: The effects in lever arm length upon isokinetic torque values during knee extension and flexion (abstract). Phys Ther 68:779, 1988.

81. Johnson D: Controlling anterior shear during isokinetic knee extension. J Orthop Sports Phys Ther 4:23, 1982.

82. Malone TR: Clinical use of the Johnson anti-shear device: How and why to use it. J Orthop Sports Phys Ther 7:304, 1986.

83. Jurist KA, Otis JC: Anteropostior tibiofemoral displacements during isometric extension efforts. The roles of external load and knee flexion angle. Am J Sports Med 13:254, 1985.

84. Timm KE: Validation of the Johnson anti-shear accessory as an accurate and effective clinical isokinetic instrument. J Orthop Sports Phys Ther 7:298, 1986.

85. Malone TR, Garrett WE: Commentary and historical perspective of anterior cruciate ligament rehabilitation. J Orthop Sports Phys Ther 7:304, 1992.

86. Shelbourne KD, Nitz P: Accelerated rehabilitation after anterior cruciate ligament reconstruction. Am J Sports Med 18:292, 1990.

87. Fillyaw M, Bevins T, Fernandez L: Importance of correcting isokinetic peak torque for the effect of gravity when calculating knee flexor to extensor muscle ratios. Phys Ther 66:23, 1986.

88. Nisell R, Ericson MO, Nemeth G, et al.: Tibiofemoral joint forces during isokinetic knee extension. Am J Sports Med 17:49, 1989.

89. Barr AE, Duncan DU: Influence of position on knee flexor peak torque. J Orthop Sports Phys Ther 9:279, 1988.

90. Perrin DH, Haskvitz EM, Weltman A: Effect of gravity correction on isokinetic average force of the quadriceps and hamstring muscle groups in women runners. Isokin Exer Sci 1:99, 1991.

91. Figoni SF, Morris AF: Effects of knowledge of results on reciprocal, isokinetic strength and fatigue. J Orthop Sports Phys Ther 6:190, 1984.

92. Hald RD, Bottjen EJ: Effect of visual feedback on maximal and submaximal isokinetic test measurements of normal quadriceps and hamstrings. J Orthop Sports Phys Ther 9:86, 1987.

93. Baltzopoulos V, Williams JG, Brodie DE: Sources of error in isokinetic dynamometry: Effects of visual feedback on maximum torque measurements. J Orthop Sports Phys Ther 13:138, 1991.

94. Wilk KE, Arrigo CA, Andrews JR: Standardized isokinetic testing protocol for the throwing shoulder: The throwers' series. Isokin Exer Sci 1:63, 1991.

95. Davies GJ, Ellenbecker TS: Eccentric isokinetics. Orthop Phys Ther Clin North Am 1:297, 1992.

96. Ariki P, Davies GJ, Siewert MW, et al.: Optimum rest interval between isokinetic velocity spectrum rehabilitation sets. Phys Ther 65:733, 1985.

97. Davies GJ: A Compendium of Isokinetics in Clinical Usage, 3rd ed. Onolaska, WI, S&S Publishers, 1987.

98. Wilk KE: Isokinetic testing: Goals, standards and knee test interpretation. Isokinetic Source Book. Biodex System 2 Manual, 1992.

99. Tutorial for Biodex System 2 Multi-Joint Testing and Rehabilitation system. Isokinetic Source Book. Biodex System 2 Manual, 1992.

100. Wilk KE, Keirns MA, Andrews JR, et al.: Anterior cruciate ligament reconstruction rehabilitation: A six month follow up of isokinetic testing in recreational athletes. Isokin Exer Sci 1:36, 1991.

101. Noyes FR, Barber SD, Mangine RE: Abnormal lower limb symmetry determined by function hop tests after anterior cruciate ligament rupture. Am J Sports Med 19:513, 1991.

102. Sapega AA: Muscle performance evaluation in orthopaedic practice. J Bone Joint Surg 72:1562, 1990.

103. Giove TP, Miller SJ, Kent BE, et al.: Non-operative treatment of the torn anterior cruciate ligament. J Bone Joint Surg 65A:184, 1983.

104. Walla DJ, Albright JP, McAuley E, et al.: Hamstring control and the unstable anterior cruciate ligament-deficient knee. Am J Sports Med 13:34, 1985.

105. Wojtys EM, Huston LJ: Neuromuscular performance in normal and anterior cruciate ligament-deficient lower extremities. Am J Sports Med 22:89, 1994.

106. Wyatt MP, Edward AM: Comparison of quadriceps and hamstring torque values during isokinetic exercise. J Orthop Sports Phys Ther 3:48, 1981.

107. Murray SM, Warren RF, Otis JC, et al.: Torque-velocity relationships of knee extensor and flexor muscles in individuals sustaining injuries of the anterior cruciate ligament. Am J Sports Med 12:436, 1984.

108. Stafford MG, Grana WA: Hamstrings/quadriceps ratios in college football players: A high velocity evaluation. Am J Sports Med 12: 209, 1984.

109. Klopfer DA, Greij SD: Examining quadriceps/hamstrings performance at high velocity isokinetics in untrained subjects. J Orthop Sports Phys Ther 10:18, 1988.

110. Ghena DR, Kurth AL, Thomas M, et al.: Torque characteristics of the quadriceps and hamstring muscles during concentric and eccentric loading. J Orthop Sports Phys Ther 14:149, 1991.

111. Kannus P, Jarvinen M, Johnson R, et al: Function of the quadriceps and hamstrings muscles in knees with chronic partial deficiency of the anterior cruciate ligament. Am J Sports Med 20:162, 1992.

112. Burdett RG, Van Swearingen J: Reliability of isokinetic muscle endurance tests. J Orthop Sports Phys Ther 8:484, 1987.

113. Lumex, Inc.: Cybex II testing protocol. Bay Shore, NY, Cybex division of Lumex, Inc., 1983.

114. Montgomery LC, Douglass LW, Deuster PA: Reliability of an isokinetic test of muscle strength and endurance. J Orthop Sports Phys Ther 10:315, 1989.

115. Seto JL, Orofino AS, Morrissey MC, Medeiros JM, et al: Assessment of quadriceps/hamstring strength, knee ligament stability, functional and sports activity levels five years after anterior cruciate ligament reconstruction. Am J Sports Med 16:170, 1988.

116. Anderson MA, Gieck JH, Perrin D, et al: The relationship among isometric, isotonic, and isokinetic concentric and eccentric quadriceps and hamstring force and three components of athletic performance. J Orthop Sports Phys Ther 14:114, 1991.

117. Delitto A, Irrang JJ, Harner CD, et al: Relationship of isokinetic quadriceps peak torque and work to one legged hop and vertical jump in ACL reconstructed subjects. Phys Ther 73:S85, 1993.

118. Swarup M, Irrang JJ, Lephart S: Relationship of isokinetic quadriceps peak torque and work to one legged hop and vertical jump. Phys Ther 72:S88, 1992.

119. Barber SD, Noyes FR, Mangine RE, et al: Quantitative assessment of functional limitations in normal and anterior cruciate ligament-deficient knees. Clin Orthop Rel Res 255:204, 1990.

120. Tegner Y, Lysholm J, Lysholm M, et al: A performance test to monitor rehabilitation and evaluate anterior cruciate ligament injuries. Am J Sports Med 14:156, 1986.

121. Lephart SM, Perrin DH, Fu FH: Relationship between selected physical characteristics and functional capacity in the anterior cruciate ligament

insufficient athlete. J Orthop Sports Phys Ther 16:174, 174.

122. Greenberger HB, Paterno MV: Relationship of knee extensor strength and hopping test performance in the assessment of lower extremity function. J Orthop Sports Phys Ther 22:202, 1995.

123. Tibone JE, Antich TJ, Fanton GS, et al.: Functional analysis of anterior cruciate ligament instability. Am J Sports Med 14:276, 1986.

124. Wilk KE, Romaniello, Soscia SM: The relationship between subjective knee scores, isokinetic testing, and functional testing in the ACL-Reconstructed knee. J Orthop Sports Phys Ther 20:60, 1994.

125. Barber SD, Noyes FR, Mangine R, et al: Rehabilitation after ACL reconstruction: Function testing. Orthopedics 15:969, 1992.

126. Sachs RA, Daniel DM, Stone ML, et al.: Pattelofemoral problems after anterior cruciate ligament reconstruction. Am J Sports Med 17:760, 1989.

127. Hart DL, Barber DC, Davis H: Cybex II-Data aquisition system. J Orthop Sports Phys Ther 2:177, 1981.

128. Thompson MC, Shingleton LG, Kegerreis ST: Comparison of values generated during testing of the knee using the Cybex II Plus and Biodex model B-2000 isokinetic dynamometers. J Orthop Sports Phys Ther 11:108, 1989.

129. Gross MT, Huffman GM, Philips CN, et al.: Intramachine and intermachine reliability of the Biodex and Cybex II for knee flexion and extension peak torque and angular work. J Orthop Sports Phys Ther 13:329, 1991.

130. Francis K, Hoobler T: Comparison of peak torque values of the knee flexor and extensor muscle groups using the Cybex II and Lido 2.0 isokinetic dynamometers. J Orthop Sports Phys Ther 8:480, 1987.

131. Bandy WD, McLaughlin S: Intrareliability and interreliability of the Cybex 6000 and Cybex II isokinetic dynamometers. J Orthop Sports Phys Ther 17:65, 1993.

132. Barbee J, Landis D: Reliability of Cybex computer measures. Phys Ther 64:R-140, 1984.

133. Molczyk L, Thigpen LK, Eickoff J, et al.: Reliability of testing the knee extensors and flexors in healthy adult women using a Cybex II isokinetic dynamometer. J Orthop Sports Phys Ther 14:37, 1991.

134. Levene JA, Hart BA, Seeds RH, et al.: reliability of reciprocal isokinetic testing of the knee extensors and flexors. J Orthop Sports Phys Ther 14:121, 1991.

135. Mawdsley RH, Knapik JJ: Comparison of isokinetic measures with test repetitions. Phys Ther 62:169, 1982.

136. Byl NN, Wells L, Grady D, et al.: Consistency of repeated isokinetic testing: Effect of different examiners, sites, and protocols. Isokin Exer Sci 1:122, 1991.

137. Feiring DC, Ellenbecker TS, Derscheid GL: Test-retest reliability of the Biodex isokinetic dynamometer. J Orthop Sports Phys Ther 11:298, 1990.

138. Rathfon JA, Matthews KM, Yang AN, et al.: Effects of different acceleration and deceleration rates on isokinetic performance of the knee extensors. J Orthop Sports Phys Ther 14:161, 1991.

139. Hanten WP, Lang JC: Reliability and validity of the kinetic communicator for the measurements of torque, work, and power. Phys Ther 68:825, 1988.

140. Tredinnick TJ, Duncan PW: Reliability of measurements of concentric and eccentric isokinetic loading. Phys Ther 68:656, 1988.

141. Snow CJ, Johnson K: Reliability of two velocity controlled tests for the measurement of peak torque of the knee flexors during resisted muscle shortening and resisted muscle lengthening. Phys Ther 68:781, 1988.

142. Harding B, Black T, Bruulsema A, et al.: Reliability of a reciprocal test protocol performed on the kinetic communicator: An isokinetic test of knee extensor and flexor strength. J Orthop Sports Phys Ther 10:218, 1988.

143. Patterson LA, Spivey WE: Validity and reliability of the LIDO active isokinetic system. J Orthop Sports Phys Ther 15:32, 1992.

144. Lord J, Aitkens S, McCrory H, et al.: Reliability of the Lido isokinetic system for the measurement of muscular strength. Phys Ther 67:757, 1987.

145. Aitkens S, Lord J, Pernauer E, et al.: Analysis of the validity of the Lido digital isokinetic system. Phys Ther 67:756, 1987.

146. Greenfield BH, Catlin PA, George TW, et al.: Intra- and interrater reliability of reciprocol, isokinetic contractions of the quadriceps and hamstrings as measured by the MERAC. Isokin Exer Sci 1:207, 1991.

147. Timm KE: Reliability of Cybex 340 and Merac isokinetic measurements of peak torque, total work, and average power at five test speeds. Phys Ther 69:389, 1990.

148. FASTEX. Functional Activity System for Testing and Exercise. User's Guide. CYBEX Division of Lumex, Inc., 1994.

149. Paine R, Losey KM, Olson S: Reliability of knee function tests as measured by the functional active system for testing and exercise (FASTEX). Submitted for publication J Orthop Sports Phys Ther, 1997.

150. Paine R, Brownstein B, Macha D: Functional outcomes and measuring function. In Brownstein B, Bronner S (eds): Evaluation Treatment and Outcomes: Functional Movement in Orthopaedic and Sports Physical Therapy. New York, Churchill Livingstone, 1997.

4—A Knee Ligament Arthrometers

KT-1000, KT-2000

Degrees of freedom: one—anteroposterior
translation
Forces: 15-lb (67 N), 20-lb (89 N), 30-lb
(134 N). Detected by audible "beeps";
also able to perform manual maximum
test (maximum displacement by exam-
iner's hand)
Estimated side-to-side test time: 5 minutes
Advantages:
Good reproducibility with extensive re-
search to verify obtained results
Ease of operation
Portable
5-minute test time
Disadvantages:
Measures only one degree of freedom
Unable to effectively perform weight-bear-
ing tests
Not computerized

GENUCOM KNEE ANALYSIS SYSTEM

Degrees of freedom: six
Rotations:
Flexion-extension
Internal-external
Mediolateral
Translations:
Abduction-adduction
Compression-distraction
Anteroposterior
Forces: 150 N
Estimated side-to-side test time: 20 minutes
Advantages:
Proposed measurement of all six degrees
of freedom
Computerization
Proposed soft tissue compensation
Disadvantages:
Cost
Difficult learning curve

Questionable reliability
Not portable
No longer manufactured

CA-4000 (KNEE SIGNATURE SYSTEM)

Degrees of freedom: four
Rotations:
Internal-external
Mediolateral
Translations:
Anteroposterior
Abduction-adduction
Forces: 20-lb (89 N) and 40-lb (178 N).
Forces applied using force applicator
housing strain gauge. Records up to
200 N.
Estimated side-to-side test time: 15 minutes
Advantages:
Proposed measurement of four degrees of
freedom
Closed kinetic chain measurement
Greater flexibility with active measure-
ments
Computerization
Disadvantages:
Slight learning curve
Semiportable

KLT (KNEE LAXITY TESTER)

Degrees of freedom: one—anteroposterior
translation
Forces: 15-lb (67 N) and 20-lb (89 N)
Estimated side-to-side test time: 5 minutes
Advantages:
Ease of operation
Portable
Cost
Disadvantages:
Measures only one degree of freedom
Active measurements not possible

CYBEX-NORM (Ronkonkoma, LI, New York)

Dynamometer:

Modes	Speeds/Sec	Torque
Concentric	5–500 degrees/sec	500 ft-lb
Eccentric	5–500 degrees/sec	500 ft-lb
Active Assist/CPM	5–500 degrees/sec	500 ft-lb
Isometrics		500 ft-lb
Isotonics	5–500 degrees/sec	500 ft-lb

Floor space requirements:
4 ft. × 7 ft. (28 square feet)
Software:
Windows-based software
Windows for Workgroups 3.11
Integrated networking capabilities
English or metric software
Multiple languages available
Computer:
IBM-compatible 486 DX2-66MHz
8 megabytes RAM
500+ megabytes formatted fast access hard disk drive
megabyte 3.5″ floppy diskette
Extended keyboard with light pen input
28.8 Kbps Internal fax/modem
Streamer tape back-up kit
HP Color Deskjet printer
Graphics:
High resolution Super VGA 15″ color graphic monitor
800 × 600 pixels resolution in 256 colors
Electrical:
Input voltage: 220 VAC
Input frequency: 50/60 Hz
Independent 20 amp dedicated circuit
International writing standards
Uninterruptible power supply
Special features:
Provides multiple accessories for testing of all joints. System includes trunk extension/flexion (TEF) modular component and work simulation adapters with 360 degrees' rotation.

CYBEX 6000

Dynamometer:

Modes	Speeds/Sec	Torque
Concentric	15–300 degrees/sec	500 ft-lb
Eccentric	15–300 degrees/sec	300 ft-lb

Active Assist/CPM	1–300 degrees/sec	300 ft-lb
Isotonics	0–300 degrees/sec	250 ft-lb

Floor space requirements:
9 ft. 9 in. × 7 ft. 8 in.
Software:
English or metric software
Multiple languages available
Computer:
IBM-compatible 486 SX
2 megabytes RAM
127 megabytes formatted fast access hard disk drive
megabyte 3.5″ floppy diskette
250 megabytes streamer tape back-up kit
101 key extended keyboard
Panasonic KX-P2180 with color kit
Graphics:
High-resolution VGA color graphics
640 × 480 pixels resolution in 16 simultaneous colors
Electrical:
Input voltage: 220 VAC
Input frequency: 60Hz
Independent 20 amp dedicated circuit
International writing standards
Uninterruptible power supply
System includes integral EMI/RFI and surge suppression
Special features:
Provides multiple accessories for testing of all joints. System includes TEF modular component and work simulation adapters with 360 degrees rotation.

BIODEX—MULTIJOINT SYSTEM 2 (Shirley, New York)

Dynamometer:

Modes	Speeds/Sec	Torque
Concentric	30–450 degrees/sec	450 ft-lb
Eccentric	5–150 degrees/sec	300 ft-lb
Active Assist/CPM	2–150 degrees/sec	300 ft-lb
Isometrics		450 ft-lb
Isotonics	2–150 degrees/sec	300 ft-lb

Floor space requirements:
8 ft. × 8 ft. (64 square feet) for single chair
Software:
Windows-based software

Windows for Workgroups 3.11
Integrated networking capabilities
English or metric software
Multiple languages available
Software:
BIODEX Advantage Software
English or metric software
Multiple languages available
Computer:
IBM-compatible 486 SX
2 megabytes RAM
127 megabytes formatted fast access hard
  disk drive
megabyte 3.5″ floppy diskette
250 megabytes streamer tape back-up kit
101 key extended keyboard
Panasonic KX-P2180 with color kit
Graphics:
High resolution VGA color graphics
640 × 480 pixels resolution in 16 simulta-
  neous colors
Electrical:
Input voltage: 200 VAC
Input frequency: 60 Hz
Independent 20 amp dedicated circuit
International writing standards
Uninterruptible power supply
Special features:
Provides multiple accessories for testing
  of all joints. Offers back, lift, and work
  simulation options. Monitor stand is
  mobile.

KIN-COM (Chattanooga Group Inc., Hixson, TN)

Dynamometer:

Modes	Speeds/Sec	Torque
Concentric	1–250 degrees/sec	450 ft-lb
Eccentric	1–250 degrees/sec	450 ft-lb
Active Assist/CPM	1–250 degrees/sec	300 ft-lb
Isometrics		450 ft-lb
Isotonics	1–250 degrees/sec	450 ft-lb

Floor space requirements:
8 ft × 8 ft (64 square feet) for single chair
Software:
Lab Master analog to digital controller
  and processing system
Kin-Com Key Touch operating software or
  SCREENTOUCH operating software

ROM Software
Automatic Voice Instruction system
AutoPositioning software and interface
  circuitry
Computer:
Pentium computer
Color laser quality printer
Graphics:
14-inch touch-screen monitor
On-line positioning graphics
SVGA color monitor
Electrical:
Input voltage: 220/240 VAC
Input frequency: 50Hz
Independent 10 amp dedicated circuit
Special features:
Provides multiple accessories for testing
  of all joints. Offers dual-channel EMG
  system activated simultaneously with
  force, velocity, and angle signals. Pro-
  vides calibrated footplates with balance
  station option kit. Also offers trunk ex-
  tension-flexion testing for strength and
  exoskeletal lumbar motion assessment.

LIDO ACTIVE (No longer manufactured)

Dynamometer:

Modes	Speeds/Sec	Torque
Concentric	1–400 degrees/sec	400 ft-lb
Eccentric	1–250 degrees/sec	250 ft-lb
Active Assist/CPM	1–120 degrees/sec	2500 ft-lb
Isometrics		400 ft-lb
Isotonics	1–999 degrees/sec	400 ft-lb

Floor space requirements:
10 ft × 10 ft (100 square feet)
Software:
IBM-compatible
Special Features:
Multiple accessories for testing of all
  joints. Offers standing and seated
  trunk/spinal flexion/extension testing
  and work simulation attachments. Provides sliding cuff or handle with most
  attachments to minimize joint compres-
  sion/distraction while allowing automatic adjustment of axis and extremity
  lengths.

4–C Fastex System Configurations

FASTEX I SYSTEM:

The 6 ft × 8 ft floor space system includes:
8 Force platform field
CPU with electronics interface
Monitor selection

FASTEX II SYSTEM:

The 10 ft × 12 ft floor space system includes:
14 Force platform field
CPU with electronics interface
Monitor selection

FASTEX III SYSTEM:

The 13 ft × 16 ft floor space system includes:
20 Force platform field
CPU with electronics interface
Monitor selection
 CPU Specifications:
IBM-compatible 486SX-25, 128K
Cache, 4 MB RAM, 214MB hard drive, 3.5″
  1.44 MB floppy, 101 keyboard, DOS 6.2,
  MS Windows
 Monitor Selections:
14-inch SVGA monitor
26-inch multiscan monitor
35-inch multiscan monitor
100-inch projection system
120-inch projection system
 Printer Options:
Panasonic KX-p2180, black and white
Deskjet printer

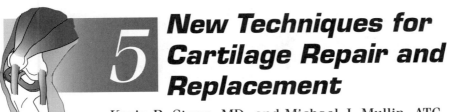

5 New Techniques for Cartilage Repair and Replacement

Kevin R. Stone, MD, and Michael J. Mullin, ATC, PTA

*I*njury to the cartilage of the knee joint is one of the most common orthopaedic presentations. Few orthopaedic problems have received more attention in recent years than the latest advances in cartilage repair, regeneration, and replacement. Surgical procedures have advanced to such a stage that patients now expect there to be alternatives to artificial joint replacement in the treatment of their arthritic condition. Patients also recognize that the techniques of yesterday will be improved upon tomorrow, and question whether to delay current treatment options in anticipation of promising new ones.

A number of the newer surgical techniques being utilized have shown promising results in the short-term treatment of cartilage dysfunction in the knee. These, as well as an improved understanding of postoperative treatment programs, have restored function and diminished symptoms in an increasingly large number of people. For many of these newer techniques, however, there is a lack of long-term follow-up.

This chapter presents a brief description of structure, biomechanics, and evaluation of articular cartilage injuries and presents some of the surgical techniques designed to stimulate cartilage repair and regeneration.

ARTICULAR CARTILAGE

Articular cartilage covers the ends of bones in joints. The smoothness and thickness of the cartilage determines the load-bearing characteristics and mobility of joints. Lesions on the chondral surfaces of joints interfere with the smooth motion of the joint. This type of damage can cause mild to significant symptoms of pain, instability, and stiffness. In the mid-1700s, Hunter first recognized that damaged articular carti-

lage does not have the capacity to repair itself.[1] This observation has led to a wide variety of treatment approaches for focal chondral defects in the knee, with varying levels of success. Treatments such as drilling, abrasion, microfracture, and débridement have been shown to provide symptomatic pain relief and improved function,[2–24] although there are very few prospective controlled comparative studies. Most of these techniques have shown the repair process to be dominated by the production of fibrocartilage instead of normal hyaline cartilage. The fibrous component of the repair is believed to be produced by fibrocytes carried to the repair site by blood introduced to the lesion by surgical or traumatic means. Other treatment options such as periosteal grafting, osteochondral autografts and allografts, and autogenous chondrocyte cell transplantation[2–4, 6, 13, 14, 22, 25–35] have also shown promising results in the reduction of pain and dysfunction. Normal hyaline articular cartilage has never been successfully or reliably reproduced by any technique to date.

ANATOMY

Articular cartilage is a thin, smooth, low-friction gliding surface with a remarkable resiliency to compressive forces. It is a material only a few millimeters thick yet with excellent wear characteristics. Its mechanical and structural capacity is dependent on the integrity of its extracellular matrix. Chondrocytes sparsely distributed throughout a matrix of structural macromolecules work together with hydrated extracellular glycosaminoglycans to attract and then sequentially extrude water. Extracellular components of collagen, such as proteoglycans, noncollagenous proteins, and water provide the shear, compressive, and permeability

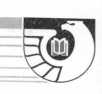

Depository
Libraries

Your Source
for Government
Information

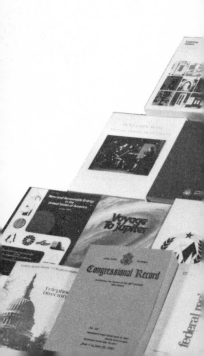

The Federal Depository Library Program

- [ ] an information link between the Federal Government and you

- [ ] free access

- [ ] more than 1,370 sites across th U.S.A.

- [ ] selections tailored to local needs

- [ ] dynamic and constantly grow ing collections

A few of the many publications avail able:

Statistical Abstract of the United States

Survey of Current Business

United States Government Manua

Public Papers of the Presidents

Monthly Labor Review

Information on:

Federal Government

Nutrition

Environment & Weather

Careers

Science & Technology

Business Opportunities

Health Care

Energy

Education

Contact your local library for mor information about the Depository Library Program.

characteristics of cartilage.[9, 14, 36–39] This charged mechanical interaction permits cartilage to perform its mechanical functions without appreciable wear.[9, 36–38] It is the composition and highly complicated interaction of these components that make regeneration and replacement techniques challenging.

Water constitutes between 65 and 80 percent of the entire wet weight of articular cartilage[36, 37] and is about 15 percent more concentrated at the surface than in the deeper zones.[36] *Chondrocyte cells* produce the extracellular matrix. Distributed throughout the matrix, chondrocytes make up less than 5 percent of the wet weight and are the derivative of pluripotential mesenchymal cells that are able to give rise to bone, fat, skin, cartilage, and tendon.[31, 36–38]

Collagen makes up about 15 to 22 percent of the wet weight and contains 90 to 95 percent type II collagen fibers with a small percentage of types IX and XI.[36–39] This is what provides the high tensile stiffness, strength, and resiliency of the tissue. *Proteoglycans* constitute about 4 to 10 percent of the total wet weight and are a mix of large aggregating (50–85%) and large nonaggregating (10–40%) proteoglycans.[36, 38] They are responsible for pressure elasticity and charged interactions with water.[9, 40, 51] *Noncollagenous proteins, elastins, integrins,* and other *macromolecules of protein* are responsible for the matrix organization and maintenance.[37] The functions of articular cartilage include load transmission and distribution, smooth articulation, and aid in lubrication.[14, 30, 36] Load transmission and distribution are due to the ability of the structural matrix to deform, which leads to increased joint contact areas and distributed mechanical stresses.[36] The structural matrix also has the ability to respond to applied loads through fluid exudation and redistribution within the interstitial tissue.

HEALING AND VASCULARITY

The combination of lack of blood supply and few cells distributed widely among a dense extracellular matrix leads to a limited ability of the articular cartilage to heal.[1, 6, 14, 15, 36] The usual inflammatory response of hemorrhage, formation of fibrin clot, cellular production, and migration of mesenchymal cells is absent.[14, 36] Other factors such as age, depth and degree of damage, traumatic or chronic conditions, associated instability, previous total meniscectomy, malalignment, and genetic predisposition also affect healing of cartilage.[6, 31, 36, 37] Age affects healing, in part, because in newborns the multifunctioning mesenchymal stem cells needed for healing account for 1 in every 10,000 cells in bone marrow, and this number reduces to 1 in 100,000 in teenagers, 1 in 400,000 by age 50, and 1 in 2 million by age 80.[31] Depth of the lesion is a factor in healing because surface defects that do not penetrate the subchondral bone have to rely on sparsely populated chondrocytes for matrix remodeling, whereas deeper lesions may introduce a blood supply from the well-vascularized subchondral bone. With the blood comes fibrocytes that modulate to fibrochondrocytes. These cells produce a relatively disorganized lattice of collagen fibers partially filling the defect with structurally weak tissue. Traumatic isolated lesions typically heal better than areas with more degenerative, global defects. Structural instability or other associated pathology also causes uneven and often excessive forces on the articulating surfaces.[38, 41–43]

EVALUATION

A careful assessment and clinical evaluation of the injured area is critical for accurately diagnosing an injury to the articular surfaces. Some of the more important questions to consider when evaluating a cartilage injury are the following: Was it of acute and/or traumatic nature? Are there other predisposing factors? Is it a chondral or subchondral lesion? Is there any associated osteoarthrosis indicating progressive loss, attempted repair, and structural remodeling? Are there indications of degenerative osteoarthrosis or indications of chronic changes from overuse or malalignment? Was any other pathology condition created at the time of injury?

Terry was the first to describe the incidence of isolated chondral fractures in 1988.[16, 44] With the advent of magnetic resonance imaging (MRI) and improved techniques, chondral or subchondral bone bruises are seen in about 80 percent of acute anterior cruciate ligament ruptures.[14, 15] Whether these bone bruises represent forces that have exceeded the lethal threshold for the overlying chondrocytes and therefore will lead to eventual frank lesions is unknown. Patients typically complain of nonspecific episodes of catching, locking, joint-line pain, and low-grade swelling.[14, 15] Pain is not the primary subjective complaint unless the lesion has penetrated subchondral bone or there is associated synovial irritation.[4, 6, 14] Symptomatic catching on the chondral edges, degradative debris, and distension of the joint causing synovitis contribute to pain production.[4] Obtaining a careful history, noting the exact mechanism and other predisposing factors, is essential. However, although some studies note a 94 percent correlation of specific incidence and tenderness to palpation,[16] others have found only a 25 to 40 percent correlation of episode and joint line tenderness.[47]

Radiography and MRI can aid in improving the diagnostic findings. Sensitivity and specificity of MRI techniques have improved in detection of chondral lesions greater than 3 mm in diameter.[45] MRI has a low sensitivity for chondral delamination injuries of about 21 percent.[47] MRI is very operator and field strength sensitive, and its utility is a function of the pulse sequences and imaging technique used.[14] Radiographs are preferred for documenting sclerotic changes, osteophytic formation, compromised joint space (in total and non-weight-bearing positions), and angle of alignment.

CLASSIFICATION

Classifying chondral lesions is difficult, frustrating, and probably totally unreliable. The most common classification system used is the Outerbridge system,[17] developed as a means for assessing chondral damage to the articular surface of the patella. There are five levels of degeneration: grade 0 is normal articular cartilage; grade I is softening and swelling; grade II is partial thickness and early fissuring on the surface, 1 cm or less in diameter; grade III is fissuring of more than 1 cm in diameter to the level of subchondral bone, but with the bone not visibly exposed; grade IV is erosion down to subchondral bone.[17] However, there is very poor interobserver correlation between surgeons in describing cartilage lesions. Also, many lesions are a mixture of types. Surface-only classifications fail to consider the underlying damage seen with MRI.

TREATMENT

Treatment of articular cartilage defects in the knee has been attempted in numerous studies, all with varying levels of success.[2–12, 13–16, 19–24] Success of these approaches has generally diminished over time, possibly due to the formation of fibrocartilage, inadequate development of repair tissue, poor cell differentiation, and poor bonding to the surrounding articular cartilage borders.[4, 12, 48] Although these techniques can result in symptomatic pain relief and improvement in functional status, the long-term results remain mixed. When comparing different conventional therapeutic options, it is important to recognize the goal of surgical intervention. Treatment can be directed either at treating the symptoms or at trying to effect articular repair or regeneration.[4] Repair refers to the restoration of a damaged chondral surface with new tissue that resembles but does not duplicate the structure, biochemical make-up, function, and durability of articular cartilage. Regeneration denotes the formation of new tissue indistinguishable from normal articular cartilage.[6, 35, 36, 49] Several investigators have also reported the efficacy of continuous passive motion following these techniques in improving the visual and chemical appearance of the defect.[20, 21, 36, 43]

There is also the component of another associated pathologic condition in conjunction with focal articular cartilage damage. Personal observations and select studies have suggested that isolated chondral defects heal and recover more slowly functionally than do those combined with other ligamentous injury or surgery.[50] This could be attributed to the increased cellular activity and cytokine stimulation with combined lesions.[50] A few of the more common treatment methods are noted here.

Treatment Methods

LAVAGE
Lavage rids the knee of loose articular debris and inflammatory mediators that are

known to be formed by damaged synovial joints. Jackson found a 45 percent symptomatic improvement in patients at 3½ years. When arthroscopic lavage was performed in conjunction with mechanical débridement, there were improved results with about 88 percent short-term improvement.[4] The degree of improvement varied widely, however, as did the duration.

SUBCHONDRAL BONE MARROW STIMULATION TECHNIQUES

Cartilage penetration techniques have also received recent favor. The goal of such procedures is to mobilize the mesenchymal stem cells to differentiate into cartilaginous repair tissue. Once disruption of the vascularized cancellous bone has occurred, a fibrin clot is formed and pluripotent cells are introduced into the area. These cells eventually differentiate into "chondrocyte-like"[14] cells that secrete type I, II, and other collagen types as well as cartilage-specific proteoglycans after receiving mechanical and biological cues. The cells produce a fibroblastic repair tissue that on appearance and initial biopsy can have a hyaline-like quality.[3, 14, 31, 36] Unfortunately, over time, the histologic characteristics change into more predominantly fibrocartilaginous tissue.[3, 4, 6, 9, 12–14, 28, 36]

Abrasion arthroplasty is one such technique that consists of débriding the articular defect to a normal tissue edge so that fresh collagen can be produced in the fibrin clot. The surface of the subchondral bone is exposed and penetrated to a depth of about 1 mm.[3, 10, 12] Various reports show 12 to 53 percent reduced pain postoperatively.[3, 5] One of the potential problems with abrasion arthroplasty is the cell death produced by the heat of the abrasion burr.[14] Additionally, the destruction of the normal subchondral anatomy handicaps any future repair or regeneration efforts.

Subchondral drilling consists of drilling through the defect to penetrate the subchondral bone. The technique was first popularized in the late 1950s by Pridie,[8, 18, 19] and subsequent findings suggest that repair tissue introduced into the area can look grossly like hyaline cartilage but histologically resembles fibrocartilage (KR Stone and AW Walgenbach, unpublished research, 1997). Drilling also increases the possibility of cell death through heat necrosis.

Microfracture is another such technique in which the lesion is exposed and débrided, and a series of small fractures about 3 to 4 mm in depth are produced with an awl. Adjacent cartilage is débrided to a stable cartilaginous rim, and any loose fragments and fibrous tissue are removed. Popularized by Steadman,[22, 23] microfracture has a few advantages over drilling. There is no heat necrosis, the awl creates more exposed surface area for clot formation, and the structural integrity of the subchondral bone is maintained.[14, 22, 23] However, fibrocartilage is produced. The clinical results are mixed, as reported by Rodrigo et al.[23]

SOFT TISSUE AND OSTEOCHONDRAL GRAFTS

Stimulating articular cartilage growth through the use of various grafting techniques has recently been reported. With the use of either autologous tissue or allografts, these procedures are designed to provide a suitable environment for stimulation of the mesenchymal cells to produce type II collagen fibers. The success of such approaches is at least in part related to the severity of the abnormalities, graft and technique utilized, age of the patient, correction of associated pathology, weight-bearing restrictions, and the use of postoperative continuous passive motion (Stone and Walgenbach, unpublished research, 1997).[3, 4, 6, 9, 20, 21, 23, 25–27, 36, 41–43, 50] Intact full-thickness grafts suffer the problems of mismatched sizes, immunologic rejection, and tissue structural weakening during the process of revascularization. Prolonged protection of intact grafts has been recommended, although this is accompanied by significant disuse osteolysis.

Perichondral and Periosteal Grafts

Attempts to provide the damaged articular cartilage with a viable durable surface have led to the introduction of soft-tissue grafts consisting of periosteum, perichondrium, fascia, joint capsule, and tendinous structures into the defect.[3, 6] Introduced by Rubak in the early 1980s following his experiments with tibial periosteal grafts in rabbit knees,[32] this technique appears to be most effective in a younger population. This finding reinforces the notion that age has an adverse effect on the growth and production of pluripotent stem cells and chondrocytes as well as on their ability to differentiate into the necessary articular chondrocytes. Recently, encouraging results have also been reported with the use of periosteal grafts in isolated chondral and osteochondral defects.[28] A critical component for success with these techniques is that the cambium layer must be placed facing into the joint and the surface must be secured adequately to avoid being knocked loose with joint motion. The potential benefits of the technique include the introduction of a new cell population along with an organic matrix, a decrease in the possibility of degeneration of the tissue before a new articular surface can be produced, and an increased protection of the graft from damage due to excessive loading.[3, 4, 6, 32, 36, 38]

Osteochondral Autograft

This technique consists of harvesting a bone-cartilage graft from the posterior aspect of the femoral condyle and transplanting it into the defect. The technique is also referred to as "mosaic-plasty" because of the mosaic fashion in which the grafts are implanted into the defect.[3, 4, 9, 52] A possible attraction is the placement of implants with fully formed articular cartilage matrix with viable chondrocytes into the area of the lesion.[6] First performed earlier this decade, the chondral plugs are harvested from the lateral intercondylar notch. Several authors have reported good to excellent results with 70 to 92 percent reduction of symptoms and improvement of function in short-term observations.[3, 4, 9, 26, 27, 52] This technique has also been shown to restore subchondral bone, improve joint incongruity, and actually restore an articular surface.[3, 9, 13, 20, 27] However, there is a risk of surface incongruity, donor site morbidity, insufficient stability of the graft, and problems with mechanical overload.[9] There are a limited number of possible donor sites from which grafts can be harvested. Correction of malalignment is a crucial factor in the long-term success of this procedure. Whether osteophytes will be formed from the harvest sites remains an unknown risk.

Osteochondral Allograft

The small number of available graft sites and donor site morbidity could be avoided by the use of fresh or cryopreserved allografts. However, there are additional problems of allograft rejection, disease transmission, mismatch in sizes and congruity, and sparse supply. Patients suffering from primary degenerative arthrosis or those with patella defects do not seem to benefit.[3, 4, 6, 9]

Despite these problems, some investigators have found a 63 to 77 percent good result ranging from 2 to 10 years.[9] Patient selection (i.e., younger, more compliant), correction for any malalignment, and matching size and inlay fixation may contribute to higher success rates.[3] However, allografting requires an open exposure of the joint; severe morbidity occurs if the allograft fails.[3, 4, 9] With the recent increase in hepatitis C transmission, we do not believe that widespread allografting will be popular.

AUTOLOGOUS CHONDROCYTE CELL TRANSPLANTATION

The limited ability of chondrocyte cells to effectively differentiate, proliferate, and regenerate hyaline cartilage has increased the interest in transplanting live cells into chondral defects.[3, 4, 6, 33, 35, 48, 53] Peterson et al.[54] performed experiments in rabbits and reported successful results with transplanting cultured autologous chondrocytes onto patellar defects. This technique consisted of injecting the cultivated chondrocytes under a periosteal flap that was sutured over the lesion.[52, 91] Oddly, the technique requires that *no* penetration of the subchondral bone occur, to prevent the introduction of blood and the circulating fibrocytes. Short-term follow-up (6 months) revealed newly formed "cartilage-like tissue"[33] covering about 70 percent of the transplanted area in animals. However, the results deteriorated significantly by 1 year. Despite this, the investigators proceeded to perform the same technique on 23 patients with cartilage defects in the knee.[3, 33, 35] Healthy chondrocytes obtained from an uninvolved area were isolated and cultured for 14 to 21 days in a lab. The cells were then injected into the defect through an open incision and covered with a periosteal flap excised from the proximal medial tibia.[6, 33, 35] Postoperative care consisted of 48 hours of continuous passive motion use and partial weight-bearing for the first 6 weeks, followed by full weight-bearing at 10 to 12 weeks.[33] Twenty-three patients underwent the experimental procedure, 16 with femoral lesions and seven with patellar defects. At 3 months post-transplant, a second-look arthroscopy revealed similar appearance, color, texture, and level borders to the surrounding undamaged cartilage.[6, 28, 33, 35] Probing the transplanted area produced a wave-like or spongy appearance, suggesting only the beginning stages of early healing. Two years after transplantation, 14 of 16 patients with femoral condyle transplants had good to excellent results, with histologic examination showing that 11 of 15 had the appearance of hyaline-like cartilage.[4, 6, 28, 33, 35] Two of the seven patients with patellar transplants had good to excellent results subjectively and only one had the histologic appearance of hyaline cartilage. The main reason stated for the poor patellar response was noncorrection of underlying joint abnormalities such as malalignment and lateral subluxation of the patella. This technique has received recent widespread attention, both in the medical journals and in the media, which has stimulated patients to request cartilage transplantation. The initial study and subsequent research have shown encouraging results regarding the use and efficacy of this technique for focal chondral defects, but not for osteoarthritic joints. It is believed that the degradative enzymatic synovial fluid of the arthritic knee is not conducive to cell transfer by this technique.

Articular Cartilage Transplantation

AUTHOR'S PREFERRED TREATMENT

Because of the limited ability of any technique to stimulate the growth of type II collagen fibers, we have sought a new approach. We had noted that following notchplasty to reduce graft impingement during anterior cruciate ligament surgery, the notchplasty area in the intercondylar groove regenerated hyaline-appearing cartilage. Subsequently, we hypothesized that if cartilage had the ability to regenerate in that area, then it should be possible for it to regrow if transferred to an articular cartilage lesion. The combination of the extracellular matrix present in articular cartilage and the undifferentiated pluripotent stem cells found in cancellous bone should be able to provide an adequate host environment for stimulation of growth of hyaline-like cartilage. We felt that microfracturing the base of the defect to stimulate blood flow and to release the growth factors, limiting weight-bearing following surgery, and utilizing continuous passive motion postoperatively could produce a new articular repair surface. The development of a paste of articular cartilage and cancellous bone would also aid in reducing the problems associated with surface incongruity of the implanted area, oddly shaped lesions, and inlay fixation techniques as encountered in previous findings.[3, 9, 13, 26] We also felt that it was important to be able to develop a technique that could be performed arthroscopically to aid in diminishing potential postoperative complications such as soft tissue fibrosis.

The surgical procedure consists of initially identifying the lesion, débriding impinging scar tissue, repairing or resecting torn meniscal cartilages, and performing any ligament repair or reconstruction. Alignment is corrected by medial opening wedge osteotomy for varus deformities using a resorbable wedge (Bionx, Blue Bell, PA) (Figs. 5–1, 5–2,

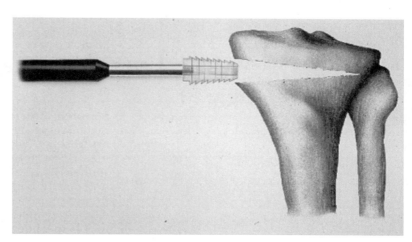

Figure 5–1. Opening wedge tibial osteotomy.

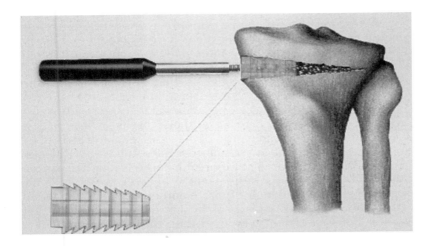

Figure 5–2. Implanting the Bionx Stone resorbable osteotomy wedge.

and 5–3). The criterion for transplantation is arthroscopic confirmation of an osteochondral lesion at the site where the patient subjectively has the worst symptoms or failed treatment of an already existing defect through previous surgery at the site of pain. The lesion is then débrided back to a stable base, and loose or fibrillated cartilage is resected (Figs. 5–4 through 5–7). The base

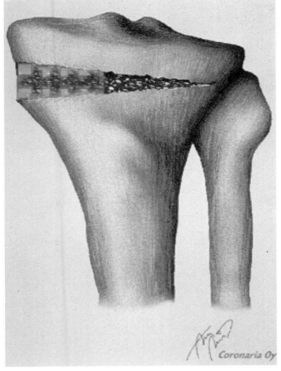

Figure 5–3. Completed medial opening wedge osteotomy.

is then microfractured until bleeding occurs from the subchondral bone. A trephine (DePuy Orthotech, Inc., Tracy, CA) is introduced into the intercondylar notch and care is taken to impact it into the margin of the articular cartilage and capture the deeper cancellous bone. The graft is morselized manually in a bone graft crusher, mixing the articular cartilage and subchondral bone to form a paste. The graft is then redirected into the area of the defect and pushed into the lesion and held in place for 1 to 2 minutes, allowing the adhesive properties of the bleeding bone to secure the graft in place (Figs. 5–8, 5–9, and 5–10).

Over the past 5 years, more than 130 patients have had articular cartilage transplantation surgery by this procedure performed by one of us (K.R.S.). Clinical follow-up evaluations in 57 patients noted an improvement in pain complaints in 94% of patients from 7 preoperatively to 3 postoperatively (on a scale of 1 to 10), reduction in swelling from 0.9 preoperatively to 0.4 postoperatively (scale of 0 to 3), improvement in giving way from 1 preoperatively to 0.3 postoperatively (scale of 0 to 3), and a decreased incidence of locking, from 0.4 preoperatively to 0.1 postoperatively (scale of 0 to 3) (Stone and Walgenbach, unpublished research, 1997).[55] No patient's condition was made worse by the procedure. Second-look arthroscopy with biopsy was performed at least 6 months post-transplant in 34 patients. Hyaline-like articular cartilage was noted in 12 biopsy samples, indicating early healing and some degree of chondrocyte cloning. Hyaline and fibrocartilage was seen in 14 specimens and purely fibrocartilage

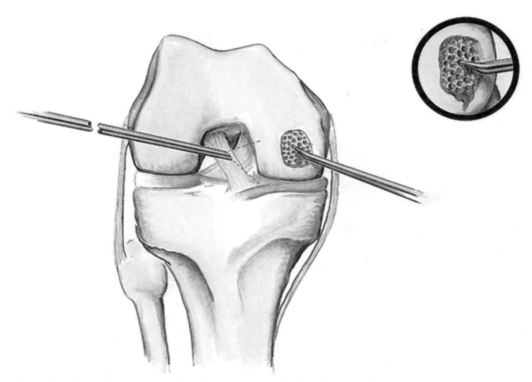

Figure 5–4. Morselization of a full-thickness articular cartilage lesion.

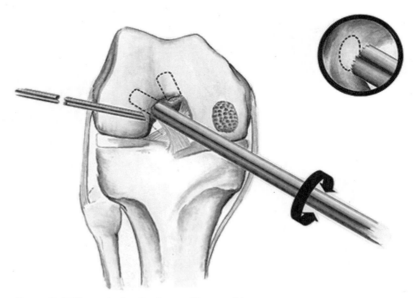

Figure 5–5. Harvest of articular cartilage and bone.

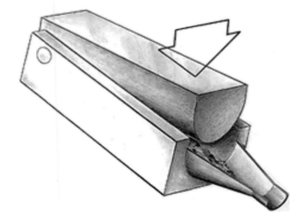

Figure 5–6. Manual crusher used to make paste graft.

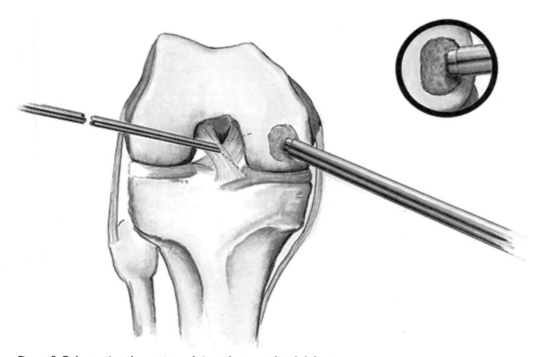

Figure 5–7. Impacting the paste graft into the morselized defect.

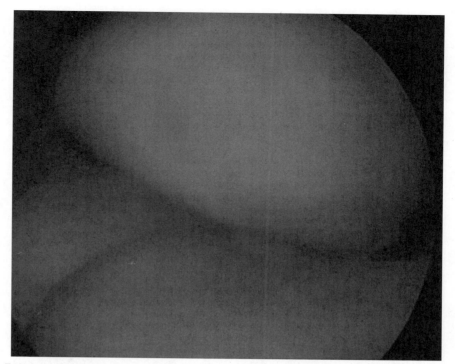

Figure 5–8. Failed abrasion arthroplasty with full-thickness cartilage loss on the medial femoral condyle in a 40-year-old volleyball player.

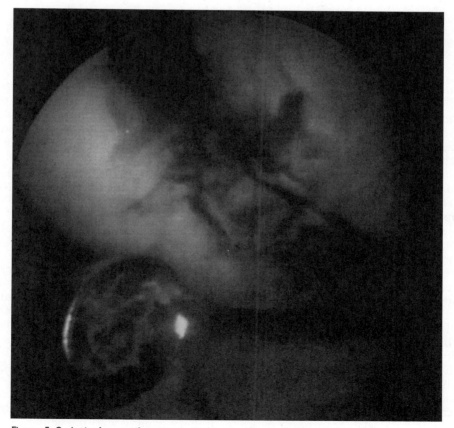

Figure 5–9. Articular cartilage paste grafting to the medial femoral condyle.

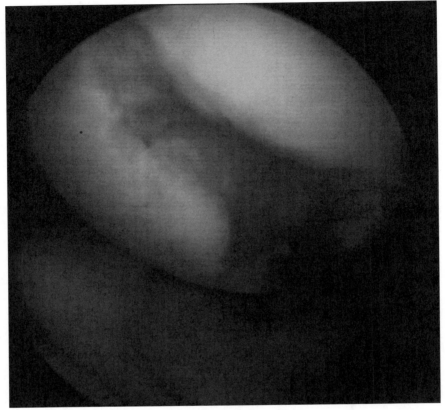

Figure 5–10. Healed medial femoral condyle 6 months after articular cartilage paste grafting.

was noted in 8 patients, with 3 of those patients demonstrating severe preoperative osteoarthritis with bone-on-bone changes (Figs. 5–11 through 5–16) (Stone and Walgenbach, unpublished research, 1997).[55, 56]

This technique has shown significant benefits, in particular in lesions of the anterior femoral condyle, trochlear groove, and tibial plateau. These areas are easily accessible arthroscopically and will have an improved ability to stabilize the impacted graft due to location and instrumentation. Posterior femoral, posterior tibial, and patellar defects pose more of a problem in that they are hard to reach arthroscopically, and proper instrumentation is still in development. The ability of the fibrin clot to adequately hold and stabilize the graft after implantation is a potential limiting factor in complete success of this technique. An added component of an adhesive nature is expected to improve the overall results of this procedure.

The results of this study have shown that articular cartilage transplantation is a viable option for patients with traumatic or ar-thritic chondral defects. It is performed as an outpatient, single arthroscopic procedure and offers the possibility of significant pain relief and a reduction of associated symptoms. The utilization of the extracellular matrix inherent in articular cartilage and cancellous bone seems to provide an adequate healing environment for cartilage regeneration. However, normal hyaline articular cartilage is still not produced.

Postoperative Rehabilitation

A critical component of the success of this procedure is careful adherence to a postoperative rehabilitation program. Patients are kept on non-weight-bearing status for 4 weeks and use a continuous passive motion machine for 6 hours a day for those first 4 weeks. A hinged knee brace is typically used to remind patients not to bear weight. They are instructed on a non-weight-bearing program of isometrics, hip exercises, leg raises, deep water pool work-outs, and well-leg stationary cycling with particular emphasis on

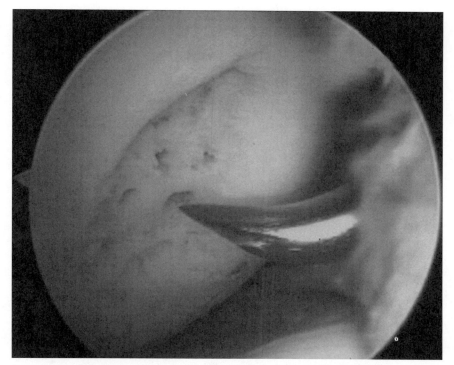

Figure 5–11. Full-thickness lesion medial femoral condyle in a 44-year-old skier.

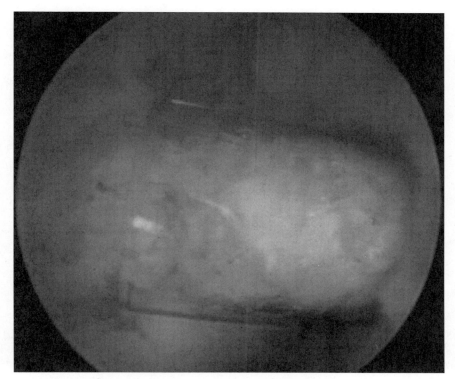

Figure 5–12. Articular cartilage paste grafting to medial femoral condyle.

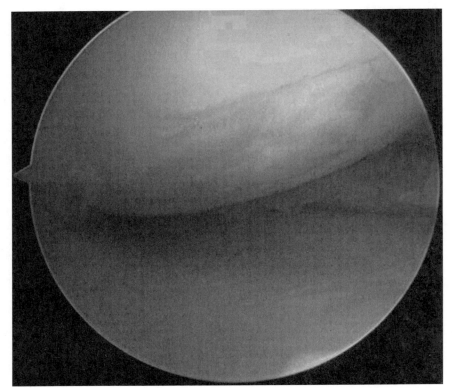

Figure 5–13. Healed medial femoral condyle 4 months after articular cartilage paste grafting.

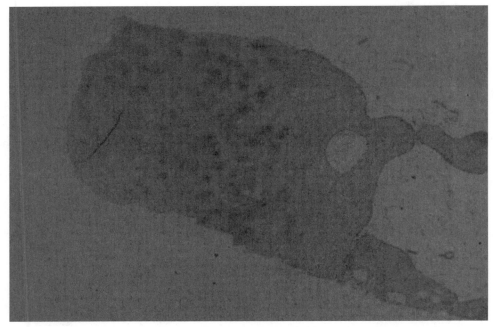

Figure 5–14. Histology showing hyaline-like cartilage in healed medial femoral condyle lesion after paste grafting.

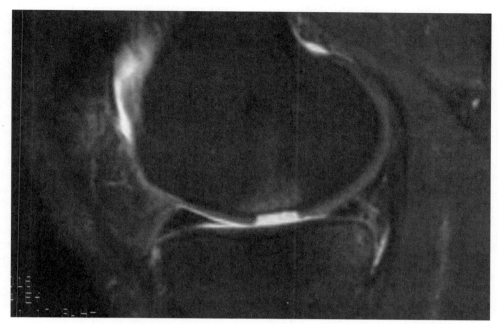

Figure 5–15. Preoperative MRI of medial femoral condyle lesion in a 44-year-old skier.

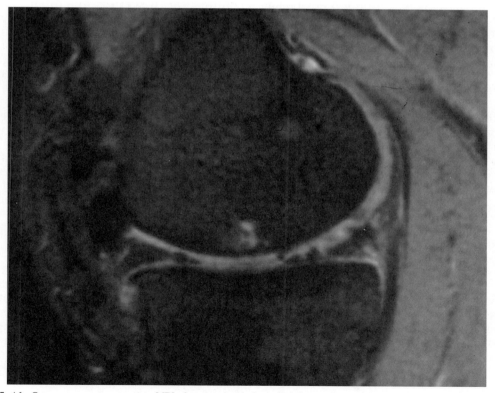

Figure 5–16. One year post-operative MRI showing healed medial femoral condyle lesion after articular cartilage paste grafting.

quadriceps recruitment. If the lesion is in the trochlear groove, then full weight-bearing in extension is allowed. At 2 weeks, two-legged stationary cycling is started with low to no resistance. Four weeks postoperatively, full weight-bearing is started along with an increasing intensity strength program of closed-chain focused, non-ballistic exercises. Double knee bends, hamstring exercises, weight training, a flexibility program, and balance and proprioceptive exercises are initiated and incorporated into a daily routine. Non-impact sports and activities such as pool work-outs, outdoor bicycling, cross-country skiing, and use of assorted cardiovascular machines are permitted for the next 2 months. Ballistic and impact sports are delayed until after the third month and upon completion of a functional strength test.

OTHER ASSOCIATED PATHOLOGY

When assessing treatment options and surgical intervention for articular cartilage damage, it is imperative that the clinician take into careful consideration predisposing risk factors that may affect healing. Is there advanced arthrosis of the tibiofemoral joint? Is there ligamentous instability? Does the patient have a collapsed joint space because of the absence of meniscal tissue? Are there clinical symptoms or degeneration in the hip or ankle? What is the patient's age and activity level? These are all important things to take into consideration when deciding to perform other associated procedures. Prioritizing by subjective and objective findings helps the clinician develop a logical progression for the course of treatment. Ligamentous or structural instability should be repaired if the patient is symptomatic. Absence of a joint space due to previous total meniscectomy may need to be addressed by osteotomy or meniscal transplantation to protect the cartilage graft. The size and age of the lesion, clinical findings of other joint pathology suggesting an underlying disease process, and the patient's weight, motivation, and compliancy should also be taken into consideration.

Osteotomy (High Tibial or Distal Femoral)

Several studies have shown that alignment correction by osteotomy in conjunction with other marrow-stimulation techniques shows improved results over performance of any technique independently.[3, 4, 6, 12, 30, 53, 57] Correcting structural varus or valgus deformities decreases the focal stresses on the involved compartment and distributes the weight-bearing component. The most common technique is a high tibial osteotomy to improve the varus knee malalignment. The effects of malalignment may be seen by taking standing radiographs, examining the gait pattern, a clinical examination, or by subjective symptoms.[57] A new technique developed at our clinic utilizes a resorbable lactide wedge and bone graft inserted in a medial opening wedge tibial osteotomy to realign the leg. The wedge is subsequently replaced by bony ingrowth. The technique may eliminate donor site morbidity and reduce the possibility of intra-operative overcorrection.

Unloading Braces

Nonoperative management of the malalignment of unicompartment arthritis includes the insertion of unloading shoe wedges or knee braces. Clinical experience has also found that proper application of a varus or valgus unloading brace (DePuy Orthotech, Inc., Tracy, CA) can provide symptomatic relief as well as improved ability to tolerate functional activity. We have also found that patients with standing uniaxial malalignment have difficulty effectively recruiting the appropriate musculature to maintain strength of the involved leg. These braces reduce the pain-inhibition cycle and allow for more effective muscular development. Unloading braces are typically fit preoperatively for use during exercise and activity and are also used postoperatively to protect the repaired articular surface.

Meniscus Implantation and Replacement

Once it has been determined that joint space compromise is a factor in the patient's complaint, then meniscal treatment options should be considered. Allografts, autografts, and synthetic polymeric structures have been used previously in numerous models with varying degrees of success.[58] Owing to the complexity of the tissue, meniscus shape and function have never been able to be modeled or reproduced effectively. It is this inherent intricacy that has eluded prac-

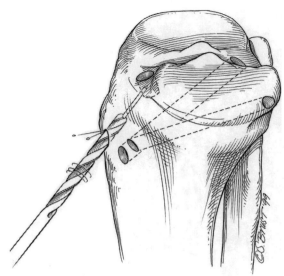

Figure 5–17. Three hole placement for meniscus allograft insertion. (With permission of the artist, Susan E. Brust, CMI.)

titioners' ability to provide effective treatment for this condition. The most common and relatively successful technique to date is the use of allograft meniscal transplanta-

tion surgery using a frozen meniscus. Over 3000 such implants have been performed nationwide with only minimal follow-up studies conducted on their use and efficacy. The most common problem post-implantation is shrinkage of the meniscal tissue, yet the results are currently encouraging. There has been no reported benefit from cryopreservation of meniscal cartilages, and therefore we now use fresh frozen menisci from our tissue transplant bank.

The surgical technique of meniscus transplantation consists of removal of almost all of the remaining meniscus and preparation of the capsular bed for suturing. The allograft meniscus is prepared with bone slivers attached. Three tunnels are made; one for the posterior horn of the meniscus, one for the anterior horn, and one at the posterior one-quarter of the meniscus (Figs. 5–17 through 5–20).[59] The implant is introduced arthroscopically with sutures at both horns extending into the tunnels for proper fixation. Zone-specific meniscus repair sutures are then brought into place and the outer rim of the meniscus is then captured and the knots are tied directly over the capsule.[59]

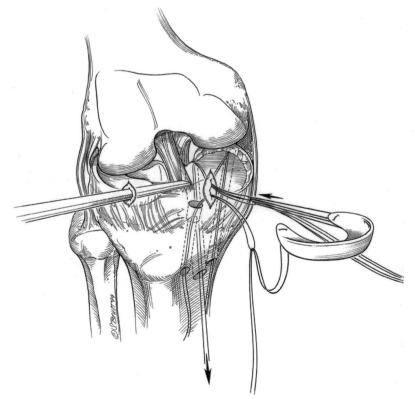

Figure 5–18. Insertion of medial meniscus allograft. (With permission of the artist, Susan E. Brust, CMI.)

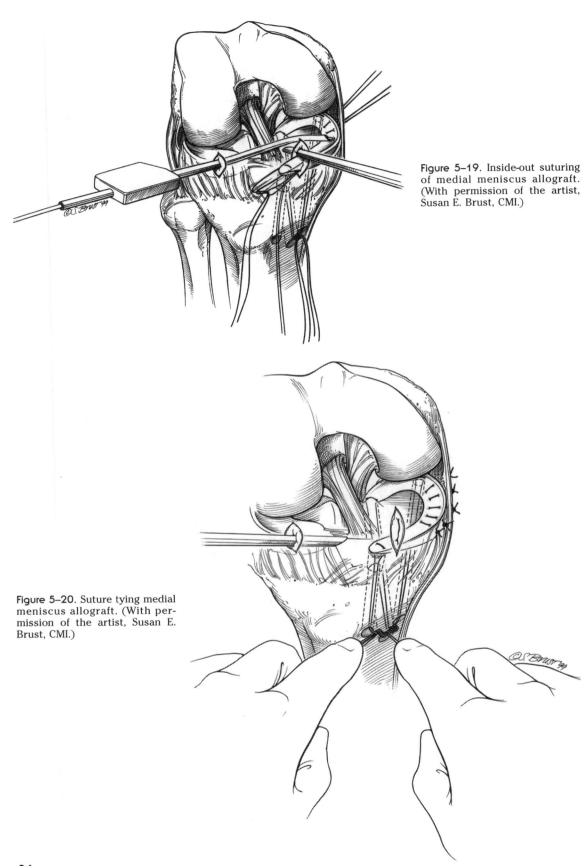

Figure 5–19. Inside-out suturing of medial meniscus allograft. (With permission of the artist, Susan E. Brust, CMI.)

Figure 5–20. Suture tying medial meniscus allograft. (With permission of the artist, Susan E. Brust, CMI.)

Partial weight-bearing postoperatively is encouraged for 1 month as long as there is no associated articular cartilage surgery. The use of a continuous passive motion machine and a good strengthening program are also critical for success following this procedure.

SUMMARY

New techniques and treatments for articular cartilage injuries are progressing at a rate that make true regeneration of hyaline cartilage a near possibility. At this time, our recommendations for patients with traumatic or arthritic lesions (excluding drug therapy) include operative procedures designed to preserve the underlying bone, repair the defect with newly grown tissue, and replace missing meniscus cartilages. Our recommendations also include nonoperative treatments such as unloading braces and wedges to diminish destructive biomechanical forces, and exercises to strengthen surrounding muscles, increase joint motion, tune up proprioception, improve cardiovascular conditioning, and improve the patient's mental outlook.

References

1. Hunter W: On the structure and diseases of articulating cartilages. Philos Trans Roy Soc 42B:514–521, 1743.
2. Jackson RW: Arthroscopic treatment of degenerative arthritis. In: McGinty JB (ed): Operative Arthroscopy. New York, Raven Press, 1991, pp. 319–323.
3. Minas T, Nehrer S: Current concepts in the treatment of articular cartilage defects. Orthopaedics 20:525–538, 1997.
4. Minas T, Raskind JR: Treatment of chondral defects in the knee. Orthop Spec Ed 33:69–74, 1997.
5. Johnson LL: Arthroscopic abrasion arthroplasty. In: McGinty JB (ed): Operative Arthroscopy. New York, Raven Press, 1991, pp. 341–360.
6. Buckwalter JA, Mankin HJ: Articular cartilage. Part II: Degeneration and osteoarthrosis, repair, regeneration and transplantation. J Bone Joint Surg Am 79A:612–;632, 1997.
7. Ficat RP, Ficat C, Gedeon P, Toussaint JB: Spongialization. A new treatment for diseased patellae. Clin Orthop 144:74–83, 1979.
8. Pridie KH: A method of resurfacing osteoarthritic knee joints. J Bone Joint Surg Br 41B:618, 1959.
9. Wirth CJ, Rudert M: Techniques of cartilage growth enhancement: A review of the literature. Arthroscopy J Arthroscop Rel Surg 12:300–308, 1996.
10. Johnson LL: Arthroscopic abrasion arthroplasty historical and pathologic perspective: present status. Arthroscopy J Arthros Rel Surg 2(1):54–69, 1986.
11. Magnuson PB: Joint debridement surgical treatment of degenerative arthritis. Surg Gynecol Obstet; 73:1–9, 1941.
12. Akizuki S, Yasukawa Y, Takizawa T: Does arthroscopic abrasion arthroplasty promote cartilage regeneration in osteoarthritic knees with eburnation? A prospective study of high tibial osteotomy with abrasion arthroplasty versus high tibial osteotomy alone. Arthroscopy J Arthros Rel Surg 13:9–17, 1997.
13. Buckwalter JA, Lohmander S: Current concepts review. Operative treatment of osteoarthrosis: Current practice and future development. J Bone Joint Surg Am 76A:1405–1418, 1994.
14. Allen AA, Fealy S, Panariello R, et al.: Chondral injuries. Sports Med Arthroscop Rev 4:51–58, 1996.
15. Mankin HJ: The response of articular cartilage to mechanical injury. J Bone Joint Surg Am 64A:460–466, 1982.
16. Terry GC, Flandry F, Van Manen JW, et al.: Isolated chondral fractures of the knee. Clin Orthop 234:170–177, 1988.
17. Outerbridge RE: The etiology of chondromalacia patellae. J Bone Joint Surg Br 43B:752–767, 1961.
18. Pridie KH: Proceedings of the British Orthopaedic Association: A method of resurfacing osteoarthritic knee joints. J Bone Joint Surg Br 41:618–619, 1959.
19. Insall J. The Pridie debridement operation for osteoarthritis of the knee. Clin Orthop 101:61–67, 1974.
20. Rodrigo JJ, Steadman RJ, Silliman JF, et al.: Improvement of full-thickness chondral defect healing in the human knee after debridement and microfracture using continuous passive motion. Am J Knee Surg 7:109–116, 1994.
21. Salter RB, Simmonds DF, Malcolm BW, et al.: The biological effect of continuous passive motion on the healing of full-thickness defects in articular cartilage. An experimental investigation in the rabbit. J Bone Joint Surg Am 62:1232–1251, 1980.
22. Kim HK, Moran ME, Salter RB: The potential for regeneration of articular cartilage in defects created by chondral shaving and subchondral abrasions. J Bone Joint Surg Am 73:1301–1315, 1991.
23. Rodrigo JJ, Steadman JR, Silliman JF: Osteoarticular injuries of the knee. In Chapman MW (ed): Operative Orthopaedics, Vol. 3, 2nd ed. Philadelphia, Lippincott, 1993, pp. 2077–2082.
24. Tippet JW: Articular cartilage drilling and osteotomy in osteoarthritis of the knee. In McGinty JB (ed): Operative Arthroscopy. New York, Raven Press, 1991, pp. 325–339.
25. McDermott AGP, Langer F, Pritzker KPH, et al.: Fresh small-fragment osteochondral allografts: Long-term follow-up on first 100 cases. Clin Orthop 197:96–101, 1985.
26. Gross AE, Beaver RJ, Mohammed MN: Fresh small-fragment osteochondral allografts used for post-traumatic defects in the knee joint. In Finerman GAM, Noyes FR (ed): Biology and Biomechanics of the Traumatized Synovial Joint: The Knee as a Model. Rosemont, IL, The American Academy of Orthopaedic Surgeons, 1992, pp. 123–141.
27. Czitrom AA, Keating S, Gross AE: The viability of articular cartilage in fresh osteochondral allografts after clinical transplantation. J Bone Joint Surg Am 72:574–579, 1990.
28. Buckwalter JA: Cartilage researchers tell of prog-

ress: Technologies hold promise, but caution urged. Bull Am Acad Orthop Surg 44:24–26, 1996.

29. Homminga GN, Bulstra SK, Bouwmeester PM, Van der Linden AJ: Perichondral grafting for cartilage lesions of the knee. J Bone Joint Surg 72B:1003–1007, 1990.

30. Freeman PM, Natarajan RN, Kimura JH, et al.: Chondrocyte cells respond mechanically to compressive loads. J Orthop Res 12:311–320, 1994.

31. Friend T: Making high tech human repairs. USA Today. Sec 6D:1, August 12, 1997.

32. Rubak JM: Reconstruction of articular cartilage defects with free periosteal grafts: An experimental study. Acta Orthop Scand 53:175–180, 1982.

33. Brittberg M, Lindahl A, Nilsson A, et al.: Treatment of deep cartilage defects in the knee with autologous chondrocyte transplantation. N Engl J Med 331:889–895, 1994.

34. Peterson L, Lindahl A: Chondrocyte transplantation technique described. Orthop Today 16(8):1,9, 1996.

35. Chen FS, Frenkel SR, Di Cesare PE: Chondrocyte transplantation and experimental treatment options for articular cartilage defects. Am J Orthop 6:396–406, 1997.

36. Ratcliffe A, Mow VC: The structure, function, and biologic repair of articular cartilage. In Friedlaender GE, Goldberg VM (ed): Bone and Cartilage Allografts. Park Ridge, IL, American Academy of Orthopaedic Surgeons, 1991, pp. 123–154.

37. Buckwalter JA, Mankin HJ: Articular cartilage. Part I: Tissue design and chondrocytematrix interactions. J Bone Joint Surg Am 79A:600–611, 1997.

38. Mow VC, Ateshian GA, Ratcliffe A: Anatomic form and biomechanical properties of articular cartilage of the knee joint. In Finerman GAM, Noyes FR (ed): Biology and Biomechanics of the Traumatized Synovial Joint: The Knee as a Model. Rosemont, IL, American Academy of Orthopaedic Surgeons, 1992, pp. 55–81.

39. Finerman GAM, Noyes FR: Overview: Section two. In Friedlander GAM, Noyes FR (ed): Biology and Biomechanics of the Traumatized Synovial Joint: The Knee as a Model. Rosemont, IL, American Academy of Orthopaedic Surgeons, 1992; pp. 53–54.

40. Athanasion KA, Rosenwasser MP, Buckwalter JA, Malinin TI, Mow VC: Interspecies comparisons of in situ intrinsic mechanical properties of distal femoral cartilage. J Orthop Res 9:330–340, 1991.

41. Guilak F, Ratcliffe A, Lane N, et al.: Mechanical and biochemical changes in the superficial zone of articular cartilage in canine experimental osteoarthritis. J Orthop Res 12:474–484, 1994.

42. Setton LA, Mow VC, Muller FS: Mechanical properties of canine articular cartilage are significantly altered following transection of the anterior cruciate ligament. J Orthop Res 112:451–463, 1994.

43. Kiviranta I, Tammi M, Muller FS: Articular cartilage thickness and glycosaminoglycan distribution in the young canine knee joint after remobilization of the immobilized limb. J Orthop Res 12:161–167, 1994.

44. Hopkinson WJ, Mitchell WA, Curl WW: Chondral fractures of the knee. Cause for confusion. Am J Sports Med 13:309–312, 1985.

45. Wojtys E, Wilson M, Buckwalter K, et al.: Magnetic resonance imaging of knee hyaline cartilage and intraarticular pathology. Am J Sports Med 15:455–463, 1987.

46. Messner K, Maletius W: The long-term prognosis for severe damage to weight-bearing cartilage of the knee. Acta Orthop Scand 67(2):165–168, 1996.

47. Levy AS, Lohnes J, Sculley S, et al.: Chondral delamination of the knee in soccer players. Am J Sports Med 24:634–639, 1996.

48. Shapiro F, Koide S, Glimcher MJ: Cell origin and differentiation in the repair of full thickness defects of articular cartilage. J Bone Joint Surg 75A:532–553, 1993.

49. Woo SLY, Buckwalter JA: Preface. In Woo SLY, Buckwalter JA (ed): Injury and Repair of the Musculoskeletal Soft Tissues. Park Ridge, IL, American Academy of Orthopaedic Surgeons, 1988, pp. 465–482.

50. Rodrigo JJ, Steadman JR, Silliman J, et al.: Isolated chondral defects of the knee recover slower than defects combined with anterior cruciate ligament and/or meniscus pathology after debridement and microfracture (abstract). Presented at the American Academy of Orthopaedic Surgeons 64th Annual Meeting, San Francisco, CA, 1997.

51. Mow VC, Rosenwasser MP: Articular cartilage: Biomechanics. In Woo SLY, Buckwalter JA (ed): Injury and Repair of the Musculoskeletal Soft Tissues. Park Ridge, IL, American Academy of Orthopaedic Surgeons, 1988, pp. 427–463.

52. Hangody L, Kish G, Karpati Z, et al.: Mosaic plasty for the treatment of articular cartilage defects: Application in the clinical practice. Presented at the SICOT meeting.

53. Thornhill TS: Evolving technologies: New answers or new problems? Cartilage resurfacing: Facts, fictions, and facets. Orthopaedics 20:819–920, 1997.

54. Peterson L, Menche D, Grande D, et al.: Chondrocyte transplantation: An experimental model in the rabbit (abstract). Trans Orthop Res Soc 9:218, 1984.

55. Stone KR: My technique: "The bone paste," compared to abrasion chondroplasty and microfracture. A critical review. Presented at 2nd Fribourg International Symposium on Cartilage Repair. Fribourg, Switzerland, Oct. 29–31, 1997.

56. Stone KR, Walgenbach AW: Surgical technique for articular cartilage transplantation to full thickness cartilage defects in the knee joint. Operative Techniques in Orthopedics 7(4):305–311, 1997.

57. Noyes FR, Roberts CS: High tibial osteotomy in knees with associated chronic ligament deficiencies. In Jackson DW (ed): Master Techniques in Orthopedic Surgery. New York, Raven Press, 1995, pp. 185–210.

58. Stone KR: Meniscus replacement. In Sherman OH (ed): Clinics in Sports Medicine: Meniscal Repair. Philadelphia, W.B. Saunders, 1986, pp. 557–571.

59. Stone KR, Rosenberg T: Surgical technique of meniscal replacement. Arthroscopy J Arthros Rel Surg 9(2):234–237, 1993.

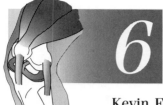

6 Assessment and Treatment of Medial Capsular Injuries

Kevin E. Wilk, PT, William G. Clancy, Jr, MD,
James R. Andrews, MD, and Gregory M. Fox, MD

*L*igamentous injuries to the knee joint are a very common occurrence in sports and account for 25 to 40 percent of all knee injuries sustained.[1, 2] Sprains of the medial collateral ligament (MCL) occur most frequently, and this is the most frequently injured ligament of the knee.[3–5] The MCL can be injured in isolation or in combination with other knee ligaments. Thus, the MCL, also referred to as the tibial collateral ligament, is a structure that has received much attention from clinicians and researchers in recent years.

Although the MCL has been the focus of increased attention by clinicians, because of the high incidence of injuries, there exists considerable controversy regarding the terminology and function of the MCL and surrounding capsular structures (posterior oblique ligament). In this chapter, we provide a discussion of the anatomy, biomechanics, mechanism of injury, and clinical examination of the medial capsular structures. Additionally, a thorough discussion of the treatment options (nonoperative and operative) as well as postoperative rehabilitation is conducted.

ANATOMY

The literature has produced significant confusion concerning the functional anatomy of the medial capsule. Some authors have described the posterior oblique ligament as a separate ligament and report that this structure plays a significant role in medial stability of the knee.[5] Conversely, Warren et al.[6] noted that the capsule was thickened in the posteromedial corner of the knee joint.

Warren and Marshall[7] have described the anatomy of the medial compartment of the knee joint and have divided the anatomic structures into three layers (Fig. 6–1). Layer one, the superficial layer, consists of the deep fascia that overlays the pes anserinus tendons and is continuous with the fascia that overlies the gastrocnemius muscle. Additionally, the medial patellar retinaculum and sartorius muscles are located in layer one (Fig. 6–2). Layer two consists of the superficial MCL and structures anterior to the MCL, which include the patellofemoral ligament, the patellotibial ligament, and the semimembranous muscle (Fig. 6–3). The deep layer, layer three, consists of the medial capsule, the deep MCL ligamentous fibers, and the meniscotibial (coronary) and meniscofemoral ligaments (Fig. 6–4). Approximately 2 cm posterior to the superficial edge of the MCL, layers two and three blend, forming the posteromedial capsule. As these two layers blend, they create an oblique orientation to the capsular fibers. Thus, the medial compartment is constructed of vertically and obliquely oriented collagen fibers. The fibers of the oblique bundle lie posterior to the vertical group and insert with the capsule into the posteromedial aspect of the tibia. Hughston and Eilers[5] have described the oblique band as the posterior oblique ligament and have stated that it is functionally independent of the MCL. The posteromedial aspect of the knee is thoroughly discussed in the biomechanics section of this chapter.

The superficial portion of the MCL (layer two) is a delta-shaped structure with a wide origin just below the adductor tubercle of the medial femoral condyle (Fig. 6–5). The superficial MCL extends inferiorly and narrows to insert distally 3 to 4 cm below the tibial plateau beneath the tendons of the pes anserinus. The MCL and pes anserinus are separated by the pes anserinus bursa. Brantigan and Voshell[8] have referred to this bursa as the bursa of Voshell. The superficial MCL fibers are vertical and contain a band

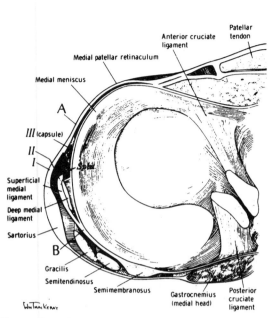

Figure 6-1. Cross section demonstrating layered approach to the medial side of the knee. (From Warren LF, Marshall JL: The supporting structures and layers on the medial side of the knee. J Bone Joint Surg 61A:56–62, 1979.)

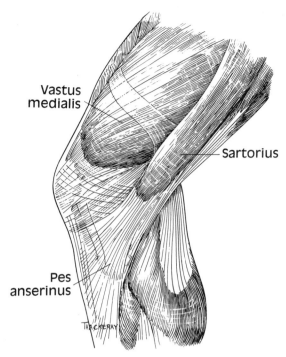

Figure 6-2. Layer one of the medial side of the knee demonstrating fascia running from vastus medialis inferiorly to and including sartortius tendons.

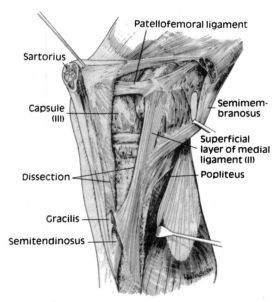

Figure 6-3. Layer two, consisting of the superficial medial collateral ligament and medial patellofemoral ligament.

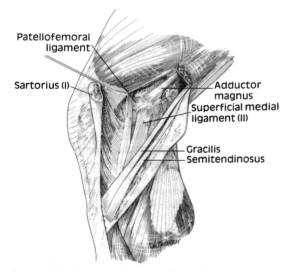

Figure 6-4. The superficial medial collateral ligament has been reflected to demonstrate the capsular structures (layer three).

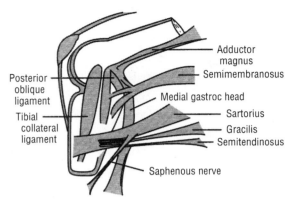

Figure 6–5. The superficial medial collateral ligament is illustrated. (From Engle RP: Knee Ligament Rehabilitation. New York, Churchill Livingstone, 1991, p. 72.)

that runs obliquely to join with several fibrous slips from the semimembranous muscle. This serves to reinforce the posteromedial corner of the knee joint.

The posteromedial capsule of the knee and the relationship to the semimembranous muscle have been described by Fowler.[9] The semimembranous has five main insertions (Fig. 6–6). It attaches (1) to the oblique fibers of the MCL, (2) to the posteromedial aspect of the tibia, (3) into the superficial MCL, (4) into the tibia just beneath the MCL, and (5) into the oblique popliteal ligament. Because of the numerous points of insertion of the semimembranous, the muscle functions are vast. The semimembranous functions to flex and internally rotate the tibia on the femur, tightens the posteromedial capsuloligamentous structures of the knee joint, and pulls the medial meniscus posteriorly during active knee flexion.

The deep portion of the MCL has a firm attachment to the medial meniscus. This attachment is most significant in the posteromedial aspect. The capsular attachments to the menisci have been referred to as the meniscofemoral and meniscotibial ligaments (Fig. 6–7). Müller[10] reported an attachment from the superficial MCL to the vastus medialis oblique muscle. Additionally, mechanoreceptors have been described located within the MCL to provide joint position sense and to provide a protective reflex against injury.[11]

BIOMECHANICS

Numerous articles have been published that thoroughly discuss the function and biomechanics of the MCL.[6, 10, 12–15] The superficial portion of the MCL acts as a primary restraint against valgus stress to the knee at both full extension and 25 degrees of knee

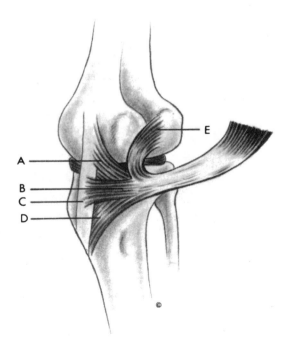

Figure 6–6. Semimembranous muscle attachments along the medial compartment of the knee joint. (From Greenfield BH: Functional anatomy of the knee. In Greenfield BH: Rehabilitation of the Knee. A Problem Solving Approach. Philadelphia, FA Davis, 1993, p. 25.)

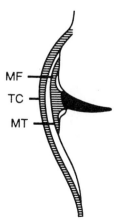

Figure 6–7. Meniscofemoral (MF) and meniscotibial (MT) portion of the medial capsular ligaments. Tibial collateral (TC) ligament. (From Engle RP: Knee Ligament Rehabilitation. New York, Churchill Livingstone, 1991, p. 72.)

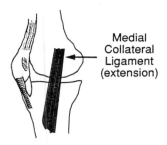

Medial
Collateral
Ligament
(extension)

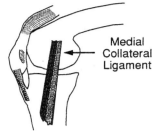

Medial
Collateral
Ligament

Figure 6–8. The effects of joint motion on the superficial MCL. (From Engle RP: Knee Ligament Rehabilitation. New York, Churchill Livingstone, 1991, p. 75.)

90° flexion anterior
5 mm of the MCL
remains taut in flexion

flexion.[6, 12] Warren et al.[6] noted that the anteriormost 5 mm of the MCL tightens when the knee is flexed and relaxes when the knee is extended, indicating that it is just anterior to the instant center of the knee (Fig. 6–8).

Grood et al.[12] demonstrated through selective tissue sectioning studies that the MCL affords 78 percent of the valgus restraint when the knee is flexed to 25 degrees (Fig. 6–9). The secondary restraints to the valgus stress are the anterior and posterior cruciate ligaments (13%), and the medial and posteromedial capsule provides 7 percent of the restraint. When the knee is placed near full extension (0–5 degrees), the MCL provides 57 percent of the valgus restraint, the medial and posteromedial capsule provides 25 percent, and the anterior and posterior cruciate ligaments contribute 15 percent (Fig. 6–10). In addition, Kennedy and Fowler,[13] Markolf et al.,[15] and Mains et al.[14] have reported significant increases in valgus laxity after sectioning of the MCL. Furthermore, these authors document that as knee extension increases, the posteromedial aspect of the knee capsule becomes taut and provides increased stability. Warren et al.[6] reported that the amount of knee joint opening on valgus stressing of the knee following excision of the superficial MCL alone was only 4 to 5 mm, with the knee flexed 30 to 40 degrees. Furthermore, when the deep MCL was sectioned, following sectioning of the superficial MCL, only a slight increase in valgus opening was noted, approximately 1 to 2 mm. This increase was statistically insignificant.

The second function of the medial capsular structures is to prevent external rotation of the tibia on the femur.[6, 10] Following sectioning of the deep portion of the MCL, only a minimal increase in external rotation of the tibia was noted.[6] With sectioning of the superficial portion of the MCL, external rotation of the tibia on the femur was nearly doubled with the knee positioned in full ex-

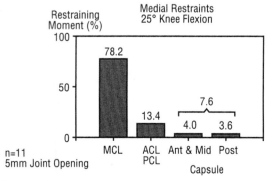

Figure 6–9. Medial soft tissue restraints to valgus stress testing at 25 degrees of knee flexion. (From Grood ES, Noyes FR, Butler DL, et al.: Ligamentous and capsular restraints preventing straight medial and lateral laxity on intact human cadaver knees. J Bone Joint Surg 63A:1257, 1981.)

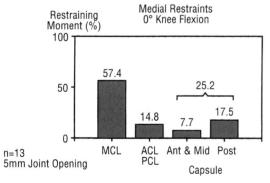

Figure 6–10. Medial soft tissue restraints to valgus stress testing in full knee extension. (From Grood ES, Noyes FR, Butler DL, et al.: Ligamentous and capsular restraints preventing straight medial and lateral laxity on intact human cadaver knees. J Bone Joint Surg 63A:1257, 1981.)

tension, resulting in approximately 6 degrees of external rotation. When the knee was flexed to 90 degrees, external rotation of the tibia on the femur tripled to 18 degrees. Sectioning of the posteromedial capsule had minimal effect on external rotation of the tibia on the femur.

A third function of the MCL is as a secondary restraint against anterior tibial translation, if the anterior cruciate ligament (ACL) was absent. Sullivan et al.[16] noted that sectioning all of the structures of the medial side of the knee, including the superficial MCL, oblique fibers, deep MCL, and capsule, will not increase anterior tibial translation if the ACL is intact. Conversely, if the ACL is sectioned first and then the superficial MCL, the result will be a significant increase in anterior tibial translation. These findings have significant treatment implications, which are discussed later. The functions of the MCL are as follows:

• Primary restraint to valgus stress
• Prevention of external rotation of tibia on the femur
• Secondary restraint to anterior tibial translation (when ACL is absent)

In summary, the superficial MCL is the primary static restraint against valgus stress to the knee joint. It also serves as an important restraint to external rotation of the tibia on the femur. Additionally, it acts as a secondary restraint against anterior tibial translation when the ACL is completely absent. The oblique portion and the deep portion of the MCL appear to play no role in preventing anterior tibial translation with or without an intact ACL. These structures contribute minimally to valgus restraint and only after the superficial MCL is sectioned. The deep portion of the MCL appears to resist further valgus opening if both the superficial MCL and ACL were injured.

MECHANISMS OF INJURY

The MCL is most often injured as a result of a valgus force or combined valgus and external rotation forces. The MCL can be injured by an external force, such as a direct blow to the lateral aspect of the knee. This type of injury is often associated with contact sports, such as football and hockey, in which there are frequent blows to the lateral side of the knee. Additionally, this mecha-

nism of injury can occur in a non-contact situation; a valgus force is applied from a fall to the side with the ipsilateral leg kept firmly fixed. Frequently, this type of injury results in a combined injury of the MCL and ACL.

O'Donoghue[17] identified the MCL-ACL–medial meniscus injury as the "unhappy triad of O'Donoghue." Shelbourne and Nitz[18] reported on patients who sustained a combined injury of the ACL and MCL. The investigators noted that 71 percent of the patients exhibited a tear of the lateral meniscus, whereas only 11 percent sustained an injury to the medial meniscus. Most of the lateral meniscal tears were middle-third radial or posterior-third peripheral tears, whereas most of the medial meniscal tears were posterior-third peripheral tears. Shelbourne and Nitz[18] went on to report that the classic O'Donoghue triad is an unusual clinical entity among athletes with acute knee injuries, and that such an injury might be more accurately described as a triad consisting of ACL, MCL, and lateral meniscus. They noted that the medial meniscus is more commonly involved in combined ACL and incomplete or second-degree MCL sprains.

Some investigators believe that the medial meniscus may become injured secondary to an MCL injury because of the anatomic configuration. The deep portion of the MCL attaches to the periphery of the medial meniscus, and this firm attachment may cause a peripheral tear owing to a significant valgus force. One of us (W.G.C.) has documented through arthroscopic examination that in an isolated MCL injury, the medial meniscus is rarely injured (unpublished data). The tear most often occurs in the meniscotibial or meniscofemoral portion of the deep capsule. These deep capsular injuries do not require surgery or post-injury immobilization because of excellent healing potential from increased vascularity in this region.

Maturation also has effects on the site of MCL failures. Tipton et al.[19] and Woo et al.[20] demonstrated changes in the structural properties of the MCL–bone complex during maturation in animals. Their findings indicated that the ligamentous attachment site was weak until the epiphyses closed. Thus, the MCL is affected by the proximity of the tibial growth plate. In their studies, the MCL failed by tibial avulsion in skeletally immature people. Conversely, after epiphyseal closure, only 12 percent of failures were due to tibial avulsion.[20] Additionally, in older individuals (older than 50 years of age), there appears to be a higher incidence of bony avulsion failure than in younger individuals.[21] Thus, when examining the skeletally immature patient or the older patient, the clinician must be sure to clinically evaluate (by radiography) for avulsion fractures. In individuals whose epiphysis is closed to approximately 50 years of age, mid-substance tears of the ligamentous tissue are most prevalent. Most commonly, the MCL is injured from the femoral origin, or at the mid-substance. In contrast, distal MCL injuries are less common but occasionally may occur. The location of the MCL injury has implications on the rehabilitation and are discussed later.

CLINICAL EXAMINATION

The clinical examination begins with a careful and thoroughly detailed subjective history, including a complete description of the mechanism of injury. It is important for the clinician to know the exact knee position when the injury was sustained; this will help to direct and guide the clinical examination. In addition, the clinician should ask the patient if he or she felt or heard a pop or tearing in the knee, whether the knee felt as if it shifted apart, whether the patient was able to continue to play, and, whether the patient noticed any swelling of the knee within 1 to 2 hours following the injury. Also, a thorough history of any previous knee injuries must be thoroughly discussed. The location of pain or tenderness, present activity level, and intended sports activities for the future are all germane items of information to gather at this point.

The physical examination starts with the assessment of swelling as determined by placing one hand on each side of the anterior surface of the knee and applying gentle pressure with one of the hands. If swelling is present, the relaxed hand will feel the fluid move into it. The quantification of swelling is determined by estimation of the amount of fluid present; mild swelling indicates about 25 mL or less; moderate swelling indicates 26 to 55 ml; and severe swelling represents 56 mL or more. Significant swelling of the knee following an isolated grade I or II MCL sprain is rare. If the ACL is injured,

then significant swelling is common. In the case of grade III MCL injuries in which the capsular integrity is disrupted, joint effusion may be minimal.

The goal of the physical examination is to identify the injured structures, detect the degree of injury, and establish an accurate diagnosis. Examination of the knee begins with the patient's leg relaxed and comfortable so that the knee can be accurately examined. In some cases, an examination with the patient under spinal or general anesthesia may be required to obtain adequate muscle relaxation; this is very unusual. When a ligamentous knee injury is suspected, the first structures that should be carefully examined to determine structural integrity are the posterior and anterior cruciate ligaments. The authors recommend a step-off test[22, 23] (Fig. 6–11) and the gravity test to determine the integrity of the posterior cruciate ligament. The anterior cruciate ligament can be accurately assessed with a Lachman test with the knee flexed to 20 to 25 degrees. Once the posterior and anterior

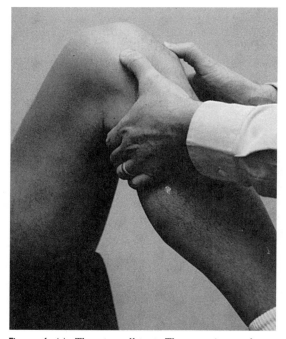

Figure 6–11. The step-off test. The examiner palpates the medial femoral condyle and then runs the palpating fingers inferiorly into the medial tibial plateau. If the posterior cruciate ligament (PCL) is intact, the tibial plateau will be slightly anterior. In the presence of a PCL injury, the medial tibial plateau will be even with or posterior to the femoral condyle.

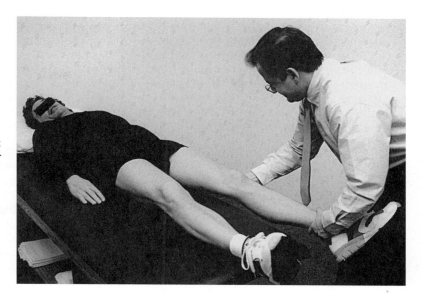

Figure 6–12. Valgus stress test with the patient's knee positioned in full extension.

cruciate ligaments have been examined, then the clinician can focus his attention specifically on the MCL.

The knee examination should be performed with the patient supine and the thigh supported by the table, which assists in relaxation of the thigh musculature. The MCL integrity is first assessed with the knee in full extension (Fig. 6–12), and then in 30 degrees of flexion (Fig. 6–13). The knee is positioned in the desired knee flexion angle, and a gentle valgus stress is applied with the opposite hand, which is positioned on the lateral side of the lateral femoral condyle near the joint line. The amount of medial opening is compared with that of the contra-

lateral knee to determine the extent of the injury. The amount of valgus opening is assessed and classified to document the degree or severity of the injury. Additionally, the clinician should assess the endfeel while evaluating the amount of joint displacement.

Medial laxity with applied valgus stress with the knee in full extension indicates an injury to the MCL, medial capsule, and posteromedial capsule. If there is gross or severe laxity (instability) noted at full extension, injury to the cruciate ligaments should be suspected (although it is not always present), and specific cruciate tests should be performed at that time. With the knee flexed to 30 degrees, the posteromedial and poste-

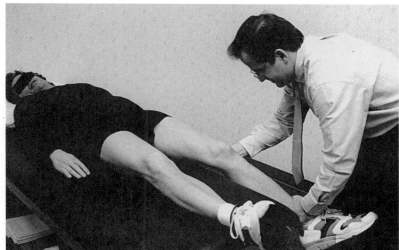

Figure 6–13. Valgus stress test with the patient's knee positioned at 25 to 30 degrees of knee flexion.

rior capsule are placed on slack. Medial laxity with applied valgus is indicative of injury to the MCL.

In addition, the examiner should attempt to quantify the amount of medial laxity noted during the valgus stress testing. The medial joint space opening is estimated, and the endfeel or endpoint is also assessed to determine severity of the injury. The findings are compared with those for the patient's contralateral normal knee. Ideally, the normal knee is evaluated first to familiarize the patient with the test and minimize patient apprehension, and to establish the normal baseline for knee laxity for that specific patient.

In a first-degree MCL sprain, there is no joint opening to approximately 2 mm, and there exists a firm endpoint. In a second-degree sprain, the opening is from 3 to 5 mm compared with the opposite side, and the endpoint has a slight give to it. In a third-degree injury, the endpoint is soft or open, and the joint space opens 5 mm more than that of the contralateral knee.[24] Grood et al.[12] reported that a 5-mm increase in laxity compared with the contralateral knee indicates a major or significant MCL injury.

When performing valgus stress testing of the knee, the clinician should be careful to control and prevent axial rotation of the tibia and femur. This rotary motion may be misinterpreted as increased medial laxity. Care should be taken to perform single-plane testing to ensure specific isolated ligamentous structural testing.

In addition, careful and meticulous palpa-tion of bony and soft tissue anatomy should be part of a comprehensive clinical examination. Careful palpation along the course of the MCL to locate the tear is extremely important in designing the rehabilitation program. In association with MCL injuries, tenderness is often elicited over the adductor tubercle of the medial femoral condyle (the origin of the MCL) (Fig. 6–14). Also associated with mid-substance MCL injuries is tenderness on the MCL just above the joint line. Point tenderness over the adductor tubercle can be also associated with lateral patellar subluxation or dislocation. The medial patellofemoral ligament inserts onto the adductor tubercle, and this ligament is often injured with lateral patellar subluxation or dislocation. To differentiate patellar subluxation from minor sprains of the MCL, palpation of the medial patellofemoral ligament (MPFL), MCL, and patellar facets, along with ligamentous tests, can clarify the precise lesion. MCL injuries are usually associated with pain during valgus stress testing, valgus laxity, tenderness along the MCL, and a slight loss of motion. Conversely, patellar subluxation is associated with pain on palpation of the MPFL, patellar facet pain or tenderness, and no change in laxity during valgus stress testing. Additionally, pain from the MPFL can occur during valgus stress testing and often can be misleading to the clinician. Lastly, tenderness distally near the insertion of the MCL into the tibia can be identified with careful palpation.

When evaluating for an MCL injury, care must be taken to evaluate the medial menis-

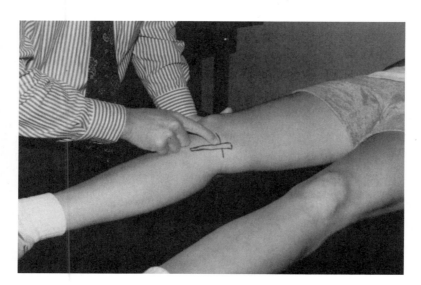

Figure 6–14. Palpation of the medial collateral ligament. (From Engle RP: Knee Ligament Rehabilitation. New York, Churchill Livingstone, 1991, p. 78.)

cus and ACL for possible injury. Persistent joint line pain on or near the MCL should be carefully evaluated for medial meniscus pathology. The traditional McMurray test and Apley compression test have been used for evaluation of meniscal pathology. Unfortunately, however, these two tests are not reliable when performed on patients with MCL injury because the rotary movement performed by the examiner on the tibiofemoral joint can create stress on the MCL structure. The use of magnetic resonance imaging may be most beneficial. If any question exists as to whether there is a first-degree MCL sprain or a medial meniscal tear, magnetic resonance imaging should be considered.

HEALING CONSTRAINTS

There has been some controversy about the treatment for isolated MCL injuries. O'Donoghue[25] reported that if a primary repair is not performed, the ends of the ligament may not remain in closed opposition and thus healing will be biomechanically inferior and delayed. Several investigators have reported biomechanically stronger MCLs in sutured compared with unsutured canine knees.[26–28] Based on these clinical studies, some surgeons have advocated surgical repair for the injured MCL. Conversely, most recent studies strongly suggest that nonoperative treatment of the MCL is indicated for most injuries.

Woo et al.[3] reported their results after sectioning canine MCLs. The investigators studied three effects: (1) no repair and immediate motion; (2) repair and immobilization for 3 weeks; and (3) repair and immobilization for 6 weeks. The results indicated that the biomechanical properties of the nonrepaired ligaments exhibited the best results at 6, 12, and 48 weeks post-sectioning. The investigators also reported that the longer immobilization period exhibited the weakened healing response.

The results of several clinical studies have provided the basis for nonoperative treatment of MCL injuries.[29–41] These clinical studies have demonstrated excellent results using a treatment approach of immediate motion without surgical intervention for isolated MCL injuries. Ellsasser et al.[29] reported on clinical findings in 64 professional foot-

ball players who sustained partial MCL sprains. All players were treated nonoperatively and with mobilization; all patients returned to play in 3 to 8 weeks. Derscheid and Garrick[30] reported on partial MCL sprains treated with motion and strengthening. The authors reported a return to participation in 10.6 days for grade I sprains, and 19.5 days in grade II cases. Wilk and Corzatt[31] reported on 52 MCL sprains in athletes who were treated with immediate motion, early weight-bearing, and immediate exercise. The results indicated a return to sport activities after 9.2 days following a grade I sprain and 17.8 days after a grade II injury. Sandberg et al.,[32] in a prospective randomized study of operative treatment compared with nonoperative treatment of both acute isolated MCL injuries and combined injuries of the MCL and ACL, noted no benefit associated with operative treatment of the torn MCL in either situation. Additionally, Mok and Good[33] and Ballmer et al.[34] have noted satisfactory healing and stabilizing of the MCL in patients with combined injuries treated with ACL reconstruction and nonoperative treatment of the MCL.

Based on these studies, consisting of treatment guidelines for isolated grade I:grade II MCL sprains, most clinicians advocate immediate motion and strengthening.[27–35] It is well accepted that isolated MCL injuries can heal with stability and excellent functional results after nonoperative treatment. Additionally, several authors have reported an enhanced healing response of the injured MCL by immediate motion and exercise.[19, 35, 41–43] Immediate motion and exercise provide the stimulus to the medial capsule, thus facilitating earlier and enhanced healing of the injured structures.

The healing rates and mechanical properties of the injured MCL are altered and slowed in the presence of a complete ACL injury. Investigators have reported that the MCLs in knees with totally sectioned ACLs showed less recovery than knee joints with an intact ACL.[44–46] In the past, several clinicians suggested that the acute treatment of such injuries should include the repair of all damaged structures.[47, 48] However, acute operative treatment of both the MCL and ACL can result in a high prevalence of postoperative knee stiffness.[49] Shelbourne and Patel[50] have suggested a treatment approach for athletically active patients that consists of treating the injury of the MCL nonoperatively and performing a delayed ACL reconstruction after the knee has normalized its motion and inflammation has subsided.

The stages of MCL healing have been explained by several authors.[51–54] These three stages include phase I, the acute inflammation, which occurs in the first 72 hours; phase II, the repair and regeneration process, which begins at 48 to 72 hours after injury and lasts up to 6 weeks (collagen production); and phase III, the remodeling, which lasts 52 weeks. During this last phase, the healing ligament continues to become stronger. The maximal return in strength appears to be approximately 70 to 75 percent of the pre-injury level. The process is expedited by motion and controlled stress to the healing ligament.

The optimal conditions for MCL healing are (1) maintenance of the torn fibers in close continuity, (2) an intact and stable ACL and other supporting ligamentous structures of the knee, (3) immediate controlled motion and stresses to the healing ligament, and (4) protection of the MCL against deleterious stresses (valgus and external rotation).

REHABILITATION PROGRAM

The complete rehabilitation following an isolated MCL sprain can be divided into a four-phase rehabilitation program (Table 6–1). The rehabilitation program is based on five basic rehabilitation principles:

1. The effects of immobilization must be minimized.
2. Healing tissue must never be overstressed, but controlled stress is beneficial.
3. The patient must fulfill criteria to progress from one phase to another.
4. The rehabilitation program should be based on current clinical and scientific research.
5. The rehabilitation program must be adaptable to each patient.

These principles must be understood and followed as a treatment philosophy to ensure proper and complete healing. Additionally, in the case of isolated MCL injuries, another key treatment philosophy is the importance of motion to facilitate the healing response.

In phase I, the goals are to initiate motion in a nonpainful arc of motion so that the deleterious effects of immobilization can be prevented and collagen synthesis and organization can be accelerated. Too aggressive stretching may cause the healing collagen to be traumatized again and thus retard the healing process. Occasionally, a brace can be used to protect the healing ligament against valgus stress. Immediate weight-bearing is performed to stimulate the healing of the ligament and provide nourishment to the articular cartilage and subchondral bone. In addition, immediate quadriceps femoris muscle strengthening exercises are initiated to prevent muscular atrophy. The quadriceps muscle tends to atrophy at a faster rate than the other muscles about the knee following a knee injury.[55, 56] Electrical muscle stimulation to the quadriceps muscle is used to facilitate an enhanced muscular contraction, retard muscle atrophy, and provide re-education to the muscle.[56–59] The muscle re-education is designed to prevent "quadriceps muscle shutdown," which is the patient's inability to perform an isolated quadriceps femoris muscle contraction. In addition, a warm whirlpool, use of the bicycle, passive range of motion (ROM), and active assistive ROM exercises are used to increase ROM.

In phase II, the goals are to re-establish full nonpainful ROM and to enhance muscular strength in the entire lower extremity. In this phase, most patients exhibit nearly full ROM, although terminal knee extension and full flexion may still be limited because of pain. During this time frame, full motion is emphasized. Stretching exercises, such as low-load, long-duration stretches to improve knee extension can be implemented at this time. The strengthening exercises are accelerated. Isotonic exercises are implemented in the form of knee extensions, leg presses, hip exercises, calf raises, and especially hip adductions and hamstring curls. The authors also emphasize closed kinetic chain (CKC) exercises, such as squats, lateral step-ups, front step-downs, wall squats, and lateral lunges (Figs. 6–15 and 6–16). Through some of the CKC exercises and specific balance drills, the goal is to restore and enhance proprioception and neuromuscular control. The bicycle and stair climber machine are employed for endurance training. Additionally, pool exercises and pool running may be initiated to improve total body

Table 6–1. **Rehabilitation Program for Grade I or II Isolated Medial Collateral Ligament (MCL) Sprains**

This program can be accelerated for grade I MCL sprains or can be extended depending on the severity of the injury. The following schedule serves as a guideline to help in the expediency of returning an athlete to his or her pre-injury state.

Please note that if there is any increase in pain or swelling or loss of range of motion, these serve as signs that the progression of the patient may be too rapid.

I. MAXIMAL PROTECTION PHASE

Goals: Early protected ROM
      Prevent quadriceps atrophy
      Decrease effusion/pain

A. Time of Injury: Day 1
- Ice, compression, elevation
- Knee hinge brace, nonpainful ROM; if needed
- Crutches, weight-bearing as tolerated
- Passive ROM/active assistive ROM to maintain ROM
- Electrical muscle stimulation to quads (8 hours a day)
- Isometric quadriceps exercises: quadriceps sets, straight-leg raises (flexion)

B. Day 2
- Continue above exercises
- Quadriceps sets
- Straight-leg raises (flexion, abduction)
- Hamstring isometric sets
- Well leg exercises
- Whirlpool for ROM (cold for first 3–4 days, then warm)
- High-voltage galvanic stimulation to control swelling

C. Days 3–7
- Continue above exercises
- Crutches, weight-bearing as tolerated
- ROM as tolerated
- Eccentric quadriceps work
- Bicycle for ROM stimulus
- Resisted knee extension with electrical muscle stimulation
- Initiate hip adduction and extension
- Initiate mini-squats
- Initiate leg-press isotonics
- Brace worn at night, brace during day as needed

II. MODERATE PROTECTION PHASE

Criteria for Progression:
1. No increase in instability
2. No increase in swelling
3. Minimal tenderness
4. Passive ROM 10–100 degrees

Goals: Full painless ROM
      Restore strength
      Ambulation without crutches

A. Week 2
- Continue strengthening program with progressive resistive exercise (PRE)
- Continue electric muscle stimulation to quads during isotonic strengthening
- Continue ROM exercise
- Emphasize closed kinetic chain exercises; lunges, squats, lateral lunges, wall squats, lateral step-ups
- Bicycle for endurance
- Water exercises, running in water forward and backward

- Full ROM exercises
- Flexibility exercises, hamstrings, quadriceps, iliotibial band, etc.
- Proprioception training (balance drills)
- StairMaster endurance work

B. Days 11–14
- Continue all exercises in week 2
- PREs emphasis on quadriceps, medial hamstrings, hip abduction
- Initiate isokinetics, submaximal → maximal fast contractile velocities
- Begin running program if full painless extension and flexion are present

III. MINIMAL PROTECTION PHASE

Criteria for Progression:
1. No instability
2. No swelling or tenderness
3. Full painless ROM

Goals: Increase strength and power

A. Week 3
- Continue strengthening program
  - Wall squats
  - Vertical squats
  - Lunges
  - Lateral lunges
  - Step-ups
  - Leg press
  - Knee extension
  - Hip abduction and adduction
  - Hamstring curls
  - Emphasis:
    - Functional exercise drills
    - Fast speed isokinetics
    - Eccentric quadriceps
    - Isotonic hip adduction, medial hamstrings
- Isokinetic test
- Proprioception training
- Endurance exercise
- Stationary bike 30–40 minutes
- NordicTrac, swimming, etc.
- Initiate agility program, sport-specific activities

IV. MAINTENANCE PROGRAM

Criteria for return to competition:
1. Full ROM
2. No instability
3. Muscle strength 85% of contralateral side
4. Proprioception ability satisfactory
5. No tenderness over MCL
6. No effusion
7. Quadriceps strength; torque/body weight ratios
8. Lateral knee brace (if necessary)

Maintenance Program

Continue isotonic strengthening exercises
Continue flexibility exercises
Continue proprioceptive activities

ROM = range of motion.
  Developed by Kevin E. Wilk, PT; revised 1/98.

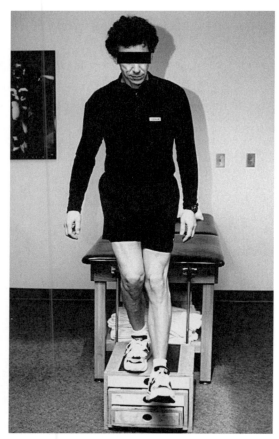

Figure 6–15. Front step-downs are utilized to re-establish neuromuscular control of the quadriceps muscle during eccentric muscle loading.

conditioning and facilitate functional progression while minimally stressing the joint.

Phase III is referred to as the minimal protection phase. All exercises are progressed with a particular focus on CKC, endurance exercises, proprioception activities, and functional drills. A running program is initiated with an emphasis on drills and agility activities specific to the demands of the patient-athlete's lifestyle and sport. Agility drills are begun to enhance coordination, balance, and neuromuscular control.

In the last phase, the return to activity phase, maintenance exercises are used when the athlete returns to his or her sport. The exercise program should be designed to continually increase the patient's strength and function, not merely to maintain strength. This continued exercise program should emphasize quadriceps strengthening, hip and hamstring muscular control, proprioception,

endurance, and functional drills and activities.

The rehabilitation program just discussed has been utilized since 1987, with excellent success. Results from an ongoing clinical study for 311 isolated grade I MCL sprains is 7.3 days, and for a grade II isolated injury, 17.8 days. The success rate is significantly affected by concomitant injuries to the posteromedial capsule or ACL. Most of these individuals sustained their knee injuries during participation in the following sports: football (71%), skiing (12%), wrestling (11%), and soccer (4%).

Variation of Rehabilitation Based on Injury Location

The nonoperative rehabilitation program may vary slightly depending on the location of the injury to the MCL. MCL injuries that occur at the femoral origin or in its midsubstance tend to become stiff and may develop loss of motion more readily. Thus, in these cases, the program emphasizes immediate motion with restoration of full motion within 2 to 3 weeks. Conversely, knees in which the MCLs have been injured at the tibial insertion site have a tendency to heal with residual valgus laxity.[50] Thus, Shelbourne and Patel[50] have recommended a brief period (usually 2 to 4 weeks) of immobilization in a brace or cast with the knee immobilized in approximately 30 degrees of flexion, which assists in healing of the MCL without residual laxity. We allow early motion with a restriction of full extension and excessive flexion. In most cases, restoration of full motion is rarely a problem after a distal injury of the MCL. Conversely, stiffness has been common following proximal injuries to the MCL.

If an injury to the posterior oblique ligament has occurred with concomitant injury to the MCL and ACL, then laxity will be noted with valgus applied stress when the knee is fully extended. Post-injury, early motion is recommended, although full extension is not permitted for the first 1 to 2 weeks to allow the posteromedial structures to heal. Occasionally, surgery is required for treatment of these injuries.

The key points of the nonoperative rehabilitation program are first to establish an accurate diagnosis and to ensure that an

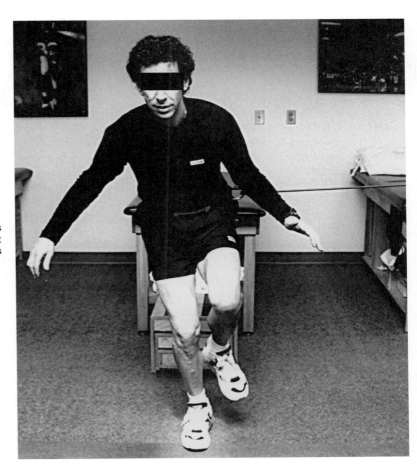

Figure 6–16. Lateral side lunges are employed to train the patient to co-contract the hamstrings and quadriceps muscles.

isolated lesion has been sustained and second to identify the location of the lesion. Next, immediate motion must be initiated to promote collagen synthesis and organization within the injured MCL and to prevent the negative effects of immobilization.[60, 61] Additionally, immediate weight-bearing and muscle training must begin to prevent atrophy and neuromuscular deficits.

SURGICAL MANAGEMENT

In cases of severe (grade III) MCL injuries, a primary surgical repair should be performed. Surgical treatment begins with a thorough examination under anesthesia. Since these injuries are usually associated with ACL injuries, valgus stress with the knee in full extension will reveal a marked increase in medial joint opening. Thus, the clinician should suspect not only superficial and deep MCL injury, but also posteromedial capsule injury. A diagnostic arthroscopy is performed next. The deep portion of the torn MCL can be visualized and often is flipped into the joint underneath the medial meniscus. Once identified, the MCL is then repaired. Performing the medial repair first creates a water-tight seal of the knee, preventing fluid extravasation and facilitating subsequent meniscal repair and ACL reconstruction.

The medial structures are approached through a small incision centered over the superficial MCL. A careful dissection is performed to identify the rupture planes. If the MCL is avulsed from bone, it can be directly reattached with suture anchors. Mid-substance tears are reapproximated with absorbable sutures. The posteromedial capsule and the oblique fibers of the MCL must be visualized and included in the repair. Care must be taken not to overtighten the medial structures. There should be consistent tension of the superficial MCL through the full arc of motion.

Additionally, the menisci must be visualized and carefully evaluated to determine their status. It is not uncommon for a meniscus injury to be sustained in combination with an MCL-ACL injury. We agree with Shelbourne and Nitz,[62] who have reported a higher rate of lateral meniscus injuries in association with combined ACL-MCL injuries. This report contradicts the "Unhappy Triad of the Knee" proposed by O'Donoghue, who stated that the medial meniscus is the most commonly involved with an ACL-MCL injury.[17] Once the meniscal lesion is identified, it is then determined whether a repair or partial meniscectomy will be performed. The decision is based on the size of the tear, its location, the length of time since the injury, and the patient's age. When the meniscal pathology has been addressed, the ACL reconstruction is performed using an autologous bone–patella tendon–bone graft.

When the surgery is completed, an intra-articular hemovac is applied to control swelling in the first 24 hours. In addition, a bulky dressing is applied with a compression wrap and a knee brace locked in full extension.

POSTOPERATIVE MANAGEMENT

The postoperative rehabilitation following primary MCL repair and ACL reconstruction must be aggressive in restoring motion, particularly full passive knee extension. It has been reported that acute operative treatment of both components of combined ACL-MCL injury can result in an unacceptably high prevalence of postoperative stiffness of the knee[49]; thus, it is our aim to prevent these postoperative complications.

The initial goal in rehabilitation is to restore motion, particularly full passive knee extension. Additional goals are to decrease swelling and inflammation, protect the knee with limited weight-bearing, and initiate quadriceps strengthening exercises. Immediately following surgery, the patient is placed in full passive knee extension (often slight hyperextension, approximately 3 to 5 degrees is encouraged), while flexion is gradually increased. Flexion should progress to 90 degrees by day 5, 105 degrees by week 2, 115 degrees by week 3, and 125 degrees by week 4. Additionally, a knee brace is used to provide support until the patient has restored dynamic stability of the knee joint while ambulatory. Immediately postoperatively, the patient's knee is wrapped with a compressive wrap and cold appliance (Polarcare, Breg Corporation, Vista, CA) (Fig. 6–17). We have found the use of cold and compression to be extremely beneficial in the reduction of postoperative pain, reduction of swelling, and regaining of quadriceps muscle control. The patient is progressed on a rehabilitation program that emphasizes quadriceps muscle strengthening, closed kinetic chain exercises, proprioception and neuromuscular training, and functional drills.

The clinician must remember that the initial 2 to 3 weeks are the most important when treating the patient with an acutely

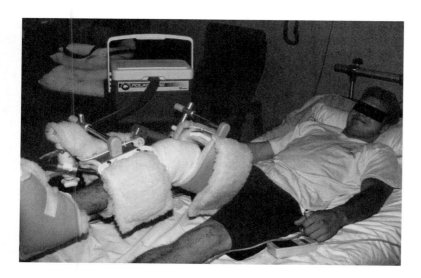

Figure 6–17. Postoperatively, the patient is immediately wrapped with a compressive wrap and cold appliance (Polarcare, Breg Corp, Vista, CA) to minimize swelling and inflammation.

repaired or reconstructed MCL-ACL. The clinician must restore full passive knee extension in an expedient fashion, and gradually improve flexion, to prevent the most common postoperative complication, knee stiffness.

Often clinicians utilize a lateral knee hinged brace to provide support against valgus stress. Numerous braces are available from numerous manufacturers. The efficiency and effectiveness of these braces remain controversial. The published research reports present conflicting data and a somewhat confusing picture. Hewson et al.[63] found no change in the MCL injury rate between athletes playing with braced knees and those playing with unbraced knees. Conversely, Rovere et al.[64] and Teitz et al.[65] reported an overall increase in MCL injuries for those wearing braces. Recently, Albright et al.[66] studied the effectiveness of preventive knee braces on MCL knee sprains among collegiate football players. The investigators concluded that preventive knee braces were effective for all players except skill position players (backs, receivers, and kickers). The data indicated a slight increase in the number of MCL injuries in the unbraced group in game-related activities only. Sitler et al.[67] published their knee results of 700 West Point cadets participating in eight-player tackle football. There were a total of 71 knee injuries, of which 37 were MCL sprains, with 25 (67%) occurring in the unbraced cadets.

Paulos et al.[68] studied the biomechanical forces on the knee joint with lateral knee bracing. The investigators noted that no significant protection could be documented with the use of these braces. They also noted four potentially adverse effects of the braces: MCL preload, center axis shift, premature joint line contact, and brace slippage. They noted that in individuals whose knees were aligned in neutral to varus alignment, the effects of the brace caused the femur and tibia to be pulled toward the brace, thus distracting the medial joint line, causing the ligaments to be tightened. In this situation, referred to as ligamentous preload, time to rupture would be reduced, thus making not only the MCL but also the ACL more susceptible to injury. Therefore, the alignment of the lower extremity must be carefully evaluated when considering the application and use of a lateral knee brace.

SUMMARY

The treatment of MCL injuries has significantly changed in the last 10 years. In the past, the emphasis was on immobilization, which often led to motion complications. Today, knowledge of the medial capsular structures has expanded extensively. The treatment for isolated MCL sprains is nonoperative, with emphasis on aggressive rehabilitation, especially in restoring motion. Additionally, most commonly the treatment of combined MCL-ACL injuries is reconstruction of the ACL and nonoperative treatment of the MCL. After the clinician has identified an injury to the medial capsular structures, the rehabilitation program must focus on restoring motion, full passive knee extension, immediate strengthening, and weightbearing. This approach will assist in improving the successful treatment and minimizing the post-injury complication rate.

References

1. Powell J: 636,000 injuries annually in high school football. Athletic Trn 22:19–26, 1987.
2. Dehaven KE, Litner DM: Athletic injuries: Comparison by age, sport and gender. Am J Sports Med 14:218–224, 1986.
3. Woo SL-Y, Inoue M, McGuik-Burleson E, et al.: Treatment of the medial collateral ligament injury: II. Structure and function of the canine knee in response to differing treatment regimens. Am J Sports Med 15:22–29, 1987.
4. Nicholas JA, Hershman EB: The Lower Extremity and Spine in Sports Medicine. St. Louis, CV Mosby, 1986, p. 657.
5. Hughston JC, Eilers AF: The role of the posterior oblique ligament in repairs of acute medial ligament tears of the knee. J Bone Joint Surg 55A:923–940, 1973.
6. Warren LF, Marshall JL, Girgis F: The prime static stabilizer of the medial side of the knee. J Bone Joint Surg 56A:665–670, 1974.
7. Warren LF, Marshall JL: The supporting structures and layers on the medial side of the knee. J Bone Joint Surg 61A:56–62, 1979.
8. Brantigan OC, Voshell AF: The mechanics of the ligaments and menisci of the knee joint. J Bone Joint Surg 23A:44–49, 1941.
9. Fowler PJ: Functional anatomy of the knee. In Hunter LY, Funk FJ (eds): Rehabilitation of the Injured Knee. St Louis, CV Mosby, 1984, pp. 16–20.
10. Müller W: The Knee: Form, Function, and Ligament Reconstruction. New York, Springer-Verlag, 1983.
11. Fetto JF, Marshall JL: Medial collateral ligament injuries of the knee: A rationale for treatment. Clin Orthop 132:206–212, 1978.
12. Grood ES, Noyes FR, Butler DL, et al.: Ligamentous and capsular restraints preventing straight medial

and lateral laxity in intact human cadaver knees. J Bone Joint Surg 63A:1257, 1981.

13. Kennedy JC, Fowler PJ: Medial and anterior instability of the knee: An anatomical and clinical study using stress machines. J Bone Joint Surg 53A:1257–1261, 1971.

14. Mains DB, Andrews JG, Stonecipher T: Medial and anterior posterior ligament stability of the human knee measured with stress apparatus. Am J Sports Med 5:144–147, 1977.

15. Markolf KL, Mensch JS, Amstutz HC: Stiffness and laxity of the knee: The contribution of supporting structures. J Bone Joint Surg 58A:583–588, 1976.

16. Sullivan DJ, Levy IM, Shesikier S, et al.: Medial restraints to anterior-posterior motion of the knee. J Bone Joint Surg 6A:930–939, 1984.

17. O'Donoghue DH: Surgical treatment of injuries to the ligaments of the knee. JAMA 169:1423–1431, 1959.

18. Shelbourne KD, Nitz PA: The O'Donoghue triad revisited: Combined knee injuries involving anterior cruciate and medial collateral ligament tears. Am J Sports Med 19:474–477, 1991.

19. Tipton CM, Mathies RD, Martin RK: Influence of age and sex on strength of bone-ligament junctions in knee joints of rats. J Bone Joint Surg 60A:230–234, 1978.

20. Woo SL-Y, Orlando CA, Gomez MA, et al.: Tensile properties of the medial collateral ligament as a function of age. J Orthop Res 4:133–136, 1986.

21. Noyes FR, Grood ES: The strength of the anterior cruciate ligament in humans and rhesus monkeys: Age-related and species-related changes. J Bone Joint Surg 58A:1074, 1976.

22. Clancy WG Jr: Repair and reconstruction of the posterior cruciate ligament. In Chapman MW (ed): Operative Orthopaedics, 2nd ed. Philadelphia, JB Lippincott, 1993, pp. 2093–2107.

23. Wilk KE, Clancy WG, Andrews JR: The posterior cruciate ligament. In Mangine RE (ed): Physical Therapy of the Knee, 2nd ed. New York, Churchill Livingstone, 1995, pp. 263–288.

24. Daniel D, Akeson W, O'Connor J: Knee Ligaments: Structure, Function, Injuries and Repair. New York, Raven Press, 1990.

25. O'Donoghue DH: Surgical treatment of fresh injuries to the major ligaments of the knee. J Bone Joint Surg 32A:721, 1950.

26. Clayton ML, Weir CR: Experimental investigations of ligamentous healing. Am J Surg 98:373–379, 1959.

27. Clayton ML, Miles J, Abdulla M: Experimental investigation of ligamentous healing. Clin Orthop 61:148–153, 1968.

28. Korkala O, Rusanen M, Groblad M: Healing of experimental ligament rupture. Arch Orthop Trauma Surg 102:179–184, 1984.

29. Ellsasser JC, Reynolds FC, Omohundro JR: The non-operative treatment of collateral ligament injuries of the knee in professional football players. J Bone Joint Surg 56A:1185, 1974.

30. Dersheid GL, Garrick JG: Medial collateral ligament injuries in football: Non-operative management of grade I & II sprains. Am J Sports Med 9:981, 1981.

31. Wilk KE, Corzatt RD: Non-operative rehabilitation of grade I & II sprains on the medial collateral ligament in athletes. Presented at the Combined Sections Meeting of the American Physical Therapy Association, Washington, DC, 1988.

32. Sandberg R, Balkfors B, Nilsson B, et al.: Operative versus non-operative treatment of recent injuries to the ligaments of the knee. A prospective randomized study. J Bone Joint Surg 69A:1120–1126, 1987.

33. Mok DW, Good C: Non-operative management of acute grade III medial collateral ligament injury of the knee: A prospective study. Injury 20:277–280, 1989.

34. Ballmer PM, Ballmer FT, Jakob RP: Reconstruction of the anterior cruciate ligament alone in the treatment of a combined instability with complete rupture of the medial collateral ligament: A prospective study. Arch Orthop Trauma Surg 110:139–141, 1991.

35. Vailas AC, Tipton CM, Matthes RD, et al.: Physical activity and its influence on the repair process of medial collateral ligaments. Connect Tissue Res 9:225, 1981.

36. Goldstein WM, Barmada R: Early mobilization of rabbit medial collateral ligament repairs: Biomechanic and histologic study. Arch Phys Med Rehabil 65:239, 1984.

37. Frank C, Woo SL-Y, Amiel D, et al.: Medial collateral ligament healing: A multidisciplinary assessment in rabbits. Am J Sports Med 11:379, 1983.

38. Indelicato PA: Non-operative treatment of complete tears of the medial collateral ligament of the knee. J Bone Joint Surg 65A:323, 1983.

39. Indelicato PA: Injury to the medial capsuloligamentous complex. In Feagin JA (ed): The Crucial Ligaments. Churchill Livingstone, New York, 1988, p. 197.

40. Fetto JF, Marshall JL: Medial collateral ligament injuries of the knee: A rationale for treatment. Clin Orthop 132:206, 1978.

41. Woo SL-Y, Gomez MA, Sites TJ, et al.: The biomechanical and morphological changes in the medial collateral ligament of the rabbit after immobilization and remobilization. J Bone Joint Surg 69A:1200, 1987.

42. Tipton CM: The influence of physical activity on ligaments and tendons. Med Sci Sports Exerc 7:165–171, 1975.

43. Woo SL-Y, Orlando CA, Gomez MA, et al.: Tensile properties of the medial collateral ligament as a function of age. J Orthop Res 4:133–139, 1986.

44. Woo SL-Y, Young EP, Ohland KJ: The effects of transection of the anterior cruciate ligament on healing of the medial collateral ligament. J Bone Joint Surg 72A:382, 1990.

45. Ohland KJ, et al.: The effects of partial and total transection of the anterior cruciate ligament on medial collateral ligament healing in the canine knee. Trans Orthop Res Soc 14:322–325, 1989.

46. Forbes I, et al.: The biomechanical effects of combined ligament injuries on the medial collateral ligament. Trans Orthop Res Soc 13:186–191, 1988.

47. Larson RL: Combined instabilities of the knee. Clin Orthop 147:68–75, 1980.

48. O'Donoghue DH: Reconstruction for medial instability of the knee. Technique and results in sixty cases. J Bone Joint Surg 55A:941–955, 1973.

49. Shelbourne KD, Baele JR: Treatment of combined anterior cruciate ligament and medial collateral ligament injuries. Am J Knee Surg 1:56–58, 1988.

50. Shelbourne KD, Patel DV: Management of combined injuries of the anterior cruciate and medial collateral ligaments. J Bone Joint Surg 77A:800–806, 1995.

51. Frank CB, Schachar N, Dittrich D: Natural history of healing in the repaired medial collateral ligament. J Orthop Res 1:179, 1983.

52. Woo SL-Y, Tkach LV: The cellular and matrix response of ligaments and tendons to mechanical injury. In Leadbetter WB, Buckwalter JA, Gordon SL (eds): Sports Induced Inflammation: Clinical and Basic Science Concepts. Chicago, AAOS, 1989, pp. 189–204.
53. Jack ER: Experimental rupture of the medial collateral ligament of the knee. J Bone Joint Surg 32B:396, 1950.
54. Laws G, Walton M: Fibroblastic healing of grade III ligament injuries. J Bone Joint Surg 70B:390, 1988.
55. Hastings DE: Non-operative treatment of complete tears of the medial collateral ligament of the knee joint. Clin Orthop 147:22, 1980.
56. Eriksson E, Haggmark T: Comparison of isometric muscle training and electrical stimulation supplementing isometric muscle training in the recovery after major knee ligament surgery. Am J Sports Med 7:169, 1979.
57. Delitto A, Rose SJ, McKowca JM: Electrical stimulation vs voluntary exercise in strengthening thigh musculature after anterior cruciate ligament surgery. Phys Ther 68:660, 1988.
58. Lossing I, Grimby G, Jonsson T, et al.: Effects of electrical muscle stimulation combined with voluntary contractions—after knee ligament surgery. Med Sci Sports Exerc 20:93, 1988.
59. Manal TJ, Snyder-Mackler L: Practice guidelines for anterior cruciate ligament rehabilitation: A criteria-based approach. Op Tech Orthop 6:190–196, 1996.
60. Dehne E, Tory R: Treatment of joint injuries by immediate mobilization—based upon the spinal adoption concept. Clin Orthop 77:218, 1971.
61. Haggmark T, Eriksson E: Cylinder of mobile cast brace after knee ligament surgery: A clinical analysis and morphologic and enzymatic studies of changes in the quadriceps muscle. Am J Sports Med 7:48, 1979.
62. Shelbourne KD, Nitz PA: The O'Donoghue triad revisited. Combined knee injuries involving anterior cruciate and medial collateral tears. Am J Sports Med 19:474–477, 1991.
63. Hewson GF, Mendini RA, Wang JB: Prophylactic knee bracing in college football. Am J Sports Med 14:262–266, 1986.
64. Rovere GD, Haupt HA, Yates CS: Prophylactic knee bracing in college football. Am J Sports Med 15:111–116, 1987.
65. Teitz CC, Hermanson BK, Kronmal RA, et al.: Evaluation of the use of braces to prevent injury to the knee in collegiate football players. J Bone Joint Surg 69A:2–9, 1987.
66. Albright JP, Powell JW, Smith W, et al.: Medial collateral ligament knee sprains in college football. Effectiveness of preventive braces. Am J Sports Med 22:12–18, 1994.
67. Sitler M, Ryan J, Hopkinson WJ, et al.: The efficacy of a prophylactic knee brace to reduce knee injuries in football: A prospective randomized study at West Point. Am J Sports Med 18:310–315, 1990.
68. Paulos LE, France EP, Rosenberg TD, et al.: The biomechanics of lateral knee bracing: Part I: Response of the valgus restraints to loading. Am J Sports Med 15:419–429, 1987.
69. Wilk KE, Andrews JR, Clancy WG Jr: Nonoperative and postoperative rehabilitation of the collateral ligaments of the knee. Op Tech Sports Med 4:192–201, 1996.

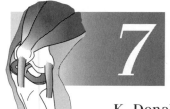

7 Anterior Cruciate Ligament Reconstruction: Evolution of Rehabilitation

K. Donald Shelbourne, MD, and Rocci V. Trumper, MD

*R*ehabilitation following anterior cruciate ligament (ACL) reconstruction has changed dramatically over the past decade. Conventional postoperative management emphasizes early protection of the ACL graft by restricting knee motion, weight-bearing, and the rate of return to functional activities.[1–4] The high rate of postoperative complications, most notably permanent knee stiffness, has brought about a number of changes in most postoperative rehabilitation protocols.[5–11]

This chapter examines the evolution of the perioperative rehabilitation that has occurred in our clinic over a 15-year period. We are limiting our presentation to the rehabilitation of patients with ACL-deficient knees reconstructed with an autogenous patellar tendon graft. Specifically, we focus on the decreased incidence of surgical morbidity and the increased patient success in returning safely to functional activities. By maintaining an extensive prospective database and retrospectively analyzing the results, our program has evolved in response to what we have learned from our patients. We emphasize, in our program and in this paper, the influence of the surgical technique and perioperative rehabilitation activities designed to optimize long-term knee stability.

SURGICAL PROCEDURE

All patients are examined under general anesthesia to confirm the preoperative diagnosis. Since 1984, we have performed arthroscopic examination of the joint routinely to evaluate for associated injuries. ACL reconstruction is performed by using a modified Clancy technique, as described elsewhere.[12] A 6-cm medial mini-arthrotomy is utilized for precise notch preparation and tunnel placement. Both the tibial and femo-

ral tunnels are drilled with cannulated reamers over guide pins placed in a free-hand manner. A 10-mm autogenous patellar tendon graft is harvested in all patients with 25-mm bone plugs from both the patellar and tibial ends. Graft fixation is secured with three ligatures of No. 2 Ethibond tied over a 19-mm polyethylene button on both the tibial and femoral tunnels. Before closure, the knee is placed through a full range of motion, including full hyperextension and full flexion equal to that of the contralateral knee. Additional notchplasty or retensioning of the graft is performed as indicated.

Changes in the surgical procedure have been few during the period of this report. However, three specific modifications are noteworthy: (1) discontinuation of the extra-articular procedure for chronic reconstructions, (2) inclusion of notchplasty as part of the routine procedure, and (3) increased emphasis on precise graft position, that is, tunnel placement.

Before 1985, chronic reconstructions were augmented with an extra-articular procedure.[13] At that time, this procedure was believed to be necessary owing to associated laxity of the secondary restraints with chronic ACL-deficient knees. We observed that, by avoiding early extension activities to protect the extra-articular procedure, a number of patients subsequently developed a permanent knee flexion contracture and anterior knee symptoms. As we became more aware of the importance of regaining extension postoperatively, we reasoned that early emphasis on extension would doom the extra-articular procedure anyway, so we began to eliminate this portion of the procedure in some patients. These patients revealed no change in KT-1000 arthrometer stability testing, so we discontinued the extra-articular procedure altogether in 1986.

Before 1988, a notchplasty was performed only to increase visualization of the intercondylar area. However, we noticed that the lateral aspect of the graft was frequently frayed when we had the opportunity to view the graft during a subsequent arthroscopy. To address this problem of lateral graft impingement, we began performing a notchplasty on most patients. To ensure adequate space for the 10-mm graft, the notchplasty was routinely performed to provide at least 11 mm from the lateral border of the posterior cruciate ligament (PCL) to the medial wall of the lateral femoral condyle.

During the mid-1980s, the third modification, our emphasis on precise tunnel placement, escalated. As we became more aware of the importance of precise graft position, we more closely evaluated our postoperative KT-1000 arthrometer measurements and how they were influenced by gradual changes in tunnel placement. As a result, our ability to reproduce the ideal femoral tunnel position improved and we gradually moved our tibial tunnel to a more posterior position.

We have elected to continue performing the surgical technique, as described, for a number of reasons. By utilizing a less rigid means of graft fixation and placing the knee through a full range of motion before closure, we allow the knee to tension the graft itself. This is the first step in preventing motion problems or graft "stretch" when motion is regained. Isometricity and adequate graft tensioning are ensured by measuring the amount the button relaxes on the tibial cortex after placing the knee through a full range of motion. This is quantified by pulling the sutures attached to the tibial bone plug distally and measuring the laxity of the button at 0, 30, and 90 degrees of flexion. Button fixation has proved to be a very reliable means of securing the graft position while allowing for a tight bone-to-bone fit in the graft tunnels. Our femoral tunnel is typically 50 to 80 mm long, depending on the length of the patellar tendon, and the tibial tunnel is usually 30 to 40 mm in length. This provides an overall tunnel length of 110 to 140 mm, which is adequate for all patellar tendon lengths (range, 34 to 67 mm in our experience). The extra length of the graft is easily taken up by the excess femoral tunnel without concern for graft tunnel mismatch. Also, straight line placement of the patellar tendon graft has also been a positive aspect of this surgical technique.

A complete description of our surgical technique for ACL reconstruction was published previously.[14]

PATIENT EVALUATION AND DATA COLLECTION

As we became increasingly aware of the value of patient follow-up for improving the quality of our medical care, we upgraded our data collection system. Following initiation of our accelerated rehabilitation protocol, data were prospectively gathered on patients with emphasis on close postoperative follow-up. Patients are routinely seen at 7 days, 2 weeks, 4 to 5 weeks, 3 and 6 months, and 1, 2, and 5 years after the surgical procedure. KT-1000 arthrometer stability examination and isokinetic strength testing is performed at all visits with the exception of the first two. Although data collected during the first 3 to 4 years of this report were recorded in a similar manner, patient follow-up was less emphasized and less frequent. Since 1984, our clinic has employed a full-time research staff responsible for research data collection. This has improved our ability to analyze our results, make clinical changes, and evaluate the subsequent clinical outcome.

EVOLUTION OF PERIOPERATIVE MANAGEMENT

Although patients generally have been pleased with the ultimate stability, we have been concerned about the morbidity associated with using the patellar tendon as the graft source for the ACL reconstruction. With this in mind, we have focused much of our attention on identifying ways to minimize surgical morbidity. As a result, several key variables that directly influence the incidence and severity of these postoperative complications have been identified. Some of these observations have seemed contrary to conventional rehabilitation dictums based on earlier reconstruction procedures and basic science studies.[1–3, 6, 7, 15–18] Therefore, many of the changes implemented have been introduced cautiously and gradually with a vigilant eye on how they ultimately affect knee stability.

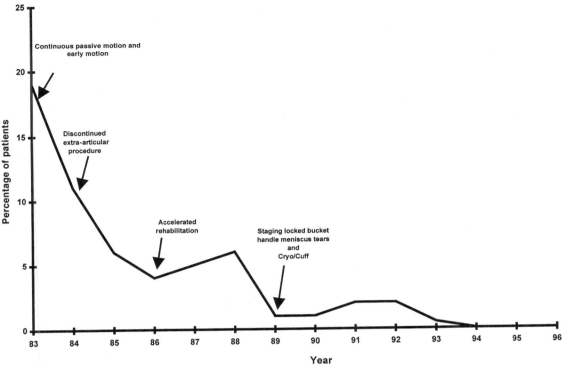

Figure 7–1. After chronic anterior cruciate ligament reconstruction, the number of patients who required a scar resection for extension loss has continued to decrease.

Initial Observations

In 1982, the surgical leg was placed in a cast at 30 degrees of flexion after ACL reconstruction to avoid excessive graft stress. Weight-bearing without a brace was not allowed for 6 to 8 weeks following surgery and most patients were restricted from full participation in sporting activities for the first year. Although knee stability was restored with the use of this protocol, we were concerned by the large number of motion problems that followed, most notably the loss of knee extension. In an effort to minimize the problems of regaining extension, we modified the postoperative protocol by eliminating casting, by emphasizing earlier restoration of extension, and by using continuous passive motion (CPM). Patients were given a 30-degree flexed splint to be worn when they were not performing motion exercises or using the CPM. Although these changes were successful in decreasing motion problems, most patients seemed to lose ground whenever they put the knee back in the splint. Therefore, the splinting was progressively changed over the next 2 years

from a 30-degree splint to a 0-degree splint. By 1985, our patients were using only the full-extension splint.

Although in retrospect our changes may seem minor, collectively our earlier emphasis on restoring knee motion noticeably decreased the incidence of motion problems in chronic reconstructions (Fig. 7–1). However, patients with acute reconstructions continued to struggle with regaining motion and were requiring surgical intervention for scar resection or manipulation significantly more often than patients with chronic reconstructions (Fig. 7–2). Stability results remained good for both groups, despite these modifications, and KT-1000 arthrometer results remained superior for patients with acute reconstructions. Therefore, despite the higher rate of motion problems, we still believed it was best to perform the reconstruction as early as possible following the injury.

During this time period, we also became more cognizant of our patients' unhappiness with the extensive time period recommended before their return to normal daily activities. Many patients missed several months of work and were frustrated by the

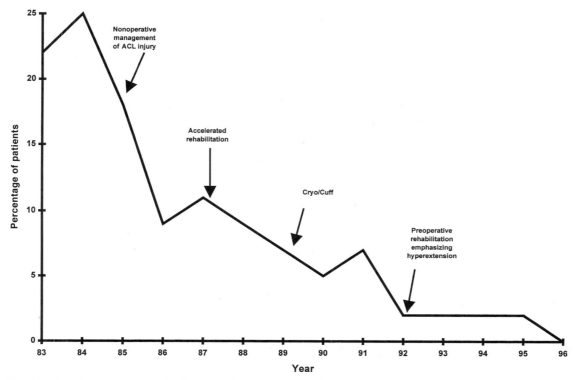

Figure 7–2. With improvements in the rehabilitation program, the incidence of patients requiring a scar resection after acute anterior cruciate ligament (ACL) reconstruction reduced.

lengthy rehabilitation required before returning to sports. It was not uncommon for patients to require 6 months or more to regain knee motion and even though we were allowing them to return to sports at 9 months after surgery, most competitive school athletes were unable to successfully compete during the season following their ACL reconstruction. For some, these considerations were sufficient to dismiss reconstruction as a treatment option. For fear that faster rehabilitation would result in graft failure, we complied with the best of published practices and continued to restrict weight-bearing and the time before returning to full participation in sporting activities.[2, 4, 13]

Increasing Awareness of Noncompliant Patients

By 1985, patients were no longer wearing rigid protection for the knee. Many patients admitted to being noncompliant with following the restrictions and we were concerned

that these patients might be progressing too rapidly in their return to activities and could be losing long-term graft stability. To examine this, we conducted a study in 1985 comparing compliant patients with those who progressed more rapidly than we recommended (noncompliant patients). To our surprise, the noncompliant patients demonstrated fewer long-term knee motion problems and fewer subjective complaints than their compliant counterparts, without a difference in long-term stability.[10, 19–21]

As a result of these findings, we became even more diligent in monitoring compliance, postoperative activities, and results by actively pursuing close follow-up of all patients. Through this process, we quickly learned that our patients had a lot to teach us concerning the rehabilitation process. Specifically, we learned that (1) an early loss of extension often led to long-term loss of extension accompanied by subjective symptoms, (2) patients who failed to regain early leg control often struggled with regaining full quadriceps muscle strength later on, and (3) patients who returned to sporting activities before recommended had similar knee stability to patients who were compliant with our restrictions.

A large number of noncompliant patients returned to sport-specific activities during the time period when we felt the graft would be the weakest.[16, 22] Initially, it appeared that some patients who regained full knee motion and returned to sporting activities early had increasing KT-1000 arthrometer values. However, on closer examination, we found that KT-1000 results did not change with time after full motion was restored.[14] The KT-1000 arthrometer stability changes observed in some patients were not a result of increased activities, but secondary to regaining full motion and eliminating postoperative stiffness. This was consistent with our observation that patients with a flexion contracture were stable, but often subjectively dissatisfied. Long-term KT-1000 arthrometer results following restoration of full knee motion were not declining, but actually improving despite increased early activities (Table 7–1). These findings not only pointed out the possible association between our postoperative restrictions and surgical morbidity, but also led us to question the in vivo strength of an autogenous patellar tendon graft. It appeared that the strength of the graft was greater than once thought and that conventional rehabilitation restrictions designed to protect the graft might be more restrictive than necessary.

During this time period (1985–1987), we also became more aware of the differences between acute and chronic reconstructions. Our observations supported the presumption that patients with acute reconstructions were more likely to have a stable knee following surgery than patients with chronic reconstructions, and were more likely to return to competitive sports successfully. We also noted, however, that patients with chronic reconstructions were less likely to develop motion problems postoperatively. We reasoned that the optimal situation would be to combine the benefits of acute reconstruction, stability, with the benefits of chronic reconstruction, less morbidity, for a better clinical result. When we began looking at how we could do this, the group of patients that stood out had combined ACL/medial collateral ligament (MCL) injuries treated with early repair of the MCL and reconstruction of the ACL. Motion problems in these patients were particularly dramatic and difficult to deal with. Inspired by Indelicato's report demonstrating that isolated MCL injuries could be effectively treated nonoperatively, we began reconstructing the ACL while allowing the MCL to heal without surgical repair.[23, 24] We hoped this might lead to decreased motion problems postoperatively. This new approach to combined ACL/MCL injuries was a key factor in decreasing the incidence of scar resection and manipulation in acute reconstructions from 25 percent in both categories to 9 percent and 6 percent, respectively, from 1984 to 1986. Stability results continued to be good for both the ACL and MCL injuries.

Accelerated Rehabilitation

As we became more critical in examining our rehabilitation protocol, we noted that most of our recommendations were negatively based. We were telling patients that they could not bear weight, could not go without crutches, could not take the splint off, and so on. It seemed to us that patients were adversely affected by these negative-type instructions for rehabilitation and that they would benefit from a protocol that was based on a more positive approach. With this in mind, we modified our rehabilitation protocol to reflect what we learned from our

Table 7–1. KT-1000 Manual Maximum Difference Between the Reconstructed and Normal Knee After Anterior Cruciate Ligament Reconstruction

Years	Acute		Chronic	
	Cases, N	*Mean Difference ± SD, mm*	*Cases, N*	*Mean Difference ± SD, mm*
1982–86	87	2.0 ± 2.1	149	2.6 ± 2.4
1987–89	160	2.2 ± 1.5	267	2.6 ± 1.9
1990–92	180	1.9 ± 1.5	265	1.9 ± 1.4
1993–95	235	1.9 ± 1.2	288	2.0 ± 1.2
1996–97	165	2.1 ± 1.2	164	2.2 ± 1.1

postoperative patients. We placed emphasis on factors felt to be of primary importance. These included (1) restoration of full hyperextension equal to the contralateral knee, (2) regaining of good quadriceps muscle leg control, and (3) allowing for early wound healing. Our goal was to force patients to do things that other patients had found beneficial (but patients were unlikely to do on their own) while allowing them to progress as tolerated in areas where compliance did not seem to influence results. However, we were still unsure of the limits of graft strength and were worried that returning to activity too early might result in graft failure. Therefore, we were careful not to push patients toward an early return to sport-specific activities, but allowed them to return on their own terms (as they were tending to do anyway) while we closely observed and learned from their experience.

During the first few months of the accelerated rehabilitation protocol in 1987 we quickly discovered the importance of limiting knee swelling. Initially, we allowed patients to get up and around as early as the first postoperative day. Unfortunately, this frequently resulted in significant swelling that retarded the rate of postoperative recovery. This increased swelling may be partly responsible for the small increase in scar resections and manipulations recorded during the initial year of this protocol. In response to this problem, we initiated several changes to limit postoperative swelling. In addition to the CPM, which serves to elevate the knee, we began limiting out-of-bed activities for the first 10 to 14 days following surgery. Combined with the addition of cold compression (Cryocuff, Aircast, Inc., Summit, NJ), introduced in 1989, these changes successfully reduced short- and long-term swelling, which helped decrease pain, improve wound healing, and increase the ease with which patients were able to reach postoperative goals.

Regaining early leg control following the surgical procedure also distinguished itself as an important variable in the postoperative rehabilitation. Early restoration of quadriceps leg control through straight leg raises and short arc quadricep contractions improved the rate of strength return and appeared to help prevent postoperative contractures. Past experience taught us that patients who were allowed to develop a tight patella struggled with regaining motion,

which in turn delayed strength recovery and return to sport-specific activities. By placing a high priority on early leg control, we observed a dramatic decline in the number of patients who were unable to regain quadriceps muscle strength.

Although we suspected that regaining hyperextension equal to the opposite knee might be important for preventing postoperative morbidity, not until the early 1990s did we fully appreciate the importance of this variable. One of the first indications of the vital nature of hyperextension was evident in patients who were treated for a symptomatic extension block with arthroscopic scar resection and restoration of knee hyperextension.[25] Although these patients continued to have more anterior knee symptoms than patients who had avoided motion problems, regaining hyperextension decreased the severity of their complaints. This group of patients not only re-enforced the importance of preventing problems in lieu of treating them after they occur, but also propelled us to look at hyperextension more closely.

Two studies were initiated to evaluate the effect of regaining full knee hyperextension on ultimate knee stability. Klootwyk reported KT-1000 arthrometer manual maximum results immediately following restoration of full knee motion (within 3 months) and again at more than 2 years postoperatively in the same group of patients. No differences were noted in values, with averages of 2.06 and 2.10, respectively,[14] which indicated that knee stability was not deteriorating with time despite early restoration of knee hyperextension and early return to sporting activities. Rubinstein examined a group of patients with extreme hyperextension (more than 8 degrees) and compared them with a group with less than 5 degrees of full hyperextension.[26] These two groups were chosen to evaluate the role of hyperextension on postoperative knee stability. KT-1000 arthrometer stability results following restoration of full hyperextension were similar for both groups. Collectively, these two studies confirmed our impression that regaining full hyperextension equal to the contralateral knee is not a threat to ultimate knee stability if the patellar tendon graft is precisely placed and tensioned.

To determine the incidence and severity of anterior knee symptoms in patients who regained full knee hyperextension postoperatively, we evaluated a group of 592 patients at 1 year or more after ACL reconstruction who followed our protocol emphasizing early restoration of full hyperextension.[27] We evaluated symptoms during different activities, including strenuous work or sports, and assigned a total patellofemoral score for each patient. The severity of symptoms and total patellofemoral scores in our postoperative patients were similar to those of a control group. This study, in conjunction with the observed association of anterior knee symptoms in patients who failed to regain even a few degrees of terminal extension, led us to conclude that restoration of full hyperextension is the key to minimizing postoperative anterior knee symptoms. Accordingly, we have continued to place a high emphasis on this goal in our rehabilitation protocol.

As we became more and more aware of the importance of regaining full knee hyperextension, we began noticing several factors that made regaining full knee motion more difficult. Initially, we were impressed by the incidence of motion problems in patients with acute reconstructions as compared with patients who delayed their surgery for reasons of convenience. Closer evaluation revealed that patients who delayed surgery for 3 weeks or more had fewer problems regaining motion in both the short and long term.[33] In response to this (in 1990), we began performing ACL reconstructions in acute knee injuries on a semi-acute basis. Although this generally improved the ease with which patients were obtaining motion following reconstruction, it was not until we realized that the important variable was restoration of full hyperextension prior to surgery and not the time from injury. Subsequently, we saw an optimal decrease in the incidence of patients requiring arthroscopic scar resection postoperatively for symptomatic anterior knee pain with extension loss. Secondarily, we observed an additional benefit of delaying surgery. Patients who underwent ACL reconstruction after regaining full hyperextension preoperatively were able to schedule their surgery around work or school and had sufficient time to recover from the period of depression, denial, and anger that often followed injury.[28] Overall, by accepting their injury preoperatively, patients have been in a frame of mind more conducive to a smooth postoperative course.

Increased emphasis on meniscal repair led us to find a subgroup of chronic ACL reconstruction patients who had an increased risk of developing range of motion problems. Patients who presented with locked bucket-handle meniscal tears and chronic ACL-deficient knees were demonstrating inordinate difficulty in regaining motion after simultaneous management of both injuries.[29] Based on our desire to save more menisci, and not knowing which ones could be repaired successfully, we reasoned that if we could repair the meniscus first and not add a major reconstruction on an acutely injured knee, we could possibly obtain two benefits: (1) save more menisci by repairing tears we would not ordinarily repair and could remove at the time of reconstruction if the repair failed to heal, and (2) perform the ACL reconstruction on a more "quiescent" knee less likely to develop motion problems postoperatively. In changing our care from simultaneous management of both injuries to a two-staged approach, we observed a decrease in long-term problems in regaining knee motion (see Fig. 7–1). Additionally, this two-staged approach has allowed us to salvage 88 percent of the locked meniscal tears, compared to 44 percent prior to the change.

As evidenced by the changes we have made in our perioperative rehabilitation protocol since 1987, our clinical experience has convinced us that restoration of full hyperextension is paramount. Our current rehabilitation protocol is a reflection of our increasing emphasis on this variable. By optimizing preoperative factors and controlling postoperative variables that directly influence the patient's ability to regain full hyperextension, we have achieved a decrease in postoperative morbidity without a decline in long-term knee stability.

Return to Sports

Although the changes in our rehabilitation protocol have been aimed at reducing postoperative morbidity, secondarily, we have observed that patients may return to sporting activities much earlier than previously thought. Initially, we were concerned to learn that some patients were returning to sport-specific activities at the time when we expected an autogenous patellar tendon graft to be its weakest.[16, 22] However, we were unable to demonstrate a loss of long-term knee stability in these patients.[10, 19–21] They actually seemed to do better than patients who followed our recommendations. As a result, we gradually relaxed the restrictions regarding return to sport-specific activities to allow patients to dictate their own return as they progress in their rehabilitation and become more comfortable and confident on their reconstructed knee. Most patients were encouraged to use a brace during sporting activities until their strength returned to 80 percent and for the first competitive season postoperatively. Neither the type of brace used nor the patients' compliance in wearing the brace correlated with the ultimate outcome.

When patients returned to sport-specific activities before regaining 65 percent of their preinjury strength, they often had problems with knee swelling and soreness. These patients often favored the reconstructed knee, and a continued increase in activities was not followed by improved strength. Patients returning with greater than 65 percent strength did so with few problems, and their strength increased as they increased their activity level. We observed that a return to competitive sports was well tolerated when patients regained 75 percent or more of quadriceps muscle strength, whereas patients returning earlier without 75 percent strength did not appear to progress as quickly. In general, these strength levels closely corresponded to the time when patients on their own began feeling ready for a return to sporting activities. The average patient returned to sport-specific activities at 10 weeks and full competitive sports 6 months following their surgical procedure. Patients who were highly motivated to return to competitive sports were often able to return at 6 weeks to sport-specific activities, and at 10 to 12 weeks to competitive sports. These patients reported a need for 3 to 4 months of competitive sporting activities before they felt fully comfortable in game situations. For example, a college basketball player who had his knee reconstructed in May needed to be playing full-court basketball by early August if he expected to compete well in games in early November. Athletes who returned to the court for the first time at the beginning of the practice season were seldom capable of competing successfully during that first year.

Many of our observations and results seem contrary to research findings in animal and cadaver models.[15, 16, 22, 30] As a result, we have become skeptical about the ability to transfer this basic science research to the human knee. This skepticism was fueled when we reviewed a series of graft biopsies on patients undergoing arthroscopic procedures for other reasons.[31] Although based on a limited number of patients, our review revealed that the autogenous patellar tendon graft is viable at 3 weeks following reconstruction. Kleiner et al.[18] also noted that at 3 weeks after implantation, the fibroblast that repopulated the graft had a high synthetic capacity. The presence of living fibroblast at this stage, and our clinical experience, indicates that this autogenous tissue is functioning more like a biologic graft than a necrotic scaffolding as early as 3 weeks following surgery. These findings are supported by Hannafin et al.,[32] who reported that graft stress appears to be a positive influence and perhaps necessary component for optimal graft healing and collagen formation. In summary, we have been unable to identify any activities that resulted in graft failure during any time period following our reconstructive procedure. Stability results appear to be solely a function of the technique used to stabilize the knee. It seems that rehabilitation restrictions are only necessary to guide the patient through a smooth postoperative course by obtaining range of motion early while limiting knee swelling and soreness.

Knee Stability

Restoration of knee stability using an autogenous patellar tendon graft and our rehabilitation protocol has been very predictable. Despite emphasis on restoration of full hyperextension and allowing patients to return to sporting activities without time restrictions, our stability results have actually improved.

Analysis of KT-1000 arthrometer values reveal improved stability for both acute and chronic reconstructions. As shown in Table 7–1, the mean manual maximum side-to-side difference for chronic reconstructions and standard deviation for both groups has improved steadily since 1982. Improvement is also reflected in the increased number of patients who demonstrate a manual maxi-

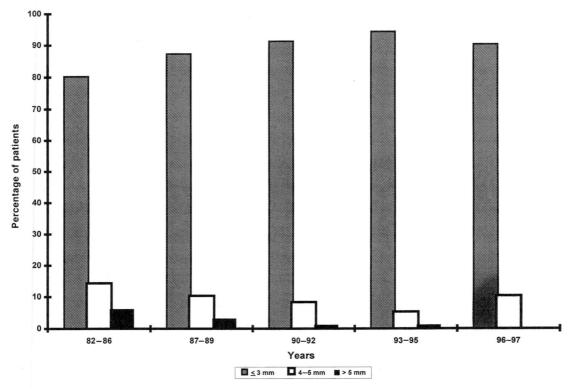

Figure 7–3. Acute anterior cruciate ligament reconstructions. The percentage of patients with a KT-1000 manual maximum difference greater than 5 mm has consistently decreased.

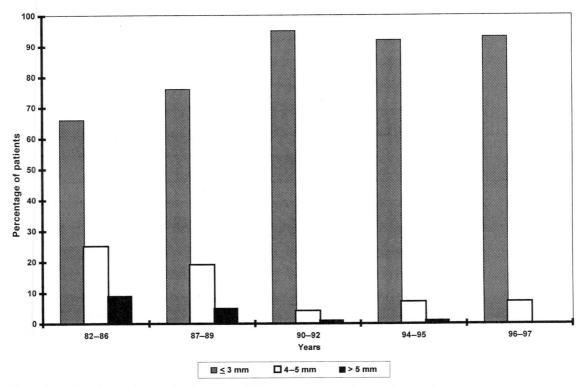

Figure 7–4. Chronic anterior cruciate ligament (ACL) reconstructions. Since 1990, the distribution of KT-1000 manual maximum scores has matched the results of patients with acute ACL reconstructions.

● Table 7–2. **Subjective Questionnaire Results After Anterior Cruciate Ligament Reconstruction**

Years	Acute		Chronic	
	Patients, N	*Mean Difference ± SD*	*Patients, N*	*Mean Difference ± SD*
1982–86	119	91 ± 10.0	180	86 ± 16.9
1987–89	171	93 ± 12.6	258	91 ± 11.9
1990–92	173	94 ± 9.3	225	93 ± 7.7
1993–95	128	92 ± 8.5	141	93 ± 9.9
1996–97	60	93 ± 7.2	70	91 ± 8.9

mum side-to-side difference of 3 mm or less (Figs. 7–3 and 7–4). Similar values for acute and chronic groups indicate that precise graft placement can restore near-normal stability regardless of the amount of preoperative laxity or the rehabilitation protocol utilized.

To supplement the arthrometry measurements, modified Noyes questionaires[20] were used to evaluate subjective satisfaction (Table 7–2). The number of patients reporting less than a perfect score of 20 for stability declined steadily through the period of this report from 9 to 10 percent in the 1980s to 4 to 5 percent in the 1990s.

CURRENT ACCELERATED REHABILITATION PROTOCOL

Our current accelerated rehabilitation protocol is a reflection of the observations we made following our patients postoperatively. From these observations, we believe that a precisely placed and tensioned autogenous patellar tendon graft has sufficient strength to allow for unrestricted rehabilitation activities without fear of graft failure. In fact, it appears the graft is viable and capable of responding to stress in a positive manner very early after the reconstructive procedure. This concept of early graft viability and positive response to graft stress is the central focus for our rehabilitation protocol. Emphasis is placed on factors that we believe are critical to avoiding postoperative morbidity. A complete description of our rehabilitation program can be found in Chapter 8 of this book.

SUMMARY

Our perioperative management of the ACL-deficient knee has changed significantly over the past several years. Most of our changes have been in response to what we have learned from observing our postoperative patients. Some of our observations have seemed contrary to conventional rehabilitation principles and have therefore been implemented cautiously as we monitor the influence of these changes on long-term results. In many respects, our rehabilitation protocol has completely changed focus. Whereas our initial concern was for graft strength and avoiding graft stress, our protocol is now designed to rehabilitate the graft donor site and knee itself without fear of injuring the newly reconstructed patellar tendon graft.

Management of postoperative rehabilitation will continue to evolve as we learn more from our postoperative patients. Our ultimate goal remains offering each patient one procedure, performed at the right time, resulting in normal subjective stability, without surgical complications.

References

1. Arms SW, Pope MH, Johnson RJ, et al.: The biomechanics of anterior cruciate ligament rehabilitation and reconstruction. Am J Sports Med 12:8–18, 1984.
2. Bilko TE, Paulos LE, Feagin JA, et al.: Current trends in repair and rehabilitation of complete (acute) anterior cruciate ligament injuries. Am J Sports Med 14:143–147, 1986.
3. Grood ES, Suntay WJ, Noyes FR, Butler DL: Biomechanics of the knee extension exercises: Effect of cutting the anterior cruciate ligament. J Bone Joint Surg 66-A:725–734, 1984.
4. Paulos L, Noyes FR, Grood E, Butler DL: Knee rehabilitation after anterior cruciate ligament reconstruction and repair. Am J Sports Med 9:140–149, 1981.
5. Fullerton LR, Andrews JR: Mechanical block to extension following augmentation of the anterior cruciate ligament: A case report. Am J Sports Med 12:166–168, 1984.
6. Harner CD, Irrgang JJ, Paul J, et al.: Loss of motion after anterior cruciate ligament reconstruction. Am J Sports Med 20:499–506, 1992.

7. Mohtadi NGH, Webster-Bogaert S, Fowler PJ: Limitation of motion following anterior cruciate ligament reconstruction: A case control study. Am J Sports Med 19:620–625, 1991.

8. Paulos LE, Rosenberg TD, Drawbert J, et al.: Intrapatellar contracture syndrome: An unrecognized cause of knee stiffness with patella entrapment and patella infera. Am J Sports Med 15:331–341, 1987.

9. Sachs RA, Daniel DM, Stone ML, Garfein RF: Patellofemoral problems after anterior cruciate ligament reconstruction. Am J Sports Med 17:760–765, 1989.

10. Shelbourne KD, Klootwyk TE, DeCarlo MS: Update on accelerated rehabilitation after anterior cruciate ligament reconstruction. J Orthop Sport Phys Ther 15:303–308, 1992.

11. Strum GM, Friedman MJ, Fox JM, et al.: Acute anterior cruciate ligament reconstruction: Analysis of complications. Clin Orthop 253:184–189, 1990.

12. Shelbourne KD, Klootwyk TE: The miniarthrotomy technique for anterior cruciate ligament reconstruction. Op Tech Sports Med 1:26–39, 1993.

13. Clancy WG, Nelson DA, Reider B, Narechania RG: Anterior cruciate ligament reconstruction using one-third of the patellar ligament, augmented by extra-articular tendon transfers. J Bone Joint Surg 64-A:352–359, 1982.

14. Shelbourne KD, Klootwyk TE, Wilckens JH, DeCarlo MS: Ligament stability 2 to 6 years after ACL reconstruction with autogenous patellar tendon graft and participation in accelerated rehabilitation program. Am J Sports Med 23:575–579, 1995.

15. Akeson WH: The response of ligaments to stress modulation and overview of the ligament healing response. In Daniel DM, Akeson WH, O'Connor JJ (eds): Knee Ligaments: Structure, Function, Injury and Repair. New York, NY, Raven Press, 1990, pp. 315–327.

16. Arnoczky SP, Tarvin GB, Marshall JL: Anterior cruciate ligament replacement using patellar tendon. An evaluation of graft revascularization in the dog. J Bone Joint Surg 64-A:217–224, 1982.

17. Fulkerson JP, Berke A, Parthasarathy N: Collagen biosynthesis in rabbit intraarticular patellar tendon transplants. Am J Sports Med 18:249–253, 1990.

18. Kleiner JB, Amiel D, Harwood FL, Akeson WH: Early histologic, metabolic, and vascular assessment of anterior cruciate ligament autografts. J Orthop Res 7:235–242, 1989.

19. Shelbourne KD, Klootwyk TE, DeCarlo MS: Clinical development of preoperative and postoperative ACL rehabilitation. In Feagin JA Jr (ed): The Crucial Ligaments, 2nd ed. New York, Churchhill Livingstone, 1994, pp. 737–750.

20. Shelbourne KD, Nitz P: Accelerated rehabilitation after anterior cruciate ligament reconstruction. Am J Sports Med 18:292–299, 1990.

21. Shelbourne KD, Wilckens JH: Current concepts in anterior cruciate ligament rehabilitation. Orthopedic Review 19:957–964, 1990.

22. Clancy WG, Narechania RG, Rosenberg TD, et al.: Anterior and posterior cruciate ligament reconstruction in rhesus monkeys: A histological, microangiographic, and biomechanical analysis. J Bone Joint Surg 63-A:1270–1284, 1981.

23. Indelicato PA: Non-operative treatment of complete tears of the medial collateral ligament of the knee. J Bone Joint Surg 65-A:323–329, 1983.

24. Shelbourne KD, Porter DA: Anterior cruciate ligament–medial collateral ligament injury: The results from non-operative management of medial collateral ligament tears with anterior cruciate ligament reconstruction. A preliminary report. Am J Sports Med 20:283–286, 1992.

25. Fisher SE, Shelbourne KD: Arthroscopic treatment of symptomatic extension block complicating anterior cruciate ligament reconstruction. Am J Sports Med 21:558–564, 1993.

26. Rubinstein RA, Shelbourne KD, Vanmeter CD, et al.: Effect on knee stability if full hyperextension is restored immediately after autogenous bone–patellar tendon–bone anterior cruciate ligament reconstruction. Am J Sports Med 23:365–368, 1995.

27. Shelbourne KD, Trumper RV: Preventing anterior knee pain after anterior cruciate ligament reconstruction. Am J Sports Med 25:41–47, 1997.

28. Smith A, Scott SG, O'Fallon WM, Young ML: Emotional responses of athletes to injury. Mayo Clinic Proc 65:35–50, 1990.

29. Shelbourne KD, Johnson GE: Locked bucket-handle meniscal tears in knees with chronic anterior cruciate ligament deficiency. Am J Sports Med 21:779–782, 1993.

30. Amiel D, Ing D, Kleiner JB, Akeson WH: The natural history of the anterior cruciate ligament autograft of patellar tendon origin. Am J Sports Med 14:449–462, 1986.

31. Rougraff B, Shelbourne KD, Gerth PK, Warner J: Arthroscopic and histologic analysis of human patella tendon autografts used for anterior cruciate ligament reconstruction. Am J Sports Med 21:277–284, 1993.

32. Hannafin JA, Arnoczky SP: Effect of stress deprivation and cyclic tensile loading on the material and morphologic properties of canine flexor digitorum profundus tendon: An in vitro study. J Orthop Res 13:907–914, 1995.

33. Shelbourne KD, Wilckens JH, Mollabashy A, DeCarlo M: Arthrofibrosis in acute anterior cruciate ligament reconstruction: The effect of timing of reconstruction and rehabilitation. Am J Sports Med 19:332–336, 1991.

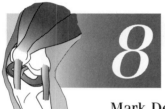

8 Anterior Cruciate Ligament

Mark DeCarlo, MHA, PT, SCS, ATC, Thomas Klootwyk, MD, and Kathy Oneacre, MA, ATC

PRIMARY GOALS OF ANTERIOR CRUCIATE LIGAMENT SURGERY AND REHABILITATION

Rehabilitation following anterior cruciate ligament (ACL) reconstruction is notably different than it was even in the early 1990s. The evolution of our current surgical technique and rehabilitation program is described elsewhere. This chapter, however, focuses on how we carry out our current ACL rehabilitation program.

The rehabilitation program is divided into four phases: phase I, preoperative; phase II, immediate postoperative; phase III, 2 to 4 weeks postoperative; and phase IV, advanced rehabilitation and return to athletics (Table 8–1). Although a timeline is given for progression in the rehabilitation program, movement from one phase to another is actually based on the patient's meeting goals outlined in each phase. With a properly placed autogenous patellar tendon graft, we believe there is sufficient strength to allow for advanced rehabilitation activities without fear of graft failure, even very early after the reconstructive procedure.[1–3] The central focus of our rehabilitation program is the concept of early graft viability and the positive response of the graft to appropriate levels of stress.

The primary goals of ACL reconstruction and rehabilitation include restoration of knee stability, preservation of menisci and articular surfaces, safe and expedient return to normal activities including athletics, and early recognition of potential complications. The knee should be in a quiescent state before the reconstruction is performed. Specific preoperative goals include decreasing swelling and restoring full range of motion (ROM), including hyperextension. Normal gait and adequate strength are also prerequisites for ACL reconstruction. Specific postoperative goals include controlling pain and swelling, restoring full ROM and strength, and going through a functional progression to make a safe and expedient return to athletics while maintaining stability of the knee.

To achieve these goals, a team effort is employed between the athlete, physician, physical therapist, athletic trainer, and coach. After surgery, the athlete returns for limited yet educational and purposeful visits to both the physician and the physical therapy staff. These visits typically occur at 1 and 2 weeks; 1, 2, and 4 months; and again at 1 year after surgery. It has been found that patients who are seen an average of only seven times for structured physical therapy visits following ACL reconstruction have similar results in terms of ROM, strength, and ligament stability to those who are seen more frequently.[4] Rather than having patients come into the clinic on a weekly basis to perform their exercises, it is our philosophy to give the patient an individualized home exercise program based on the equipment and facilities available to them. Formal physical therapy visits are used to monitor the progress of rehabilitation and to update the rehabilitation program as clinical goals are met. If complications occur during the rehabilitation process, the patient can be seen on a more frequent basis to assess and correct the problem. Throughout the postoperative period, communication is maintained between the members of the medical team and the athlete.

We have demonstrated more favorable clinical outcomes with our current rehabilitation approach than with earlier rehabilitation protocols, noting a decrease in complications while maintaining ligamentous stability.[3, 5] One component of our approach to ACL rehabilitation that is significant in achieving excellent results is a strict dedication to clinical research. In addition to their

117

●━ Table 8–1. Anterior Cruciate Ligament (ACL) Reconstruction Rehabilitation Program

Phase I: Preoperative
Clinical Goals
- Control swelling prior to ACL reconstruction
- Restore full ROM, normal gait, and normal strength prior to ACL reconstruction
- Ensure complete understanding of the basic principles of accelerated rehabilitation including
  Full terminal knee extension
  Early weight bearing
  Closed and open chain strengthening
Testing
- Bilateral ROM including full terminal knee extension
- KT-1000 ligament stability test
- Isokinetic evaluation at 180 degrees/sec
- Isometric leg press test
- Single leg hop on non-involved leg
Exercises
- Prone hangs and hyperextension device for extension
- Heel slides for flexion
- Closed kinetic chain strengthening
  Leg press
  One-quarter squats
  Step-downs
  Bicycle
  StairMaster

Phase II: 1 to 6 Days
Discharge Goals
- Full passive terminal knee extension and 110 degrees of flexion
- Independent straight leg raise
- Weight-bearing as tolerated
Testing
- Bilateral ROM
Exercises
- Continuous passive motion machine set from 10 degrees hyperextension to 30 degrees flexion
- Cryo/Cuff (AirCast, Inc., Summit, NJ)
- Extension
  Pillow extensions
- Flexion
  Rest knee in CPM machine, set at 110 degrees, and hold for 10 minutes, 4×/day
  Continue to increase bend beyond 110 degrees by pulling leg further to buttocks with hands
- Leg control
  Active quadriceps contraction with quadriceps sets
  Straight leg raises
  Active heel height
- Full weight-bearing as tolerated when going to the bathroom
Clinical Follow-up
- Patient will report to physical therapy one week after surgery and should have:
  Full terminal extension and flexion to 110 degrees
  Minimal swelling and soft tissue healing
  Normal gait

Phase II: 7 to 14 Days
Clinical Goals
- Full terminal extension and flexion to 110 degrees
- Minimal swelling
- Soft tissue healing
- Normal gait without assistive devices
- Demonstrate ability to lock knee with weight shifted to ACL leg
Testing
- Bilateral ROM
Exercises
- Extension
  Towel extensions
  Prone hangs
  Wall slides
  Heel slides
- Single leg stance
- Partial to full weight-bearing without crutches
- Strengthening
  Bilateral one-quarter knee bends
  Calf raises
  StairMaster 4000 workouts on manual control
Clinical Follow-up
- The patient will return 2 weeks following surgery
- The patient should have full terminal extension and full flexion to 130 degrees

Phase III: 2 to 4 Weeks
Clinical Goals
- Full terminal extension and full flexion to 130 degrees

- Consistent weight room and moderate speed strengthening
- Early return to agility and sport-specific drills
Testing
- Bilateral ROM
Exercises
- Extension
  Hyperextension device
- Flexion
  Heel slides
- Weight room activities (once the patient has sufficient leg control to perform a unilateral knee bend without difficulty):
  One-quarter squats
  Unilateral leg press
  Unilateral calf raises
  StairMaster 4000 continued at greater intensity levels
  Unilateral step-downs
  Unilateral leg extensions
  Bicycling workouts are started. Initially the bicycle is used as a mechanical means of attaining flexion. Once the patient has gained 120 degrees flexion, it can be used for moderate-speed strengthening workouts.
  Swimming and other hydrotherapy exercises can be started once the incisions have healed
Agility
- If full ROM and other goals have been met, sport-specific and agility drill may be initiated:
  Jump rope
  Single-leg hop
  Easy position drills
Clinical Follow-up
- After phase III, the patient will return to physical therapy every 4–6 weeks until 6 months, then again at 9, 12, and 24 months following surgery.
- At the 4-week follow-up visit the patient will work on:
  Full terminal extension and full flexion to 135 degrees
  Improved quadriceps tone
  70% strength

Phase IV: 4 Weeks on
Clinical Goals
- Full ROM including terminal extension
- Quadriceps tone continues to improve with noticeable quadriceps definition
- Return to full activity
- At least 60% strength
- Proprioceptive/agility-specific program
- Complete a sport-specific functional progression
Testing
- Isokinetic evaluation at 180 degrees per second
- Isometric leg press test
- Bilateral ROM
- Subjective questionnaire
- KT-1000 ligamentous stability testing
- Beginning with the 2-month follow-up visit: single-leg hop test
Exercises
- Full squat as tolerated
- Unilateral leg press
- Unilateral leg extensions
- Unilateral step-downs
- Unilateral calf raises
- Lunges
- StairMaster
- Bicycle
Agility
- Fast speed strength and confidence
  Jump rope
  Lateral slides
  Backward running
  Shooting baskets, dribbling soccer ball, and other sport-specific drills
Clinical Follow-up
- From this point forward, the patient will return to physical therapy every 4–6 weeks until 6 months, then again at 9, 12, and 24 months following surgery for:
  ROM
  KT-1000
  Isokinetic strength testing
  Isometric strength testing
  Single-leg hop
  Subjective assessment

ROM = range of motion.

postoperative visits in the first year following surgery, patients return to the clinic 2, 5, 10, and 15 years after reconstruction for follow-up and prospective data collection. The specific data collected at these visits include results of KT-1000 stability assessment, isometric and isokinetic strength testing, functional testing, and subjective questionnaire. The resulting database enables us to constantly update and revise the rehabilitation program as needed, based on clinical data and what we learn from our patients.

PHASE I: PREOPERATIVE

Initial Evaluation

Regardless of the decision for reconstructive surgery, the injured knee needs to be rehabilitated beginning immediately after the ACL injury. The first component of phase I is the initial evaluation, which includes assessment of swelling, range of motion, and gait. Knee extension is measured with a goniometer with the patient in a supine position and the heel propped to allow for full hyperextension (Fig. 8–1). Knee ROM is recorded as A-B-C, with A being the degrees of hyperextension, B indicating lack of extension, and C documenting degrees of flexion. For example, for a patient with 8 degrees of hyperextension and 120 degrees of flexion, ROM would be recorded as 8–0-120. The importance of recording preoperative range of

motion, especially knee hyperextension, cannot be overstated. A recent study found that in the normal population of high school–aged athletes, 97 percent had at least 1 degree of knee hyperextension. Normal knee ROM, on average, was 6–0-140 for girls and 5–0-140 for boys.[6] This finding is in contrast to typical, normal range for knee extension, which is generally given as 0 degrees. To restore the knee to a normal state postoperatively, full ROM must be restored, including full hyperextension; therefore, normal ROM must be restored and recorded prior to the ACL reconstruction.

Rehabilitation Instructions

At the time of the initial evaluation, rehabilitation instructions are given to the patient on how to decrease swelling, increase ROM, and normalize gait. A component of restoring the knee to a more normal state prior to surgery includes pain modulation and controlled swelling. A CryoCuff (AirCast, Inc., Summit, NJ) is used for cold and compression. The patient is instructed to wear it as much as possible when in a relaxed position with the knee elevated. During the day, when the CryoCuff is not being worn, the patient wears a Tubigrip elastic sleeve to provide compression to the knee. The patient should be cautioned against wearing the CryoCuff and Tubigrip together because of the possibility of vascular compromise.[7]

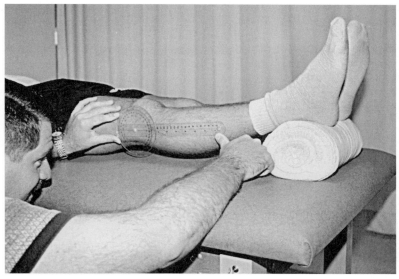

Figure 8–1. Measuring knee extension. The patient is in a supine position with the heel adequately propped to allow for full hyperextension.

It has been found that returning full symmetric knee ROM prior to surgery decreases complications such as arthrofibrosis.[8-10] To restore full ROM, the patient is instructed in several exercises, including heel props, prone hangs, and towel extensions for extension, and wall slides and heel slides for flexion. These exercises are described later in the chapter. If the patient has problems attaining full terminal extension with the exercises, he or she may be given a hyperextension device to assist in gaining full hyperextension (Fig. 8–2).

Encouraging the patient to move from partial to full weight-bearing as tolerated stresses the importance of restoring a normal gait. The emphasis of gait instruction is on achieving full knee extension at heel strike with full weight-bearing on the involved side. The patient is expected to be walking normally prior to surgery.

To encourage early strengthening, the patient is instructed in several closed kinetic chain exercises, including leg press, one-quarter squats, step-downs, bicycling and StairMaster (Tri-tech, Inc., Tulsa, OK). These exercises will be introduced after swelling from the injury has decreased and ROM has been restored.

Preoperatively, three methods are used to assess strength: isokinetic strength test, closed kinetic chain isometric leg-press test, and single-leg hop test. Isokinetic strength evaluation is performed at 180 degrees per second. Closed kinetic chain isometric strength assessment is performed using a Cybex (division of Lumex, Ronkonkoma, NY) leg press machine attached to the Jackson Evaluation System (Lafayette Instruments, Lafayette, IN) (Fig. 8–3). The testing procedure for the isometric leg press involves the patient isometrically contracting against a footplate, yielding an isometric peak displayed on the control unit. Three repetitions are performed with each leg and a percentage of involved compared with noninvolved is determined.[11] Single-leg hop test is also performed on the noninvolved leg to get a measure of functional strength and ability.[12, 13]

In addition to these strength measures, ligament stability is assessed with a KT-1000 ligament arthrometer (MEDmetric Corporation, San Diego, CA). A manual maximum side-to-side difference is recorded in millimeters. Range of motion, strength, and ligament stability measurements are collected prospectively and maintained in a data base for future analysis.

During the initial evaluation, the functional demands of the patient are assessed, including activities of daily living (ADLs) and athletic and recreational activities. School, work, and family schedules are also examined to determine when the most appropriate time to schedule surgery would be.

Patient Counseling

Phase I also includes patient counseling on the concepts of our approach to rehabilitation, the timing of the surgery with details

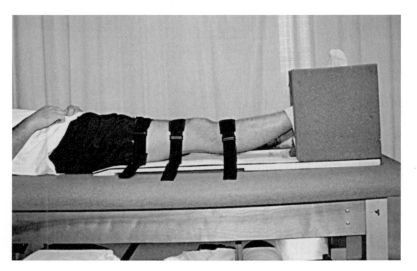

Figure 8–2. A hyperextension device is used preoperatively or postoperatively when patients are having trouble obtaining full hyperextension equal to that of the noninvolved knee.

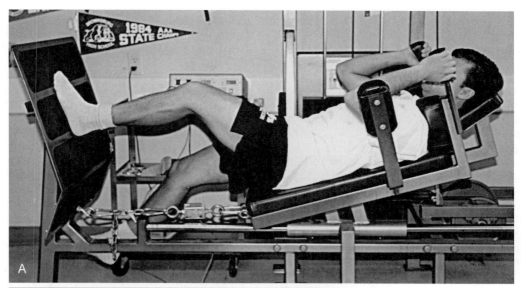

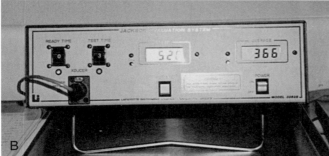

Figure 8–3. *A,* Isometric leg press evaluation assists in determining closed kinetic chain strength. *B,* The Jackson Evaluation System is attached to the leg press machine to display isometric peak.

of the reconstructive procedure, and specific postoperative rehabilitation goals and expectations. Because mental preparation is a very important aspect of success of the surgical reconstruction and rehabilitation, it is essential that the patient understands the goals of the rehabilitation process and how these goals will be achieved.[14–16]

Before a course of treatment is decided on, the physician discusses treatment options with the patient. Indications for ACL reconstruction are discussed as well as risk factors associated with both surgical and nonsurgical treatment. The most important factor for deciding on a treatment approach is the functional demands of the patient. Functional demands include ADLs, employment, and involvement in athletic and recreational activities. The most predictable treatment option for those patients who want to return to the demands of athletic activities is to have an ACL reconstruction. Those who may benefit from a nonoperative treatment plan include patients who are

skeletally immature or are not involved in high-risk activities that include side-to-side twisting or jumping maneuvers.

Activity modification is the key for nonoperative treatment. Recurrent instability represents failure of conservative treatment, which must be addressed with more stringent activity modification, or surgical reconstruction.

The incidence of ACL injuries among the adolescent population has risen over the past few years. Originally, ACL tears in this group of patients were reported to be rare.[17–20] With an increase in adolescent participation in organized sports, improved diagnostic modalities, and greater awareness of adolescent sports injuries, however, recent reports of ACL injuries have shown the incidence to be higher than was once thought. Current literature shows that overall the incidence is between 3 and 4 percent in skeletally immature patients.[21, 22] Treatment for the adolescent with a mid-substance tear to the ACL remains controversial. Currently, nonoperative treatment is recommended if the following criteria are present[23–25]:

- Posterolateral and lateral radiographs show "wide-open" physes
- Patient has not undergone adolescent growth spurt
- Patient is shorter than older sibling and parents
- Patient is at Tanner stage 1 or 2

Nonoperative treatment includes rehabilitation with an emphasis on quadriceps and hamstring strengthening, bracing if needed for ADLs only, and counseling for activity modification. Even with a brace, participation in high-risk sports such as football, basketball, and soccer should be avoided to reduce the risk of giving-way episodes, which can lead to menisci and articular cartilage damage. An algorithm for the treatment of ACL tears in adolescents has been developed that takes into account the following variables when dealing with patients in this age group:

- This population is often not compliant with activity restriction.
- Intra-articular reconstruction through growth plates has not been recommended because of the potential for growth disturbances.
- Functional instability places the young child at a high risk for meniscal tears and very early degenerative arthritis.

The management system that has been developed aims to protect the menisci and delay surgery so that one definitive stabilizing procedure is performed for the knee. The algorithm for this process can be seen in Figure 8–4.

Once the medical team has decided that a surgical course of action will take place, it is very important to develop a comprehensive plan of care that includes appropriate timing of the ACL reconstruction procedure.[26] Rather than delaying surgery a set amount of time, the preoperative condition of the knee, including no swelling and full ROM, as well as the mental preparedness of the patient serve as a better indicator for the timing of the surgery. It typically takes 3 to 4 weeks from the time of the ACL injury until the knee is ready. The patient who is ready for surgery has a knee with full ROM, no swelling, normal gait, and adequate strength. The surgical procedure and postoperative rehabilitation program will be explained in detail to the patient. In addition, the patient

has arranged his or her school, work, and family schedules so that he or she can be compliant with the early rehabilitation guidelines.

Advantages of timing the surgery appropriately include preoperative rehabilitation and patient preparation.[16] We have demonstrated that delaying surgery allows the knee to return to normal, decreasing the risk of potential complications.[13] Shelbourne and Foulk[15] also found that by delaying surgery for more than 21 days, quadriceps muscle strength returned more quickly than if surgery was performed immediately following the injury (<11 days).

SURGICAL PROCEDURE

Our technique involves harvesting the graft from the central one-third of the patellar tendon with a miniarthrotomy visualization and button fixation. With proper graft placement and fixation, patients are able to follow an aggressive rehabilitation program without the development of graft laxity.[14, 27]

PHASE II: IMMEDIATE POSTOPERATIVE

Postoperative rehabilitation begins in the operating room, confirming full knee ROM after the graft is in place and properly fixed. With the properly positioned graft, full knee hyperextension will place the ligament perfectly into the intercondylar notch without impingement. Confirming full knee flexion ensures that graft placement and fixation have not captured the knee and will not prevent the patient from obtaining full ROM during postoperative rehabilitation. We have demonstrated that restoring full hyperextension does not adversely affect ligamentous stability.[8]

The clinical goals of phase II include decreasing swelling and obtaining full passive knee extension and flexion to 110 degrees. Additional variables include performing an independent straight leg raise and restoring normal gait.

Immediate Postoperative Rehabilitation (1–6 Days)

Our patients are placed in 23-hour observation postoperatively. This overnight hos-

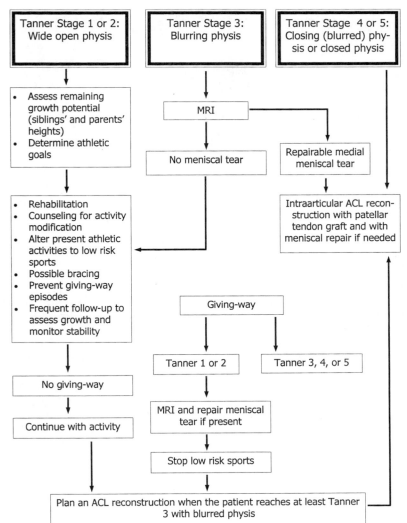

Figure 8–4. Algorithm for management of adolescent athletes with an anterior cruciate ligament tear. (From Shelbourne KD, Patel DV, McCarroll JR: Management of anterior cruciate ligament injuries in skeletally immature adolescents. In Knee Surgery, Sports Traumatology, Arthroscopy, vol. 4. New York, Springer Verlag, 1996, pp. 68–74.)

pital stay allows for excellent pain control and provides for a predictable, consistent start to postoperative rehabilitation. A self-contained CryoCuff (AirCast, Inc., Summit, NJ) is placed on the patient's knee immediately following the operation (Fig. 8–5). Continuous passive motion (CPM) is initiated following discharge from the recovery room and the machine is set to 10–0-30 degrees. The CPM machine is to remain on, with the patient's leg in it at all times, except when the patient is doing motion exercises or going to the bathroom.

Rehabilitation exercises are started upon the patient's arrival to the hospital room after surgery. Pillow extensions are performed, allowing the knee to relax into full hyperextension every hour for 10 minutes.

Quadriceps muscle contraction and full knee extension exercises are emphasized, including active heel height (Fig. 8–6), to promote leg control and to minimize the potential for a patellar contracture. Patients also start to work on flexion the day of reconstructive surgery. On the evening of the surgery, the reconstructed knee is flexed to 110 degrees in the CPM machine. When the machine reaches 110 degrees of flexion, it is placed on pause for 10 minutes. To increase flexion even more, the patient takes his or her leg out of the CPM machine and pulls it further to the buttocks with his or her hands. The following day the patient does these flexion exercises four or five times along with the hourly extension exercises. During the first week, the patient is to remain reclining as

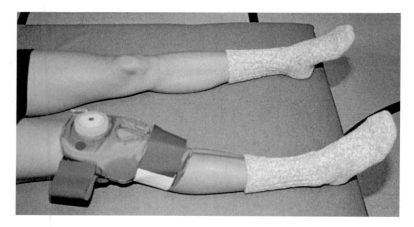

Figure 8–5. A self-contained Cryo-Cuff (AirCast, Inc., Summit, NJ) is used as a form of cold and compression for control of swelling.

much as possible to control swelling. However, when getting up to go to the bathroom, the patient is encouraged to be full weight-bearing as tolerated. Crutches are discarded when the patient can resume a normal gait pattern. It is our opinion that these activities provide the graft with an appropriate level of stress in the initial stages of healing.

The patient is discharged from the hospital the morning after surgery. Goals at discharge are minimal swelling, full extension, good quadriceps leg control, and flexion to 110 degrees. Weight-bearing as tolerated with crutches is encouraged. The exercises that the patient started in the hospital are continued on the same schedule at home during the first week after surgery.

First Clinic Visit (7 Days)

The goal of our protocol is to avoid complications rather than treat problems after

they occur. Routine follow-up postoperatively ensures that the patient is on the correct clinical course. The first follow-up visit takes place 1 week after surgery. Clinical concerns at this visit include swelling, ROM including full passive hyperextension, leg control, soft tissue healing, and gait. Along with measuring ROM with a goniometer, extension is evaluated by performing a passive heel lift.[28] The patient lies supine on the examination table. The examiner stabilizes the distal femur with the top hand above the patella and grasps the forefoot with the lower hand. An extension force is then applied to the knee by stabilizing the distal femur while lifting the foot off the table with gradual and gentle motion (Fig. 8–7). The distances the heels can be raised off the table are compared to provide an estimate of extension difference.

The patient is evaluated at the 1-week visit by both the surgeon and the physical therapist. The patient's rehabilitation program is

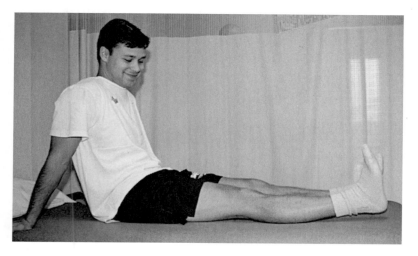

Figure 8–6. The patient contracts the quadriceps to actively lift the heel off the table or bed to promote leg control and strength.

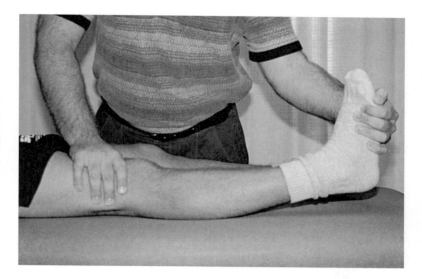

Figure 8–7. The passive heel height is used to measure hyperextension by holding the thigh stationary just above the knee with one hand, while the other hand lifts the foot to pull the knee into passive hyperextension.

advanced, concentrating on swelling control, ROM, quadriceps leg control, and gait. Full hyperextension is maintained with heel prop and prone hang exercises. Heel prop exercises are performed with the patient in a long sitting position with a towel roll under the heel. The towel roll should be high enough to elevate the thigh off the table or floor and allow the knee to fully extend. A prone hang is performed with the patient lying in a prone position with the involved knee and lower leg hanging off the edge of the table in a gravity-assisted position. A light weight is placed across the ankle to assist with full knee extension (Fig. 8–8). As in the preoperative phase, if the patient has problems maintaining full hyperextension, a

hyperextension device may be used. The CPM is discontinued at 1 week. Flexion is progressed with wall slides and heel slides (Fig. 8–9). The CryoCuff is used on a regular basis to control swelling when the patient is not performing exercises.

Restoration of normal gait is also a goal of the second week of the rehabilitation process. Gait-training activities involve heel-to-toe walking, retrowalking, and high-knee activities. The focus with retrowalking is to fully extend the knee when going from toe to heel. We have found that having patients practice walking in front of a mirror greatly aids in the return of a normal gait pattern. The mirror gives patients an immediate visual clue as to how they are walking. By the

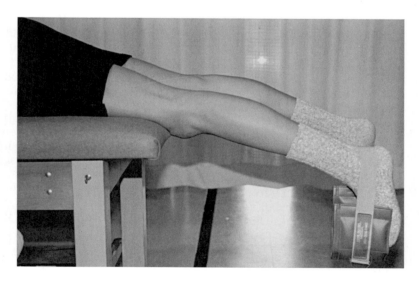

Figure 8–8. Prone hang exercises are used to help the patient regain full hyperextension as in the opposite leg. A light weight may be placed across the ankle to assist with extension.

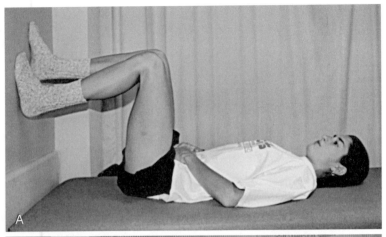

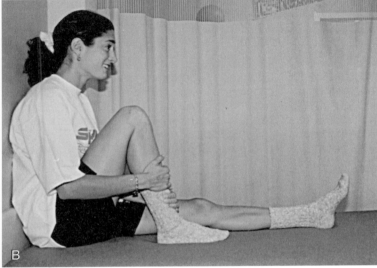

Figure 8–9. When the continuous passive motion is discontinued, wall slides *(A)* and heel slides *(B)* are used to promote gaining full flexion.

end of the second week, our goal is to have the patient walking normally without crutches. It is very important to emphasize leg control early in the rehabilitation program. Through early extension and normal gait, the patient is able to regain good quadriceps tone and leg control. This combination of clinical variables will set the pace for the entire rehabilitation program and a successful outcome.

One exercise that is beneficial for maintaining full terminal extension, improving leg control, and regaining a normal gait is to have the patient lock the knee out by standing with the weight shifted to the ACL-reconstructed leg so that extension is full and the knee is fully locked. This is referred to as single-leg stance (Fig. 8–10). The patient is encouraged to concentrate on this whenever standing. Too often, the patient will stand on the contralateral leg for comfort and the

ACL-reconstructed leg will be in a slightly flexed position. Single-leg stance on the involved leg is an effective method of working on full ROM and leg control, while giving the patient confidence in standing on the injured leg to begin to do functional activities.

Instructions on quadriceps strengthening exercises of one-quarter double-leg squats and step-downs (Fig. 8–11) are also given at this visit. The goals of the second week of postoperative rehabilitation are to maintain full hyperextension, increase activity by returning to school or sedentary work, control swelling, increase flexion to 120 degrees and restore normal gait.

PHASE III: 2 TO 4 WEEKS

Rehabilitation Emphasis

Phase III begins at the second postoperative visit 2 weeks after surgery. The empha-

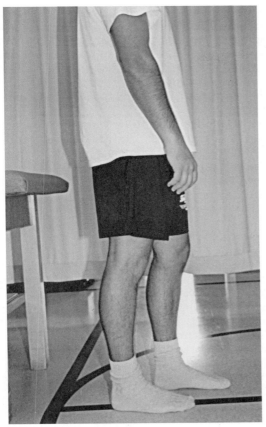

Figure 8–10. When standing, the patient is encouraged to stand on the anterior cruciate ligament–reconstructed leg with the knee fully extended. This is referred to as a single-leg stance.

to return to full-time sedentary work, school, and normal activities of daily living by the beginning of the third postoperative week.

Functional strengthening is initiated in this phase, including knee bends, step-ups, leg presses, squats, and using a StairMaster and stationary bicycle. Closed kinetic chain (CKC) exercises are preferred for functional strengthening of the lower extremity. This form of exercise has been shown to reduce shear forces across the tibiofemoral joint.[29] Caution must be exercised when utilizing full arc open kinetic chain (OKC) exercises, owing to patellofemoral compressive forces being distributed over a small contact area in the terminal end of knee extension. CKC exercises stress function whereas OKC exercises facilitate isolated quadriceps muscle strengthening. Our preferred exercise progression includes OKC and CKC exercises, including short arc quadriceps from 90 to 30 degrees, knee bends, step-ups, and leg presses. These are started with lower weight

sis in this phase is on gaining full flexion, return to normal daily activities, and early strengthening. At this time, the patient should have full passive extension and flexion to 130 degrees.

Exercise Instruction

Maintaining full knee extension is continued, with exercises including prone hangs, passive and active heel lift, and, if needed, a hyperextension device. These exercises are performed three to four times per day. Increasing knee flexion is achieved by the patient's performing exercises such as heel slides and active assistive flexion in a sitting position and using a stationary bike to facilitate flexion ROM. The patient should be full weight-bearing without the use of crutches and without a limp. Usually patients are able

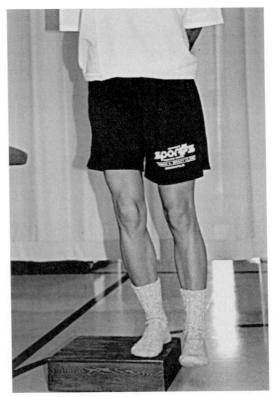

Figure 8–11. Step-downs are performed by having the patient stand on a step on the anterior cruciate ligament–reconstructed knee and slowly lowering the contralateral leg to the floor and then returning to starting position.

and then gradually progressed to higher weight with lower repetitions.

PHASE IV: ADVANCED REHABILITATION

Rehabilitation Emphasis

The emphasis in phase IV is on advanced strengthening and return to sports. To advance into the final phase of the rehabilitation program, the patient needs to have nearly full ROM. Our goal is to reach this phase by 4 to 5 weeks after surgery. However, if the patient has not achieved the previous phase's goals, advanced agility and sport-specific activities are not yet initiated. Exercise instruction includes an increase in weight room and home strengthening activities. Patients are encouraged to progress from high repetition/low weights to low repetition/high weights. Also, some type of moderate speed strength and cardiovascular activity should be continued, such as bicycling, swimming, or using a StairMaster.

The patient's first visit during phase IV is 4 weeks after surgery. This visit will include the first isokinetic evaluation, a CKC leg press evaluation,[11] and KT-1000 ligament arthrometer evaluation. The first isokinetic evaluation includes testing at 180 degrees per second with a 20-degree extension block.

Exercise Instruction

If the patient's strength ratio is at least 60 percent, agility activities are started. These activities include lateral shuffles, cariocas, cross-over drills, and backward running. Patients may also begin solo sports activities such as shooting a basketball or hitting a racquetball. These early agility activities promote patient confidence, facilitate moderate-speed strength, and redevelop quickness, agility, and sport-specific skills. As the patient progresses, agility workouts become more vigorous, to include activities such as figure-of-eights and half- to full-speed running. The speed of progression is based on the specific athletic and recreational desires of the patient. Sport-specific activities are incorporated into the progression with specific focus on athletic goals.

Although many patients ask, "When can I start running again?" at the beginning of phase IV, running for conditioning or rehabilitation actually is the final step in the rehabilitation process. We prefer that the patient work on agility drills and sport-specific skills instead of running 2 to 3 miles. Running long distances at this time leads to swelling and therefore can cause a delay in the rehabilitation process.

It is important to have the athlete participate in sport-specific activities. It can take 2 to 3 months of these sport-specific activities before the athlete will feel completely comfortable with the knee and recover the rest of his or her quickness.

Periodic Follow-Up

The patient is followed every 4 to 6 weeks for up to 6 months. Specific testing strategies at each visit consist of isokinetic evaluation, CKC isometric leg press evaluation, and the single-leg hop test as well as KT-1000 ligament arthrometer evaluation. The isokinetic evaluation at 9 to 10 weeks is conducted at 180 degrees per second with the 20 degree extension block removed. The third isokinetic evaluation at 14 to 16 weeks includes the addition of a 60-degree per second test. With the single-leg hop test, the patient is instructed to hop for distance, with take-off and landing completed on the same leg. At 6 months postoperatively, patients are given a Modified Noyes assessment questionnaire (Appendix VIII), which measures subjective outcomes. The questionnaire is repeated at 12 and 18 months, and 2, 5, 10, and 15 years. The Modified Noyes assessment is one of the most important tools we have to collectively measure how the patients feel long-term about the function and status of their knees. It examines such variables as stability, swelling, pain, and function. After 6 months, the patient is seen again at the 1-year postoperative mark and again at 2, 5, 10, and 15 years for continual, long-term assessment and collection of postoperative data.

SUMMARY

Rehabilitation after ACL reconstruction continues to be examined and discussed. Our current rehabilitation program has evolved over the past 12 years by our collecting and analyzing data and listening to what our patients tell us about their experience with the rehabilitation process. The four-phase rehabilitation program involves a preoperative stage that emphasizes returning the knee to a normal state and mentally preparing the patient for surgery and the rehabilitation that will follow. Immediately postoperatively, the focus is on decreasing swelling, restoring full passive hyperextension and flexion to 110 degrees, and gaining leg control and normal gait. Two to 4 weeks after surgery, the emphasis is on gaining full flexion, returning to normal activities and beginning early strengthening. Advanced rehabilitation focuses on increasing strength and returning to sports.

Our goal with the rehabilitation process is not to rapidly return an athlete to the field of play, but to emphasize the return to normal ADL level with full knee ROM and adequate strength. Once patients arrive at this goal, if they desire to rapidly return to athletic activities, we will assist them and monitor their return. We encourage our patients to reach the stage of full ROM and normal gait, but we do not push patients back onto the athletic field. Likewise, if they are ready, we do not hold them back.

References

1. Hannafin JA, Arnoczky SP, Hoonjan A, Torzilli PA: Effect of stress deprivation and cyclic tensile loading on the material and morphologic properties of canine flexor digitorum profundus tendon: An in vitro study. J Ortho Res 13:907, 1995.
2. Rougraff B, Shelbourne KD, Gerth PK, Warner J: Arthroscopic and histologic analysis of human patellar tendon autografts used for anterior cruciate ligament reconstruction. Am J Sports Med 21:277, 1993.
3. Shelbourne KD, Gray T: Two- to nine-year results after anterior cruciate ligament reconstruction with autogenous patellar tendon graft and accelerated rehabilitation. Am J Sports Med 25:786, 1997.
4. De Carlo MS, Sell K: The effects of the number and frequency of physical therapy treatments on selected outcomes of treatment in patients with ACL reconstruction. J Orthop Sports Phys Ther 26:332, 1997.
5. De Carlo MS, Shelbourne KD, McCarroll JR, Rettig AC: Traditional versus accelerated rehabilitation following ACL reconstruction: A one-year follow-up. J Orthop Sports Phys Ther 15:309, 1992.
6. De Carlo MS, Sell K: Normative data for range of motion and single leg hop in high school athletes. J Sport Rehab 6:246, 1997.
7. Mindrebo N, Shelbourne KD: Knee pressure dressings and their effect on lower extremity venous capacitance and venous outflow. Orthop Int 2:273, 1994.
8. Rubinstein RA, Shelbourne KD, Van Meter CD, et al: Effect on knee stability if full hyperextension is restored immediately after autogenous bone-patellar tendon-bone anterior cruciate ligament reconstruction. Am J Sports Med 23:365, 1995.
9. Shelbourne KD, Patel DV, Martini DJ: Classification and management of arthrofibrosis of the knee following anterior cruciate ligament reconstruction. Am J Sports Med 24:857, 1996.
10. Shelbourne KD, Wilckens JH, Mollabaashy A, et al: Arthrofibrosis in acute anterior cruciate ligament reconstruction. Am J Sports Med 19:332, 1991.
11. De Carlo MS, Sell K, Shelbourne KD, Klootwyk TE: Current concepts on accelerated ACL rehabilitation. J Sport Rehab 3:304, 1994.
12. Booher LK, Hench KM, Worrell TW, et al: Reliability of three single leg hop tests. J Sports Rehab 2:165, 1993.
13. Kramer JF, Nusca D, Fowler P, et al: Test-retest reliability of the one-leg hop test following ACL reconstruction. Clin J Sports Med 2:240, 1992.
14. Klootwyk TE, Shelbourne KD, De Carlo MS: Perioperative rehabilitation considerations. Op Tech Sports Med 1:22, 1993.
15. Shelbourne KD, Foulk AD: Timing of surgery in acute anterior cruciate ligament tears on the return of quadriceps strength after reconstruction using autogenous patellar tendon graft. Am J Sports Med 23:686, 1995.
16. Shelbourne KD, Patel DV: Timing of surgery in anterior cruciate ligament-injured knees. Knee Surg Sports Traum Arthroscopy 3:148, 1995.
17. Bradley GW, Shives TC, Samuelson KM: Ligament injuries in the knees of children. J Bone Joint Surg 61:588, 1979.
18. Clanton TO, DeLee JC, Sanders B, et al.: Knee ligament injuries in children. J Bone Joint Surg 61:1195, 1979.
19. DeLee JC, Curtis R: Anterior cruciate ligament insufficiency in children. Clin Orthop 172:112, 1983.
20. Matz SO, Jackson DW: Anterior cruciate ligament injury in children. Am J Knee Surg 1:59, 1988.
21. Lipscomb AB, Anderson AF: Tears of the anterior cruciate ligament in adolescents. J Bone Joint Surg 68:19, 1986.
22. McCarroll JR, Rettig AC, Shelbourne KD: Anterior cruciate ligament injuries in young athletes with open physes. Am J Sports Med 16:44, 1988.
23. McCarroll JR, Shelbourne KD, Porter DA, et al.: Patellar tendon graft reconstruction for midsubstance anterior cruciate ligament rupture in junior high school athletes. Am J Sports Med 22:478, 1994.
24. Shelbourne KD, Patel DV, McCarroll JR: Management of anterior cruciate ligament injuries in skeletally immature adolescents. Knee Surg Sports Traumatol Arthroscopy 4:68, 1996.
25. Mizuta H, Kubota K, Shiraishi M, et al.: The conservative treatment of complete tears of the anterior cruciate ligament in skeletally immature patients. J Bone Joint Surg 77-B:890, 1995.
26. Johnson GE, Shelbourne KD: Patient selection for anterior cruciate ligament reconstruction. Op Tech Sports Med 1:16, 1993.
27. Rubinstein RA, Shelbourne KD: Graft selection, placement, fixation, and tensioning for ACL reconstruction. Op Tech Sports Med 1:10, 1993.
28. Shelbourne KD, Johnson G: Evaluation of knee extension following ACL reconstruction. Ortho 17:205, 1994.
29. Beynnon BD, Fleming BC, Johnson RJ, et al.: ACL strain behavior during rehabilitation exercise in vivo. Am J Sports Med 23:24, 1995.

VIII ACL Knee: Postoperative Questionnaire

Please check the statement that best describes the condition of your knee.

Pain

20 _____ I experience no pain in my knee.

16 _____ I have occasional pain with strenuous sports or heavy work. Limitations are mild and tolerable.

12 _____ There is occasional pain in my knee with light recreational sports or moderate work.

8 _____ I have pain brought on by sports, light recreational activities, or moderate work. Occasional pain is brought on by daily activities such as standing or kneeling.

4 _____ The pain I have in my knee is a significant problem with activities as simple as walking. The pain is relieved by rest. I can't participate in sports.

0 _____ I have pain in my knee at all times, even during walking, standing, or light work.

Intensity: A. ( ) Mild B. ( ) Moderate C. ( ) Severe

Frequency: A. ( ) Constant B. ( ) Intermittent

Location: A. ( ) Medial (Inner side) B. ( ) Lateral (Outer side) C. ( ) Anterior (Front) D. ( ) Posterior (Back) E. ( ) Diffuse (All over)

Occur: A. ( ) Kneel B. ( ) Stand C. ( ) Sit D. ( ) Stairs

Type: A. ( ) Sharp B. ( ) Aching C. ( ) Throbbing D. ( ) Burning

Swelling

10 _____ I experience no swelling in my knee.

8 _____ I have occasional swelling in my knee with strenuous sports or heavy work.

6 _____ There is occasional swelling with light recreational activities or moderate work.

4 _____ Swelling limits my participation in sports and moderate work. Occurs frequently with simple walking or light work—about three times a year.

2 _____ My knee swells after simple walking activities and light work. The swelling is relieved by rest.

0 _____ I have severe swelling with simple walking activities. The swelling is not relieved by rest.

Stability (referring to actual shifting of the joint)

20 _____ My knee does not give out.

16 _____ My knee gives out only with strenuous sports or heavy work.

12 _____ My knee gives out occasionally with light recreational activities or moderate work.

8 _____ Because my knee gives out, it limits all sports and moderate work. It occasionally gives out with walking or light work.

4 _____ My knee gives out frequently with simple activities such as walking. I must guard my knee at all times.

0 _____ I have severe problems with my knee giving out. I can't turn or twist without my knee giving out.

Stiffness: A. ( ) None B. ( ) Occasional C. ( ) Frequent

Grinding: A. ( ) None B. ( ) Mild C. ( ) Moderate D. ( ) Severe

Locking: A. ( ) None B. ( ) Occasional C. ( ) Frequent

Overall Activity Level

20 _____ No limitations. I am able to do everything including strenuous sports and/or heavy labor.

16 _____ I can partake in sports including strenuous ones but at a lower level. I must guard my knee and limit the amount of heavy labor or sports.

12 _____ Light recreational activities are possible. Walking activities are pos-

sible with RARE symptoms. I am limited to light work.

8 _____ No sports or recreational activities are possible. Walking activities are possible with RARE symptoms. I am limited to light work.

4 _____ Walking activities and daily living cause moderate problems and persistent symptoms.

0 _____ Walking and other daily living activities cause severe problems.

Walking

10 _____ Normal, unlimited.
8 _____ Slight, mild problems.
6 _____ Moderate problems, flat surfaces up to half a mile.
4 _____ Severe problems, only 2 to 3 blocks possible.
2 _____ Severe problems, need cane or crutches.

Stairs

5 _____ Normal, unlimited.
4 _____ Slight, mild problems.
3 _____ Moderate problems, only 10 to 15 steps possible.
2 _____ Severe problems, require banister for support.
1 _____ Severe problems, only 1 to 5 steps with support.

Running

10 _____ Normal, unlimited, fully competitive.
8 _____ Slight, mild problems, run at half speed.
6 _____ Moderate problems, only about 1 mile possible.
4 _____ Severe problems, only 1 to 3 blocks possible.
2 _____ Severe problems, only a few steps.

Jumping and Twisting

5 _____ Normal, unlimited, fully competitive.
4 _____ Slight, mild problems, some guarding.
3 _____ Moderate problems, gave up strenuous sports.
2 _____ Severe problems, affects all sports, always guarding.
1 _____ Severe problems, only light activity possible (golf/swim).

Courtesy of Frank R. Noyes, MD.

Please circle one answer for each question.

How does your current level of activity compare with that before your injury?

A. I have increased my level of activity.
B. I am fully competitive. I have returned to the full level of work or sport.
C. I can take part in the same type of work or sport as before the injury, but I must work or compete at a lower level. I do have some limitations.
D. I am able to participate in light recreational activities or work but I must be careful.
E. I have not been able to return to sports or work activities but I have no problem with daily activities.
F. I have difficulties with daily activities or light work.

Why have you limited your activities?

A. I have not limited my activities.
B. I have decreased my activity level in order to decrease wear and tear on my knee.
C. I have no desire to participate in activities at a higher level than before surgery, but I feel that I could if I wanted to.
D. I am in a rehabilitation program that limits my activities.
E. I have significant symptoms when I increase my activity level.
F. I have another injury or problem not related to my knee injury which will not allow me to increase my activity level.

Do you believe that your knee has recovered to the level that you expected? In other words, have you achieved your goal?

A. Yes.
B. No—Due to pain.
C. No—Due to swelling.
D. No—Due to lack of stability.
E. No—I no longer have the same goal.

Do you wear a functional brace for sports? (e.g.: Indiana Knee Orthosis, McLight II brace, CTI Brace, etc.)

A. Yes, I do wear a brace.
B. No, I do not wear a brace.

If I had to give my knee a grade from 1 to 100, with 100 being the best, I would give my knee a _____.

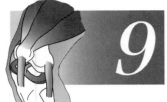

9 Autogeneic and Allogeneic Anterior Cruciate Ligament Rehabilitation

Timothy P. Heckmann, PT, ATC, Frank R. Noyes, MD, and Sue D. Barber-Westin, BS

*R*ehabilitation following anterior cruciate ligament (ACL) reconstruction has undergone dramatic changes over the past 2 decades. Concepts such as immediate knee motion and immediate or early weight-bearing following reconstruction, endorsed by current literature, are actually less than 20 years old. We first described the use of immediate knee motion after ACL patellar tendon autogenous reconstruction in 1983[1] and subsequently published in 1987[2] the effects of an early partial weight-bearing program on ACL allograft reconstructions. Subsequent clinical studies reported that this progressive approach was not deleterious to ACL allografts or autografts, or concomitant procedures such as meniscal repairs or other ligament reconstructions.[3–8]

Treatment today faces difficult challenges due to managed care and insurance restrictions concerning the number of patient visits, bracing, modalities, and use of specialized equipment. In some instances, rehabilitation after ACL reconstruction consists of a home exercise program with only a few follow-up visits to the therapist covered under the patient's plan. Even so, clinicians must continue to provide patients with quality medical care and outcome without increasing complication or failure rates. Prior studies have shown that ACL autogenous and allogeneic reconstruction restores stability in over 80 percent of knees with few complications.[9, 10] We believe that to continue to provide these results with less direct patient contact, rehabilitation programs must incorporate a balance between the immediate implementation of certain exercises and a delay of strenuous activities for at least 4 months postoperatively. Additionally, we advocate a minimum of seven to eight physical therapy clinic visits during the first 3 months after surgery to ensure that initial

knee motion, muscle strength, and neuromuscular goals have been achieved.[10]

The rehabilitation protocols described in this chapter consist of a careful incorporation of exercise concepts supported by scientific data and clinical experience.[11–14] The goal is to progress a patient through the program at a rate that takes into account sports and occupational goals, condition of the articular surfaces and menisci, and postoperative healing, graft remodeling, and joint effusion. Two different protocols are provided based on these factors, both which incorporate a home self-management program along with an estimated number of formal physical therapy visits (Table 9–1). For the majority of patients, a range of 11 to 21 postoperative visits is expected to produce a desirable result. A few more visits may be required between the sixth and twelfth postoperative months for certain patients who desire to return to strenuous activities for advanced training. For all patients, the following signs are continually monitored postoperatively: joint swelling, pain, gait pattern, knee motion, patellar mobility, muscle strength, flexibility, and anteroposterior (AP) knee displacement. Any individual who experiences difficulty progressing through the protocol or who develops a complication is expected to require additional supervision in the formal clinic setting.[15]

We developed discharge criteria following ACL reconstruction based on patient goals for athletics and occupations, the rating of symptoms, KT-1000 testing, muscle strength testing, and function testing (Table 9–2). First, patients complete the Cincinnati Sports Activity Scale[16] (Appendix IX–1) and Occupational Rating Scale[17] to provide sports and occupational levels that are desired after surgery. Upon completion of the

Table 9–1. Physical Therapy Visit Timeline Following Anterior Cruciate Ligament Reconstruction*

Weeks Postoperative	Minimum Visits	Maximum Visits
1 to 2	2	4
3 to 4	2	4
5 to 6	1	2
7 to 8	1	2
9 to 12	1	2
13 to 26	2	3
27 to 52	2	4
Total	11	21

*Patients desiring to return to sports or strenuous work activities may require 4 to 6 more physical therapy visits during postoperative weeks 25 to 52 for advanced neuromuscular, strength, and activity-specific training to prevent reinjury.

protocol, pain, swelling, and giving-way are rated on the Cincinnati Symptom Rating Scale[16] (Appendix IX–2). The patient must not experience symptoms at the level of activity that they wish to participate in prior to discharge. Knee joint arthrometer testing is performed at 134 N of total AP force and must be within normal limits (less than 3 mm difference between limbs[18]) prior to allowance of return to strenuous activities. Muscle strength testing is performed with a Biodex isokinetic dynamometer (Biodex Corporation, Shirley, NY) to ensure that adequate strength exists prior to the initiation of the running and cutting programs. At least two functional tests are completed and limb symmetry calculated as previously described[19, 20] prior to the final discharge.

SURGICAL TECHNIQUE

The arthroscopically assisted ACL operative procedures that we use for allografts[6] and autografts[10] have been described in detail. For the autograft procedure, an endoscopically or arthroscopically assisted procedure is performed as indicated. Diagnostic arthroscopy is performed, with assessment of menisci and articular surfaces. Meniscal repairs are performed as indicated for both simple and complex tears.[5, 21–23] Any remaining ACL fibers are excised and a limited notchplasty is performed as required. A 4-cm incision is made medial to the tibial tubercle and a 9- to 10-mm-wide central one-third patellar tendon graft is removed. The femoral graft tunnel is drilled over a guide pin placed endoscopically. The graft hole is oriented into a 1 o'clock or 11 o'clock position. The graft is placed at the normal femoral and tibial ACL insertion sites without use of an isometric device. After endoscopic internal femoral graft fixation is accomplished, the knee is flexed 15 times with tension placed on the tibial bone plug by previously placed sutures to ensure that no more than 2 mm of proximal or distal graft displacement occurs from 0 to 120 degrees. The tibial portion of the graft is internally fixed with an interference screw with the knee at 10 degrees of flexion at approximately 20 N of force. The patellar tendon defect is closed and a bone graft of the patellar and tibial graft sites is performed from bone preserved from the tibial and femoral drilling procedures.

Table 9–2. Discharge Criteria Following Anterior Cruciate Ligament Reconstruction

Sports/Occupation Level	Symptom Rating* (pain, swelling, giving-way)	KT-1000 Total AP (I-N, 134 N) (mm)	Biodex Isokinetic Test (% deficit)	Function Testing (limb symmetry) (%)
Sports: I (jumping, pivoting, cutting) Occupation: heavy/very heavy	None level 10	<3	≤15	≥85
Sports: II (running, turning, twisting) Occupation: moderate	None level 8	<3	≤20	≥85
Sports: III (swimming, bicycling) Occupation: light	None level 6	3–5	≤30	≥75
Sports: IV (none) Occupation: very light	None level 4	3–5	≤30	≥75

*Level 10, normal knee, no symptoms with strenuous work/sports with jumping, hard pivoting; level 8, no symptoms with moderate work/sports with running, turning, twisting; level 6, no symptoms with light work/sports with no running, twisting or jumping; level 4, no symptoms with activities of daily living.

REHABILITATION PROTOCOL FOR ANTERIOR CRUCIATE LIGAMENT PATELLAR TENDON AUTOGENOUS RECONSTRUCTION

We developed a rehabilitation protocol for patients who have ACL autogenous reconstruction and desire to return to strenuous sports or work activities early postoperatively (Table 9–3). Any of the following criteria exclude a patient from this protocol: concomitant meniscal repair, concomitant ligament reconstruction, concomitant patellofemoral realignment procedure, prior ACL reconstruction that has failed, residual muscular atrophy with chronic instability, or magnetic resonance imaging (MRI) or arthroscopic evidence of articular cartilage damage. Patients who develop complications or problems postoperatively (such as patellofemoral symptoms) are placed into

Table 9–3. Cincinnati Sportsmedicine and Orthopaedic Center Rehabilitation Protocol for Anterior Cruciate Ligament Patellar Tendon Autogenous Reconstruction

	Postoperative Weeks			Postoperative Months	
	1 to 4	*5 to 8*	*9 to 12*	*4 to 6*	*7 to 12*
Brace: immobilizer for patient comfort	X				
Range of motion (degrees)					
Minimum goals 0–90	X				
0–120	X				
0–135		X			
Weight-bearing					
Toe touch to one-quarter of body weight	X				
Full	X				
Patella mobilization	X	X			
Modalities					
Electrical muscle stimulation (EMS)	X				
Pain/edema management (cryotherapy)	X	X	X	X	X
Stretching					
Hamstring, gastroc/soleus, iliotibial band, quadriceps	X	X	X	X	X
Strengthening					
Quadriceps isometrics, straight-leg raises, active knee extension	X	X			
Closed-chain (gait retraining, toe raises, wall sits, mini-squats)	X	X	X		
Knee flexion hamstring curls (90 degrees)	X	X	X	X	X
Knee extension quads (90–30 degrees)	X	X	X	X	X
Hip abduction-adduction, multi-hip	X	X	X	X	X
Leg press (70–10 degrees)	X	X	X	X	X
Balance/proprioceptive training	X	X	X	X	X
Weight-shifting, mini-trampoline, BAPS, KAT, plyometrics					
Conditioning					
UBE	X	X			
Bicycling (stationary)	X	X	X	X	X
Aquatic program	X	X	X	X	X
Swimming (kicking)			X	X	X
Walking			X	X	X
Stair-climbing machine		X	X	X	X
Ski machine		X	X	X	X
Running: straight			X	X	X
Cutting: lateral carioca, figure-of-eights				X	X
Full sports				X	X

our second protocol, in which delays are instituted to protect articular cartilage surfaces and to avoid exacerbation of patellofemoral or tibiofemoral symptoms. Additionally, all patients are warned that the return to strenuous activities early postoperatively carries the definite risk of a repeat injury or the potential of compounding the original injury. These risks cannot always be scientifically predicted, and patients are cautioned to return to strenuous activities carefully and to avoid any activity in which pain, swelling, or a feeling of instability is present.

Brace

Postoperative bracing represents a controversial area in the management of the reconstructed ACL. Historically, the standard of care has been to issue either a rigid knee immobilizer or a long-leg range of motion brace postoperatively. With advances in surgical techniques (including improved fixation and stronger grafts), bracing is becoming less of a major component in the immediate postoperative phase. Screening patients for personality type, pain tolerance, and program compliance may provide insight into the individual who will require brace protection postoperatively.

Our primary indication for the use of a knee immobilizer immediately postoperatively is protection of the patient during weight-bearing in the event of a fall and for the initiation of early, more comfortable weight-bearing during the first 2 postoperative weeks. The brace should be rigid, with the knee held at 0 degrees. As long as a strong intra-articular graft is used, immediate full extension is emphasized and a knee immobilizer is a useful tool to reinforce this concept. Periodic evaluation of the immobilizer and its position on the leg must occur to ensure that maximal benefit is achieved from the device.

Range of Motion

We have shown that early range of knee motion is an absolute requirement to avoid postoperative complications.[2] The goal for the first postoperative week is to obtain 0 degrees extension and 90 degrees of flexion. The use of continuous passive motion (CPM) is a valid concept, but there is considerable debate about the necessity of CPM machines for patients who do not experience complications or difficulty regaining knee motion. The preoperative evaluation often provides insight into patients who may require a CPM device versus those who will probably regain normal flexion and extension using self-directed active and passive motion techniques. Our patients are instructed to perform motion exercises in a seated position for 10 minutes a session, approximately four to six times per day. Range of motion programs can be initiated both in passive and active modes from 0 to 90 degrees as long as a strong graft is used with excellent internal fixation. If there is any question concerning the quality of the graft or the internal fixation, active motion should be avoided in the terminal range (0–30 degrees).

Full passive knee extension must be obtained immediately. Early instruction and emphasis on positioning of the leg to maintain 0 degrees is critical with intra-articular grafts, to avoid excessive scarring in the intercondylar notch. The patient is instructed to prop the foot and ankle on a towel to elevate the hamstrings and gastrocnemius, which allows the knee to drop into full extension. This position is maintained for 10 minutes and repeated approximately six times per day. If full extension is not achieved with this passive method, a hanging weight program is initiated. Using the same propped leg position, a 10-pound weight is added to the distal thigh and knee to provide overpressure to stretch the posterior capsule. Full knee extension should be obtained by the second to third postoperative week. If this is not accomplished, or if the clinician notes a firm endfeel, then a serial casting program (Fig. 9–1) may be required. Even though we advocate regaining 0 degrees of knee extension, we do not encourage achieving hyperextension, as this can place the graft at increased risk for failure in the initial 3 to 4 weeks after surgery.

Our program allows for a gradual increase in knee flexion to 120 degrees by the fourth postoperative week and then 135 degrees by the fifth postoperative week. Early work on passive knee flexion typically occurs in the traditional seated position, using the opposite lower extremity to provide overpressure. Other methods to assist in achieving flexion greater than 90 degrees include chair rolling (Fig. 9–2), wall sliding, and passive

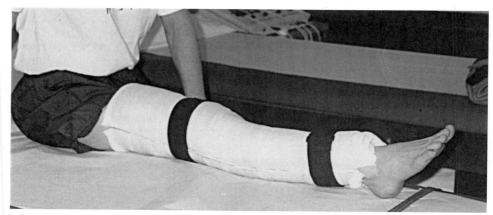

Figure 9–1. Extension casting. Patients with knees that do not respond to our extension overpressure program and do not regain full extension are placed into a serial extension cast program. This program is most successful if performed within the first 4 to 12 weeks postoperatively when the extension deficit is less than 10 degrees and there exists a soft endpoint to terminal extension. Casting is not recommended in knees that have greater than 12- to 15-degree extension deficits, or in those that demonstrate a hard block to terminal extension. The cylinder cast extends from the proximal thigh to the ankle and is well padded to prevent skin breakdown. Either a closing anterior wedge or an open posterior wedge is used every 12 to 24 hours to gradually achieve extension. Cast applications last from 36 to 48 hours and are followed by active knee flexion and extension exercises. Once extension is regained, the cast is converted into a posterior night splint, which is used for an additional 7 to 10 days to maintain extension. If loss of extension recurs, then a second cast program is initiated.

quadriceps stretching exercises. Patients who have difficulty achieving these flexion goals may undergo a gentle manipulation under anesthesia. We perform this procedure early postoperatively (an average of 6 weeks after reconstruction) and have found that a normal range of motion can be re-established with very little pressure applied to the knee. The adhesions that have formed by this time, although painful to the patient, have not matured to the point that a significant block exists. Any patient who demonstrates a hard resistant block to this gentle manipulation of the knee under anesthesia is treated with an arthroscopic release of tissues.[15]

Weight-Bearing

One of the most prominent areas of change in postoperative management of the ACL reconstructed knee is the institution of early or immediate weight-bearing. With the use of a high-strength graft and adequate fixation, early ambulation is advocated, but care must be taken to ensure its safety and efficacy. We allow partial weight-bearing as soon as pain and swelling are minimal, quadriceps tone is good, passive knee extension is 0 to 5 degrees, and the amount of anterior translation is estimated to be equal to or

less than that found in the opposite knee. These qualifications are typically met within the first week postoperatively. Initially, bilateral crutches are used and 25 percent body weight is placed on the involved foot. The amount of weight the patient is allowed to place on the involved limb is progressed approximately 25 percent each week as long as the patient continues to meet the evaluation criteria. Patients are usually weaned from crutches by the fourth postoperative week.

We initiate and progress weight-bearing using a normal gait technique that avoids a locked knee position and encourages normal knee flexion throughout the gait cycle. This technique allows for normal patterning of heel to toe ambulation, quadriceps contraction during midstance, and hip and knee flexion during the gait cycle. We avoid the locked knee position whenever possible because of the potential for development of a quadriceps avoidance gait pattern.[24] Preoperative gait training may be beneficial in certain patients in determining how quickly they can discontinue crutch support postoperatively by regaining sufficient quadriceps control.

Patellar Mobilization

This exercise is critical in the promotion of a full range of knee motion. The loss of

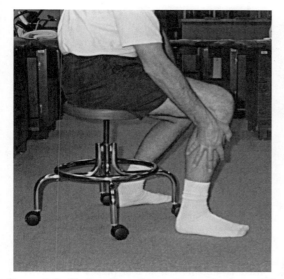

Figure 9–2. Chair rolling. For patients who have difficulty regaining more than 90 degrees of knee flexion, the chair-rolling exercise is an effective method to passively stretch tissues in a relaxed and controlled manner under the patient's control, but not to induce pain or tearing of tissues, which could promote an inflammatory response. With the patient seated on a small stool close to the ground, the knee is flexed to the maximum position possible. This position is held for 1 to 2 minutes while the patient is asked to tolerate mild discomfort. Then, the patient rolls the stool forward maintaining the same foot position on the floor to achieve a few more degrees of flexion. The procedure is repeated for a total of 10 to 12 minutes.

patellar mobility is often associated with knee motion complications and, in extreme cases, the development of patella infera.[25] Patellar glides are performed in all four planes (superior, inferior, medial, and lateral) with sustained pressure applied to the appropriate patellar border for at least 10 seconds (Fig. 9–3). This exercise is performed for 5 minutes whenever range of motion exercises are completed. Caution is warranted if an extensor lag is detected, as this may be associated with poor superior migration of the patella, indicating the need for additional emphasis on this exercise. Patellar mobilization is performed for approximately 5 to 6 weeks postoperatively.

Modalities

The use of therapeutic modalities after ACL reconstruction is usually minimal. The initiation of electrical muscle stimulation (EMS) for quadriceps facilitation is based on the evaluation of quadriceps and vastus medialis obliquus (VMO) muscle tone. A fair or poor muscle tone rating is our indication for EMS. One electrode is placed over the VMO and the second electrode is placed on the central to lateral aspect of the upper one-third of the quadriceps muscle belly. Treatment times are 20 minutes in length. The patient is taught to actively contract the quadriceps muscle simultaneously with the machine's stimulation. This technique is used as an adjunct to the active exercise program. The use of a home EMS machine may be required in individuals whose muscle rating is poor. We continue to use EMS until the muscle grade is rated as good.

Biofeedback therapy also has a pivotal role in facilitating postoperative quadriceps muscle contraction. The surface electrode is placed over the selected muscle component to provide positive feedback to the patient and clinician regarding the quality of active or voluntary quadriceps contraction. Biofeedback is also useful in enhancing hamstring relaxation if the patient experiences difficulty achieving full knee extension secondary to knee pain or muscle spasm. The electrode is placed over the belly of the hamstring muscle while the patient performs range of motion exercises.

Probably the most widely used modality after ACL reconstruction is cryotherapy. This treatment method can be applied through a variety of techniques. We institute cryotherapy in the recovery room after surgery. Although many insurance carriers currently view cold modalities as convenience items, the use of immediate cryotherapy combined with compression has been shown to have an impact on the ability to begin an early approach to aggressive rehabilitation.[26] Cost and patient compliance are two major factors in the success of cryotherapy for postoperative management of pain and swelling. Patient feedback regarding commercially available cold therapy units tends to favor the motorized cooler units (e.g., Polar Care, Breg, Inc., Vista, CA). These units maintain a constant temperature and circulation of ice water through a pad, which provides excellent pain control. One potential drawback with these units is their cost, quoted by a recent study to be approximately $225.00 to the patient.[27]

Gravity flow units (e.g., CryoCuff, AirCast, Summit, NJ) also provide effective pain management. Temperature maintenance with

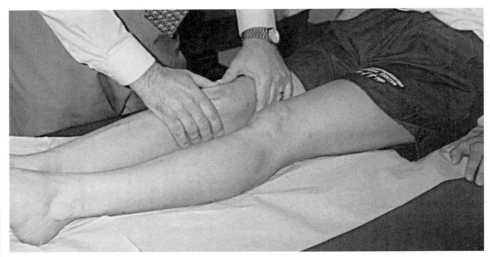

Figure 9–3. Patellar mobilizations. Patellar mobilization is performed to assist in promoting a full range of knee motion and to avoid the complication of patella infera. The patella is mobilized in all four planes with sustained pressure applied to the appropriate border for at least 10 seconds. This exercise is maintained for 5 minutes whenever range of motion exercises are performed.

these units is a little more difficult compared with the motorized cooler units. We have found that the temperature can be controlled by using gravity to backflow and drain the water, refilling the cuff with fresh ice water as required. The standard method of cold therapy is still an ice bag or commercial cold pack, which is kept in the freezer until required. Standard treatment times are 20 minutes and are performed from three times a day to every waking hour, depending on the extent of pain and swelling. In some cases, the treatment time can be extended based on the thickness of the buffer used between the skin and the device. The motorized units contain a thermostat, which is helpful when cold therapy is used for an extended treatment time. Cryotherapy is typically used after exercise or when required for control of pain and swelling, and is maintained throughout the entire postoperative rehabilitation protocol.

Stretching

Flexibility exercises are performed both before and after the ACL reconstruction. Hamstring and gastroc/soleus stretches are initiated the day following surgery. A standard procedure of sustained static stretching is advocated, with the stretch held for 30 seconds and repeated five times. The most common hamstring stretch is the modified hurdler stretch, and the most common gastroc/soleus stretch is the towel pull. These stretches assist in controlling pain, which occurs due to the reflex response created in the hamstrings when the knee is kept in the flexed position. The towel pulling exercise can also help lessen discomfort in the calf, Achilles tendon, and ankle. Additionally, these stretches represent critical components of the knee extension range of motion program. The ability to relax these two muscle groups is imperative to achieve full passive knee extension.

Quadriceps and iliotibial band stretches are performed to assist in achieving full knee flexion and controlling lateral hip and thigh tightness. Complete evaluation of the lower extremity kinetic chain will reveal deficit areas that should be corrected. Other factors to consider when designing a flexibility program include examination of the particular sport or activity the individual wishes to return to, as well as the position or physical requirements of that activity. The stretching program is performed prior to strengthening exercises and before initiating functional or sports activities. Flexibility is incorporated in the maintenance program the individual performs once he or she returns to his or her sport or occupation.

Strengthening

The strengthening program is begun on the first postoperative visit. Early emphasis on the quadriceps muscle group is critical for a successful and safe return to functional activity. In the acute postoperative phase of rehabilitation, initiation of a good voluntary quadriceps contraction sets the tone for the progression of the strengthening program. Isometric quadriceps contractions are completed on an hourly basis following the repetition rules of 10-second holds, 10 repetitions, 10 times per day. Adequate evaluation by both the therapist and patient of this contraction is critical. Patients can monitor contractions by visual or manual means, comparing the quality of the contractions to those achieved by the contralateral limb. They can also assess the superior migration of the patella during the contraction, which should be approximately 1 cm, and the inferior migration of the patella during the initial relaxation of the contraction.

Other exercises included in the acute phase are straight leg raises in the four planes of hip movement. The adduction straight-leg raise has a beneficial effect on the VMO. Supine straight leg raises must include a sufficient isometric quadriceps contraction to benefit the quadriceps. Straight-leg raises in the other two planes are also important for proximal stabilization. As these exercises become easy to perform, Velcro ankle weights are added to progress muscle strengthening. Initially, 1 to 2 pounds of weight are used, and eventually up to 10 pounds is added as long as this is not more than 10 percent of the patient's body weight. Active-assisted range of motion can also be used to facilitate the quadriceps muscle if poor tone is observed during isometric contractions. Primary utilization of these exercises occurs in the first 2 postoperative months, during which time emphasis is placed on controlling pain and swelling, regaining full range of motion, achieving early quadriceps control and proximal stabilization, and resuming a normal gait pattern.

Once partial weight-bearing is initiated, closed kinetic chain (CKC) exercises may begin. Numerous studies have assessed both the safety of these exercises on the healing ACL graft and the benefits incurred to the lower extremity musculature.[28–30] Cup walking is the first CKC exercise we implement (Fig. 9–4). This activity is designed to facilitate adequate quadriceps control during midstance of gait to prevent knee hyperextension from occurring. If necessary, bio-

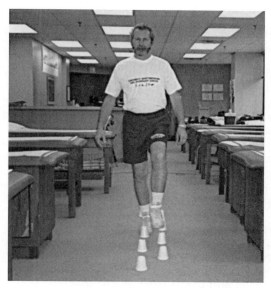

Figure 9–4. Cup walking. Cup walking is begun as soon as the patient is allowed to bear weight and is designed to facilitate quadriceps control during midstance of gait to prevent knee hyperextension.

feedback can also be used to reinforce a good quadriceps contraction.

When the patient progresses to 50 to 75 percent weight-bearing, toe raises for gastroc/soleus strengthening, wall sitting isometrics for quadriceps control, and mini-squats for quadriceps strengthening are begun. The goal of wall sitting is to improve quadriceps contraction by performing the exercise to muscle exhaustion. These exercises can be modified to decrease patellar pain or place additional stress on the quadriceps muscle. Patellar pain can be decreased by either altering the knee flexion angle of the sit or by subtly changing the toe out/toe in angle by no more than 10 degrees. Wall sitting isometrics can be made more challenging by modifying the exercise technique. First, patients can voluntarily set the quadriceps muscle once they reach their maximum knee flexion angle, which is typically between 30 and 45 degrees. This contraction and knee flexion position are held until muscle fatigue occurs, and the exercise is repeated three to five times. In a second modification, the patient performs a hip adduction contraction by squeezing a ball between the distal thighs. This modification promotes a stronger VMO contraction. In a third variation, the patient holds dumbbell weights in his or her hands to increase body weight, which promotes an even stronger quadriceps contraction. Finally, patients can shift their body weight over the involved side to stimulate a single-leg contraction.

The last CKC exercise we recommend is the mini-squat. Initially, the patient's body weight is used as resistance. Gradually, theraband or surgical tubing is employed as resistance mechanisms. The depth of the squat is controlled to protect the patellofemoral joint. Quick, smooth, rhythmic squats are performed to a high set/high repetition cadence to promote muscle fatigue. It is important to monitor hip position to emphasize the quadriceps.

We also include open kinetic chain (OKC) exercises in our rehabilitation program. One advantage of the OKC concept is muscle group isolation. Hamstring curls are initiated with Velcro ankle weights within the first few weeks and eventually weight machines (e.g., (Nautilus, Body Masters, Cybex Eagle) are employed. The advantage of weight machines is the muscle isolation obtained as the machine provides stability to the knee joint. The patient is encouraged to exercise the involved limb alone, as well as both limbs together. If the lightest amount of weight on the machine is too heavy to be lifted by the involved limb alone, the exercise can be performed as an eccentric contraction in which the patient lifts the weight with both legs and lowers the weight with the involved side. Eccentric contractions can also be used in the advanced stages of strength training when tendinitis or overuse syndromes develop from overtraining. Hamstring strength is critical to the overall success of the rehabilitation program because of the complementary role that this musculature plays in the dynamic stabilization of the knee joint. Function of the hamstrings, knee flexion, and hip extension are all emphasized. Weight training is used throughout the advanced program and continues in the return to activity and maintenance phase of rehabilitation.

Knee extension exercises are used to further develop quadriceps muscle strength. Caution is warranted because of the potential problems these exercises may create for the healing graft and the patellofemoral joint. Resisted knee extension is begun with Velcro ankle weights in the first few weeks postoperatively in the range of 90 to 30 degrees. We avoid the range of 30 to 0 degrees where anterior tibial translation forces are highest.[31] Many patients have an unsatisfactory outcome based on persistent anterior or patellofemoral knee pain, which can occur because of improper training in the terminal phase of extension. Therefore, our recommendations for knee extension exercises include emphasis on patellofemoral protection (monitoring for changes in pain, swelling, and crepitus), protection against high anterior tibial translation forces, and a gradual progression of weight to avoid overuse syndromes.

A full lower extremity strengthening program is critical for early and long-term success of the rehabilitation program. Other muscle groups included in this routine are the hip abductors, hip adductors, hip flexors, and hip extensors. These muscle groups can be exercised on either the multi-hip machine or the hip abductor/adductor machine. Gastroc/soleus strength is a key component for both early ambulation and the running program. In addition, an upper extremity and torso strength program is important for safe return to work or sports. These exercises are included as part of general conditioning, and general strength training concepts are emphasized. Sport and position specificity are taken into account when devising the program to maximize its benefits.

Balance/proprioceptive Training

Balance and proprioceptive training are initiated as soon as the patient begins partial weight-bearing. The first exercise involves weight shifting from side to side and front to back. This activity encourages patient confidence in the leg's ability to withstand the pressures of weight-bearing and initiates the stimulus to knee joint position sense. A second exercise begun with partial weight-bearing is cup walking. This activity is designed to develop symmetry between the surgical and uninvolved limbs. Cup walking helps develop hip and knee flexion, quadriceps control during midstance, hip and pelvic control during midstance, and adequate gastroc/soleus control during push-off. This exercise also helps to control hip hiking. These components of gait control are critical in the early phases of rehabilitation to decrease the stresses to the healing graft. One other activity for balance control is the single-leg balance exercise. The stance position is key to making this exercise beneficial. The patient is instructed to point the foot straight ahead, flex the knee approximately 20 to 30 degrees, extend the arms outward to horizontal, and position the torso upright with the shoulders above the hips and the hips above the ankles. The object of this activity is to stand in position until balance is disturbed. A mini-trampoline can be used to make this exercise more challenging. The unstable position the trampoline creates with the soft surface requires greater dynamic limb control than that used to stand on a flat surface.

The progression of balance training leads to the use of more sophisticated systems. There are many balance systems available, with a wide cost variance. Some of the lower-end technical devices include styrofoam half rolls, whole rolls, and the Biomechanical Ankle Platform System (BAPS, Camp, Jackson, MI). Clinically, we feel that these devices help to develop balance, coordination, and proprioception; however, there are few data in the literature to assess their efficacy. In the early phases of full, unassisted weight-bearing, half foam rolls are used as part of the gait retraining program. Walking on half rolls helps the patient develop balance and dynamic muscular control required to maintain an upright position and be able to walk from one end of the roll to the other. Developing a center of balance, limb symmetry, quadriceps control in midstance, and postural positioning are benefits obtained from this type of training. Use of the BAPS board in double-leg and single-leg stance provides another proprioceptive exercise.

The use of more sophisticated devices adds another dimension to the proprioception program, as certain units objectively attempt to document balance and dynamic control. Three of the more common units include Breg's Kinesthetic Awareness Trainer (Breg, Inc., Vista, CA), Biodex's Stabilometry System (Biodex Corporation, Shirley, NY), and Neurocom's Balance System (Neurocom, Clackamas, OR). While these systems may provide objective information, more research is required to justify the cost and reliability of each unit.

In the later phases of rehabilitation, plyometric exercises are initiated to provide a functional basis for return to activity. The first exercise is level-surface box hopping. A four-square grid is created with tape on the floor of four equally sized boxes. The patient is instructed to first hop from box 1 to box 3 (front-to-back), and then from box 1 to box 2 (side-to-side). Several instructions are very important to ensure safety of this exercise. The drill is initially performed using both legs. The patient is instructed to keep the body weight on the ball of the foot, to hop with the knees bent, and to land in flexion to avoid knee hyperextension. It is also important for the patient to understand that the exercise is a reaction and agility drill; therefore, speed is emphasized. It is important for the patient to focus on limb symmetry during this exercise. One way to measure improvement is to count the number of hops in a defined time period. The initial exercise time period is 15 seconds. The patient is asked to complete as many hops between the squares as possible in 15 seconds. Three sets are performed for both directions and the number of hops is recorded. An assistant is present to count and time the exercise. Progression of the program occurs as the number of hops, as well as patient confidence, improves. This exercise has four levels. The first level includes front-to-back and side-to-side hopping previously described. The second level incorporates both of the directions in level one into one sequence, and also includes hopping in both right and left directions (i.e., box 1 to box 2 to box 4 to box 2 to box 1). Level three progresses to diagonal hops, and level four includes pivot hops in a 180-degree direction. Once the patient can perform level four double-leg hops, we initiate similar exercises using single-leg hops.

The next phase of plyometric exercises utilizes vertical box hops. It is important to stress that plyometric exercise is intense and adequate rest must be included in the program. Individual sessions can be performed in a manner similar to interval training. Initially, the rest period lasts two to three times the length of the exercise period and is gradually decreased to one to two times the length of the exercise period. Also, plyometric hopping is performed two to three times each week and is incorporated into the strength and cardiovascular endurance program.

Other parameters to consider when performing plyometric exercises include surface, footwear, and warm-up. This program should be performed on a surface that is firm yet forgiving, such as a wooden gym floor. Very hard surfaces like concrete should be avoided. A cross-training or running shoe should be worn to provide adequate shock absorption, as well as adequate stability to the foot. Checking wear patterns and outer sole wear will help avoid overuse injuries. Finally, an adequate warm-up should include exercises and a light cardiovascular workout.

Conditioning

Depending on accessibility, a cardiovascular program can be initiated as soon as the patient can sufficiently tolerate the upright position with an upper body ergometer (UBE). A neutrally supported position of the surgical limb should be encouraged to minimize lower extremity swelling. This exercise can be performed to tolerance. Stationary bicycling can be initiated as soon as partial weight-bearing begins and the range of motion is adequate to allow completion of repetitions. Water walking is begun based on wound care and weight-bearing status. Early goals of these programs include facilitation of full range of motion, gait retraining, and cardiovascular reconditioning. To improve cardiovascular endurance, the program should be performed at least three times per week for 20 to 30 minutes, and the exercise performed to at least 60 to 85 percent of maximal heart rate. It is generally thought that performing in the higher levels of percentage of maximal heart rate achieves greater cardiovascular efficiency and endurance.

Gradually, cross-country ski and stair climbing machines are incorporated. Protection against high stresses to the patellofemoral joint is strongly advocated in patients with symptoms or articular cartilage deterioration. During bicycling, the seat height is adjusted to its highest level based on patient body size and a low resistance level is used during the workout. If a stair climbing machine is tolerated, we suggest maintaining a short step and using lower resistance levels. Monitoring heart rate will ensure that work levels are sufficient to improve cardiovascular fitness.

A complete cardiovascular exercise program is an important component of the later phases of rehabilitation. In addition to the previously described exercises, an aquatic program that includes lap work using freestyle or flutter kicking, water walking, water aerobics, and deep water running is initiated. Determining which cardiovascular exercises are appropriate is based on each individual patient. Factors to assess include concomitant operative procedures, secondary injuries, access to specific equipment, individual preferences, and prior experience. The primary consideration for the conditioning program throughout the rehabilitation protocol is to stress the cardiovascular system without compromising the joint.

Running and Return to Sports Activities

To initiate the running program, the patient must demonstrate no more than a 30 percent deficit in average torque for the quadriceps and hamstrings on isometric testing, have no more than 3 mm of increase in AP displacement on arthrometer testing, and be at least 12 weeks postoperative. The majority of our patients begin straight running between the fourth and sixth month postoperatively. The design of the running program is based on the sport the patient desires to return to, as well as the particular position or physical requirements of the activity. For instance, an individual returning to short-duration, high-intensity activities participates in a sprinting program rather than a long-distance endurance program.

As previously stated, the beginning level running program is first performed with a straight ahead walk/run combination. Running distances are 20, 40, 60, and 100 yards in both forward and backward directions. Initially, running speed is approximately one-quarter to one-half of the patient's normal speed, and gradually progresses to three-quarters and full speed. An interval training-rest approach is applied by which the rest phase is two to three times the length of the training phase. The running program is performed three times per week, on opposite days to the strength program. Since the running program may not reach aerobic levels initially, a cross-training program is used to facilitate cardiovascular fitness. The cross-training program is performed on the same day as the strength workout.

After the patient is able to run straight ahead at full speed, the program progresses to include lateral running and crossover maneuvers. Short distances, such as 20 yards, are used to work on speed and agility. Side-to-side running over cups may be used to facilitate proprioception. At this time, sport-specific equipment is introduced to enhance skill development (e.g., a soccer ball for a soccer player to work on dribbling and passing activities). These variations are useful to motivate the patient and minimize training boredom.

Another level of the running program incorporates figure-of-eight running drills. These drills begin with long and wide movement patterns to encourage subtle cutting. The training distance initially is 20 yards; as speed and confidence improve, the distance is decreased to approximately 10 yards. Progression through this phase is similar to that used in the lateral side-to-side program just described. Speed and agility are emphasized and equipment is introduced to develop sport-specific skills.

The fourth phase in the running program introduces cutting patterns. These patterns include directional changes at 45- and 90-degree angles, which allow the patient to progress from subtle to sharp cuts. Once the patient has completed the functional program and the strength, displacement, and function testing reach normal values, return to sports is allowed. A trial of function is encouraged in which the patient is monitored for overuse symptoms or giving-way episodes. Upon successful return to activity, the patient is encouraged to continue with a maintenance program. During the in-season, a conditioning program of two workouts a week is recommended. In the off-season or pre-season, this program should be performed three times a week to maximize gains in flexibility, strength, and cardiovascular endurance.

REHABILITATION PROTOCOL FOR ANTERIOR CRUCIATE LIGAMENT ALLOGRAFT, REVISION, OR COMPLEX PATELLAR TENDON AUTOGENOUS RECONSTRUCTION

We also developed a rehabilitation protocol for patients who have had ACL allograft reconstructions, ACL revision reconstructions (with either allogeneic or autogeneic tissue), or complex patellar tendon autogenous reconstructions in which concomitant meniscal repair, ligament reconstruction, or patellofemoral realignment procedures were performed, or in whom significant articular cartilage lesions were found during the operation (Table 9–4). Delays in return of full knee flexion, weight-bearing, initiation of certain strengthening and conditioning exercises, and initiation of running and return to full sports activities are incorporated. These delays are advocated to protect the healing concomitant meniscal or ligament repairs or to avoid exacerbating articular cartilage deterioration or symptoms.

Weight-bearing is delayed for approximately 3 to 4 weeks to allow for sufficient healing as well as evaluation of postoperative pain and swelling, quadriceps muscle control, and range of motion. The amount of weight is then progressed approximately 25 percent of the patient's body weight each week as long as the patient reaches the goals set forth and evaluations of the postoperative radiographs show adequate healing. The patients are weaned from crutches by the eighth week postoperatively.

Range of motion represents the second area modified in this protocol. Knees that undergo a concomitant lateral or posterolateral procedure are placed into either a bivalved long leg cast or long leg postoperative brace locked at 15 degrees of flexion. The patient removes the device to perform range of motion exercises several times a day and is instructed to reach 0 degrees of extension, but to avoid hyperextension. In individuals who have a hyperelastic tissue type, knee extension is limited to -15 degrees for approximately 3 weeks to allow for sufficient healing before stress is applied to push for 0 degrees. Hyperextension is avoided during both range of motion exercises and ambulation.

Knee flexion is protected in patients who have concomitant proximal patellar realignment. These knees are allowed 0 to 90 degrees for the first 2 postoperative weeks. Then, the flexion goals are to reach 110 degrees by the fourth week, and 135 degrees by the sixth week. Additional range of motion beyond 135 degrees is expected to be obtained gradually over time as the patient's activity level increases. Knee flexion is also limited in knees that have a concomitant PCL reconstruction. In these cases, the PCL protocol takes precedence, owing to the significant increase in force that is created on

Table 9–4. Cincinnati Sportsmedicine and Orthopaedic Center Rehabilitation Protocol for Anterior Cruciate Ligament Allograft, Revision, or Complex Patellar Tendon Autogenous Reconstruction

	Postoperative Weeks			Postoperative Months	
	1 to 4	*5 to 8*	*9 to 12*	*4 to 6*	*7 to 12*
Brace: postoperative and functional	X	X	X	X	X
Range of motion (degrees)					
Minimum goals 0–90	X				
0–120		X			
0–135		X			
Weight-bearing					
Toe touch to one-quarter of body weight	X				
Full		X			
Patella mobilization	X	X			
Modalities					
Electrical muscle stimulation (EMS)	X	X			
Pain/edema management (cryotherapy)	X	X	X	X	X
Stretching					
Hamstring, gastroc/soleus, iliotibial band, quadriceps	X	X	X	X	X
Strengthening					
Quadriceps isometrics, straight-leg raises, active knee extension	X	X	X		
Closed-chain (gait retraining, toe raises, wall sits, mini-squats)	X	X	X	X	
Knee flexion hamstring curls (90 degrees)		X	X	X	X
Knee extension quads (90–30 degrees)		X	X	X	X
Hip abduction-adduction, multi-hip		X	X	X	X
Leg press (70–10 degrees)		X	X	X	X
Balance/proprioceptive training		X	X	X	X
Weight-shifting, mini-trampoline, BAPS, KAT, plyometrics					
Conditioning					
UBE	X	X			
Bicycling (stationary)		X	X	X	X
Aquatic program		X	X	X	X
Swimming (kicking)			X	X	X
Walking			X	X	X
Stair-climbing machine			X	X	X
Ski machine			X	X	X
Running: straight				X	X
Cutting: lateral carioca, figure-of-eights					X
Full sports					X

the PCL past 90 degrees of flexion. These knees are therefore kept at 90 degrees for approximately 3 weeks postoperatively, and then flexion is gradually progressed over the next 6 weeks. Knee flexion is protected in patients who have a concomitant meniscus repair. Flexion in these individuals is limited to 90 degrees for 2 weeks to protect the meniscus repair site.

The final modification of this protocol is return to activity, which is delayed until at least the sixth postoperative month. In these knees, additional time is required for healing of all repaired and reconstructed tissues, and return of joint and muscle function. Evaluation is a key component to allow initiation of the functional program, which includes the subjective questionnaire and examination of knee motion, muscle strength, and ligament stability. It should be the sum of the evaluation that determines return to function, not just one parameter. In these knees, return to full activity is not expected to occur until the ninth to twelfth postoperative month. It should also be noted that return to full activity does not guarantee return to pre-injury activity levels.

CLINICAL OUTCOME STUDIES

We have completed several patient outcome studies following ACL patellar tendon autogenous and allogeneic reconstructions that support the rehabilitation programs described in this chapter (Table 9–5).[2–10, 32–37] All of these studies incorporated serial knee joint arthrometer testing throughout the postoperative course to assess the effect of various exercises on AP displacements. Additionally, all used the Cincinnati Knee Rating System to determine outcome. The following are brief summaries of some of these studies; the reader is encouraged to seek the original references for detailed information. We currently prefer patellar tendon autografts as our first choice for ACL reconstructions, reserving allografts for knees requiring multiple ligamentous reconstructive procedures or revision operations where suitable autogenous graft material does not exist.

A prospective study of 94 consecutive patients who received ACL patellar tendon autogenous reconstruction between August 1990 and July 1992 was conducted to determine whether differences in outcome existed between patients who had the reconstruction for acute ACL ruptures and those who had chronic ruptures.[10] Eighty-seven patients returned for follow-up a mean of 28 months postoperatively. Normal or partial ACL function (≤5 mm difference between limbs) was restored in 97 percent of the knees in both acute and chronic rupture subgroups. Only one patient had a knee motion complication. In the patient rating of the overall knee condition, 69 percent of the knees with chronic ruptures and 100 percent of the knees with acute ruptures scored in the normal or very good range.

An investigation was conducted to determine whether differences existed in outcome and complications between men and women who received ACL patellar tendon autogenous reconstruction between January 1991 and September 1993.[4] Forty-seven patients of each sex, matched for chronicity of injury, age, preoperative sports activity levels, articular cartilage condition, and months of follow-up, were studied. All returned a mean of 26 months postoperatively. No significant differences were found between men and women for stability, complications, or outcome. Women required an average of six more rehabilitation visits than

● ▬▬ **Table 9–5. Stability and Complication Rates from Cincinnati Sportsmedicine's Prospective Studies on ACL Allogeneic and Autogeneic Reconstruction Using Protocols Described in Tables 9–3 and 9–4**

Study	Population Description	KT-1000 Testing (%) Normal/Partial ACL Function Restored (≤5 mm I-N)	Failure (≥6 mm I-N)	Knee Motion Complications (manipulations, surgical releases) (%)
Noyes et al.[6]	47 allografts, acute	95	5	17
Noyes & Barber[9]	64 allografts alone, chronic	88	12	3
	40 allografts + EA, chronic	96	4	8
Noyes & Barber[32]	64 allografts alone, chronic	87	13	3
	46 allografts + LAD, chronic	83	17	2
Noyes & Barber-Westin[33]	65 allografts, revisions, chronic	83	17	6
Noyes & Barber-Westin[7]	46 allografts + MCL, acute	89	11	22
Noyes & Barber-Westin[8]	68 allografts, acute, some + MCL	97	3	24
Noyes & Barber-Westin[36]	40 allografts, chronic arthrosis	76	24	0
Noyes & Barber-Westin[10]	87 autografts, acute vs chronic	96	4	1
Barber-Westin et al.[4]	94 autografts, men vs women	91	9	1
Noyes & Barber-Westin[37]	38 autografts, WC vs no WC	97	3	0
Noyes & Barber-Westin[35]	53 autografts, chronic arthrosis	95	5	4

I = involved, N = noninvolved, EA = extra-articular, LAD = ligament augmentation device, MCL = medial collateral ligament, WC = Workers' Compensation.

men; however, none required additional surgery for knee motion complications and the rate of patellofemoral crepitus conversion was only 7 percent, lower than that found for men (15 percent). Normal or partial ACL function was restored in 94 percent of the women and 96 percent of the men.

We studied the efficacy of ACL reconstruction in knees with symptomatic arthrosis determined by direct arthroscopic visualization using both allografts[36] and autografts.[35] Patients selected for these studies had advanced articular cartilage lesions—fissuring and fragmentation extending greater than one-half of the depth of the cartilage or subchondral bone exposure. Using the delayed protocol defined in this chapter, both studies showed statistically significant reductions in pain, swelling, and functional limitations with daily and sports activities. In the allograft population of 40 patients followed for a mean of 37 months, no patient had a knee motion complication, and normal or partial ACL stability was restored in 70 percent. At follow-up, 42 percent rated their knee condition as normal/very good, 24 percent as good, 21 percent as fair, and 13 percent as poor. In the patellar tendon autograft population of 53 patients followed an average of 27 months postoperatively, only 2 patients had a knee motion complication, and normal or partial ACL stability was restored in 94 percent. At follow-up, 79 percent had returned to sports activities—mostly light recreational based on our recommendations—without symptoms.

Sixty-eight patients who received allogeneic ACL reconstruction between November 1982 and April 1987 for acute ruptures returned for an early postoperative evaluation (2- to 4-year) and a later evaluation (5- to 9-year) to assess whether there were any changes in results over time.[8] There were no significant changes in AP displacement, patellofemoral crepitus, the pain or jumping scores, or the overall knee rating over the time period studied. Three knees (4 percent) required a reoperation for knee arthrofibrosis and 13 knees required a gentle manipulation under anesthesia for limitations of flexion. A full range of motion (0 to 135 degrees) was restored in all but 6 knees that lacked 1 to 5 degrees of full extension. At the most recent follow-up evaluation, 93 percent of the grafts were rated as functional or partially functional.

To directly assess the effect of the rehabilitation program designed for patients who received allogeneic ACL reconstructions, we sequentially measured AP displacements with the KT-1000 on 84 patients who were followed for at least 2 years postoperatively.[3] This study allowed us to determine whether correlations existed between the initial onset of abnormal displacements (greater than 2.5 mm increase between limbs) and time from surgery or the phase of rehabilitation. Fifty-two patients received only an allograft; 78 percent of these had normal or partial stability restored. Thirty-two patients received an allograft and an iliotibial band extra-articular procedure; 97 percent of these had normal or partial stability restored postoperatively. The study showed that the rehabilitation program did not result in an increased incidence of abnormal displacements in the early phases after surgery. The abnormal displacements typically occurred during intensive strength training or after return to sports activities. Approximately one-third of the abnormal displacements occurred more than 2 years postoperatively.

Two investigations were conducted regarding the outcome of revision ACL surgery using allografts[33] and autografts[34] and the delayed rehabilitation protocol described in this chapter. The allograft group consisted of 65 patients followed a mean of 42 months postoperatively and the autograft group was composed of 20 patients followed an average of 27 months postoperatively. No patient in either group required a reoperation for a knee motion complication. Four patients in the allograft group and one patient in the autograft group required gentle manipulations under anesthesia for limitations in knee motion. All but one regained a normal range of motion. Normal or partial stability was restored in 67 percent of the allograft group and 73 percent of the autograft group. Significant improvements were noted in both groups for symptoms, functional limitations, AP displacements, and the overall rating scores. Although we prefer patellar tendon autogenous grafts for revision cases, allografts can be used because they offer reasonable success rates for patients who are symptomatic with daily activities.

Using the rehabilitation protocols described in this chapter, we have found that 94 percent of patients will regain a normal range of knee motion without additional measures, and that 98 percent of patients will eventually regain full motion by 1 year postoperatively. In a recent investigation, we followed 443 patients who returned an average of 25 months (range, 12 to 86 months) after ACL autogenous reconstruction. We assessed the effect of several variables on the final motion achieved, including concomitant operative procedures, gender, injury chronicity, condition of the articular cartilage surfaces, location of physical therapy, prior surgery, and prior failed ACL reconstructions.

At follow-up, a normal range of motion was found in 385 of the 436 patients (88 percent). Twenty-three individuals required additional treatment for motion limitations, all of whom demonstrated at least 0 to 135 degrees of motion at follow-up. The treatment interventions included extension casting in nine patients, gentle manipulations in nine patients, arthroscopic débridement in three patients, and intensive in-patient physical therapy in two patients.

Seven other patients in whom additional treatment measures were not used had a limitation of extension of −3 to −5 degrees at follow-up.

A concomitant medial collateral ligament repair had a significant clinical effect on motion complications as two of the nine patients (22 percent) who had such a repair required treatment intervention. None of the other variables assessed influenced motion complications.

Knee arthrometer testing at follow-up showed that the program was safe in terms of AP displacements, as 272 of 312 patients tested (87 percent) had less than 3 mm of increased displacement, 27 patients (9 percent) had 3 to 5.5 mm of increase, and 13 patients (4 percent) had 6 mm or more of increase.

SUMMARY

Amid controversy regarding rehabilitation after ACL reconstruction, we provide two postoperative protocols based on extensive research, clinical outcome investigations, and experience that provide either a progressive or a delayed approach to the management of various patient populations. Both protocols follow similar early postoperative concepts of immediate knee motion and early weight-bearing—concepts that we

have used successfully for 2 decades. The progressive program was designed for patients who undergo autogenous reconstruction and who desire to return to strenuous athletics or occupations early postoperatively. Strict criteria are detailed for inclusion in this protocol, as well as cautions for problems that may occur postoperatively which would necessitate delays in exercise progression and return to activity. The second protocol was developed for patients who undergo allograft, revision, or complex reconstructions in which major concomitant procedures are performed, or for patients who have significant articular cartilage deterioration. This program delays the return of full weight-bearing, initiation of certain strengthening and conditioning exercises, and return to running and sports activities. The results of several clinical outcome studies are provided to demonstrate the effectiveness of these protocols in various patient populations.

References

1. Noyes FR, Butler DL, Paulos LE, Grood ES: Intra-articular cruciate reconstruction. I: Perspectives on graft strength, vascularization, and immediate motion after replacement. Clin Orthop 172:71, 1983.
2. Noyes FR, Mangine RE, Barber SD: Early knee motion after open and arthroscopic anterior cruciate ligament reconstruction. Am J Sports Med 15:149, 1987.
3. Barber-Westin SD, Noyes FR: The effect of rehabilitation on anterior/posterior knee displacements following anterior cruciate ligament reconstruction. Am J Sports Med 21:264, 1993.
4. Barber-Westin SD, Noyes FR, Andrews MA: A rigorous comparison between the sexes of results and complications after anterior cruciate ligament reconstruction. Am J Sports Med 25:514, 1997.
5. Buseck MS, Noyes FR: Arthroscopic evaluation of meniscal repairs after anterior cruciate ligament reconstruction and immediate motion. Am J Sports Med 19:489, 1991.
6. Noyes FR, Barber SD, Mangine RE: Bone-patellar ligament-bone and fascia lata allografts for anterior cruciate ligament reconstruction. J Bone Joint Surg 72A:1125, 1990.
7. Noyes FR, Barber-Westin SD: The treatment of acute combined ruptures of the anterior cruciate and medial ligaments of the knee. Am J Sports Med 23:380, 1995.
8. Noyes FR, Barber-Westin SD: Reconstruction of the anterior cruciate ligament with human allograft. Comparison of early and later results. J Bone Joint Surg 78A:524, 1996.
9. Noyes FR, Barber SD: The effect of an extra-articular procedure on allograft reconstructions for chronic ruptures of the anterior cruciate ligament. J Bone Joint Surg 73A:882, 1991.

10. Noyes FR, Barber-Westin SD: A comparison of results in acute and chronic anterior cruciate ligament ruptures of arthroscopically assisted autogenous patellar tendon reconstruction. Am J Sports Med 25:460, 1997.
11. DeMaio M, Mangine RE, Noyes FR, Barber SD: Advanced muscle training after ACL reconstruction: Weeks 6 to 52. Orthopedics 15:757, 1992.
12. DeMaio M, Noyes FR, Mangine RE: Principles for aggressive rehabilitation after reconstruction of the anterior cruciate ligament. Orthopedics 15:385, 1992.
13. Mangine RE, Noyes FR, DeMaio M: Minimal protection program: Advanced weight bearing and range of motion after ACL reconstruction—Weeks 1 to 5. Orthopedics 15:504, 1992.
14. Noyes FR, DeMaio M, Mangine RE: Evaluation-based protocols: A new approach to rehabilitation. Orthop 14:1383, 1991.
15. Noyes FR, Mangine RE, Barber SD: The early treatment of motion complications after reconstruction of the anterior cruciate ligament. Clin Orthop 277:217, 1992.
16. Noyes FR, Barber SD, Mooar LA: A rationale for assessing sports activity levels and limitations in knee disorders. Clin Orthop 246:238, 1989.
17. Noyes FR, Mooar LA, Barber SD: The assessment of work-related activities and limitations in knee disorders. Am J Sports Med 19:178, 1991.
18. Daniel DM, Malcolm LL, Losse G, et al.: Instrumented measurement of anterior laxity of the knee. J Bone Joint Surg 67A:720, 1985.
19. Barber SD, Noyes FR, Mangine RE, et al: Quantitative assessment of functional limitations in normal and anterior cruciate ligament-deficient knees. Clin Orthop 255:204, 1990.
20. Noyes FR, Barber SD, Mangine RE: Abnormal lower limb symmetry determined by function hop tests after anterior cruciate ligament rupture. Am J Sports Med 19:513, 1991.
21. McLaughlin JR, Noyes FR: Arthroscopic meniscus repair: Recommended surgical techniques for complex meniscal tears. Tech Orthop 8:129, 1993.
22. Rubman MH, Noyes FR, Barber-Westin SD: Technical considerations in the management of complex meniscus tears. Clin Sports Med 15:511, 1996.
23. Rubman MH, Noyes FR, Barber-Westin SD: Arthroscopic repair of meniscus tears that extend into the avascular zone: A review of 198 single and complex repairs. Am J Sports Med 26:, 1998.
24. Noyes FR, Dunworth LA, Andriacchi TP, et al: Knee hyperextension gait abnormalities in unstable knees: Recognition and preoperative gait retraining. Am J Sports Med 24:35, 1996.
25. Noyes FR, Wojtys EM, Marshall MT: The early diagnosis and treatment of developmental patella infera syndrome. Clin Orthop 265:241, 1991.
26. Shelbourne K, Rubinstein R, McCarroll J: Postoperative cryotherapy for the knee in ACL reconstructive surgery. Orthop Int 2:165, 1994.
27. Konrath GA, Lock T, Giotz HT, Scheidler J: The use of cold therapy after anterior cruciate ligament reconstruction. A prospective, randomized study and literature review. Am J Sports Med 24:629, 1996.
28. Bynum EB, Barrack RL, Alexander AH: Open versus closed chain kinetic exercises after anterior cruciate ligament reconstruction: A prospective randomized study. Am J Sports Med 23:401, 1995.
29. Lutz GE, Palmitier RA, An KN, Chao EYS: Comparison of tibiofemoral joint forces during open-kinetic-chain and closed-kinetic-chain exercises. J Bone Joint Surg 75A:732, 1993.
30. Yack HF, Collins CE, Whieldon TJ: Comparison of closed and open kinetic chain exercise in the anterior cruciate ligament-deficient knee. Am J Sports Med 21:49, 1993.
31. Grood ES, Suntay WJ, Noyes FR, Butler DL: Biomechanics of the knee-extension exercise: Effect of cutting the anterior cruciate ligament. J Bone Joint Surg 66A:725, 1984.
32. Noyes FR, Barber SD: The effect of a ligament augmentation device on allograft reconstructions for chronic ruptures of the anterior cruciate ligament. J Bone Joint Surg 74A:960, 1992.
33. Noyes FR, Barber-Westin SD: Use of allografts after failed treatment of rupture of the anterior cruciate ligament. J Bone Joint Surg 76A:1019, 1994.
34. Noyes FR, Barber-Westin SD: Revision anterior cruciate ligament surgery with allograft and autograft tissues: Experience from Cincinnati. Clin Orthop 325:116, 1996.
35. Noyes FR, Barber-Westin SD: Anterior cruciate ligament reconstruction with autogenous patellar tendon graft in patients with articular cartilage damage. Am J Sports Med 25:626, 1997.
36. Noyes FR, Barber-Westin SD: Arthroscopic-assisted allograft anterior cruciate ligament reconstruction in patients with symptomatic arthrosis. Arthrosc J Arthrosc Rel Surg 13:24, 1997.
37. Noyes FR, Barber-Westin SD: A comparison of results of arthroscopic-assisted anterior cruciate ligament reconstruction between Worker's Compensation and noncompensation patients. Arthroscopy 13:474, 1997.

IXA Cincinnati Sports Activity Scale

LEVEL	FREQUENCY RATING
	I (participates 4–7 days/week)
100	Jumping, hard pivoting, cutting (basketball, volleyball, football, gymnastics, soccer)
95	Running, twisting, turning (tennis, racquetball, handball, ice hockey, field hockey, skiing, wrestling)
90	No running, twisting, jumping (cycling, swimming)
	II (participates 1–3 days/week)
85	Jumping, hard pivoting, cutting (basketball, volleyball, football, gymnastics, soccer)
80	Running, twisting, turning (tennis, racquetball, handball, ice hockey, field hockey, skiing, wrestling)
75	No running, twisting, jumping (cycling, swimming)
	III (participates 1–3 times/month)
65	Jumping, hard pivoting, cutting (basketball, volleyball, football, gymnastics, soccer)
60	Running, twisting, turning (tennis, racquetball, handball, ice hockey, field hockey, skiing, wrestling)
55	No running, twisting, jumping (cycling, swimming)
	IV (no sports)
40	I perform activities of daily living without problems
20	I have moderate problems with activities of daily living
0	I have severe problems with activities of daily living; on crutches, full disability

From Noyes FR, Barber SD, Mooar LA: A rationale for assessing sports activity levels and limitations in knee disorders. Clin Orthop 246:238, 1989.

IXB Cincinnati Symptom Rating Scale*

SCALE DESCRIPTION

10	Normal knee, able to do strenuous work/sports with jumping, hard pivoting
8	Able to do moderate work/sports with running, turning, and twisting; symptoms with strenuous work/sports
6	Able to do light work/sports with no running, twisting, or jumping; symptoms with moderate work/sports
4	Able to do activities of daily living alone; symptoms with light work/sports
2	Moderate symptoms (frequent, limiting) with activities of daily living
0	Severe symptoms (constant, not relieved) with activities of daily living

*Symptoms rated are pain, swelling, partial giving-way, and full giving-way.

From Noyes FR, Barber SD, Mooar LA: A rationale for assessing sports activity levels and limitations in knee disorders. Clin Orthop 246:238, 1989.

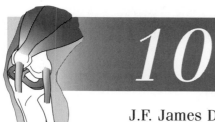

10 Synthetic Ligaments in Anterior Cruciate Ligament Reconstruction

J.F. James Davidson, MD, and H. Royer Collins, MD

Synthetic ligaments have been used in anterior cruciate ligament (ACL) reconstructions for nearly a century. In 1914, Connor described the use of a loop of silver wire to reconstruct the ACL, stating that the patient was "much pleased."[1, 2] Problems with existing synthetic ligaments and reproducibly good results with autogenous grafting make autogenous grafts the current choice in most ACL reconstructions.[3–5] However, synthetics may play a role in some special circumstances. The role of synthetic ligaments may expand in the future, and worthwhile investigation is currently underway.

DEVELOPMENT

The impetus for synthetic ligaments remains the same as it began. Synthetics offer obvious advantages: no donor site morbidity, no disease transmission, infinite availability, immediate maximum strength, more rapid rehabilitation, smaller incisions, and shorter operating room time. Unfortunately, numerous complications have been reported with most existing synthetic ligaments. Synovitis, effusion, mechanical loosening, re-rupture, tunnel osteolysis, and accelerated arthritis have been reported.[6–22] On the other hand, many complications have also been reported with autogenous grafting. Patellar tendon rupture, patellar fracture, chondromalacia patella, patellar capture, arthrofibrosis, failure of graft incorporation, and re-rupture have been described.[23–40] Similarly, the use of allografts carries complication potential as well. Rerupture, delayed incorporation, gradual lengthening, immunologic reactions, persistent inflammatory response, and communicable disease transmission are documented in the literature.[3, 26, 41–46] Moreover, lack of availability, relatively complicated storage, and transportation procedures are also drawbacks.

An ideal ACL substitute would capitalize on the potential benefits of the synthetic ligament while avoiding its pitfalls. The goal is a graft that provides no donor site morbidity, immediate high tensile strength, minimal fatigue or creep properties, inert nature, reproduction of normal knee biomechanics, simple implantation, and ready availability.[3, 26, 47, 48] Furthermore, once implanted, the ligament would be replaced by remodeling autogenous tissue with characteristics similar to those of the natural ACL.[3, 48] Jackson et al.[3] proposed that a synthetic ligament in the form of a collagen matrix scaffold might fulfill these characteristics. They summarized that "a biologic substitute that is either bioengineered or remodeled by the host to the point of duplicating the original ACL remains the goal for investigators."

CATEGORIZATION OF FAILURE OF AUTOGENOUS GRAFTS

Numerous authors have attempted to categorize failures of ACL reconstructions.[4, 26, 27] The University of Pittsburgh grouped recurrent patholaxity into three categories: (1) errors in surgical technique, (2) failure of incorporation, and (3) trauma.[27]

Error in Surgical Technique
- Initially incompletely recognized or addressed complex ligament injuries[4, 6, 49, 50]
- Inadequate notch plasties[50–53]
- Improper tunnel placement[54–58]
- Improper graft tensioning[59, 60]
- Insufficient fixation[60, 62]

Failure of Incorporation
- Failure of graft to mature and remodel[27, 29, 61, 63, 64]

Trauma
- Insufficient or excessive rehabilitation[4, 27]
- Recurrent injury (the knee abuser)[4, 6, 27, 55]

Recognition of these problems and refinement in techniques have led to improved results with autogenous ACL reconstruction. Accelerated rehabilitation programs have lessened the time necessary to safely return to sports and activities.[65, 66] In spite of better recognition and avoidance of pitfalls in ACL reconstruction, there remain graft failures following reconstruction. Revision in most circumstances relies on recognizing the mistake leading to the failure and avoiding it in the revision. For example, recognizing and addressing a concurrent instability pattern, revising the location of tunnels, or avoiding recurrent trauma in the revision may prevent recurrent failure with the second attempt.

BIOLOGIC FAILURE

Some failures occur when no mistakes were made on the part of the surgeon and no recurrent trauma was sustained by the patient. One reason for recurrent instability is failure of incorporation of the graft by the host. Why this occurs is not fully understood. Noyes et al.,[67] Arnoczky et al.[68], Johnson[69] and others[63] have described the process of revascularization and maturation with development of new remodeling collagenous tissue that occurs after successful autogenous ACL reconstruction. Conversely, failure of incorporation and remodeling in some failed reconstructions has been reported by multiple authors.[4, 27, 29, 61, 63] Many have recognized and characterized the problem of failure of maturation without an underlying technical or mechanical cause. At the time of second-look arthroscopy, some reconstructed ligaments show little revascularization, with disorganization of the collagen structure.[41, 63] Resorption zones at the tunnels in both allografts and autografts have been demonstrated.[70] The question of how to revise the reconstruction that occurs secondary to a failure of incorporation remains. No errors were made by the surgeon or the patient that can actively be avoided in the second attempt. If an autogenous graft fails to incorporate or mature for intrinsic reasons in a primary reconstruction, why will it mature with a revision also performed with autogenous tissue? How can a revision successfully be performed in this situation?

The answer may rest in part with the synthetic ligament, and consideration and further study of prosthetic ligaments remain relevant in this situation.

CLASSIFICATION OF SYNTHETIC LIGAMENTS

Friedman[71] classified synthetic ligaments into three types: permanent prostheses, stents, and scaffolds. Collins has described a fourth type, the composite.[63] Prosthetic ligaments stand alone as a permanent and immediate replacement of the ruptured ligament. This type of ligament relies on the inherent strength of the synthetic to withstand long-term forces across the joint. No ingrowth of autogenous tissue is expected to augment the graft.

Stents are synthetic ligaments designed to initially share the loads placed across the autogenous graft or allograft during maturation and remodeling. These synthetic grafts protect the autograft or allograft from excessive forces during the healing phase, until the natural graft is strong enough to bear the full load.

Scaffolds are synthetic ligaments designed to promote autogenous fibrous ingrowth. The scaffold provides initial stability to the reconstruction while creeping substitution of autogenous fibrous tissue is relied upon to provide long-term stability and remodeling potential to the graft.[1]

Composite grafts are a combination of a true prosthetic and an autogenous graft. Unlike the temporary stent, the prosthetic portion of the reconstruction is designed to be a long-term stabilizer functioning in tandem with the autograft.

Prosthetics

Examples of prosthetics are the Gore-Tex, Dacron, and PolyFlex graft.

Gore-Tex. The Gore-Tex graft (Fig. 10–1) showed early promise, but later reports showed increased complication rates. The Gore-Tex graft was initially produced to serve as a salvage procedure for the knee that had undergone multiple operations with previous failed reconstruction. The graft is a braided chain made from a single strand of polytetrafluoroethylene.[72] Polytetrafluoroethylene was chosen as a synthetic liga-

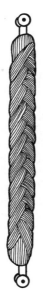

Figure 10–1. Gore-Tex ligament.

ment because of its inert nature and high tensile strength.[72, 73] Simulated Gore-Tex wear particles exposed to human synovial cells created no cytotoxicity.[73] Material testing demonstrated a tensile strength of approximately 5000 N, 2.8 times that of the human ACL.[72, 74] Animal studies showed bony ingrowth into the tunnels. Indelicato and others showed good early results in human patients[10, 75, 76]; however, the percentage of graft failures increased over time.[11, 12, 20, 21] Another concern was the incidence of sterile effusion in reconstructed knees with Gore-Tex grafts.[10, 15] Links were made to polytetrafluroethylene wear debris, but synovial analysis did not demonstrate a direct relationship between the degree of effusion and the number of particles seen in the synovium.[48]

The Gore-Tex II ligament was utilized primarily outside the United States as an evolution from the original graft (Fig. 10–2). The intra-articular portion was rounded and compacted and wrapped in a sheath to minimize abrasion and fray. It was an improvement over the initial design. This ligament demonstrated significantly better postoperative stability with fewer overall adverse events at 31 months.[4, 77] Despite these improvements, the W.L. Gore Company discontinued manufacture of both the Gore-Tex and Gore-Tex II ligaments in 1993 because of economic constraints.

Many of the principles currently used in autogenous reconstruction were learned in the development of the Gore-Tex graft. Smooth rounded tunnels, elimination of acute angles, and adequate notchplasty were all required in the proper use of this synthetic ligament. Furthermore, "preconditioning," taking the slack out of the ligament by cycling it prior to distal fixation, lessened subsequent loosening. These techniques have been carried over into common practice in current ACL reconstructions. Learning from past mistakes, and utilizing these techniques with future synthetic grafts, will lower complication rates and improve results.[63]

Dacron. The Dacron graft measures over 3600 N in maximal tensile strength. Early good results were reported by several investigators.[79, 80] But, as with the Gore-Tex graft, long-term studies showed deterioration of results.[13, 14, 81, 82] The Dacron ligament was shown to have considerable loss of stability in 23 percent of patients at 5 year follow-up.[9] In another report, almost 50 percent of patients had disruption or elongation at 5 to 7 years follow-up.[81] Richmond et al.[82] reported an 88 percent failure rate with Dacron grafts in the revision or complex ligament laxity setting. Other investigators have demonstrated a greater than 20 percent incidence of wear particle–induced synovitis in patients with a Dacron reconstruction.[13]

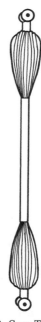

Figure 10–2. Gore-Tex II ligament.

PolyFlex. Another early prosthetic ligament was made of polyethylene and steel and produced by Richards in the late 1970s, the PolyFlex. Poor results led to its early discontinuation.[49]

Stents

The second type of ligament is the stent. The Kennedy ligament augmentation device (LAD) and the Proplast ligament are examples. The LAD is a braided polypropylene graft initially used as an augmentation for the Marshall-McIntosh reconstruction by Dr. John Kennedy (Fig. 10–3). The Marshall-McIntosh procedure is an older technique that has been replaced by current ACL techniques. In this reconstruction, a strip of patellar tendon, aponeurotic tissue peeled off the patella, and quadriceps tendon were augmented with an LAD. This graft was then used to reinforce a primary ACL repair or substitute for the ACL. The graft tissue was left attached to the tibial tubercle, pulled through a tibial tunnel and then through the intracondylar notch and "over the top" of the lateral femoral condyle where it was secured. Early studies suggested that the LAD-augmented reconstruction provided a statistically significant improvement over the nonaugmented reconstruction in the Marshall-McIntosh procedure.[83]

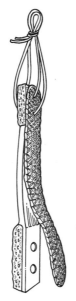

Figure 10–3. Ligament Augmentation Device (LAD) and autograft.

Later, no long-term difference was found in augmented versus nonaugmented intra-articular reconstructions using either autografts or allografts with current bone tunnel techniques.[5, 84] There has been no series reporting significant complications of wear debris or chronic synovitis with the LAD; however, results with current ACL reconstructions and rehabilitation protocols have not been improved by use of the LAD. The current role of the LAD remains unclear.[1]

Historically, another stent no longer available is the Proplast ligament introduced in 1973. This ligament was designed to act as an internal stent to protect an extra-articular repair. Ligament rupture was reported in over half the patients in the published series.[4, 13]

Scaffolds

The third type of synthetic ligament is the scaffold. Examples of this are the Leeds-Keio graft, the carbon fiber graft, and the LARS ligament. Animal research has been performed using a collagen matrix scaffold.

Leeds-Keio Ligament. The Leeds-Keio ligament was designed in a collaboration between English and Japanese investigators. This ligament is made from polyester and is designed to allow ingrowth of autogenous collagen.[17] Theoretically, autogenous tissue would gradually provide long-term structural support. Results using this synthetic ligament have been disappointing.[16–18] Dandy and Gray reported increased instability with long-term follow-up.[7] Other investigators have shown fragmentation of the graft and a chronic inflammatory response or granulomatous reaction. Ryan and Banks concluded that "chronic inflammatory response occurs as a result of the fragmentation of the graft fibers and once established inhibits production of the neoligament that is dooming it to failure."[18]

Another scaffold made from carbon fiber was taken off the market shortly after introduction because of high failure rate. The elastic modulus of carbon fibers is extremely low compared with that of the natural ACL. Intra-articular friction led to degradation and a high incidence of reactive synovitis.[15, 85]

LARS Ligament. The LARS ligament, ligament advanced reinforcement system, is currently in use on a limited basis in Europe, Canada, and the United States (Fig. 10–4).[86, 87] Also called Ligastic, it is a knitted polyester scaffold with open fibers in its central intra-articular portion to allow fibrous ingrowth. The designers proposed that the knitted design offers improved wear characteristics to previous designs. The French surgeon Laboureau[88] described the use of the LARS ligament in a two-bundled open surgical technique for reconstructing the posterior cruciate ligament (PCL) as well as an additional technique utilizing the LARS ligament in posterolateral reconstruction. He reported 6-month to 8-year follow-up in PCL reconstruction with 86 percent good results in acute cases and 70 percent good results in chronic cases. He concluded that his results are encouraging, and further study and investigation are ongoing.

In a previous study, Laboureau[87] reported on 225 patients with acute ACL rupture treated by reconstruction with the LARS ligament and suture repair of the ACL. He reported that 87 percent of patients returned to their sport at the same level. Also, he reported that postoperative cases that were re-examined arthroscopically showed that the ligament became covered with an organized fibrous tissue.

One of Laboureau's coinvestigators, Derricks,[86] advocated using the LARS ligament for ACL reconstruction. He also maintained the ACL stump, theorizing advantages as a collagen scaffold, a vascular supply, and a source of proprioceptive fibers. He reported 86 percent excellent objective and subjective results at an average of 2½ years after surgery.

Johnson,[89] a Canadian investigator, reported use of the LARS ligament in arthroscopic PCL reconstruction. He reported a 30 percent failure rate at 2 years. Johnson questioned whether his modification to an arthroscopic procedure with debridement of the PCL stump led to less tissue ingrowth and diminished results. Johnson's current limited indications are acute and chronic PCL reconstruction in older sedentary patients with multiple ligamentous injuries, and in revisions in which no other graft source is available.

At this time, some of the results reported with the LARS ligament may be promising. However, much of the published data comes from the ligament's investigating design team. Moreover, past experience with synthetic ligaments has demonstrated the importance of long-term follow-up, with declining rates of good results occurring over the years. Long-term study by multiple investigators will determine whether the LARS ligament has a role in cruciate ligament reconstruction.

Collagen Matrix. The collagen matrix scaffold is a graft with promise (Fig. 10–5). Jackson et al.[3] have studied biologic remodeling after ACL reconstruction using a collagen matrix in the goat model. The matrix is derived from demineralized bone. In vivo, the graft underwent site-specific remodeling, transforming from an initial haversian system to a ligament-like structure at 1 year. New bone filled the osseous tunnels and displaced the demineralized matrix. A ligament-like transition zone developed peripherally and a ligamentous collagen orientation with crimp developed in the intra-articular portion. There was no long-term inflammatory response. Jackson et al. concluded that optimization of this type of matrix may allow clinical application in the near future.[3]

Composite Graft

A composite graft is a combination of a permanent prosthetic and an autogenous

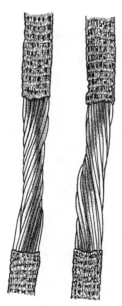

Figure 10–4. Ligament Advanced Reinforcement System (LARS) ligaments.

graft and has demonstrated better long-term results than most prosthetic grafts alone (Fig. 10–6).[63] The graft is composed of the Gore-Tex prosthesis plus a semitendinosus or patellar tendon autograft. This combination offers the immediate strength of a prosthetic and the long-term remodeling potential of the autograft. Technically, a femoral tunnel is made at the so-called isometric point on the lateral femoral condyle for the autograft. The tibial tunnel for the autograft is in the anterior medial portion of the anatomic insertion of the ACL, mimicking the anterior medial bundle of the natural ACL.

The Gore-Tex ligament is attached to the femur extra-articularly in the "over the top" position. A second tunnel is placed through the posterolateral portion of the ACL insertion on the tibia for the Gore-Tex graft. This construction provides several important features. First, the over-the-top position causes the synthetic ligament to tighten with full extension. This provides protection of the autograft from lengthening or rupture in extension during healing. But since the synthetic does completely eliminate stress in flexion, it allows maturation of the autograft. Stress sharing rather than complete stress shielding occurs.[90] Another beneficial fea-

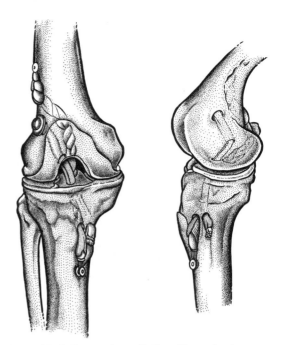

Figure 10–6. Composite graft: Gore-Tex and autogenous.

ture of this design is that the autograft is placed anterior to the synthetic to protect the synthetic ligament from notch impingement and wear. Long-term subjective and objective results of composite reconstruction have been good.[63] At 5- to 7-year follow-up, the composite graft provided significant increase in knee score, activity level, and objective stability. The composite graft had a low failure rate, no tendency toward gradual loosening, and no incidence of sterile effusion. Lack of incorporation of autogenous grafts has been recognized as an etiology of failure in ACL reconstruction in the absence of technical error or recurrent trauma. Revision of this type of failure with another autograft or allograft alone will predictably result in another failure. A composite graft offers a potential solution to this difficult problem.

SUMMARY

Many problems have been associated with most synthetic graft use up to this time. Failure by rupture, gradual elongation, and wear debris–induced synovitis have all been reported. Most of the synthetic ligaments have not stood the test of time. Enthusiasm

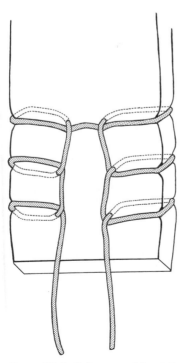

Figure 10–5. Collagen matrix graft.

for synthetic ligaments by the general orthopedic community has waned. However, some investigators remain optimistic about the future role of synthetics. Johnson[89] has questioned, "Did prosthetic ligaments fail us or did we fail the prosthetic ligament?" Many failures of synthetic ligaments occurred secondary to intrinsic flaws and insufficiencies in their designs and properties. Other failures resulted from unrefined techniques and improper indications.

Role of Synthetic Ligaments

Synthetic ligaments offer some clear advantages over autografts and allografts. At this point, refinements in autogenous ACL reconstruction and rehabilitation protocols provide reproducibly good results and make autogenous reconstruction the treatment of choice for the practicing orthopedic surgeon. Investigation is ongoing and future synthetic ligaments may be an improvement over past designs. Advocates of the LARS ligament report good, albeit limited, results. Further testing of this design is necessary and is underway. Collagen matrix scaffolding has been proposed by Jackson. So far, animal testing of this technique shows promise. The problem of failure, of incorporation of autogenous ACL grafts in the absence of surgical error or recurrent trauma, has been recognized. In this situation, revision using another autogenous tissue is likely to lead to another failure. Good results with a synthetic ligament plus autogenous tissue suggest this as one possible solution to a difficult problem. Improved synthetic grafts will likely play an expanded role in the future of ACL reconstruction. For now, the role is limited to special indications in an investigational setting.

References

1. Hunter RE: Anterior cruciate ligament reconstruction with a composite graft bone-patellar tendon-bone/ligament augmentation device. Op Tech Sports Med 10:182, 1995.
2. Corner EM: Notes from a case illustrative of an artificial anterior cruciate ligament demonstrating the action of that ligament. Proc R Soc Med 7:120, 1914.
3. Jackson DW, Simon TM, Lowery W, Gendler EL: Biologic remodeling after anterior cruciate ligament reconstruction using a collagen matrix derived from demineralized bone. Am J Sports Med 24:405, 1996.
4. Johnson DL, Fu FH: Anterior cruciate ligament reconstruction: Why do failures occur? Instructional course lectures 44:391, 1995.
5. Noyes FR, Barber SD: The effect of a ligament-augmentation device on allograft reconstructions for chronic ruptures of the anterior cruciate ligament. J Bone Joint Surg 74-A:960, 1992.
6. Barrett GR, Line LL Jr, Shelton WR, et al: The Dacron ligament prosthesis in anterior cruciate ligament reconstruction: A four year review. Am J Sports Med 21:367, 1993.
7. Dandy DJ, Gray AJ: Anterior cruciate ligament reconstruction with the Leeds-Keio prosthesis plus extraarticular tenodesis. J Bone Joint Surg 76B:193, 1994.
8. Forster IW, Malis VA, McKibbin, Jenkins B: Biologic reaction to carbon fiber implants. The formation and structure of carbon induced neotendon. Clin Orthop 131:299, 1978.
9. Gillquist J, Odenstein M: Reconstruction of old anterior cruciate ligament tears with a Dacron prosthesis. Am J Sports Med 21:358, 1993.
10. Glousman R, Sheilds C, Kerlan R, Jobe F, Yocum L, Tibone J: Gore-Tex prosthetic ligament in anterior cruciate deficient knees. Am J Sports Med 16:321, 1988.
11. Indelicato PA, Woods GA, Prevot TJ: The Gore-Tex anterior cruciate ligament prosthesis: 2 versus 3 year results. Am J Sports Med 19:48, 1991.
12. Karzel RP, Defendor DR, Fox JM, et al: Four year experience with the Gore-Tex prosthetic ligament in anterior cruciate deficient knees. Orthop Trans 14:618, 1990.
13. Kline W, Jensen KU: Synovitis in artificial ligaments. Arthroscopy 8:116, 1992.
14. Lopez-Vasquez E et al: Reconstruction of the anterior cruciate ligament with a Dacron prosthesis. J Bone Joint Surg 73A:1294, 1991.
15. Olson EJ, Kong JD, Fu FH, Georgescu AL: The biomechanical and histological effects of artificial ligament wear particles. Am J Sports Med 16:558, 1988.
16. Prescott RJ, Ryan WG, Bisset DL: Histopathological features of failed prosthetic Leeds-Keio ACL. J Clin Pathol 47:375, 1994.
17. Rading J, Peterson L: Clinical experience with the Leeds-Keio artificial ligament in anterior cruciate ligament reconstruction. Am J Sports Med 23:316, 1995.
18. Ryan WG, Banks AJ: A failure mechanism of the Leeds-Keio ligament. Injury 25:443, 1994.
19. Safran MR, Harner CD: Revision ACL surgery: Techniques and results using allografts. In Jackson DW (ed): Instructional Course Lectures Vol. 44. Parkridge, IL, American Academy of Orthopedic Surgeons, 1995, p. 407.
20. Seemann MD, Stedman JR: Tibial osteolysis associated with Gore-Tex graft. MJ Knee Surg 6:31, 1993.
21. Sledge CL, Stedman JR, Silliman JF, et al: Five year results with the Gore-Tex anterior cruciate ligament prosthesis. MJ Knee Surg 5:65, 1992.
22. Wilk RM, Richmond JC: Dacron ligament reconstruction for chronic anterior cruciate ligament insufficiency. Am J Sports Med 21:374, 1993.
23. Bonamo JL, Crinick RM, Sporn AA: Rupture of the patellar ligament after use of its central third for anterior cruciate ligament reconstruction. A report of two cases. J Bone Joint Surg 66A:1294, 1984.

24. DeLee JC, Craviotto DF: Rupture of the quadriceps tendon after central third patellar tendon anterior cruciate reconstruction. Am J Sports Med 19:415, 1991.
25. Eilerman M, Thomas J, Marsalka D: The effect of harvesting the central one third of the patella tendon on patellofemoral contact pressure. Am J Sports Med 20:738, 1992.
26. Goertzen M: Donor tissue choices in ACL revision. Sports Med Arthroscy Rev 5:128, 1997.
27. Gries PE, Johnson DL, Fu FH: Revision anterior cruciate ligament surgery: Causes of graft failure and technical considerations of revision surgery. Clin Sports Med 12:839, 1993.
28. Harner CD, Irrgang JJ, Paul J, et al: Loss of motion after anterior cruciate ligament reconstruction. Am J Sports Med 20:499, 1992.
29. Johnson DL, Coen MJ: Revision ACL surgery. Etiology, indications, techniques and results. Am J Knee Surg 8:155, 1995.
30. Jackson DW, Schaeffer RK: Cyclops syndrome: Loss of extension following intraarticular anterior cruciate ligament reconstruction. Arthroscopy 6:171, 1990.
31. Kramer J, Nusca D, Fowler P et al: Knee flexor and extensor strength during concentric and eccentric muscle actions after anterior cruciate ligament reconstruction using the semitendinosus tendon and ligament augmentation device. Am J Sports Med 21:285, 1993.
32. Langan P, Fontanetta AP: Rupture of the patella tendon after use of its central third. Orthop Rev 16:61, 1987.
33. Lephart FM, Cocher MS, Harner CD, et al: Quadriceps strength and functional capacity after anterior cruciate ligament reconstruction: Patellar tendon autografts versus allografts. Am J Sports Med 21:738, 1993.
34. McCarrol JR: Fracture of the patella during a golf swing following reconstruction of the anterior cruciate ligament. Am J Sports Med 11:26, 1983.
35. Mohtadi MG, Webstor-Bugaerts S, Fowler PJ: Limitation of motion following anterior cruciate ligament reconstruction: A case controlled study. Am J Sports Med 19:620, 1991.
36. Paulos LE et al: Infrapatellar contracture syndrome. Am J Sports Med 15:331, 1987.
37. Roth JH, Kennedy JC, Lachstad H, et al: Intraarticular reconstruction of the anterior cruciate ligament with and without extraarticular supplementation by transfer of the biceps femoris tendon. J Bone Joint Surg 69A:274, 1988.
38. Sachs RA, Daniel DM, Stone ML, et al: Patellofemoral problems after anterior cruciate ligament reconstruction. Am J Sports Med 17:760, 1989.
39. Shelbourne KD, Wilckens JH, Mollabashy A, et al: Arthrofibrosis in acute anterior cruciate ligament reconstruction: The effect of timing of reconstruction and rehabilitation. Am J Sports Med 19:332, 1991.
40. Shinow K, Nakagawa S, Inoue M, et al: Deterioration of patellofemoral articular surfaces after anterior cruciate ligament reconstruction. Am J Sports Med 21:206, 1993.
41. Buck RE, Malinin T, Brown MD: Bone transplantation and human immunodeficiency virus. An estimation of risks of AIDS. Clin Orthop 240:129, 1989.
42. Buck BE, Resnick L, Shah SM, et al: Human immunodeficiency virus cultured from bone. Implications for transplantation. Clin Orthop 251:249, 1990.

43. Fu FH, Jackson DW, Jameson J, et al: Allograft reconstruction of the anterior cruciate ligament. In Jackson DW (ed): Anterior cruciate ligament: Current and future concepts. New York, Raven Press, 1993, p. 325.
44. Rodrigo JJ, Jackson DW, Simon TM, Muto KN: The immune response to freeze dried bone, tendon bone. Trans Orthop Res 13:105, 1988.
45. Simon T, Jackson DW: Anterior cruciate ligament allografts. In Jackson DW, Drez D Jr (eds): The Anterior Cruciate Deficient Knee: New Concepts in Ligament Repair. St. Louis, Mosby, 1987, p. 211.
46. Simonds RJ, Holmberg SD, Hurwitz R, et al: Transmission of human immunodeficiency virus from a seronegative organ and tissue. N Engl J Med 326:726, 1992.
47. Tolin BS, Friedman MJ: Artificial cruciate ligament reconstruction. In Scott WN (ed): The Knee. St. Louis, Mosby, 1994, p. 839.
48. Bruchman WC, Bolton CW, Bain JR: Design considerations for cruciate ligament prosthesis. In Jackson DW, Drez D JR (eds): The Anterior Cruciate Deficient Knee: New Concepts in Ligament Repair. St. Louis, Mosby, 1987, p. 254.
49. O'Brien SJ, Warren RF, Pavlov H, et al: Reconstruction of the chronically insufficient anterior cruciate ligament with the central third of the patellar ligament. J Bone Joint Surg 73A:278, 1991.
50. Burns GS, Howell FM: Roof plasty requirements in vitro for different tibial hold placement in anterior cruciate ligament reconstruction. Am J Sports Med 21:292, 1993.
51. Howell FM, Taylor MA: Failure of reconstruction of the anterior cruciate ligament due to impingement by the intracondylar roof. J Bone Joint Surg 75A:1044, 1993.
52. Howell FM, Clark JA, Farley TE: A rationale for predicting anterior cruciate graft impingement by the intercondylar roof: A magnetic resonance imaging study. Am J Sports Med 19:276, 1991.
53. Tanzer M, Lenczner E: The relationship of intercondylar notch size and content to notchplasty requirement in anterior cruciate ligament surgery. Arthroscopy 6:89, 1990.
54. Graf B, Uhr F: Complications of intraarticular anterior cruciate ligament reconstruction. Clin Sports Med 17:835, 1988.
55. Hoogland T, Hillen B: Intraarticular reconstruction of the anterior cruciate ligament. An experimental study on length changes in different ligament reconstructions. Clin Orthop 185:197, 1984.
56. Howell FM, Clark JA: Tibial tunnel placement anterior cruciate ligament reconstructions and graft impingement. Clin Orthop 283:187, 1992.
57. Olson EJ, Fu FH, Harner CD, et al: Optimal tibial tunnel starting point in endoscopic anterior cruciate ligament reconstruction. Presented at the 60th Annual Meeting of the American Academy of Orthopedic Surgeons, San Francisco, CA, 1993.
58. Romano VM, Graf B, Keen JS, et al: Anterior cruciate ligament reconstruction: The effect of tibial tunnel placement on range of motion. Am J Sports Med 21:415, 1993.
59. Burks RT, Leland R: Determination of graft tension before fixation in anterior cruciate ligament reconstruction. Arthroscopy 4:260, 1988.
60. Gertel TH, Lew WD, Lewis JL, et al: Effective anterior cruciate ligament graft tensioning, direction, magnitude, and flexion angle on knee biomechanics. Am J Sports Med 21:572, 1993.

61. Vergis A, Gillquist J: Graft failure in intraarticular anterior cruciate ligament reconstructions: A review of the literature. Arthroscopy 11:312, 1995.

62. Matthews LS, Soffer SR: Pitfalls in the use of interference screws for anterior cruciate ligament reconstruction. Arthroscopy 5:225, 1989.

63. Davidson JF, Collins HR, Campbell ED: Composite Gore-Tex and autogenous semitendinosus anterior cruciate ligament reconstruction: Long term results an historical review. Op Tech Sports Med 3:177, 1995.

64. Shinow K, Inque M, Horibe S, et al: Maturation of allograft tendons transplanted into the knee: An arthroscopic and histologic study. J Bone Joint Surg 70BR:556, 1988.

65. Fu FH, Irrgang JJ, Harner CD: Loss of motion following anterior cruciate ligament reconstruction. In Jackson DW, Arnoczky SP, Wu Sly, et al. (eds.): The Anterior Cruciate Ligament: Current and Future Concepts. New York, Raven Press, 1993, p. 373.

66. Shelbourne KD, Nitz P: Accelerated rehabilitation after anterior cruciate ligament reconstruction. Am J Sports Med 18:292, 1990.

67. Noyes FR et al: Intraarticular cruciate reconstructions: Prospective on graft strengths, vascularization and immediate motion after replacement. Clin Orthop 172:171, 1993.

68. Arnoczky SP, Warren RF, Ahlock MA: Replacement of the anterior cruciate ligament using a patellar tendon allograft: An experimental study. J Bone Joint Surg 68A:376, 1986.

69. Johnson LL: The outcome of a free autogenous semitendinosus tendon graft in human anterior cruciate ligament surgery: A histologic study. Arthroscopy 9:131, 1993.

70. Berg EE: Tibial bone plug nonunion: A cause of anterior cruciate ligament reconstructive failure. Arthroscopy 8:380, 1992.

71. Friedman MJ: Prosthetic anterior cruciate ligaments. Clin Sports Med 10:499, 1991.

72. Bolton CW, Bruchman WC: The Gore-Tex expanded polytetrafluoroethylene prosthetic ligament. An in vitro and in vivo evaluation. Clin Orthop 196:202, 1985.

73. Thompson LA, Law FC, James KH, Rushton N: Biocompatibility of particles of Gore-Tex cruciate ligament prosthesis: An investigation both in vitro and in vivo. Biomaterials 12:781, 1991.

74. Noyes FR, Groodes: The strength of the anterior cruciate ligament in humans and rhesus monkeys: Age related and species related changes. J Bone Joint Surg 58A-1074, 1986.

75. Ahfeld SA, Larson RL, Collins HR: Anterior cruciate ligament reconstruction in the chronically unstable knee using an expanded polytetrafluoroethylene prosthetic ligament. Am J Sports Med 15:326, 1987.

76. Indelicato PA, Pascale MS, Huegel MO: Early experience with the Gore-Tex polytetrafluoroethylene anterior cruciate ligament prosthesis. Am J Sports Med 17:55, 1989.

77. Johnson DL: Gore-Tex synthetic ligament. Op Tech Sports Med 3:173, 1995.

78. Parke JP, Grana WA, Chitwood JS: A high strength Dacron augmentation for cruciate ligament reconstruction. A two year canine study. Clin Orthop 196:175, 1985.

79. Anderson HN, Brune C, Sondergard-Peterson PE: Reconstruction of chronic insufficient anterior cruciate ligament in the knee using a synthetic Dacron prosthesis: A prospective study of 57 cases. Am J Sports Med 20:20, 1992.

80. Wilk RM, Richmond JC: Dacron ligament reconstruction for chronic anterior cruciate ligament insufficiency. Am J Sports Med 21:374, 1993.

81. Barrett GR, Lawrence LL, Shelton WR, et al: The Dacron ligament prosthesis in anterior cruciate ligament reconstruction. A four year review. Am J Sports Med 21:367, 1993.

82. Richmond JC, Manseau CJ, Patz R, McConville O: Anterior cruciate reconstruction using a Dacron ligament prosthesis. A long term study. AM J Sports Med 20:24, 1992.

83. Kennedy JC: Application of prosthetics to anterior cruciate ligament reconstruction and repair. Clin Orthop 172:125, 1983.

84. Barrett GR, Field LD: Comparison of patellar tendon versus patellar tendon/Kennedy ligament augmentation device for anterior cruciate ligament reconstruction: A study of results, morbidity, and complications. Arthroscopy 9:624, 1993.

85. Forster IW, Malis ZA, McKibbin B, Jenkins B: Biologic reaction to carbon fiber implants. The formation and structure of carbon induced neotendons. Clin Orthop 131:299, 1978.

86. Derricks G: Ligament advanced reinforcement system anterior cruciate ligament reconstruction. Op Tech Sports Med 3:187, 1985.

87. Laboureau JP: Recent rupture of the anterior cruciate ligament. Suture technique on a reinforced ligament. Results of five year experience. Rev Chir Orthop Reparatrice Appar Mot 77:92, 1991.

88. Laboureau JP: Two bundle posterior cruciate ligament reconstruction: Technique and results. Op Tech Sports Med 3:206, 1995.

89. Johnson DL: Cruciate ligament reconstruction with synthetics. Presented at the Arthroscopy Association of North American 16th Annual Meeting, April 23, 1997, San Diego, CA.

90. McCarthy JA, Stedman R, Dunlap J, et al: A nonparallel, nonisometric synthetic graft augmentation of the patellar tendon anterior cruciate ligament reconstruction. Am J Sports Med 18:43, 1990.

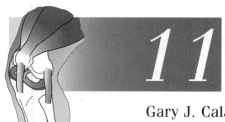

11 Posterolateral Instability

Gary J. Calabrese, PT, and John A. Bergfeld, MD

*P*osterolateral instability of the knee is described as a complex problem that is frequently misdiagnosed and can lead to severe disability.[1] Isolated posterolateral instability is considered rare and is more commonly associated with posterior cruciate ligament (PCL) or anterior cruciate ligament (ACL) injuries.[2] Posterior lateral rotary instability (PLRI) is recognized as one of the causes of poor outcomes following operative reconstruction of the ACL- or PCL-deficient knee. Therefore, recognition and management of PLRI has clinical significance in the evaluation of the traumatic knee injury.[3]

FUNCTIONAL ANATOMY OF THE POSTEROLATERAL CORNER

The posterolateral compartment of the knee is composed of capsular and extracapsular structures that combine to form a single functional structure called the arcuate complex.[4, 5] The arcuate complex is primarily composed of the arcuate ligament, lateral collateral ligament, popliteus muscle and tendon, popliteofibular ligament, fabellofibular ligament, posterior capsule, and lateral gastrocnemius head (Fig. 11–1).[6] The arcuate complex functions as a static and dynamic stabilizing structure counteracting lateral tibiofemoral rotation. Seebacher et al.[7] described the posterolateral corner as consisting of three layers. Layer I, the most superficial, is made up of the iliotibial band (ITB) and the superficial portion of the biceps, which covers the peroneal nerve. The second layer, layer II, is described as having anterior borders at the quadriceps retinaculum, adjacent to the patella, and posteriorly by the patellofemoral ligaments. Layer III, the deepest layer, is formed by the joint capsule, the meniscal attachment of the coronary ligament, and the popliteofibular ligament, which joins the popliteus tendon and

forms a Y-shaped unit to insert on the femur.[7]

Hughston et al.[8, 9] described six classifications of instability associated with acute and chronic lateral instabilities of the knee. Anterolateral rotary instability (ALRI), posterolateral rotary instability (PLRI), combined ALRI and PLRI, acute straight lateral instability (SLI), combined anteromedial rotary instability (AMRI), and combined AMRI and PLRI, and ALRI. The classification system describes the tibial movement on the femur. Thus, ALRI describes abnormal anterior rotation of the lateral tibial plateau on the axis of the intact PCL in relation to the femur and is usually associated with a combined ACL injury. PLRI is defined as posterior rota-

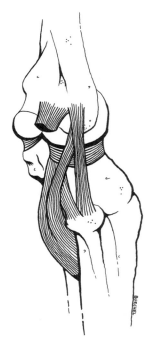

Figure 11–1. Lateral stabilizing structures of the knee demonstrating the relationship of the lateral collateral ligament, popliteofibular ligament, posterior fibula, and popliteal tendon.

tion of the lateral tibial plateau, or external tibial plateau rotation around the axis of the intact PCL in relation to the femoral condyles. PLRI is believed to occur with far less frequency than ALRI and is often missed on acute examination but manifests itself later as chronic instability of the knee. Straight lateral instability is defined as complete disruption of the entire lateral ligament complex and PCL.[10] In spite of an early attempt at a well-structured classification system, as described by Hughston et al., there continues to be confusion surrounding instability patterns of the posterolateral corner of the knee.[7, 11, 12] Many of these instability patterns are associated with combined ligament injuries involving the ACL or PCL, or both, often making early acute diagnosis difficult.

Kennedy Towler[13] and Gollehon et al.[14] have demonstrated that the axis of the knee is complex and may not center on the PCL in posterolateral ligament complex injuries. Selective ligament sectioning studies have demonstrated the importance of the posterolateral structures to overall knee stability. Grood et al.[15] described the limits of movement in the knee through sectioning studies utilizing cadaveric knees. They found that sectioning only the PCL increased posterior tibial translation without changing tibial rotation and varus or valgus angles. Posterior tibial translation increased according to the degree of knee flexion, with the least at 0 degrees and reaching maximal displacement at 90 degrees. This progressive increase in translation with knee flexion resulted from the progressive slackening of the posterior capsular structures. Sectioning of the posterolateral structures increased the amount of external tibial rotation and varus angulation, reaching its maximum at 30 degrees of knee flexion. Sequential sectioning of the PCL following the posterolateral complex revealed significant increases in tibial external rotation at 90 degrees of knee flexion.[15]

Markolf et al.[16] further demonstrated through sectioning studies that posterolateral ligament sectioning increased posterior tibial translation, varus rotation, and tibial external rotation. Skyhar et al.[17] measured the articular contact pressure within the knee after sequential sectioning of the PCL and posterolateral complex in a simulated non-weight-bearing knee extension. Medial compartment articular cartilage pressure was significantly elevated with sectioning of the PCL, whereas patellofemoral pressure and quadriceps load increased significantly after combined sectioning of the PCL and the posterolateral complex. Injury to the posterolateral structures are magnified by a primary varus knee. The examiner must determine whether the knee is a primary varus or valgus knee. Examination of the contralateral knee is often helpful.

MECHANISM OF INJURY

The primary mechanism of injury for PLRI is direct trauma to the anteromedial tibia with the knee in extension, or knee hyperextension with tibial external rotation. Many PLRI injuries occur in athletics, often in conjunction with other rotational instabilities or cruciate disruption. Numerous authors have indicated that the incidence of mild PLRI may be higher than previously reported and have observed that nonoperative treatment of individuals with these injuries has not impaired their function enough to prevent athletic participation.[18, 19] With an acute injury, the patient often complains of pain in the posterolateral region of the knee and may present with relatively minor swelling with giving-way episodes at heel strike with full knee extension.[10] The patient often ambulates with a flexed knee gait pattern to splint against the pain and instability associated with PLRI. Patients with chronic PLRI injuries of the knee complain of "buckling" episodes while ambulating or navigating stairs, lateral joint line pain, and an evident varus thrust from heel strike to mid-stance position. Peroneal nerve symptoms of dysthesias and motor weakness of the leg and foot were described by Baker et al.[18] in 2 of 17 patients with acute PLRI injuries of the knee. The clinician must remain cognizant of associated ACL and PCL injuries and symptoms that may overshadow the often subtle signs and symptoms of PLRI.

HISTORY AND CLINICAL EVALUATION

Posterolateral instability and PCL injuries often go undetected on physical examination. A detailed history usually reveals an injury associated with high-energy trauma or in contact sports. The patient may or may

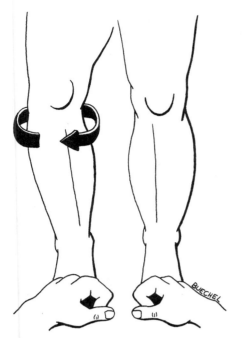

Figure 11-2. The external rotation recurvatum test for posterolateral rotatory instability of the right knee.

not have an effusion but will be unwilling to fully extend the knee at heel strike and often ambulates with a flexed knee gait. A gait analysis often reveals a varus thrust as the knee reaches the extended position. Standing limb posture and radiographic evaluation may reveal a varus knee alignment. Acutely, the examiner should be aware of posterolateral tenderness and ecchymosis or contusion at the anteromedial tibial plateau. Neurovascular status is surveyed to test for peroneal nerve injury symptoms. The examination should include testing for associated cruciate ligament disruption. In addition to the Lachman, pivot-shift, anterior drawer, and posterior drawer tests for ACL and PCL disruption, the external rotation recurvatum test, reverse pivot-shift test, and posterolateral drawer sign test are sensitive for PLRI injuries.[2] The anterior and posterior drawer tests should be performed in 30 and 90 degrees of knee flexion. An increase in tibial excursion at 30 degrees as compared with 90 degrees has a high suspicion for posterolateral instability, whereas an increase at both 30 and 90 degrees indicates a PCL disruption. Valgus and varus testing at 0, 30, and 90 degrees is performed. The integrity of the medial collateral ligament (MCL) and lateral collateral ligament (LCL) are assessed. PLRI and LCL injuries demonstrate increased varus joint line opening at 0 and 30 degrees when stress-tested. Isolated cruciate ligament injuries are not affected by varus and valgus testing.

The external rotation recurvatum test, as described by Hughston and Norwood,[6] is performed with the patient supine. The clinician lifts both feet off the table while grasping the toes. PLRI is determined by the appearance of knee hyperextension and varus alignment as the tibia rotates externally (Fig. 11-2). A second method of performing the external rotation recurvatum test entails the examiner's holding the patient's heel in one hand and placing the opposite hand on the posterolateral joint line to note side-to-side differences in hyperextension and external tibial rotation (Fig. 11-3). The reverse pivot-shift test is conducted by moving the knee from a 90-degree to a full-extension position while applying a valgus force and foot external rotation. If positive for PLRI, the lateral tibial plateau slides from a subluxed position posteriorly in relation to the femoral condyle to the normal anatomic position. This minimizes a positive pivot-shift for a deficient ACL. If positive, this subluxed position is reduced or shifts as the knee is brought in to full extension. The posterolateral drawer test is performed with the patient supine and hip flexion of 45 degrees and

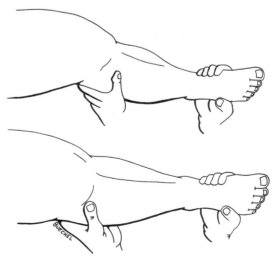

Figure 11-3. Alternate method of assessing rotatory instability of the knee. Initiating the test with the knee flexed, the examiner slowly extends the knee and feels for the external rotation and recurvatum at the posterolateral border of the knee.

knee flexion of 80 degrees. The examiner performs the drawer test in neutral, tibial external, and internal rotations. The test is considered diagnostic when the lateral tibial plateau externally rotates relative to the femur. This should be compared to the normal knee. In patients with PLRI, the posterior drawer test will be positive with external tibial rotation but negative with internal rotation.[6] If abnormal translation occurs with tibial internal rotation, the clinician must suspect an associated ACL or PCL injury.

Variability in clinical findings predominate in the literature on testing procedures for PLRI. Baker et al.[20] report a 94 percent sensitivity with the external rotation recurvatum test in surgically proven PLRI patients. Cooper[3] reported on 100 patients with normal knees who underwent an examination under anesthesia while having surgery for an unrelated problem. The Lachman, pivot-shift, anterior drawer, posterior drawer, varus stress, and external rotation recurvatum tests were negative in all subjects. The reverse pivot-shift sign was present in 35 percent of the knees tested. These findings indicate that the reverse pilot-shift sign may not be a significant finding unless the contralateral limb has negative indicators.

Plain radiographs allow for examination of the intra-articular osteoarthritic changes, such as joint line narrowing, often associated with chronic PLRI. Acute PLRI presents with the potential of fibular head fractures and tibial plateau fractures, which are also commonly associated with ACL or PCL disruption in high-velocity trauma situations.

TREATMENT OPTIONS

Isolated PLRI is uncommon, and the treatment options after meticulous examination often involve ACL and PCL disruption. Reconstruction of the knee should address all intra-articular and extra-articular ligaments and capsular and musculotendinous structures. Several studies have demonstrated dismal results from addressing only the ACL or PCL disruption and not the combined injury of the posterolateral structures.[14] The results of acute surgical reconstruction of the posterolateral structures have been reported to be better than for chronic PLRI.[21] Nonoperative management for patients with mild laxity (less than 1+ laxity without asso-

ciated intra-articular injury) is reported to yield good results. Baker et al.[18] reported on 14 of 31 patients with mild instability who were able to return to the same level of athletic participation following cast immobilization and progressive functional rehabilitation. A clinical examination of the acute or chronic knee that reveals increased laxity and associated cruciate disruption is approached surgically. Numerous surgical procedures have been developed for reconstructing the posterolateral structures. The ultimate surgical goal is the restoration of the normal anatomy and thus kinematics of the knee.

SURGICAL TECHNIQUE

Hughston and Jacobson[1] contributed significantly to the early surgical technique for reconstruction for PLRI. Their technique involves the performance of anterior and superior advancement of a bone button that includes the insertion of the LCL and popliteus tendon and repair of the joint capsule through a lateral parapatellar incision. This arcuate complex flap and bone plug is secured to the prepared lateral femoral condyle with a screw and washer, staple, or sutures (Fig. 11–4). Hughston reported on a series of 140 consecutive patients, with follow-up of 2 to 13 years, who underwent reconstruction with this procedure. Patient-reported functional outcomes were described as 77 percent good, 16 percent fair, and 4 percent poor results.

Clancy et al.[22] reported on the utilization

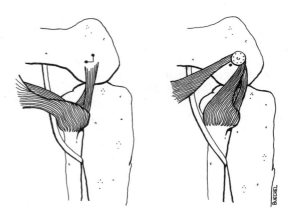

Figure 11–4. Surgical approach for biceps tenodesis. A completed tenodesis procedure is shown, using an anterior fixation point.

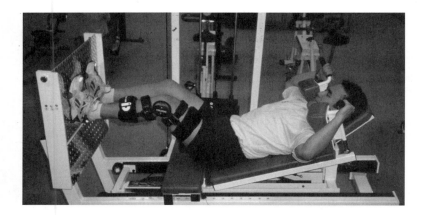

Figure 11-5. Closed kinetic chain leg press exercise with a modified range of motion.

of a biceps tenodesis to stabilize the posterolateral structures. To attempt the recreation of the LCL, the biceps is transferred anteriorly to the lateral femoral condyle. Wascher et al.[23] reported, using cadaveric specimens, on the effects of the biceps tendon tenodesis on varus and valgus laxity of the knee after sequential sectioning of the posterolateral structures. An anterior fixation point was reported to be more effective than a point 1 cm proximal to the LCL insertion, demonstrating that the biceps advancement procedure is effective in decreasing PLRI in the knee.

Our preferred technique combines the procedure of Hughston and Jacobson with an allograft reconstruction (reinforcement) of the posterior lateral cruciate complex. We have noted better results than with the Hughston-Jacobson procedure alone.

POSTOPERATIVE REHABILITATION

Postoperative rehabilitation following posterior lateral corner reconstructive surgery places greater restriction on the patient than an isolated PCL or ACL reconstruction. The patient is placed in full extension in a long leg cast or immobilizer for 6 weeks initially. There is no attempt at range-of-motion during this period. Isometric quadriceps, gluteal, and adductor exercises are performed in full extension during the first 6 weeks. Active assisted straight-leg raises in a supine position enhance protected quadriceps strengthening in this period. Active hamstring exercises are avoided for 8 to 10 weeks to protect against unwanted strain on the posterolateral structures. If an immobilizer is being used, functional electrical stimulation and patellar mobilization are included in the rehabilitation process. Elevation and the application of a commercially available cryotherapy system are used extensively in the acute postoperative period. The patient is permitted to ambulate with crutches, allowing partial weight-bearing immobilized in extension. Patients are progressed to full weight-bearing ambulation in the extension brace by the sixth postoperative week.

The immobilization is discontinued at 6 weeks postoperatively and the patient can progress off crutches when normal ambulation without gait deviation is demonstrated. Range of motion (ROM) exercises to regain flexion are initiated at postoperative week 6 with aquatic therapy, gravity-assisted active and passive ROM, and stationary cycling. Full ROM should be attained by the eighth postoperative week. If the patient has a primary varus knee, a lateral shoe wedge is prescribed. A gradual initiation of progressive resistive exercises for the quadriceps is begun. Closed kinetic chain exercises including mini-squats, modified ROM leg press (Fig. 11-5), balance and proprioceptive exercises (Fig. 11-6), and ankle- and hip-strengthening exercises allow for a functional progression of rehabilitation. Functional rehabilitation and strengthening allow a gradual return to light activity by 5 to 6 months after surgery.

A gradual return to athletic participation is dependant on successful rehabilitation, which includes continued closed kinetic chain exercises emphasizing concentric and eccentric muscular control, agility and proprioception exercises, a walk-jog-run progressive sequence from 6 to 10 months, and plyometric exercises. Generally, 8 to 12

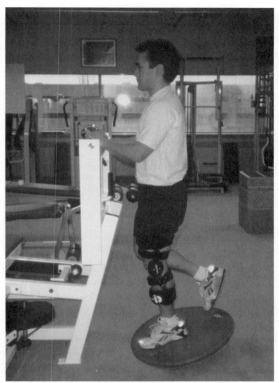

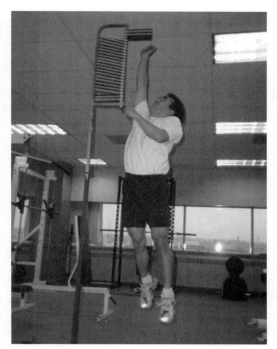

Figure 11–7. Vertical jump test.

Figure 11–6. Balance and proprioception training using a BAPS board (Biomechanical Ankle Platform System, CAMP, Jackson, MI).

months is required for adequate functional rehabilitation to occur and allow a full return to athletic participation. The criteria for returning to full participation include no pain or tenderness with associated swelling after progressive activity, no change in joint laxity and rotational testing, and demonstration of equal side-to-side functional testing measuring muscular strength, vertical jump (Fig. 11–7), one-leg hop for distance, and sport-specific movement patterns.

SUMMARY

Isolated PLRI of the knee is rare. Rotary instabilities of the knee are usually associated with cruciate ligament disruption. Conservative management of mild PLRI is reported to yield good functional results. Moderate PLRI should be addressed surgically to avoid the progressive varus deformity and medial compartment degeneration associated with these injuries. This is particularly true in the primary varus knee. Primary surgical reconstruction of the cruciate deficiency allows intraoperative assessment of the degree and direction of the associated rotatory instability common in PLRI. Restoration of the normal soft tissue anatomy, in particular the LCL and arcuate complex, will yield the best results in surgically addressing PLRI. Individualized rehabilitation must reflect a systematic approach, based on the biomechanics of the knee and a knowledge of reconstructed structures, to allow for early quadriceps activity while limiting flexion ROM, progressive weight-bearing in extension for ambulation, and a gradual functional progression utilizing open and closed kinetic chain exercises. Athletic participation is generally achieved by 8 to 12 months post reconstruction.

References

1. Hughston JC, Jacobson KE: Chronic posterolateral rotatory instability of the knee. J Bone Joint Surg 67-A(3):351–359, 1985.
2. Veltri DM, Warren RF: Anatomy, biomechanics, and physical findings in posterolateral knee instability. Clin Sports Med 13(3): 599–614, 1994.
3. Cooper DE: Tests for posterolateral instability of the knee in normal subjects. J Bone Joint Surg 73-A(1):30–36, 1991.

4. Hughston JC, Andrews JR, Cross MJ, Moschi A: Classification of knee ligament instabilities. Part I. The medial compartment and cruciate ligaments. J Bone Joint Surg 58-A: 159–172, 1976.
5. Hughston JC, Andrews JR, Cross MJ, Moschi A: Classification of knee ligament instabilities; Part II. The lateral compartment. J Bone Joint Surg 58-A:173–179, 1976.
6. Hughston JC, and Norwood LA: The posterolateral drawer test and external rotational recurvatum test for posterolateral rotatory instability of the knee. Clin Orthop Rel Res 147:82–87, 1980.
7. Seebacher J, Inglis A, Marshall J, et al.: The structure of the posterolateral aspect of the knee. J Bone Joint Surg 64:536, 1982.
8. Hughston JC, Andrews JR, Cross MJ, Moschi A: Classification of knee ligament instabilities: Part I. The medial compartment and cruciate ligaments. J Bone Joint Surg [Am] 58:159–172, 1976.
9. Hughston JC, Andrews JR, Cross MJ, Moschi A: Classification of knee ligament instabilities: Part II. The lateral compartment. J Bone Joint Surg [Am] 58:173–179, 1976.
10. Jakob RP, Warner JP: Lateral and posterolateral rotatory instability of the knee. *In* Jakob RP, and Staubli U (eds.): The Knee and the Cruciate Ligaments. Berlin: Springer-Verlag, pp. 1275–1312. 1992.
11. Sudasna S, Harnsiriwattanagit K: The ligamentous structures of the posterolateral aspect of the knee. Bull Hosp J Dis 50:35, 1990.
12. Watanabe Y, Moriya H, Takahashi K, et al.: Functional anatomy of the posterolateral structures of the knee. Arthroscopy 9:57, 1993.
13. Kennedy JC, Towler RJ: Medial and anterior instability of the knee. J Bone Joint Surg [Am] 53:1257, 1971.
14. Gollehon DL, Torzilli PA, Warren RF: The role of the posterolateral and cruciate ligament in stability of the human knee. J Bone Joint Surg [Am] 69:233–142, 1987.
15. Grood ES, Stowers SF, Noyes FR: Limits of movement in the human knee. Effect of sectioning the posterior cruciate ligament and posterolateral structures. J Bone Joint Surg 70-A(1):88–97, 1988.
16. Markolf KL, Wascher DC, Finerman GA: Direct in vitro measurement of forces in the cruciate ligaments: Part II. The effect of section of the posterolateral structures. J Bone Joint Surg 75-A(3):387–394, 1993.
17. Skyhar MJ, Warren RF, Ortiz GJ, Schwartz E, Otis JC: The effects of sectioning of the posterior cruciate ligament and the posterolateral complex on the articular contact pressures within the knee. J Bone Joint Surg [Am] 75(5):694–699, 1993.
18. Baker CL, Norwood LA, Hughston JC: Acute posterolateral rotatory instability of the knee. J Bone Joint Surg [Am] 65:614–618, 1983.
19. Nicholas JA: Acute and chronic lateral instabilities of the knee: Diagnosis, characteristics and treatment. In Evarts CM (ed.): American Academy of Orthopaedic Surgeons Symposium on Reconstructive Surgery of the Knee. St. Louis, C.V. Mosby, 1978, pp. 187–206.
20. Baker CL, Norwood LA, Hughston JC: Acute posterolateral rotatory instability of the knee. J Bone Joint Surg 65-A(5):614–618, 1983.
21. Veltri DM, Warren RF: Operative treatment of posterolateral instability of the knee. Clin Sports Med 13(3):615–627, 1994.
22. Clancy WG, Ray J, Zoltan D: Acute tears of the anterior cruciate ligament. J Bone Joint Surg 70:1483, 1988.
23. Wascher DC, Grauer JD, Markoff KL: Biceps tendon tenodesis for posterolateral instability of the knee. An in vitro study. Am J Sports Med 21(3):400–406, 1993.

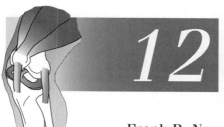

Posterior Cruciate Ligament and Posterolateral Reconstruction

12

Frank R. Noyes, MD, Timothy P. Heckmann, PT, ATC, and Sue D. Barber-Westin, BS

*A*lthough numerous studies have presented details of operative techniques and clinical outcome of patients with posterior cruciate ligament (PCL) ruptures, the rehabilitation programs used after reconstruction have only received brief mention. We first described our program of rehabilitation following allograft PCL reconstruction in 1994,[1] and then further defined the protocol in detail in 1995.[2] In those studies, we introduced for the first time the concepts of immediate knee motion and early weight-bearing after PCL reconstruction, which were proven not to be deleterious to the healing grafts. We also designed the exercise program to avoid or diminish posterior shear forces on the tibia based on the work of others who demonstrated that these forces occurred during high knee flexion angle activities.[3–6]

An even greater paucity of information exists in the literature concerning surgical reconstruction and rehabilitation for lateral collateral ligament (LCL) and posterolateral complex (arcuate ligament, fabellofibular ligament, popliteus tendon and muscle) ruptures. These rare injuries are often misdiagnosed and many times not surgically corrected. Our experience in surgically treating injuries to these structures has been discussed elsewhere and includes allograft reconstruction of the LCL,[7] proximal advancement of the posterolateral complex,[8] and autogenous graft substitution of the LCL and posterolateral complex.[9] These knees often sustain cruciate ligament ruptures, which we surgically reconstruct concomitantly with the lateral, posterolateral procedure. These knees present tremendous challenges in terms of rehabilitation and our program allows the use of immediate protected knee motion but protects the knee

against undue varus and hyperextension loads, weight-bearing, or vigorous exercises in the early postoperative period.

The two rehabilitation protocols described in this chapter consist of a careful incorporation of exercise concepts supported by scientific data and clinical experience. The goal is to progress a patient through the program at a rate that takes into account athletic and occupational goals, condition of the articular surfaces and menisci, and postoperative healing, graft remodeling, and joint effusion.

Both protocols incorporate a home self-management program along with an estimated predetermined number of formal physical therapy visits. For the majority of patients, a range of 11 to 21 postoperative physical therapy visits is expected to produce a desirable result. A few more visits may be required between the sixth and twelfth postoperative months for certain patients who desire to return to strenuous activities for advanced training. For all patients, the following signs are continually monitored postoperatively: joint swelling, pain, gait pattern, knee motion, patellar mobility, muscle strength, and flexibility. For patients who undergo PCL reconstruction, the amount of posterior tibial displacement (dropback) is monitored with stress radiography,[10] and total anteroposterior displacement is measured with the KT-2000 (Fig. 12–1). Lateral and posterolateral reconstructions are monitored with lateral stress radiographs and manual examination of lateral joint opening and external tibial rotation. Any individual who experiences difficulty progressing through the protocol or who develops a complication is expected to require additional supervision in the formal clinical setting.

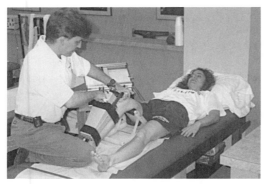

Figure 12–1. The KT-2000 is used to monitor total anteroposterior displacement following posterior cruciate ligament reconstruction.

REHABILITATION PROTOCOL FOR POSTERIOR CRUCIATE LIGAMENT RECONSTRUCTIONS

We developed a rehabilitation protocol for PCL reconstructions performed with a high strength graft (e.g., double-bundle quadriceps tendon-bone [Fig. 12–2],[9] Achilles tendon-bone allograft[1]) and secure internal fixation (Table 12–1). Important principles are the allowance of immediate knee motion and the avoidance of strenuous hamstring exercises for the first 5 to 6 postoperative months. Patients are warned to avoid any

exercises or activities that place high posterior shear forces on the tibia, such as walking down inclines, squatting, or hamstring flexion curl machines. Additionally, all patients are warned that the early return to strenuous activities postoperatively carries the definite risk of a repeat injury or the potential of compounding the original injury. These risks cannot always be scientifically predicted and patients are cautioned to return to strenuous activities, after at least 9 to 12 postoperative months, carefully and to avoid any activity in which pain, swelling, or a feeling of instability is present.

Brace

For patients who undergo PCL reconstruction without a concurrent medial or lateral ligament procedure, a long-leg hinged postoperative brace is worn for the first 8 weeks postoperatively (Fig. 12–3). The brace is worn 24 hours a day, including during sleep, to avoid sudden knee flexion motions that may occur. Initially, the device is worn in full extension for the first 4 weeks and is then opened to 0 to 90 degrees. For individuals evaluated with hyperelastic tissue type, the brace is prescribed for 12 weeks postopera-

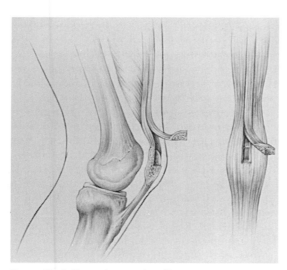

Figure 12–2. Posterior cruciate ligament reconstruction is performed with a quadriceps tendon-bone autograft. (From Noyes, FR, Barber-Westin SD: Treatment of complex injuries involving the posterior cruciate and posterolateral ligaments of the knee. Am J Knee Surg 9:200, 1996.)

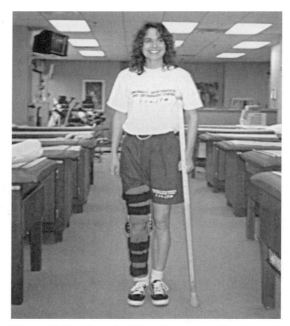

Figure 12–3. A long-leg hinged postoperative brace is worn for the first 8 weeks following posterior cruciate ligament reconstruction.

Table 12–1. **Cincinnati Sportsmedicine and Orthopaedic Center Rehabilitation Protocol for Posterior Cruciate Ligament Reconstruction**

	Postoperative Weeks			Postoperative Months	
	1 to 4	*5 to 8*	*9 to 12*	*4 to 6*	*7 to 12*
Hinged long-leg brace	X	X			
Brace (functional training, return to activity)		X	X	X	X
Range of motion goals (degrees)					
0–90	X				
0–110	X				
0–120		X			
0–135			X		
Weight-bearing					
One-quarter to one-half of body weight	X				
Full		X			
Patella mobilization	X	X			
Modalities					
Electrical muscle stimulation (EMS)	X	X	X		
Pain/edema management (cryotherapy)	X	X	X	X	X
Stretching					
Hamstring, gastroc-soleus, iliotibial band, quadriceps	X	X	X	X	X
Strengthening					
Quadriceps isometrics, straight-leg raises, active knee extension	X	X	X		
Closed-chain (gait retraining, toe raises, wall sits, mini-squats		X	X	X	
Knee flexion hamstring curls (90 degrees)			X	X	X
Knee extension quads (90–0 degrees)	X	X	X	X	X
Hip abduction-adduction, multi-hip	X	X	X	X	X
Leg press (50–0 degrees)	X	X	X	X	X
Balance/proprioceptive training					
Weight-shifting, mini-trampoline, BAPS, KAT, plyometrics		X	X	X	X
Conditioning					
UBE	X	X	X		
Bicycle (stationary)	X	X	X	X	X
Aquatic program			X	X	X
Swimming (kicking)				X	X
Walking				X	X
Stair-climbing machine			X	X	X
Ski machine			X	X	X
Running: straight				X	X
Cutting: lateral carioca, figure-of-eights					X
Full sports					X

tively. During this phase, the patient may also be measured for a functional PCL brace, which is indicated for higher level occupational or sports activities. For patients who return to lower levels of activity, or who develop patellofemoral symptoms, a patellofemoral knee sleeve may be indicated for prolonged standing and walking activities.

With complex ligament reconstructions that involve the PCL and medial or lateral ligament structures, it is not safe to use a standard hinged brace. These devices are not effective in preventing excessive medial or lateral forces (joint openings), which place the reconstruction at risk in the initial 4 weeks postoperatively. In these cases, it is necessary to use a bivalved cast to limit medial or lateral joint openings during ambulation and activities of daily living. It is still possible to design an effective range of motion program to prevent joint contracture and promote the beneficial effects of motion to the joint. The bivalved cast is removed four times a day under controlled conditions and active range of motion is allowed in a seated position. The cast is then carefully reapplied to protect the knee joint during walking activities. After the first 4 postoperative weeks, sufficient healing of the medial or lateral ligamentous reconstructive procedure should occur and the patient can then be placed in a long-leg hinged brace.

Range of Knee Motion

Passive knee motion from 0 to 90 degrees is allowed immediately postoperatively. While patients are encouraged to regain full extension as soon as possible, knee flexion is limited for the first 7 to 8 postoperative weeks to avoid high posterior shear forces. The goals for flexion are shown in Table 12–1 and include 110 degrees at postoperative week 2, 120 degrees at postoperative week 6, and 135 degrees at postoperative week 8.

The early emphasis on regaining 0 degrees is critical to avoid excessive scarring in the intercondylar notch. One exercise helpful in the early postoperative period is propping of the patient's foot and ankle on a towel, which elevates the hamstrings and gastrocnemius, allowing the knee to drop into full extension. This exercise is performed for 10 minutes and repeated approximately six times per day. If 0 degrees is not achieved,

a hanging weight program is begun. Using the same propped leg position, a 10-pound weight is added to the distal thigh and knee to stretch the posterior capsule. Care should be taken to keep the hanging weight away from the proximal tibia to avoid posterior shear stresses. Full knee extension should be obtained by the third to sixth postoperative week. If this is not accomplished, or if the clinician notes a firm endfeel, then a serial casting program may be required. Even though we advocate regaining 0 degrees of knee extension, we do not encourage achieving hyperextension, as this can place the graft at increased risk for failure.

Passive knee flexion exercises are performed in the seated position, using the opposite lower extremity to provide overpressure. Care must be taken to provide proximal tibial support to prevent posterior dropback during this exercise. A 10-pound anterior drawer is maintained on the proximal tibia during passive knee flexion, as PCL forces significantly increase after 70 degrees of flexion. Knee flexion exercises are strictly passive for the first 12 weeks. Care must be taken to avoid activating the hamstrings. Other methods to assist in gaining flexion include chair rolling, wall sliding, and passive quadriceps stretching exercises.

Weight-Bearing

Patients are allowed partial weight-bearing (25 percent of the patient's body weight) for the first 2 weeks. Progression to 50 percent of the patient's body weight is then allowed at postoperative weeks 3 to 4 when the patient demonstrates 0 to 90 degrees of flexion, pain and joint hemarthrosis are controlled, and the quadriceps tone is good. Patients are allowed to bear more weight on the limb and are usually weaned from crutches between postoperative weeks 6 and 8.

Once patients are full weight-bearing, they are warned to avoid squatting, walking down hills or ramps, or any sudden deceleration movements that may place high forces on the PCL graft. These precautions are maintained for at least the first 6 postoperative months.

Weight-bearing is progressed using a normal gait technique, avoiding a locked knee position and encouraging normal flexion throughout the gait cycle. This allows for normal patterning of heel to toe ambulation, quadriceps contraction during midstance, and hip and knee flexion during the gait cycle. The locked knee position is avoided because of the potential for developing a quadriceps avoidance gait pattern.

Patellar Mobilization

This exercise is critical in the promotion of a full range of knee motion. The loss of patellar mobility is often associated with knee motion complications and, in extreme cases, the development of patella infera.[11] Patellar glides are performed in all four planes (superior, inferior, medial, and lateral) with sustained pressure applied to the appropriate patellar border for at least 10 seconds. This exercise is performed for 5 minutes whenever range of motion exercises are completed. Caution is warranted if an extensor lag is detected, as this may be associated with poor superior migration of the patella, indicating the need for additional emphasis on this exercise. Patellar mobilization is performed for approximately 8 weeks postoperatively.

Modalities

The use of therapeutic modalities after PCL reconstruction is usually minimal. If the patient demonstrates a fair or poor rating of the quadriceps or vastus medialis obliquus (VMO) musculature, then electrical muscle stimulation (EMS) is initiated. Electrodes are placed over the VMO and on the central to lateral aspect of the upper one-third of the quadriceps muscle belly. The patient actively contracts the quadriceps muscle simultaneously with the machine's stimulation. Treatment sessions last for 20 minutes. This modality is used as an adjunct to the active exercise program. Home EMS machines may be required in individuals whose muscle rating is poor. EMS is continued until the muscle grade is rated as good.

Biofeedback therapy is also quite useful in facilitating quadriceps muscle contractions. The surface electrode is placed over the selected muscle component to provide positive feedback to the patient and clinician regarding the quality of active or voluntary quadriceps contraction. This modality can enhance relaxation of the hamstring musculature if the patient experiences difficulty achieving full knee extension secondary to knee pain or muscle spasm. The electrode is placed over the belly of the hamstring muscle while the patient performs range of motion exercises.

Cryotherapy is instituted in the recovery room after surgery. Several different cold modalities are available for use in both the clinical and home settings. Commercially available cold therapy units include the popular motorized cooler units (eg, Polar Care, Breg, Inc., Vista, CA), which maintain a constant temperature and circulation of ice water through a pad, providing excellent pain control. One potential drawback with these units is their cost, quoted by a recent study to be approximately $225.00 to the patient.[12] Gravity flow units (eg, CryoCuff, AirCast, Summit, NJ) also provide effective pain management; however, the maintenance of a constant temperature is difficult with these devices. We have found that the temperature can be controlled by using gravity to backflow and drain the water, refilling the cuff with fresh ice water as required. For most patients, cryotherapy is accomplished with an ice bag or commercial cold pack. Standard treatment times are 20 minutes and are performed from three times a day to every waking hour depending upon the extent of pain and swelling. In some cases, the treatment time can be extended based on the thickness of the buffer used between the skin and the device. Cryotherapy is typically used after exercise or when required for pain and swelling control, and is maintained throughout the entire postoperative rehabilitation protocol.

Stretching

Flexibility exercises are performed both before and after PCL reconstruction. Hamstring and gastrocsoleus stretches are begun the first postoperative day. Sustained static stretching is encouraged, with the stretch held for 30 seconds and repeated five times. The modified hurdler stretch is the most common hamstring exercise, and the towel pull is the most common gastrocsoleus stretch. These exercises assist in controlling pain that occurs due to the reflex response created in the hamstrings when the knee is kept in the flexed position. Also, the towel pulling exercise can help lessen discomfort in the calf, Achilles tendon, and ankle. These stretches represent critical components of the range of motion program, as the ability to relax these muscle groups is imperative to achieving full passive knee extension. The patient must be instructed not to perform harsh, aggressive stretching, which could result in activation of the hamstring muscles.

Quadriceps and iliotibial band stretches assist in achieving full knee flexion and controlling lateral hip and thigh tightness. Factors to consider when designing a flexibility program include examination of the particular sport or activity the individual wishes to return to, as well as the position or physical requirements of that activity. The stretching program is performed prior to strengthening exercises and before functional or sports activities and should be performed after the patient is discharged from formal care.

Strengthening

The strengthening program is begun on the first postoperative visit. Early emphasis on the quadriceps muscle group is critical for a safe return to functional activities and to prevent posterior subluxation of the tibia from occurring during activities in which the knee is flexed greater than 50 degrees. In this phase of rehabilitation, initiation of a good voluntary quadriceps contraction sets the tone for the progression of the strengthening program. Isometric quadriceps contractions are done every hour following the repetition rules of 10-second holds, 10 repetitions, 10 times per day. Adequate evaluation by both the therapist and patient of this contraction is critical. The patient can monitor contractions by visual or manual means, comparing the quality of the contractions to those achieved by the contralateral limb. They can also assess the superior migration of the patella during the contraction, which should be approximately 1 cm, and the inferior migration of the patella during the initial relaxation of the contraction.

Other exercises performed immediately postoperatively are supine straight-leg raises and active-assisted knee extension (70 to 0 degrees postoperative weeks 1 and 2, then 90 to 0 degrees). The patient must

achieve a sufficient isometric quadriceps contraction with the leg raises to benefit the quadriceps. Initially, 1 to 2 pounds of weight are used and eventually, up to 10 pounds is added as long as this is not more than 10 percent of the patient's body weight. Active-assisted range of motion facilitates the quadriceps muscle if poor tone is observed during isometric contractions. At postoperative weeks 3 to 4, adduction straight leg raises are incorporated. Abduction leg raises are begun at postoperative weeks 7 to 8, and extension leg raises are initiated at postoperative week 9. These exercises are continued through at least postoperative week 12, when emphasis is placed on controlling pain and swelling, regaining full range of motion, achieving quadriceps control and proximal hip stabilization, and resuming a normal gait pattern.

Once partial weight-bearing is initiated, closed kinetic chain (CKC) exercises are begun. Numerous studies have assessed both the safety of these exercises on the healing graft and the benefits incurred to the lower extremity musculature.[3, 13, 14] The first CKC exercise we use is cup walking, an activity designed to facilitate adequate quadriceps control during midstance of gait to prevent knee hyperextension. When the patient progresses to 50 to 75 percent weight-bearing, toe-raises for gastrocsoleus strengthening, wall sitting isometrics for quadriceps control, and mini-squats for quadriceps strengthening are begun. The goal of wall sitting is to improve quadriceps contraction by performing the exercise to muscle exhaustion. This exercise can be modified to decrease patellar pain or place additional stress on the quadriceps muscle. Patellar pain can be decreased either by altering the knee flexion angle of the sit or by subtly changing the toe out/toe in angle by no more than 10 degrees. Additional stress to the quadriceps can be accomplished by several methods. First, patients can voluntarily set the quadriceps muscle once they reach their maximum knee flexion angle, which is typically between 30 and 45 degrees. This contraction and knee flexion position is held until muscle fatigue occurs, and the exercise is repeated three to five times. In a second modification, the patient performs a hip adduction contraction by squeezing a ball between the distal thighs. This modification promotes a stronger VMO contraction. In a third variation, patients hold dumbbell weights in their hands to increase body weight which promotes an even stronger quadriceps contraction. Finally, patients can shift their body weight over the involved side to stimulate a single-leg contraction.

The last CKC exercise we recommend is the mini-squat. Initially, the patient's body weight is used as resistance. Gradually, theraband or surgical tubing is employed as resistance mechanisms. The depth of the squat is controlled to protect the patellofemoral joint. Quick, smooth, rhythmic squats are performed to a high set/high repetition cadence to promote muscle fatigue. It is important to monitor hip position to emphasize the quadriceps. Increased trunk flexion facilitates increased hamstring contractions[4] and therefore must be carefully monitored to avoid forceful hamstring contractions for a minimum of 3 to 6 months.

We include open kinetic chain (OKC) exercises in our rehabilitation program because of the advantage of muscle group isolation provided by weight machines (eg, Nautilus, Body Masters, Cybex Eagle). Initially, if the lightest amount of weight on the machine is too heavy to be lifted by the involved limb alone, the patient is instructed to lift the weight with both legs and lower it with the involved side. Eccentric contractions can also be used in the advanced stages of strength training if tendinitis or overuse syndromes develop from overtraining. Weight training is used in the latter stages of rehabilitation and continues after the patient has returned to activity.

The timing of the initiation of knee extension, hip, leg press, and hamstring curl OKC exercises is shown in Table 12–1. Knee flexion hamstring curls are delayed until the ninth postoperative week to avoid excessive posterior shear forces incurred with this activity. Leg press (50–0 degree range) exercises and hip abduction-adduction are allowed at the fourth postoperative week. Knee extension OKC exercises begin between postoperative weeks three and four. Caution is warranted because of the potential problems knee extension OKC exercises may create for the healing graft and the patellofemoral joint. Many patients have an unsatisfactory outcome based on persistent anterior or patellofemoral knee pain, which can occur due to improper training in the terminal phase of extension (0 to 30 degrees).[15] Therefore, our recommendations for knee extension exercises include empha-

sis on patellofemoral protection (monitoring for changes in pain, swelling, and crepitus) and a gradual progression of weight to avoid overuse syndromes.

A full lower extremity strengthening program is critical for long-term success of the rehabilitation program. Gastrocsoleus strength is a key component for both early ambulation and running. In addition, an upper extremity and torso strength program is important for safe return to work or sports. These exercises are included as part of general conditioning, and general strength training concepts are emphasized. Sport and position specificity are taken into account when devising the program to maximize its benefits.

Balance and Proprioceptive Training

Balance and proprioceptive training are initiated at approximately the fifth to sixth postoperative week when the patient is partial weight-bearing. The first exercise involves weight shifting from side to side and front to back. This activity encourages patient confidence in the leg's ability to withstand the pressures of weight-bearing and initiates the stimulus to knee joint position sense. A second exercise begun with partial weight-bearing is cup walking, which is designed to develop symmetry between the surgical and uninvolved limbs. Cup walking helps develop hip and knee flexion, quadriceps control during midstance, hip and pelvic control during midstance, and adequate gastrocsoleus control during pushoff, and controls hip hiking. One other activity for balance control is the single-leg balance exercise. The stance position is key to making this exercise beneficial. The patient is instructed to point the foot straight ahead, flex the knee approximately 20 to 30 degrees, extend the arms outward to horizontal, and position the torso upright with the shoulders above the hips and the hips above the ankles. The object of this activity is to stand in position until balance is disturbed. A mini-tramp can be used to make this exercise more challenging. The unstable position the tramp creates with the soft surface requires greater dynamic limb control than that used to stand on a flat surface.

The progression of balance training leads

to the use of more sophisticated systems. There are many balance systems available, with a wide cost variance. Some of the lower-end technical devices include styrofoam half rolls, whole rolls, and the Biomechanical Ankle Platform System (BAPS, Camp, Jackson, MI). Clinically, we feel that these devices help develop balance, coordination, and proprioception; however, there are few data in the literature to assess their efficacy. In the early phases of full, unassisted weight-bearing, half foam rolls are used as part of the gait retraining program. Walking on half rolls helps the patient develop balance and dynamic muscular control required to maintain an upright position and be able to walk from one end of the roll to the other. Developing a center of balance, limb symmetry, quadriceps control in midstance, and postural positioning are benefits obtained from this type of training. Use of the BAPS board in double-leg and single-leg stance provides another proprioceptive exercise. These activities can also be progressed to include partner ball catching, Body Blade (Hymanson, Inc., Playa Del Rey, CA) exercises, or the advancement to Plyoback (Functionally Integrated Technologies, Watsonville, CA) programs, depending on the patient's functional goals.

The use of more sophisticated devices adds another dimension to the proprioception program, as certain units objectively attempt to document balance and dynamic control. Three of the more common units include Breg's Kinesthetic Awareness Trainer (Breg, Inc., Vista, CA), Biodex's Stabilometry System (Biodex Corporation, Shirley, NY) and Neurocom's Balance System (Neurocom, Clackamas, OR). Although these systems may provide objective information, more research is required to justify the cost and reliability of each unit.

In the later phases of rehabilitation, plyometric exercises are initiated to provide a functional basis for return to activity. This training begins after the sixth postoperative month when the patient demonstrates no more than a 20 percent deficit for the quadriceps and hamstrings on isokinetic testing. The first exercise is level surface box hopping. A four-square grid is created with tape on the floor of four equally sized boxes. The patient is instructed to first hop from box 1 to box 3 (front-to-back), and then from box 1 to box 2 (side-to-side). Several instructions are very important to ensure safety of this

exercise. The drill is initially performed using both legs. The patient is instructed to keep the body weight on the ball of the foot, to hop with the knees bent, and to land in flexion to avoid knee hyperextension. It is also important for the patient to understand that the exercise is a reaction and agility drill; therefore, speed is emphasized. It is important for the patient to focus on limb symmetry during this exercise. One way to measure improvement is to count the number of hops in a defined time period. The initial exercise time period is 15 seconds. The patient is asked to complete as many hops between the squares as possible in 15 seconds. Three sets are performed for both directions, and the number of hops is recorded. An assistant is present to count and time the exercise. Progression of the program occurs as the number of hops improves, as well as patient confidence. This exercise has four levels. The first level includes front-to-back and side-to-side hopping previously described. The second level incorporates both of the directions in level one into one sequence, and also includes hopping in both right and left directions (box 1 to box 2 to box 4 to box 2 to box 1). Level three progresses to diagonal hops, and level four includes pivot hops in a 180-degree direction. Once the patient can perform level four double-leg hops, we initiate similar exercises using single-leg hops.

The next phase of plyometric exercises uses vertical box hops. It is important to stress that plyometric exercise is intense and adequate rest must be included in the program. Individual sessions can be performed in a manner similar to interval training. Initially, the rest period lasts two to three times the length of the exercise period and is gradually decreased to one to two times the length of the exercise period. Also, plyometric hopping is performed two to three times each week and is incorporated into the strength and cardiovascular endurance program.

Other parameters to consider when performing plyometric exercises include surface, footwear, and warm-up. This program should be performed on a surface that is firm yet forgiving, such as a wooden gym floor. Very hard surfaces like concrete should be avoided. Additionally, a cross-training or running shoe should be worn to provide adequate shock absorption as well as adequate stability to the foot. Checking wear patterns and outer sole wear will help avoid overuse injuries. Finally, an adequate warm-up should include exercises and a light cardiovascular workout.

Conditioning

Depending on accessibility, a cardiovascular program can be initiated at approximately the third to fourth postoperative week with an upper body ergometer (UBE). A neutrally supported position of the surgical limb should be encouraged to minimize lower extremity swelling. This exercise can be performed to tolerance. Stationary bicycling is begun at postoperative week 4. The goals of these early conditioning exercises include facilitation of full range of motion, gait retraining, and cardiovascular reconditioning. To improve cardiovascular endurance, the program should be performed at least three times per week for 20 to 30 minutes, and the exercise performed to at least 60 to 85 percent of maximal heart rate. It is generally regarded that performing in the higher levels of percentage of maximal heart rate achieves greater cardiovascular efficiency and endurance.

Gradually, between the ninth and twelfth postoperative weeks, cross-country skiing and stair-climbing machines are incorporated. Protection against high stresses to the patellofemoral joint is strongly advocated in patients with symptoms or articular cartilage deterioration. During bicycling, the seat height is adjusted to its highest level based on patient body size and a low resistance level is used during the workout. Toe clips should be avoided to decrease hamstring involvement. If a stair-climbing machine is tolerated, we suggest maintaining a short step and using lower resistance levels. Monitoring heart rate will ensure that work levels are sufficient to improve cardiovascular fitness.

A complete cardiovascular exercise program is an important component of the latter phases of rehabilitation. In addition to the previously described exercises, an aquatic program that includes lap work using freestyle or flutter kicking, water walking, water aerobics, and deep water running is initiated. Determining which cardiovascular exercises are appropriate is based on each individual patient. Factors to assess include concomitant operative procedures, second-ary injuries, access to specific equipment, individual preferences, and prior experience. The primary consideration for the conditioning program throughout the rehabilitation protocol is to stress the cardiovascular system without compromising the joint.

Running and Return to Sports Activities

Current studies do not allow a prediction of return of strength of PCL grafts, so conservative estimates regarding return to strenuous activities are warranted. To initiate the running program, the patient must demonstrate no more than a 30 percent deficit in average torque for the quadriceps and hamstrings on isometric testing, have no more than 3 mm of increase in anteroposterior displacement on arthrometer testing, and be at least 6 months postoperative. The running program is designed based on the sport the patient desires to return to, as well as the particular position or physical requirements of the activity. For instance, an individual returning to short-duration, high-intensity activities participates in a sprinting program rather than a long-distance endurance program.

The beginning level running program is first performed with a straight ahead walk/run combination. Running distances are 20, 40, 60, and 100 yards in both forward and backward directions. Initially, running speed is approximately one-quarter to one-half of the patient's normal speed, and gradually progresses to three-quarters and full speed. An interval training-rest approach is applied in which the rest phase is two to three times the length of the training phase. The running program is performed three times per week, on opposite days of the strength program. Since the running program may not reach aerobic levels initially, a cross-training program is used to facilitate cardiovascular fitness. The cross-training program is performed on the same day as the strength workout.

After the patient is able to run straight ahead at full speed, the program progresses to the second level to include lateral running and crossover maneuvers. Short distances, such as 20 yards, are used to work on speed and agility. Side-to-side running over cups may be used to facilitate proprioception. At this time, sport-specific equipment is introduced to enhance skill development (eg, a soccer ball for a soccer player to work on dribbling and passing activities). These variations are useful to motivate the patient and minimize training boredom.

The third level of the running program incorporates figure-of-eight running drills. These drills begin with long and wide movement patterns to encourage subtle cutting. The training distance initially is 20 yards; as speed and confidence improve, the distance is decreased to approximately 10 yards. Progression through this phase is similar to that used in the lateral side-to-side program just described. Speed and agility are emphasized and equipment is introduced to develop sport-specific skills.

The fourth phase in the running program introduces cutting patterns. These patterns include directional changes at 45- and 90-degree angles, which allow the patient to progress from subtle to sharp cuts. Once the patient has completed the functional program and the strength, displacement, and function testing results reach normal values, return to sports is allowed. A trial of function is encouraged in which the patient is monitored for overuse symptoms or giving-way episodes. Upon successful return to activity, the patient is encouraged to continue with a maintenance program. During the in-season, a conditioning program of two workouts a week is recommended. In the off-season or pre-season, this program should be performed three times a week to maximize gains in flexibility, strength, and cardiovascular endurance.

We developed discharge criteria following PCL reconstructions based on patient goals for athletics and occupations and the rating of symptoms, stress radiography, KT-2000 testing, muscle strength testing, and function testing (Table 12–2). First, patients complete the Cincinnati Sports Activity Scale[16] and Occupational Rating Scale[17] to provide sports and occupational levels that are desired after surgery. Upon completion of the protocol, pain, swelling, and giving-way are rated on the Cincinnati Symptom Rating Scale.[16] The patient must not experience these symptoms at the level of activity at which they wish to participate prior to discharge. Stress radiography is performed at 70 degrees of flexion with 89 N of force as described previously[10] and the difference between knees (average of measurements for both the medial and lateral tibial plateaus) must be within normal limits (less than 3 mm) prior to recommendation of return to strenuous activities. KT-2000 testing is also conducted at both 20 and 70 degrees of flexion (134 N at 20 degrees and 89 N at 70 degrees). Muscle strength testing is performed with a Biodex isokinetic dynamometer (Biodex Corporation, Shirley, NY) to ensure that adequate strength exists prior to the initiation of the plyometric, running, and cutting programs. At least two function tests are completed and limb symmetry calculated as previously described[18, 19] prior to the final discharge.

Table 12–2. Discharge Criteria Following Posterior Cruciate Ligament Reconstruction

Sports/Occupation Level	Symptom Rating* (pain, swelling, giving-way)	Stress Radiography (70 degrees, 89 N) (mm)	KT-2000 (Total AP, I-N) (mm)		Biodex Isometric Test (% deficit)	Function Testing (limb symmetry) (%)
			20 degrees	*70 degrees*		
Sports: I (jumping, pivoting, cutting) Occupation: heavy/very heavy	None level 10	<3	<3	<5	≤15	≥85
Sports: II (running, turning, twisting) Occupation: moderate	None level 8	<5	<3	<5	≤20	≥85
Sports: III (swimming, bicycling) Occupation: light	None level 6	<8	3–5	3–5	≤30	≥75
Sports: IV (none) Occupation: very light	None level 4	<8	3–5	3–5	>30	<75

*Level 10, normal knee, no symptoms with strenuous work/sports with jumping, hard pivoting; level 8, no symptoms with moderate work/sports with running, turning, twisting; level 6, no symptoms with light work/sports with no running, twisting, or jumping; level 4, no symptoms with activities of daily living.

AP, anteroposterior; I-N, involved-noninvolved.

LATERAL, POSTEROLATERAL GRAFT RECONSTRUCTIONS

A specific rehabilitation protocol was developed for patients who have had lateral or posterolateral major reconstructions for acute or chronic deficiencies of these tissues. In acute cases, a direct repair of the LCL with or without augmentation of a one-half biceps tendon transfer with repair of the posterolateral structures is performed (Table 12–3). In chronic injury cases in which a definitive LCL of normal width and integrity (although lax) is identified, the popliteus attachments to the fibula (popliteo-fibular ligament) and tibia are intact, and the posterolateral structures are of adequate thickness, a proximal advancement may be performed. However, many knees require a major graft reconstruction for a chronically deficient LCL and posterolateral complex from prior gross disruption and poor healing, and considerable scar tissue in the posterolateral complex structures. Frequently, a concomitant ACL or PCL ligament reconstruction is required. These ligamentous reconstructive procedures represent major operative procedures with extensive postoperative swelling, muscle weakness, and need for intensive supervised rehabilitation. The potential complication rate is high for motion limitations and extensive muscle weakness.

In cases in which the LCL is deficient and of reduced size, an LCL circle allograft reconstruction can be performed as described elsewhere in detail.[7] This procedure provides the first portion of the lateral reconstruction and replaces important lateral tensile-bearing tissues. Then, the posterolateral complex is either plicated or advanced to produce a dense collagenous plate of tissues. A straight lateral incision 12 to 15 cm in length is extended distally to allow exposure of the fibular head and proximally to expose the LCL femoral attachment site. A 6-mm drill hole is made anteriorly and posteriorly at the head-neck junction in the center of the fibula. At the LCL femoral attachment site, another 6-mm drill hole is made just anterior and posterior to the ligament insertion. This drill hole is deepened 10 mm, leaving approximately 8 mm of the LCL attachment. An Achilles tendon allograft, 6 to 7 mm in diameter and of sufficient length for the proximal and distal posterior arms of the circle graft to overlap, is inserted through bony tunnels in the femur and fibula (Fig. 12–4). The allograft is placed under slight tension with the knee at 30 degrees of flexion and neutral tibial rotation. Multiple interrupted sutures are used through the posterior overlapped arms of the allograft. The LCL is interposed between the posterior and anterior arms of the allograft, and horizontal sutures are then placed between both structures (Fig. 12–5-*A* and *B*). This procedure is followed by a proximal advancement of the posterolateral complex, previously described.[9]

In certain cases of lateral and posterolateral complex deficiency in which only scar tissues are present and active function of the popliteus is not expected, autogenous graft replacement of these structures is required. We prefer to use a 10-mm bone-patellar tendon-bone autograft to replace the LCL (Fig. 12–6). The graft is attached at the LCL femoral anatomic insertion site with two small fragment screws. A semitendinosus and gracilis two-strand autograft is used to replace the popliteus-arcuate complex (Fig. 12–7). Both tendons are brought out through the proximal lateral tibia (at the site of the popliteus-tendon junction) or through a separate drill hole in the fibula. In cases in which the distal popliteal attachments to the tibia and fibula are intact, a proximal advancement of the popliteus tendon alone can be performed. Alternative graft choices include the iliotibial band or an allograft.

We frequently see at our center failure of prior cruciate and posterolateral procedures that occur early postoperatively when wean-

---

●▬ Table 12–3. **Authors' Recommendations for Repair/Reconstruction of Lateral and Posterolateral Complex Ruptures**

Acute Injury	1. Direct repair, augment with one-half biceps tendon transfer
Chronic Injury	1. Advance: proximal or recession
	2. Augment: circle Achilles tendon allograft
	3. Replace:
	Lateral collateral ligament: bone-patellar tendon-bone autograft
	Popliteus tendon: semitendinosus and gracilis two-stranded autograft or allograft
	Posterolateral capsule: allograft

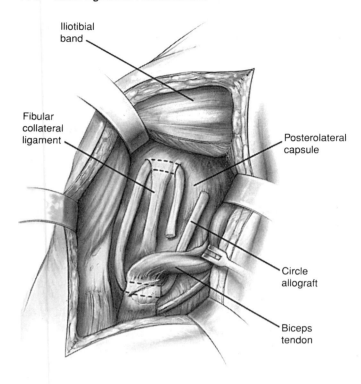

Figure 12–4. Achilles tendon circle allograft reconstruction for lateral collateral ligament (LCL) deficiency. After a drill hole is made and dilated anteriorly and posteriorly at the fibula head-neck junction, a second drill hole is made just anterior and posterior to the insertion site of the LCL on the femur. The allograft is passed through the tibial and femoral tunnels and lies adjacent to the remaining LCL tissue. (From Noyes FR, Roberts CS: High tibial osteotomy in knees with associated chronic ligament deficiencies. In Jackson DW (ed): Master Techniques in Orthopaedic Surgery: Reconstructive Knee Surgery. Philadelphia, Lippincott-Raven, 1995. Illustrations by Christy Krames.)

(Labels on figure: Iliotibial band; Fibular collateral ligament; Posterolateral capsule; Circle allograft; Biceps tendon)

ing from crutch support occurs and there has been inadequate muscle strength and conditioning to provide knee stability during ambulatory activities. In these situations, the knee musculature is unable to provide the joint compression forces required to protect against lateral compartment lift-off[20] and stretching of the lateral procedures occurs. We emphasize intensive follow-up in the early postoperative phase to detect these problems.

Protocol for Lateral, Posterolateral Graft Reconstructions

The protocol incorporates immediate protected knee motion, but also includes maximal protection against undue joint loads to prevent graft stretching and failure (Table 12–4). Patients are warned that they must avoid hyperextension and activities that would incur varus loading on the joint. Delays in return of full knee flexion, weightbearing, initiation of certain strengthening and conditioning exercises, and initiation of running and return to full sports activities are incorporated. A specific gait retraining program is implemented for patients who demonstrate an abnormal knee hyperextension gait pattern.[21] This program is begun before surgery, and the principles of avoiding a thrusting hyperextension motion at the knee and walking with the knee slightly flexed throughout stance phase are advocated postoperatively.

A Bledsoe (Bledsoe, Grand Prairie, TX) long-leg postoperative brace, locked at 0 degrees of extension, is worn for the first 4 postoperative weeks. The patient is instructed to remove the brace three to four times each day for range of motion exercises only. Then, a custom medial unloader brace is worn for at least the first postoperative year to provide protection against knee hyperextension and excessive varus loads.[22] To date, the Bledsoe unloader brace (Fig. 12–8) has been used because of its medial hinge placement. Care must be taken to avoid condylar pad or strap friction along the lateral incision.

Patients are allowed 0 to 90 degrees of flexion immediately postoperatively. Flexion is slowly advanced to 110 degrees by postoperative week 5, 120 degrees by week 8, and 130 degrees by week 12. Partial weightbearing is begun at postoperative week 4 with slow advancement to full by week 8. When working on knee flexion, care must be

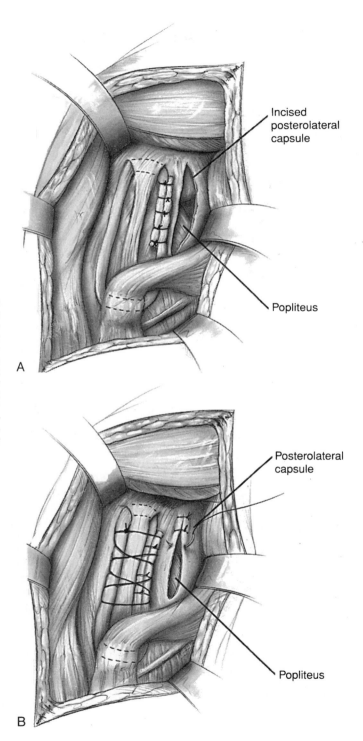

Figure 12–5. *A*, After passage of the Achilles tendon circle allograft, an incision is made in the posterolateral capsule behind the lateral collateral ligament (LCL) and anterior to the arcuate complex. *B*, A simple vest-over-pants plication of the allograft to the LCL will remove any redundancy. (From Noyes FR, Roberts CS: High tibial osteotomy in knees with associated chronic ligament deficiencies. In Jackson DW (ed): Master Techniques in Orthopaedic Surgery: Reconstructive Knee Surgery. Philadelphia, Lippincott-Raven, 1995. Illustrations by Christy Krames.)

Incised
posterolateral
capsule

Popliteus

A

Posterolateral
capsule

Popliteus

B

taken to avoid varus tensioning. The patient is taught (and the assistance of a partner is encouraged) to place a hand on the lateral aspect of the knee and to create a 10-pound valgus load to protect the lateral structures.

Patellar mobilization, flexibility exercises, modality usage, and the strengthening and conditioning programs are all similar to those described in the PCL reconstruction protocol. Regarding strengthening exercises, active knee extension is maintained in the 90- to 30-degree range throughout the rehabilitation program. The running program is not allowed to begin until at least the ninth postoperative month, and the plyometric and sport-specific training programs are delayed until at least the twelfth postoperative month. Patients must have obtained the previously described muscle strength indices, and must also demonstrate no more than 2

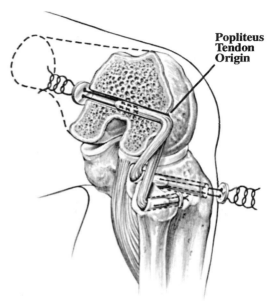

Figure 12–7. Semitendinosus and gracilis two-strand autograft substitution of the popliteus complex. Both tendons are brought through the tibia and the popliteofibular ligament is reconstructed, or a separate drill hole is added to the fibula. (From Noyes FR, Barber-Westin SD: Treatment of complex injuries involving the posterior cruciate and posterolateral ligaments of the knee. Am J Knee Surg 9:200, 1996.)

mm increase in lateral joint opening on stress radiographs, prior to being allowed to engage in stressful activity such as running and cutting.

Discharge criteria following lateral and posterolateral graft reconstructions are based on patient goals for athletics and occupations and the rating of symptoms, lateral joint opening, muscle strength testing, and function testing (Table 12–5). Lateral joint opening is assessed either by stress radiography or manual testing at 20 degrees of flexion. The remainder of the assessment is performed as previously described for PCL reconstructions.

CLINICAL OUTCOME STUDIES

We reported results of 25 patients who had PCL allograft reconstructions previously.[1] Ten patients had a PCL allograft reconstruction alone and 15 patients had the allograft augmented with a ligament augmentation device (LAD). The allograft tissues used were either bone-patellar tendon-bone

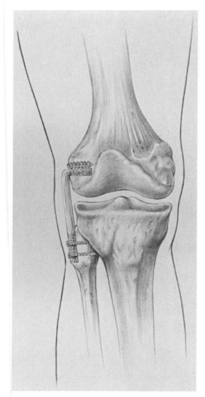

Figure 12–6. Bone-patellar tendon-bone autogenous graft substitution for deficient lateral collateral ligament (LCL). Two small fragment screws are used to fix the bone into a slot created in the proximal fibula. Interference screw fixation is used at the LCL femoral anatomic site. (From Noyes FR, Barber-Westin SD: Treatment of complex injuries involving the posterior cruciate and posterolateral ligaments of the knee. Am J Knee Surg 9:200, 1996.)

Table 12–4. Cincinnati Sportsmedicine and Orthopaedic Center Rehabilitation Protocol for Lateral, Posterolateral Ligament Reconstruction

	Postoperative Weeks			Postoperative Months	
	1 to 4	*5 to 8*	*9 to 12*	*4 to 6*	*7 to 12*
Brace					
Bledsoe 0° locked	X				
Custom medial unloader		X	X	X	X
Range of motion goals (degrees)					
0–90	X				
0–110		X			
0–120		X			
0–130			X		
Weight-bearing					
None	X				
Toe-touch to one-quarter to one-half body weight	X				
Full body weight			X		
Patella mobilization	X	X			
Modalities					
Electrical muscle stimulation (EMS)	X	X			
Pain/edema management (cryotherapy)	X	X	X	X	X
Stretching					
Hamstring, gastroc-soleus, iliotibial band, quadriceps	X	X	X	X	X
Strengthening					
Quadriceps isometrics, straight-leg raises	X	X	X		
Active knee extension	X	X	X		
Closed-chain (gait retraining, toe raises, wall sits, mini-squats	X	X	X	X	
Knee flexion hamstring curls (90 degrees)			X	X	X
Knee extension quads (90–0 degrees)		X	X	X	X
Hip abduction-adduction, multi-hip			X	X	X
Leg press (50–0 degrees)			X	X	X
Balance/proprioceptive training					
Weight-shifting, mini-trampoline, BAPS, KAT, plyometrics		X	X	X	X
Conditioning					
UBE	X	X			
Bicycling (stationary)			X	X	X
Aquatic program			X	X	X
Swimming (kicking)			X	X	X
Walking				X	X
Stair-climbing machine			X	X	X
Ski machine				X	X
Running: straight					X
Cutting: lateral carioca, figure-of-eights					X
Full sports					X

or Achilles tendon. All allografts were sterilized with 25,000 grays of gamma irradiation. Eleven patients also had a proximal advancement of the posterolateral complex for insufficiency of these structures. The results were assessed an average of 45 months (range, 23 to 73 months) postoperatively.

The results demonstrated that posterior stability was restored at lower functional knee flexion angles (20 degrees) but not uniformly at high flexion angles (70 degrees). There were no statistically significant differences in stability, symptoms, functional limitations, sports activity levels, or the overall knee rating score between the two groups of patients. A second analysis was then performed to determine whether differences existed between patients who had the recon-

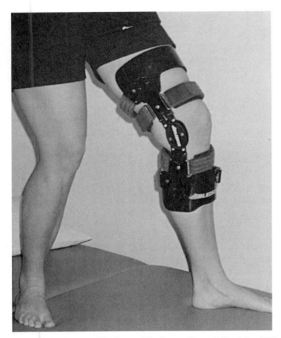

Figure 12–8. The Bledsoe (Bledsoe, Grand Prairie, TX) medial compartment unloader brace is worn for at least the first postoperative year following a major lateral or posterolateral graft reconstruction to provide protection against knee hyperextension and excessive varus loads.

creased displacement compared with 60 percent of those with chronic ruptures. At 70 degrees of flexion, partial stability (less than 5.5 mm of increased displacement) was restored in 60 percent of patients with acute ruptures and in 37 percent of patients with chronic ruptures. Based on the findings of our clinical allograft study and studies conducted in our laboratory on PCL fiber-length changes,[23-25] we currently use a double-bundle quadriceps-tendon graft for PCL reconstruction.

The results of the reconstructive procedure using Achilles tendon allograft tissue to restore LCL function were reported in 1995.[7] Twenty patients who underwent the operation for chronic lateral and posterolateral insufficiency were studied a mean of 42 months (range, 24 to 73 months) postoperatively. All received an Achilles tendon allograft reconstruction and a proximal advancement of the posterolateral complex. The majority of patients also had a concomitant cruciate ligament reconstruction. The results showed that 76 percent of the knees had a functional lateral, posterolateral reconstruction, 14 percent had partial function, and 10 percent failed. All but 1 of the 13 patients who had a concomitant ACL reconstruction had function or partial function of the ACL restored. Two of the three patients who had a concomitant PCL reconstruction had function or partial function of the PCL restored and one failed. For all patients, statistically significant improvements were found for symptoms and functional limitations between the preoperative and follow-up scores. We concluded from these data that the LCL allograft procedure

struction for acute PCL ruptures (10 patients) and those who had chronic ruptures (15 patients). Patients who had acute ruptures had significantly lower anteroposterior displacements and fewer symptoms and functional limitations than those who had chronic ruptures. For instance, at 20 degrees of knee flexion, all patients who had acute ruptures had less than 3 mm of in-

⊙▬ Table 12–5. **Discharge Criteria Following Lateral, Posterolateral Reconstructions**

Sports/Occupation Level	Symptom Rating* (pain, swelling, giving-way)	Lateral Joint Opening Increase (20 degree flexion) (mm)	Biodex Isokinetic Test (% deficit)	Function Testing (limb symmetry) (%)
Sports: I (jumping, pivoting, cutting) Occupation: heavy/very heavy	None level 10	None	≤15	≥85
Sports: II (running, turning, twisting) Occupation: moderate	None level 8	<3	≤20	≥85
Sports: III (swimming, bicycling) Occupation: light	None level 6	3–5	≤30	≥75
Sports: IV (none) Occupation: very light	None level 4	3–5	≤30	≥75

*Level 10, normal knee, no symptoms with strenuous work/sports with jumping, hard pivoting; level 8, no symptoms with moderate work/sports with running, turning, twisting; level 6, no symptoms with light work/sports with no running, twisting, or jumping; level 4, no symptoms with activities of daily living.

was effective in restoring lateral and posterolateral complex function in the majority of knees.

One of the major problems in patients with chronic injuries to the lateral and posterolateral structures is that they often develop an abnormal gait pattern, which is characterized by excessive knee hyperextension during the stance phase. These individuals complain of giving-way episodes that occur during activities of daily living. Severe quadriceps atrophy often accompanies this gait abnormality. Medial joint line pain may be experienced, which probably originates from increased compressive forces at the medial tibiofemoral compartment that are often related to varus osseous malalignment. Pain in the posterolateral soft tissues, presumed to arise from increased soft tissue tensile forces, is also a frequent complaint. The abnormal knee hyperextension gait pattern involves increased extension in the sagittal plane and is often accompanied by

a varus alignment in the coronal plane, which has been previously described as a varus recurvatum alignment.[26–28] In these patients, the degree of altered gait mechanics and the amount of knee hyperextension varies significantly. Some individuals may present with a markedly abnormal gait that severely disables the patient and limits ambulation. Others may only experience the hyperextension pattern after prolonged walking and muscle fatigue.

We recently conducted a study to examine the gait mechanics in patients who had a knee hyperextension gait pattern and combined posterolateral complex and ACL or PCL deficiency.[21] A gait analysis was conducted before and after the retraining program shown in Table 12–6. The program was designed to train patients to avoid knee hyperextension by walking with the knee slightly flexed throughout stance, maintaining ankle dorsiflexion in early stance, and maintaining an erect trunk-hip attitude

Table 12–6. Gait Retraining Program for Abnormal Knee Stance Hyperextension

Anatomical Part	Retraining Program
Trunk–Upper Body	1. Maintain erect position avoiding forward loading position, which shifts body weight anterior to knee joint during stance phase. 2. Avoid excessive medial-lateral sway during stance phase, which induces varus-valgus moments about the knee and hip.
Hip	1. Avoid excessive hip flexion during stance phase, which encourages knee hyperextension and fatigues hip extensors. 2. For valgus lower limb alignment, avoid excessive internal femoral rotation. Encourage external femoral rotation and walking on lateral foot border. Avoid "knock-knee" position (important for valgus thrusts). 3. For varus lower limb alignment, avoid external femoral rotation. Encourage internal femoral rotation, "knock-knee" position.
Knee	1. Avoid any knee hyperextension throughout stance phase by always maintaining a knee-flexion position. 2. Practice knee flexion-extension control walking in a slow manner; often, begin with crutches. Initially use an excessive knee-flexion position. 3. Gradually resume a more normal walking speed, after flexion-extension control and a more normal gait pattern are assumed. 4. Look for increase in patellofemoral pain. 5. Look for varus or valgus thrust with knee-flexion position. 6. Look for external or internal rotational tibiofemoral subluxations when flexion position resumed.
Ankle	1. Avoid excessive plantar flexion. Maintain dorsiflexion using soleus muscle to induce early heel rise (rocker-action) to encourage forward tibial progression and knee flexion. 2. Initially use excessive dorsiflexion and walking aids (elevated heel) to increase early heel-off in stance phase.
Foot	1. Encourage push-off against forefoot and toes along with early heel-off in stance phase to assist knee flexion during stance phase. 2. With associated varus alignment, encourage toe-out position. For valgus alignment, encourage toe-in position.

Reprinted with permission from Noyes FR, Dunworth LA, Andriacchi TP, Andrews M, Hewett TE: Knee hyperextension gait abnormalities in unstable knees. Recognition and gait retraining. Am J Sports Med 24:35–45, 1996.

during stance. Prior to retraining, all patients had excessive knee hyperextension during the stance phase (Fig. 12–9). After retraining, hyperextension at the knee and abnormal motion patterns at the hip and ankle were successfully reduced in four of the five patients tested to nearly normal levels. Additionally, pain during daily activities was reduced or eliminated. Based on this study, we recommend gait analysis and retraining in patients who demonstrate abnormal knee hyperextension patterns prior to ligament reconstruction. The thrusting hyperextension motion, which is associated with an abnormally high adduction moment that increases medial compartment compression forces and lateral distraction forces, will place any posterolateral reconstruction at risk for stretching out posteriorly. The failure to recognize and correct this abnormal gait pattern may lead to failure of reconstructed ligaments if the gait pattern is resumed postoperatively.

Finally, in patients in whom varus osseous malalignment exists, high tibial osteotomy is recommended prior to surgical reconstruction of severe lateral and posterolateral ligament deficiency.[7, 28–30] If the varus alignment is not corrected, lateral or posterolateral reconstructive procedures may fail because of the varus thrusting forces that will occur postoperatively. This is especially true in patients who have a high knee adduction moment measured on gait analysis,[31] or in patients who have the abnormal knee hyperextension gait pattern just described.

SUMMARY

The two rehabilitation protocols presented in this chapter describe our current criteria for postoperative management of complex reconstructive procedures of the posterior cruciate and lateral/posterolateral complex ligaments. Clinical studies demonstrated that immediate knee motion was not deleterious to these reconstructions and is recommended to prevent permanent knee arthrofibrosis. Each protocol is detailed with regard to bracing; range of knee motion exercises; progression of weight-bearing; gait retraining; use of modalities and cryotherapy; flexibility, strengthening, and conditioning programs; balance and proprioception training; and running and return to sports activity programs. Discharge criteria are detailed based on patient goals for athletics and the rating of several factors. Precautions are given for patients who demonstrate articular cartilage deterioration at surgery in regard

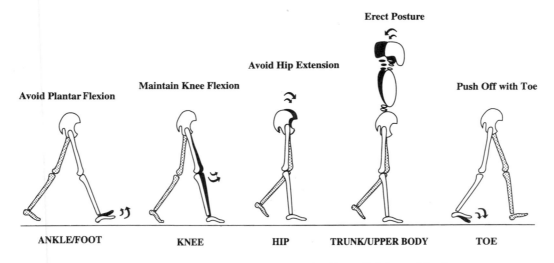

Figure 12–9. Graphic representation of gait abnormalities observed in patients before gait retraining. Filled gray anatomic structures represent the correct, retrained position at the trunk and upper body, hip, knee, foot and ankle, and toes. (From Noyes FR, Dunworth LA, Andriacchi TP, Andrews M, Hewett TE: Knee hyperextension in gait abnormalities in unstable knees: Recognition and gait retraining. Am J Sports Med 24:35–45, 1996.)

to exercise progression and realistic goals for future athletics. Outcome studies are summarized that support the use of these protocols, and recommendations are provided for various reconstructive options for chronic PCL and lateral/posterolateral ligament deficiency.

References

1. Noyes FR, Barber-Westin SD: Posterior cruciate ligament allograft reconstruction with and without a ligament augmentation device. Arthroscopy 10:371, 1994.
2. Anderson JK, Noyes FR: Principles of posterior cruciate ligament reconstruction. Orthopedics 18:493, 1995.
3. Lutz GE, Palmitier RA, An KN, Chao EYS: Comparison of tibiofemoral joint forces during open-kinetic-chain and closed-kinetic-chain exercises. J Bone Joint Surg 75A:732, 1993.
4. Ohkoshi Y, Yasuda K, Kaneda K, et al: Biomechanical analysis of rehabilitation in the standing position. Am J Sports Med 19:605, 1991.
5. Smidt GL: Biomechanical analysis of knee flexion and extension. J Biomech 6:79, 1973.
6. Yasuda K, Sasaki T: Exercise after anterior cruciate ligament reconstruction. The forces exerted on the tibia by the separate isometric contractions of the quadriceps or the hamstrings. Clin Orthop 220:275, 1987.
7. Noyes FR, Barber-Westin SD: Surgical reconstruction of severe chronic posterolateral complex injuries of the knee using allograft tissues. Am J Sports Med 23:2, 1995.
8. Noyes FR, Barber-Westin SD: Surgical restoration to treat chronic deficiency of the posterolateral complex and cruciate ligaments of the knee. Am J Sports Med 24:415, 1996.
9. Noyes FR, Barber-Westin SD: Treatment of complex injuries involving the posterior cruciate and posterolateral ligaments of the knee. Am J Knee Surg 9:200, 1996.
10. Hewett TE, Noyes FR, Lee MD: Diagnosis of complete and partial posterior cruciate ligament ruptures. Stress radiography compared with KT-1000 arthrometer and posterior drawer testing. Am J Sports Med 25:648, 1997.
11. Noyes FR, Wojtys EM, Marshall MT: The early diagnosis and treatment of developmental patella infera syndrome. Clin Orthop 265:241, 1991.
12. Konrath GA, Lock T, Giotz HT, Scheidler J: The use of cold therapy after anterior cruciate ligament reconstruction. A prospective, randomized study and literature review. Am J Sports Med 24:629, 1996.
13. Bynum EB, Barrack RL, Alexander AH: Open versus closed chain kinetic exercises after anterior cruciate ligament reconstruction. A prospective randomized study. Am J Sports Med 23:401, 1995.
14. Yack HF, Collins CE, Whieldon TJ: Comparison of closed and open kinetic chain exercise in the anterior cruciate ligament–deficient knee. Am J Sports Med 21:49, 1993.
15. Grood ES, Suntay WJ, Noyes FR, Butler DL: Biomechanics of the knee-extension exercise. Effect of cutting the anterior cruciate ligament. J Bone Joint Surg 66A:725, 1984.
16. Noyes FR, Barber SD, Mooar LA: A rationale for assessing sports activity levels and limitations in knee disorders. Clin Orthop 246:238, 1989.
17. Noyes FR, Mooar LA, Barber SD: The assessment of work-related activities and limitations in knee disorders. Am J Sports Med 19:178, 1991.
18. Barber SD, Noyes FR, Mangine RE et al.: Quantitative assessment of functional limitations in normal and anterior cruciate ligament–deficient knees. Clin Orthop 255:204, 1990.
19. Noyes FR, Barber SD, Mangine RE: Abnormal lower limb symmetry determined by function hop tests after anterior cruciate ligament rupture. Am J Sports Med 19:513, 1991.
20. Markolf KL, Bargar WL, Shoemaker SC, Amstutz HC: The role of joint load in knee stability. J Bone Joint Surg 63A:570, 1981.
21. Noyes FR, Dunworth LA, Andriacchi TP et al: Knee hyperextension gait abnormalities in unstable knees. Recognition and preoperative gait retraining. Am J Sports Med 24:35, 1996.
22. Lindenfeld TN, Hewett TE, Andriacchi TP: Decrease in knee joint loading with unloader brace wear in patients with medial compartment gonarthrosis. Clin Orthop 344:290, 1998.
23. Galloway MT, Grood ES, Mehalik JN, et al: Posterior cruciate ligament reconstruction. An in vitro study of femoral and tibial graft placement. Am J Sports Med 24:437, 1996.
24. Saddler SC, Noyes FR, Grood ES: Anatomy of the posterior cruciate ligament's femoral attachment. Orthop Trans 19:2, 1995.
25. Saddler SC, Noyes FR, Grood ES, et al: Posterior cruciate ligament anatomy and length-tension behavior of PCL surface fibers. Am J Knee Surg 9:194, 1996.
26. Baker CL, Jr., Norwood LA, Hughston JC: Acute posterolateral rotatory instability of the knee. J Bone Joint Surg 65A:614, 1983.
27. Hughston JC, Jacobson KE: Chronic posterolateral rotary instability of the knee. J Bone Joint Surg 67A:351, 1985.
28. Noyes FR, Simon R: The role of high tibial osteotomy in the anterior cruciate ligament–deficient knee with varus alignment. *In* DeLee JC, Drez D (eds): Orthopaedic Sports Medicine. Principles and Practice, vol 2. Philadelphia, W. B. Saunders, 1993, p. 1401.
29. Noyes FR, Barber SD, Simon R: High tibial osteotomy and ligament reconstruction in varus angulated, anterior cruciate ligament–deficient knees. A two- to seven-year follow-up study. Am J Sports Med 21:2, 1993.
30. Noyes FR, Roberts CS: High tibial osteotomy in knees with associated chronic ligament deficiencies. *In* Jackson DW (ed): Master Techniques in Orthopaedic Surgery. Reconstructive Knee Surgery. New York, Lippincott-Raven Publishers, 1995, p. 185.
31. Noyes FR, Schipplein OD, Andriacchi TP, et al: The anterior cruciate ligament–deficient knee with varus alignment. An analysis of gait adaptations and dynamic loadings. Am J Sports Med 20:707, 1992.

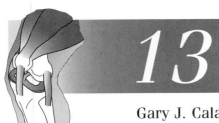

13 Posterior Cruciate Ligament Reconstruction and Rehabilitation

Gary J. Calabrese, PT, and John A. Bergfeld, MD

*C*linical recognition of the number of posterior cruciate ligament (PCL) injuries has increased over the past decade. The PCL has been described as a primary stabilizer of the knee joint.[1] The PCL is the strongest ligament of the knee and is approximately twice as strong as the anterior cruciate ligament (ACL). Injuries associated with disruption of the PCL contribute to altered kinematics of the knee joint. The PCL-deficient knee, especially if associated with capsular ligamentous injury in addition to symptoms of instability, is susceptible to adverse degenerative changes usually most prominent in the medial femoral compartment and the patellofemoral joint.[2] The primary goal of PCL reconstruction, then, is to restore near-normal anatomy to the primary ligamentous stabilizer of the knee joint, thus stabilizing the knee.

ANATOMY AND BIOMECHANICS

The PCL has an average length of 38 mm and width of 13 mm. It is named for its insertion site on the posterior tibia 1 cm inferior to the articular plateau. This posterior attachment extends distally into the posterior tibial cortex.[3-5] The size of the tibial insertion is three times the area of the midsubstance and 117 percent the size of the ACL tibial attachment. The PCL femoral attachment is on the lateral surface of the medial femoral condyle and is semilunar in shape. The size of the femoral origin is three times the area of the midsubstance and 121 percent the size of the ACL femoral attachment.[6] The PCL is described as consisting of two distinct but inseparable bands, the thick anterolateral and smaller posteromedial. The anterolateral bundle has greater linear stiffness and is taut in flexion and relaxed in extension, whereas the posteromedial bundle is taut in extension and lax in flexion.[7]

The cross-sectional area of the PCL increases from the tibia to femur, which is the opposite of the ACL. The importance of this tautness in flexion is to restrict posterior tibial translation as the secondary restraints, posterolateral complex, medial collateral ligament, and capsule become slack and biomechanically ineffective. The PCL with its complex biomechanical relationship with the ACL is further responsible for guiding the "screw home" mechanism of the knee. Guided primarily by the PCL, the "screw home," or external rotation of the tibia with terminal knee extension, is controlled by the congruity and weight-bearing capabilities of the medial femoral condyle. The ACL becomes taut in extension to stabilize the lateral femoral condyle.

Contributing to the posterior stability of the knee are the accessory and often variable meniscofemoral ligaments. The anterior ligament of Humphrey and posterior ligament of Wrisberg function as the secondary restraints to posterior tibial translation and enhance the congruence of the tibial articular surface and the lateral femoral condyle during knee flexion.[7]

The primary neurovascular supply to the cruciate ligaments arises from the middle genicular artery and the posterior tibial nerve. Little understanding exists regarding the role and prevalence of this nerve supply in functional biomechanics of the knee. Several authors have reported on the existence of Golgi-like receptors and mechanoreceptors at the origin of the PCL.[5, 8, 9] These neurologic structures are theorized to play a role in the proprioceptive reflex function of the knee.

MECHANISM OF INJURY

Various mechanisms of posterior cruciate ligament injury have been described in the literature: (1) an anterior force applied to the tibia in conjunction with knee flexion, as in the dashboard impact in an automobile accident; (2) a fall on a flexed knee with further forced hyperflexion with the foot in plantar flexion, resulting in an isolated PCL injury; and (3) knee hyperextension usually resulting in combined ligament injuries of the knee.[7, 10]

PHYSICAL EXAMINATION

A careful and detailed physical examination is essential to making an accurate diagnosis of ligamentous injury to the knee. An accurate diagnosis will guide the appropriate treatment approach. The clinician must be able to differentiate between isolated and combined ligament injuries based on the history, mechanism of injury, and physical examination of the knee.

The examination begins with a detailed history and inquiry as to the mechanism of injury. Observation of standing posture and gait are valuable to determine limb alignment and willingness to bear weight on the injured leg. Flexed knee gait patterns may indicate an unwillingness to allow the "screw home" mechanism of external rotation to occur at terminal tibial range-of-motion. With PCL insufficiency, increased flexion is also observed at mid-stance, serving as a compensatory mechanism to avoid stress to the joint and posterior capsule. The neurovascular status and signs of contusion or ecchymosis are further noted on physical examination. An acute hemarthrosis, which usually accumulates in the first 24 hours, is an indicator of significant intra-articular damage. The patient often denies hearing or feeling a "pop" or "snap," which is commonly associated with acute ACL disruption. The most common mechanism of injury in athletes is a fall on the flexed knee with further hyperflexion.

Numerous clinical testing techniques for knee ligament pathology have been described. The critical examination procedures for testing the integrity of the PCL are the posterior drawer test, posterior sag sign, and the quadriceps active test.[7, 11] The posterior drawer test assesses the comparative tibial translation and endpoint characteristics. Normally the anterior border of the tibial plateau is approximately 1 cm anterior to

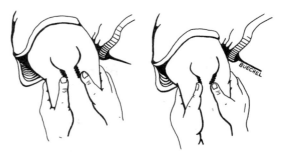

Figure 13–1. Posterolateral drawer test, starting position of 85 degrees hip flexion, with the knee flexed to 45 degrees. The examiner holds the tibia in slight external rotation with the thumbs marking the borders of the patellar tendon at the level of the tibial tubercle. Force is then applied posteriorly on the tibia. A positive test is indicated by the examiner's feeling the tibia plateau rotate posterolaterally on the femur.

the anterior border of the medial femoral condyle. Assessing the tibial step off or "starting point" prior to applying posterior directed force to the tibia is crucial for accurate testing (Fig. 13–1).[7] PCL laxity is based on a scale from 0 to 3, with the starting point being the 1 cm step-off at 90 degrees of knee flexion. Grade 1 PCL laxity is defined as 5 mm difference in step-off, grade 2 is 8 to 10 mm difference in step-off, and grade 3 is when the posterior excursion is greater than 12 mm.

The posterior sag sign is performed with the patient supine, with the knee and hip flexed to 90 degrees. Observation of the gravitational effects causing the tibia to sag posteriorly and the tibial tubercle to become less prominent are positive indicators of PCL disruption (Fig. 13–2). The quadriceps active test is also performed with the patient supine and 90 degrees of knee flexion with

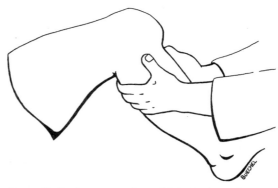

Figure 13–2. Gravitational sag. With the knee flexed to 45 degrees, the posterior tibial sag is observed.

the foot flat on the examination table. The patient is then instructed to perform a quadriceps contraction. In a PCL-deficient knee, the tibia will translate anteriorly from the posteriorly positioned starting point.[12, 13]

Other ancillary tests used in the evaluation of the injured knee include the KT-1000 knee ligament testing device (Medmetric Corporation, San Diego, CA). The KT-1000 and second generation KT-2000 are designed to obtain objective measurements of tibial translation. Although the research has indicated good reliability with the detection of ACL injuries, the results for PCL testing may be less than reliable. Daniel et al.,[12] utilizing the quadriceps active test, determined that anterior tibial displacement greater than 1 mm side-to-side difference is abnormal and probably is indicative of a PCL injury. Rubenstein and Shelbourne concluded that a single examiner had a 86 percent sensitivity in detecting grade 2 and 3 PCL tears and a 33 percent reliability detecting grade I PCL tears.[14, 15]

Radiographs are obtained to (1) investigate the potential for avulsion fractures of the PCL, which are more common from the tibial origin; (2) assess the growth plate status in the skeletally immature athlete; and (3) determine the severity of degenerative changes in the medial compartment and patellofemoral articulation in the chronic PCL patient. Magnetic resonance imaging (MRI) can easily show the status of the PCL with great accuracy.[16] The PCL, unlike the ACL, is associated with a large uniform appearance when viewed on sagittal and coronal films. Complete PCL tears are evident by a disruption of the ligament continuity, whereas partial tears often demonstrate a focal area of increased signal intensity in the mid-substance or at the bony insertion. Although MRI is not routinely used to diagnose PCL tears, it can give the clinician useful information on the status of the menisci and joint surface.

ciated with combined ligament injuries of the knee. It is widely reported that nonoperative treatment of isolated PCL-deficient knees in an athletic population results in satisfactory function in the short term.[10, 17, 18] The long-term results of nonoperative management of the PCL-deficient knee remains unclear. Parolie and Bergfeld[19] retrospectively evaluated 25 isolated PCL-injured knees, treated nonoperatively, in athletes with a mean follow-up of 6.2 years. Their finding indicated an 80 percent satisfaction rate and an 84 percent return to previous sport (68 percent at their previous level). Evaluation of mean quadriceps strength for the athletes who had returned to their previous sport and were satisfied with their results was greater than 100 percent of the uninvolved knee; conversely, those not satisfied all had values less then 100 percent of the uninvolved knee. Posterior drawer testing at follow-up ranged from 2.5 to 14.5 mm.[21]

Fowler and Messich[20] followed 12 patients with isolated PCL tears over a 2.5-year period. Of this population, all returned to their previous level of activity without limitations. All demonstrated persistent posterior laxity but had acceptable subjective and objective functional stability.

Shelbourne and Rubinstein studied the accuracy of the clinical examination of isolated chronic PCL tears. Their results demonstrated an overall accuracy rate of 96 percent for all five orthopaedic surgeons tested. Examination sensitivity for grade I injuries was 70 percent; however, grade II and grade III sensitivity was 97 percent accurate.[14] Isolated PCL physical examination of knees at 90 degrees flexion found (1) straight abnormal post laxity less than 10 mm (2+), (2) abnormal laxity decreased with internal rotation of tibia (approximately 4–5 mm), (3) no abnormal rotary laxity greater than 5 to 10 degrees, and (4) no significant valgus or varus abnormal laxity.

NATURAL HISTORY

The natural history of the PCL remains unknown and is difficult to prospectively study. An accurate diagnosis done acutely is the mainstay of determining the natural history of the PCL. Historically, many PCL injuries have gone unrecognized or are asso-

TREATMENT OF POSTERIOR CRUCIATE LIGAMENT INJURIES

The treatment of acute and chronic PCL injuries is based on an accurate diagnosis, functional symptoms, degree of laxity, and associated injuries. Most authors continue to treat the majority of acute and chronic isolated PCL-deficient knees nonoperatively. Surgical rationale is based on the symptomatic response to functional activities and the premise that restoration of normal PCL anatomy will significantly improve the biomechanics of the knee and reduce the patient's symptoms. If the injury is outside the envelope of isolated PCL injury, then surgical reconstruction of the PCL and the associated capsuloligamentous injury is called for.

Biomechanical Considerations

Ligamentous disruption equates to loss of normal biomechanical function of the knee. Stresses to the secondary static and dynamic stabilizers, namely the articular surface and patellofemoral articulation, increases dramatically with disruption of the normal joint kinematics. The rehabilitation program must take into account the biomechanical stresses placed on the knee joint and patellofemoral articulation while incorporating appropriate open and closed kinetic chain exercises. The effects of open kinetic chain (OKC) and closed kinetic chain (CKC) exercises on knee function remain an area of continued research. During OKC exercises, the distal segment of the limb is free to move in space, whereas CKC has the distal segment fixed on a movable or immovable object. OKC exercises result in isolated muscular contractions whereas CKC exercises allow coordinated co-contraction of many muscle groups in a predictable manner. Open and closed kinetic chain exercises produce different effects on the tibiofemoral and patellofemoral joint.

Lutz et al.[21] investigated the shear force development in the tibiofemoral joint with OKC isometric contractions in 30, 60, and 90 degrees of knee flexion and extension to CKC exercises. Their results indicated significantly less posterior shear force developed during the CKC exercises as compared with OKC knee flexion at 60 and 90 degrees. A maximum posterior shear force of 1780 N was reported at 90 degrees of knee flexion. These tremendous shear forces indicate that OKC knee flexion should be avoided so as not to induce posterior tibiofemoral shear. Open kinetic chain resisted knee extension produces an anterior tibial shear force and is included early in the rehabilitation of the PCL-deficient knee program. The rehabilita-

tion program must balance the intensity of the exercises to avoid irritation of the patellofemoral articulation while performing OKC knee extension exercises.

Closed kinetic chain exercises are not benign in relation to PCL shear stress. Dahlkuist et al.[22] demonstrated an increase in posterior shear up to three times body weight during squatting exercises. Other investigators have indicated that the posterior shear forces increase proportionately with increased knee flexion during front knee squats and lunges.[23–25] CKC exercises reproduce functional positioning and co-contraction muscle firing patterns, which OKC exercises cannot, that are necessary for functional activity. These activities can be used to reduce the patellofemoral joint compressive forces experienced with OKC exercises.

The current research and data presented indicate that it is important to include both OKC knee extension and CKC exercises in a comprehensive PCL rehabilitation program. Both OKC extension from 60 to 0 degrees and CKC exercises from 0 to 60 degrees appear to have a beneficial effect of decreasing posterior shear force and thus are safe to perform by PCL-deficient patients.

Nonoperative Treatment

Historically, the majority of PCL injuries have been treated nonoperatively. The rehabilitation process for the ACL reconstructed knee has changed dramatically over the past several years. Keller et al.[10] reviewed 40 patients treated nonoperatively who sustained isolated PCL ruptures. Their results indicated that a greater time from initial injury to follow-up directly correlates to lower knee questionnaire scores and increased radiographic degenerative changes even while maintaining excellent muscular strength. However, since the impetus for changes in ACL rehabilitation have surrounded the surgical reconstruction, the nonoperatively treated PCL has not had the investigational attention of clinicians in the past. Often, nonoperative treatment is described as no treatment. It is our opinion that nonoperative or operative treatment of PCL injuries should be approached with the same rehabilitation enthusiasm as for the reconstructed ACL. The rehabilitation process for

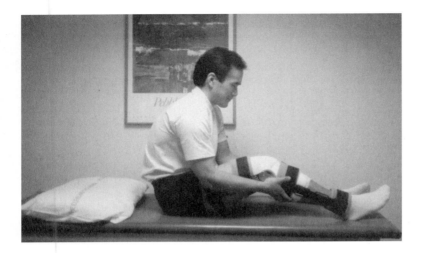

Figure 13–3. Range-of-motion exercises with postoperative brace applied. Patient-assisted flexion while maintaining the tibial plateau in neutral position.

PCL injuries remains an imprecise science and a significant challenge to the rehabilitation team of physician, physical therapist, athletic trainer, and athlete. Rehabilitation efforts must be scientifically based and geared toward the individual goals and objectives of each patient. For this reason, strict protocols are difficult to develop that would incorporate all patients. General rehabilitation guidelines with critical milestones for progression will allow the clinician to adapt the treatment approach to each patient.

Treatment of acute PCL disruption is managed by splinting or bracing in full extension for pain relief. Range-of-motion exercises are initiated immediately in the brace from 0 to 60 degrees to counteract the harmful effects of immobilization and joint effusion (Fig. 13–3). The patient is permitted to ambulate bearing weight as tolerated with crutches. The early rehabilitation emphasizes quadriceps and hip flexor strengthening. Isometric quadriceps sets, straight-leg raises (SLR), and concentric knee extension exercises from 0 to 60 degrees are initiated in the initial phase of rehabilitation. Closed kinetic chain exercises such as mini-squats and leg presses are performed in a limited range of motion of 0 to 60 degrees flexion (Fig. 13–4). Hamstring exercises are avoided in the early phases of rehabilitation because of the posteriorly directed forces on the tibia in the PCL-deficient knee. When the patient can demonstrate good leg control and ambulate without gait deviation, the crutches are discontinued. Progression to more aggressive rehabilitation is dependent upon resolution of pain and inflammation, ambulation without gait deviation, and demonstration of good quadriceps contraction and leg control. A rehabilitation program is designed to strengthen the quadriceps while protecting the patellofemoral articulation from degenerative compressive forces.

The rehabilitation program is advanced to include progressive resistive exercises (PREs) using light resistance and high repetitions to avoid inducing patellofemoral pain symptoms, bicycling, unilateral balance and proprioceptive training, aquatic therapy, and ambulation without assistive devices. CKC exercises continue, incorporating calf raises, step-up and step-down exercises

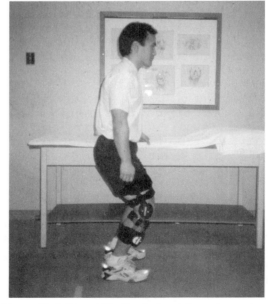

Figure 13–4. Closed kinetic chain mini-squat exercise.

starting at 2 inches and progressing to 8 to 10 inch boxes (Fig. 13–5), Stair Master, and Versa Climber progression from seated to standing positions. The drop-lock brace is discontinued at 6 to 8 weeks. The patient is progressed to a walk/jog program, running/straight sprint program, jumping vertical to horizontal program, cutting and pivoting, and acceleration/deceleration functional maneuvers. The use of a functional brace remains controversial for the PCL-deficient knee. If a functional brace is utilized, a custom-contoured combined instability design is applied (Don Joy, Smith & Nephew Corporation, Carlsbad, CA). Patients do not generally complain of functional instability during activity but are encouraged to continue a preventative exercise program three to four times per week for life.

POSTERIOR CRUCIATE LIGAMENT RECONSTRUCTION

A large variety of surgical techniques have been developed for the reconstruction of the PCL.[26–29] Many of the reconstructive procedures have mirrored the surgical approaches of the commonly reconstructed ACL; however, distinct differences exist between the ACL reconstruction and the PCL reconstruction in terms of success. The an-

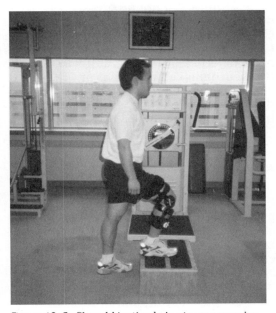

Figure 13–5. Closed kinetic chain step-up exercise.

terior approach, the oblique tibial tunnel angle impinging on the PCL graft, and attempts at suture repair of the PCL have contributed to the often variable results associated with attempts at PCL reconstruction. Our preferred technique, originally described by Berg,[30] utilizes a patellar bone–tendon–bone tibial inlay reconstructive procedure. The length of the graft is sized using lateral radiographs to measure from the anterior margin of the intercondylar line to 1 cm below the posterior tibia. The patient is draped and prepped in the decubitus position with hip flexion of 45 degrees and knee flexion to 90 degrees. This allows the surgeon to have anterior access to the knee for arthroscopic portals. The patellar bone–tendon–bone graft (1 cm) is obtained from the central third of the patellar tendon from this position. Through an anteromedial portal, a femoral jig is positioned in the femoral origin of the PCL. Guide pin placement positions a cannulated reamer to drill an interosseous medial femoral condyle tunnel.

The patient is then rotated to the prone position. A posteromedial curved incision is performed for visualization of the insertion of the PCL on the posterior tibial plateau. The posterior joint is approached medial to the medial head of the gastrocnemius muscle. Identification and ligation of the medial geniculate artery and vein permit exposure of the PCL insertion on the tibial plateau through a vertical incision of the posterior joint capsule and popliteal oblique ligament. The bone-tendon-bone graft is passed through the femoral tunnel. With the knee at 90 degrees of flexion, manual tension is used to determine where to fix the bone-tendon-bone graft on the tibia placement of the distal graft. The distal patellar tendon bone block is inlaid in a cortical window created of equal size on the posterior tibia and secured with a cancellous screw and washer.[30]

The patient is then rotated back to the supine position. The graft is then tensioned with the knee at 80 degrees of flexion and fixed in the femur with a Kurasaka screw. The patient is braced in full extension and initiates physical therapy 5 to 7 days postoperatively.

POSTERIOR CRUCIATE RECONSTRUCTION REHABILITATION

Rehabilitation following PCL reconstructive surgery has not been given adequate emphasis in the literature and has characteristically been referred to as "the ACL turned around,"[31] a perplexing situation and a clinical challenge. Hughston et al.[32] further stated, "In my estimation, rehabilitation accounts for 50 percent of a successful result following injury or operation." Reconstructive PCL procedures and rehabilitation are performed to allow functional return to previous activity and prevent further articular cartilage degeneration. The lack of research data on the graft maturation sequence, the forces imposed on the healing graft during rehabilitation, and the prospectively randomized research on isolated PCL-reconstructed knees create a significant challenge for the clinician. Using a functional progression protocol, the frequency of clinical visits for rehabilitation or re-evaluation is determined by the patient's level of function.

The goal of rehabilitation is to return the athlete to previous levels of function between 6 and 8 months. The qualification of the patient's functional status is determined by a combination of subjective patient assessment and objective evaluation of postoperative range of motion, swelling, gait abnormalities, resolution of acute postoperative symptoms such as the degree of effusion, incision healing and patella mobility, balance and proprioception deficits, muscle strength, patellofemoral pathology, and joint stability. These factors aid the clinician in determining the level of progression and can be useful in the recognition and management of potential complications early in the rehabilitation process.

General rehabilitation guidelines are as follows:

1. Minimize postoperative immobilization.
2. Allow tissue healing and remodeling to occur in a non-stressed environment.
3. Be aware of potential complications from the start.
4. Base rehabilitation progression and treatments on available basic science and applied clinical research.
5. Use a functional progression based on critical milestones and re-evaluation.
6. Individualize the rehabilitation with patient's goals as the functional targets.
7. Use a team approach to care with the patient, physician, physical therapist, athletic trainer, and coaching staff to optimize results of the surgery and rehabilitation.

Rehabilitation after PCL reconstruction is divided into overlapping phases of acute immediate postoperative, acute progressive range of motion and strengthening, and functional return to activity. During the acute immediate postoperative period, the goals of rehabilitation are to control pain and decrease joint effusion, progress range of motion from active-assisted to active to decrease the incidence of fibrosis, initiate quadriceps strengthening exercises, and educate the patient on positions that counteract gravitational stresses on the PCL graft, such as lying and sleeping prone rather than supine and the avoidance of aggressive hamstring contractions.

In the acute immediate postoperative phase, the patient is placed into a hinged brace locked at 0 degrees of extension. The patient is allowed to ambulate with crutches with partial weight-bearing (25–50 percent), and a normal heel-toe pattern is encouraged. Cryotherapy application with a commercially available continuous cold system is used in conjunction with elevation and ankle pumps. The brace is unlocked each hour for patient-assisted tibial lifts into flexion, limited to 0 to 60 degrees of knee motion. Strengthening exercises for the quadriceps are initiated using functional electrical stimulation for quadriceps sets, straight-leg raises in all directions, and knee extension 0 to 40 degrees and are progressed to 0 to 60 degrees by postoperative week 4. Functional electrical stimulation of the quadriceps in the immediate postoperative period has been reported in the literature to improve the neuromuscular control of the quadriceps.[33, 34] This should be initiated if the patient fails to obtain a good quadriceps contraction in the first week.

Acute Phase

The goals of the acute phase (weeks 1–3) include progressive weight-bearing as tolerated with crutches, emphasizing a normalized gait pattern. Range of motion is increased to 0 to 90 degrees of knee flexion both actively and assisted. Patellar mobilization is guided by the degree of knee joint effusion. Aggressive patellar mobilization is avoided if marked effusion is present because of the potential for exacerbating patel-lofemoral fibrosis that may occur with pro-longed effusion and limited range of motion. Isometric quadriceps exercises continue, to include multi-angle extensions from 60 to 0 degrees, straight-leg raises with proximal resistance transferred progressively to the ankle if quadriceps control allows no quadri-ceps lag, and knee extension from 60 to 0 degrees without resistance. CKC exercises are initiated that include mini-squats (only after 0 to 100 degrees and not before 3 weeks) for proprioceptive training; recipro-cal bicycling and weight shifts start earlier for range of motion and contralateral cycling and standing weights shifts. The patient is fit with a functional PCL brace between 5 and 6 weeks.

Progressive Range of Motion and Strengthening Phase

The progressive range of motion and strengthening phase is characterized by in-creasing the range of motion to full motion and full weight-bearing ambulation without assistive device. Exercise continues to focus on quadriceps activity with isotonic strength-ening, leg press (0–60 degrees), concentric and eccentric step drills progressing from 2 to 8 inches, resisted forward and backward walking, seated Versa Climber exercises, and bicycling. Little scientific research exists to support a progression of the rehabilitation program into truly functional stages. There-fore, progression should be based on the patient's tolerance to exercises geared to individual activities and level of function. Functional tests that estimate power and en-durance, popularized in ACL rehabilitation, should give the clinician a standard measure of total lower limb functional ability and can be utilized for the PCL-reconstructed knee. The anticipated return to full unrestricted activity following PCL reconstruction is 9 to 12 months.

SUMMARY

Posterior cruciate ligament injuries occur less frequently than ACL injuries; however, the clinical recognition of these injuries is approaching the consistency that has been achieved with ACL-deficient knees. The clini-cal examination is based on a detailed his-tory and physical examination geared to-ward assessing the stability of the knee. The PCL-deficient knee presents a clinical chal-lenge secondary to the well-documented ar-ticular cartilage degeneration of the medial compartment and patellofemoral articula-tion with altered joint kinematics. Rehabilita-tion of the PCL-deficient or PCL-recon-structed knee is dependent on resolution of the initial pain and effusion, return of normal range of motion, and increased quadriceps strength while avoiding unrestricted ham-string exercises that allow knee flexion. The natural history of the PCL-deficient knee re-mains poorly understood, with little or no prospective outcome data. Restoration of ligamentous stability of the knee through a PCL tibial inlay reconstruction, the authors' preferred technique, using a patellar bone–tendon–bone inlaid reconstruction provides a method of reconstructing near-normal anatomy of the knee. Continued research and future modifications to this recon-structive procedure for the PCL in conjunc-tion with prospectively designed outcome-based rehabilitation guidelines will provide the patient and clinician with improved sta-bility, surgical confidence, and functional re-turn to activity.

References

1. Butler DL, Noyes FR, Grood ES: Ligamentous re-straints to anterior posterior drawer in the human knee: A biomechanical study. J Bone Joint Surg 62A:259–270, 1980.
2. Dejour H, Walch G, Peyrot J, Eberhard PH: The natural history of rupture of the posterior cruciate ligament. Fr J Orthop Surg 2:112–120, 1988.
3. Girgis FG, Marshall JL, Al Monajem ARS: The cruci-ate ligaments of the knee joint: Anatomical, func-tional and experimental analysis. Clin Orthop 106:216–231, 1975.
4. Grood ES, Stowers SF, Noyes FR: Limits of move-ment in the human knee: Effect of sectioning the posterior cruciate ligament and posterolateral structures. J Bone Joint Surg 70:88–97, 1988.
5. Covey DC, Sapega AA: Anatomy and function of the posterior cruciate ligament. Clin Sports Med 13(3):509–518, 1994.
6. Race A, Amis AA: Mechanical properties of the two bundles of the human posterior cruciate ligament. Trans Orthop Res Soc 17:124, 1992.
7. Miller MD, Harner CD, Koshiwaguchi S: Acute poste-rior cruciate ligament injuries. Clin Sports Med 13:749–767, 1994.
8. O'Brien WR, Friederich NF, Muller W, Henning CE: Functional anatomy of the cruciate ligaments. In print.

9. Barton TM, Torg JS, Das M: Posterior cruciate ligament insufficiency: A review of the literature. Sports Med 1:419–430, 1984.
10. Keller PM, Shelbourne KD, McCarroll JR, Rettig AC: Nonoperatively treated isolated posterior cruciate ligament injuries. Am J Sports Med 21(1):132–136, 1993.
11. Shelbourne KD: Posterior cruciate ligament injuries. In Reider B (ed): Sports Medicine: The School-Aged Athlete. Philadelphia: W.B. Saunders, 1991.
12. Daniel DM, Stone ML, Barnett P, Sachs R: Use of the quadriceps active test to diagnose posterior cruciate-ligament disruption and measure posterior laxity of the knee. J Bone Joint Surg 70A:386–391, 1988.
13. Kannus P: Injuries to the PCL of the knee. Sports Med 12:116, 1991.
14. Rubenstein RA, Shelbourne KD, McCarroll JR, VanMeter CD, Rettig AC: The accuracy of the clinical examination in the setting of posterior cruciate ligament injuries. AJSM 22(4):550–557, 1994.
15. Rubenstein RA Jr, Shelbourne KD: Diagnosis of posterior cruciate ligament injuries and indications for nonoperative and operative treatment. Oper Tech Sports Med 1:99–103, 1993.
16. Fischer SP, Fox JM, Del Pizzo W, et al.: Accuracy of diagnoses from magnetic resonance imaging of the knee. J Bone Joint Surg 73:2, 1991.
17. Shino K, Horibe S, Nakata K, Maeda A, Hamada M, Nakamura N: Conservative treatment of isolated injuries to the posterior cruciate ligament in athletes. J Bone Joint Surg 77B:895–900, 1995.
18. Shelbourne KD, Rubenstein RA: Methodist Sports Medicine Center's experience with acute and chronic isolated posterior cruciate ligament injuries. Clin Sports Med 13(3):531–543, 1994.
19. Parolie J, Bergfeld JA: Long term results of nonoperative treatment of PCL injuries in the athlete. Am J Sports Med 13(1):35–38, 1986.
20. Fowler PJ, Messieh SS: Isolated posterior cruciate ligament injuries in athletes. Am J Sports Med 15:553–557, 1987.
21. Lutz GE, Palmitier RA, An KN, et al.: Comparison of tibiofemoral joint forces during open and closed kinetic chain exercises. J Bone Joint Surg, 1993.
22. Dahlkuits NJ, Mago P, Seedholm BB: Forces during squatting and rising from a deep squat. Engineering Med 11:69–76, 1982.
23. Morrison JB: Function of the knee joint in various activities. Biomech Engineering 4:573–580, 1969.
24. Smidt GL: Biomechanical analysis of knee extension and flexion. J Biomech 6:79–92, 1973.
25. Ohkoshi Y, Yasuda K, Kaneda K, et al.: Biomechanical analysis of rehabilitation in standing position. Am J Sports Med 19:605–611, 1991.
26. Clancy WG Jr, Smith L: Arthroscopic anterior and posterior cruciate ligament reconstruction technique. Ann Chir Gynaecol 80(2):141–148, 1991.
27. Thomas YR, Gaechter A: Dorsal approach for reconstruction of the posterior cruciate ligament. Arch Orthop Trauma Surg 113(3):142–148, 1994.
28. Insall JN, Hood RW: Bone-block transfer of the medial head of the gastrocnemius for posterior cruciate insufficiency. J Bone Joint Surg 64A:691–699, 1982.
29. Hughston JC, Degenhardt TC: Reconstruction of the posterior cruciate ligament. Clin Orthop 164:59–77, 1982.
30. Berg EE: Posterior cruciate ligament tibial inlay reconstruction. Arthroscopy 11(1):69–76, 1995.
31. Wilk KE: Rehabilitation of isolated and combined posterior cruciate ligament injuries. Clin Sports Med 13(3):649–677, 1994.
32. Hughston JC, Bowden JA, Andrews JR, et al.: Acute tears of the posterior cruciate ligament: Results of operative treatment. J Bone Joint Surg 62:438–450, 1980.
33. Morrissey MC, Brewster CE, Shields CL, et al.: The effects of electrical stimulation on the quadriceps during post-operative knee immobilization. Am J Sports Med 13:40–45, 1985.
34. Lossing I, Gremby G, Johnson T: Effects of electrical muscle stimulation combined with voluntary contractions after knee ligament surgery. Med Sci Sports Exerc 20:93–98, 1988.

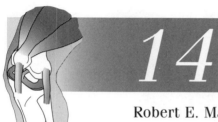

14 Nonoperative Posterior Cruciate Ligament Rehabilitation

Robert E. Mangine, MEd, PT, ATC, and Brian L. Becker, PT

*H*istorical analysis of the literature has demonstrated a concentration on the frequency of anterior cruciate ligament (ACL) injury, but over the past 20 years, there has been an increased recognition of the role of the posterior cruciate ligament (PCL). Many authors have defined the importance of the PCL as the primary stabilizer at the knee joint.[1-3] The PCL is defined as the primary restraint to posterior translation of the tibia throughout the full range of motion of knee flexion.[1, 4, 5] Injuries to the PCL were thought to be an infrequent clinical entity, yet this type of ligament injury appears to be more common than once believed.[6] Several authors reported an incidence of PCL injuries between 9 and 23 percent in their series of knee ligament injuries.[7-11] The ACL is commonly injured in sports-related activities; however, injury of the PCL has a 50 percent occurrence outside of sporting activities. PCL insufficiency may lead to altered biomechanics and eventually may lead to degenerative osteoarthritis in both the medial and the patellofemoral compartment secondary to increased laxity of the secondary stabilizing structures of the knee.

ANATOMY

The PCL lies in the origin of the intercondylar space of both the femur and the tibia. It is situated behind the ACL and in fact is the strongest ligament about the knee. Harner et al.[12] have demonstrated that the PCL cross-sectional area is approximately 50 and 20 percent greater than that of the ACL at the femur and the tibia, respectively.

The fibers of the PCL can be split into two primary bundles, the posterior medial bundle and the anterior lateral bundle.

The larger anterior lateral band is taut in knee flexion; the smaller posterior medial fibers become taut in knee extension. There are two accessory bands associated with the PCL called the meniscal femoral ligaments, once described as "the third cruciate ligament."[13] The anterior meniscal femoral ligament or the ligament of Humphrey originates on the medial femoral condyle anterior to the PCL and extends inferiorly and laterally to insert on the lateral meniscus. The posterior meniscal femoral ligament or the ligament of Wrisberg lies posterior to the PCL and inserts off the posterior lateral aspect of the lateral meniscus. This structure was reported by Heller and Langman[14] to be present in 35 percent of the knees examined. Girgis et al.[15], using calipers, determined that the average length of the PCL is 38 mm and the average width was 13 mm.

BIOMECHANICS

The tibiofemoral joint demonstrates six degrees of freedom. The PCL is responsible for controlling four motions of the knee, one translation and three rotations. Butler demonstrated that the PCL provides 95 percent of the restraint to posterior translation of the knee.[4] The posterior medial band is taut with the knee in full extension, and the greatest amount of tension is in the mid-range between 70 and 90 degrees of knee flexion. The ACL demonstrates the least amount of tension between 70 and 90 degrees. Because of this tension relationship between the ACL and the PCL, the ideal laxity testing for the PCL will occur between 70 and 90 degrees of knee flexion motion.

External tibial rotation of the knee is strongly coupled with anteroposterior translation. The degree of external rotation is dependent on the external load applied and the angle of knee flexion or extension. Isolated cutting of the PCL revealed no increase in external tibial rotation over the normal knee; however, when combined with an insufficiency of the posterior lateral structures, a significant increase in laxity is noted. Grood et al.[16] reported that an intact knee hyperextends in excess of an average of 5.6 degrees; however, the degree of hyperextension significantly increased when an isolated PCL insufficiency was present and was greatly increased with a combined PCL and posterior lateral insufficiency.[16] Thus it can be assumed that the PCL is the primary stabilizer to posterior translation and a secondary restraint to external rotation, varus rotation, and hyperextension.

PATHOMECHANICS

There are three common mechanisms of injury to the PCL. The most common is the motor vehicle "dashboard injury," in which a direct blow is given to the tibial crest with the knee in a flexed position, during which the tibia is driven posteriorly.[2, 17–20] The second most common mechanism is a fall on to a flexed knee and a plantar flexed foot in which the brunt of the fall is taken through the tibial tubercle, driving the tibia posteriorly and rupturing the PCL.[5] The third most common mechanism involves extreme internal or external rotational motions. These extreme rotational injuries generally cause complete knee dislocations, which may also incriminate the popliteal artery as well as the peroneal nerve.

PHYSICAL EXAMINATION AND CLINICAL DIAGNOSIS

Posterior cruciate ligament injuries can fall into two distinct categories; one encompassing isolated PCL tears and the other involving secondary structures that cause combined PCL injuries (Fig. 14–1). Clancy[8] observed 191 PCL injuries between 1977 and 1987 in which he noted that approximately 40 percent were isolated injuries and the other 60 percent fell into a category of combined PCL injuries. Clancy noted that in the combined category the most common injury involved the PCL and the posterior lateral knee structures, followed by combined ACL and PCL injuries, and lastly PCL and MCL combined injuries. Thus with 60 percent of

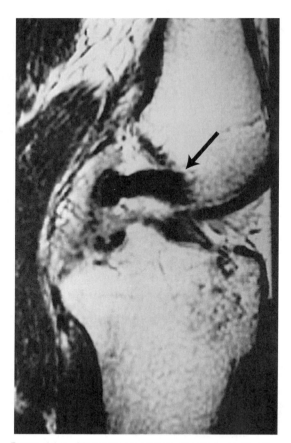

Figure 14–1. Magnetic resonance imaging examination of the knee. *Arrow* indicates a torn posterior cruciate ligament.

all PCL injuries being combined injuries, physical examination of the PCL injured knee can be difficult and confusing.

It is not uncommon for PCL laxity to be confused with ACL laxity. An anterior drawer will pull the tibia forward and reduce the posteriorly subluxed tibia, and thus it is difficult for the clinician to determine a neutral point of the tibiofemoral position. It is critical, therefore, to determine whether the knee is in a neutral position when conducting an anterior-posterior drawer test.

For this reason, we recommend that the examination begin in an anti-gravity or a drop-back position (Fig. 14–2). This is accomplished by flexing both the hip and the knee to 90 degrees of flexion and palpating the normal anterior medial and lateral tibial plateau step-off in the normal knee. The step-off in a normal knee is approximately 8 to 10 mm anteriorly. If there is no step-off and the anterior tibial crest is level with the medial and lateral femoral condyle, there is

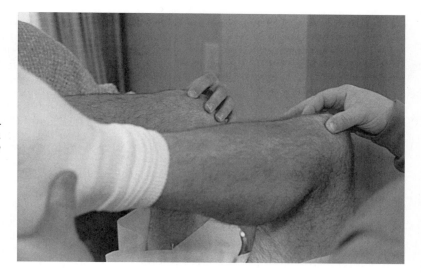

Figure 14–2. The drop-back position for evaluating laxity with both the hip and knee flexed to a 90-degree position.

at least a 2+ posterior drawer test result indicative of PCL disruption.

If the anterior tibial plateau is relatively posterior to the femoral condyles, than a 3+ drawer result is present, and if the step-off is less than that of the normal knee but is still palpable, this should be considered a 1+ posterior drawer result.

The second test we perform is between 70 and 90 degrees of flexion in the traditional drawer position while flexing the hip to a 45-degree angle. The knee ligament arthrometer test is also performed in this position, with an increase in translation showing PCL laxity. This position allows us to assess total translation, both anterior and posterior, of both the medial and anterior compartments (Fig. 14–3). The second portion of this evaluation is the unilateral compartmental drawer test, which is described as a hand placement that will only effect a translation of medial or lateral compartment of the tibiofemoral

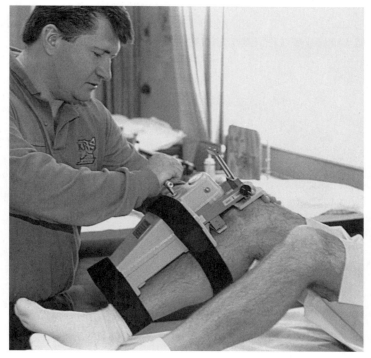

Figure 14–3. Position for KT-1000 arthrometer measurement with hip flexed to 45 degrees and the knee flexed between 70 and 90 degrees.

joint. With PCL laxity, posterior displacement of the lateral compartment is greater than posterior displacement of the medial compartment.[21] The compartmental difference in translation will result in an increase in external rotation by about 15 percent in the externally rotated position. This is because the lateral secondary restraints do not absorb tension at the same time that the medial secondary restraints do.

Daniels and associates[22] also describe the quadriceps active test. This test evaluates the integrity of the PCL. The patient is positioned supine with the hip flexed to 45 degrees and the knee flexed to 90 degrees. The foot is flat on the table. In this position, the tibia is supported by the PCL, and if the PCL is intact, the patellar tendon is oriented posteriorly as is passes from the tibia to the patella. An active quadriceps contraction will move the tibia slightly posteriorly. If the PCL is not intact, the tibia will sag posteriorly, thus the patellar tendon is oriented anteriorly as it passes from the tibial tubercle to the patella (Fig. 14–4).

NONOPERATIVE MANAGEMENT

It can be somewhat difficult to convince an acute post-injury PCL patient to undergo a major reconstructive procedure in a knee when few patients will develop functional instability following an isolated PCL injury. Consequences of PCL instability may lead to accelerated cartilage damage. A conservative approach often should be considered in an acute PCL disruption.

The conservative approach should consider the following elements:

1. Patellar protection program due to an increase in tibial drop-back.
2. Guarding of the lateral structures of the knee that serve as secondary stabilizers to posterior translation. If these structures are compromised, functional instability may result.
3. During the conservative program, reassessment of joint laxity and articular cartilage damage must be made periodically with special attention being paid to the medial femoral condyle and the patellofemoral joint surfaces.
4. Treatment of other associated pathologic conditions may need to be considered surgically such as meniscus tears, other ligament laxities, capsular damage, and patellofemoral pathology.
5. Use of a Don Joy PCL Brace for all recreational activities and sporting activities may assist the patient in maintaining normal positioning of the knee and prevent repetitive stress to posterior lateral structures.
6. There has to be a significant increase in the dynamic stability, including ratio

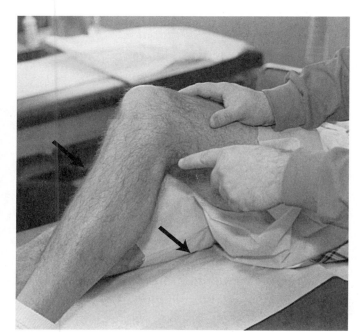

Figure 14–4. Position for the quadriceps active test as described by Daniels. *Arrows* indicate that positive test results show posterior subluxation of the tibia relative to the femur.

⬤━ Table 14–1. Nonoperative Treatment of Posterior Cruciate Ligament Injury

General Observation Evaluation	Treatment	Goals
Phase 1 (Protection Phase): Weeks 1 to 4		

• Protected ROM
• Limited weight-bearing
• Early strengthening
• Limit closed chain exercises because of risk of posterior displacement of tibia
• KT-2000 initially and every 2 weeks until the 8th week
	Day 1 to 7
	• Weight-bearing with two crutches as tolerated. Discontinue when signs/symptoms allow
	• Electrical muscle stimulator to quadriceps
	• Exercises
	  • Quadriceps sets
	  • Straight leg raises
	  • Hip abduction
	  • Hip adduction
	  • Knee extension (60–0 degrees)
	  • Multiangle isometrics (quadriceps) (60, 40, 20 degrees)
	Weeks 2 to 4
	• ROM 0–60 degrees
	• Weight-bearing with one crutch, then without at week 3
	• Progress exercises (listed above) using weight progression
	• Cycling (week 4) for ROM
	• Pool program
	• Leg press (30–90 degrees)
		• Protect ROM 0–60 degrees
		• Adequate quadriceps contraction to control gait pattern
		• Control inflammation and effusion

Phase II (Moderate Protection Phase): Weeks 5 to 8		
• Allow full pain-free ROM • Increase quadricep and hamstring strengthening • Increase neuomuscular control	**Week 5** • ROM to tolerance • Discontinue protection brace • Bicycle, StairMaster, rowing • Continue exercise in Phase I; progress weight • Knee extension (90–30 degrees) • Mini squats (45–90 degrees) • Leg press (30–90 degrees) • Step-ups • Hamstring curls (light resistance) (0–45 degrees) • Hip abduction and adduction • Toe–calf raises **Weeks 6 to 8** • Continue all exercises above • Fit for functional brace • Pool, running • KT-2000 repeated • Isokinetic testing done isometrically	
Phase III (Minimal Protection Phase): Weeks 9 to 12		

• Functional evaluation based on activity level
• Observe for patellofemoral symptoms
• Continue with isokinetic evaluations
• Observe for changes in KT-2000 score
	• Initiate running program
	• Continue all strengthening exercises
	• Gradual return to sports activities
	  Criteria for return to sports activities
	  • Isokinetic quadriceps torque to body weight ratio
	  • Isokinetic test 85 percent or greater of contralateral side, if patellofemoral symptoms do not exist
	• No change in laxity per KT-2000 repeated at the 12th week
	• No pain/tenderness or swelling
	• Satisfactory clinical examination	

of quadriceps to body weight. We must also consider an increase in strength, power, and endurance.

The post-injury rehabilitation program initially needs to emphasize immediate motion to decrease articular cartilage breakdown. Early quadriceps strengthening exercises should be initiated starting at 0 degrees of an isometric contraction.

Multiangle isometrics should also be considered between the ranges of 60 and 20 degrees of knee flexion. We should also concentrate on decreasing effusion inside the knee joint and resuming normal quadriceps function. By the third to fourth week post-injury, aggressive strengthening exercises need to be instituted (Table 14–1).

Initially, closed chain exercises are not

AGILITY AND QUICKNESS PROGRAM

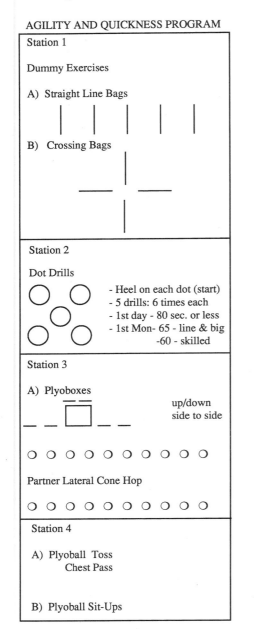

Figure 14–5. Functional duration drills used as criteria for return to play.

ceps strengthening, and neuromuscular training (see Table 14–1). Return to sports can be accomplished when full pain-free range of motion is achieved, there is no change in laxity, there is no pain or tenderness about the knee, and the patient is able to achieve a 60 to 65 percent torque-to-body weight ratio (Fig. 14–5).

SUMMARY

Injuries to the PCL occur more often than clinicians seem to realize. PCL deficiency in the knee is a difficult condition to comprehend because of the complexity of quadriceps contraction and difficulty in recognizing what is known as the neutral position in the knee joint. The anatomy, the biomechanics, and the natural history of the PCL-deficient knee are dramatically different than those of the ACL-deficient knee. Our treatment approach should be based on the biomechanics of exercise to reduce posterior shear forces of the tibia that can lead to weakening of the secondary stabilizing structures of the knee. Once the biomechanics of the PCL are better understood, it will be easier to rehabilitate patients with this condition.

References

1. Kennedy JC, Grainger RW: The posterior cruciate ligament. J Trauma 7:367–377, 1967.
2. Cain TE, Schwab GH: Performance of an athlete with straight posterior knee instability. Am J Sports Med 9:203–208, 1981.
3. Hughston JC, Degenhardt TC: Reconstruction of the posterior cruciate ligament. Clin Orthop 164:59–77, 1982.
4. Butler DL, Noyes FR, Grood ES: Ligamentous restraints to anterior-posterior drawer in the human knee. J Bone Joint Surg 62A:259–270, 1980.
5. Grood ES, Stowers SF, Noyes FR: Limits of movement in the human knee: Effects of sectioning the posterior cruciate ligament and posterolateral structures. J Bone Joint Surg 70A:88–97, 1988.
6. Wilk KE: Rehabilitation of isolated and combined posterior cruciate ligament injuries. Clin Sports Med 13(3):649–677, 1994.
7. Bianchi M: Acute tears of the posterior cruciate ligament: Clinical study and results of operative treatment in 27 cases. Am J Sports Med 11(5):308, 1983.
8. Clancy WG: Repair and reconstruction of the posterior cruciate ligament. In Chapman MW (ed): Operative Orthopaedics. Philadelphia, JB Lippincott, 1988, p. 1651.

done because of the initiation of hamstring activities, which creates a posterior displacement of the tibia. At the third to fourth week, closed chain exercises can be initiated. Knee flexion exercises, however, should be delayed until the sixth to eighth week post-injury. Return to activities can be considered during the 6- to 8-week period, depending on no changes in stability, control of effusion or swelling, an increase in quadri-

9. Clancy WG, Shelbourne KD, Zoellner GB, et al.: Treatment of knee joint instability secondary to rupture of the posterior cruciate ligament. Report of a new procedure. J Bone Joint Surg 65A:310, 1983.

10. Clendenin MD, DeLee JC, Heckman JD: Interstitial tears of the posterior cruciate ligament of the knee. Orthopedics 3:764, 1980.

11. O'Donoghue DH: Surgical treatment of fresh injuries to the major ligaments of the knee. J Bone Joint Surg 32A:721, 1950.

12. Harner CD, Xerogeanes JW, Livesay GA, et al.: The human posterior cruciate ligament complex: An interdisciplinary study: Ligament morphology and biomechanical evaluation. Am J Sports Med 23(6):736–745, 1995.

13. Palmer I: On the injuries to the ligaments of the knee joint: A clinical study. Acta Chir Scand 81(Suppl):2, 1938.

14. Heller L, Langman J: The menisco-femoral ligaments of the human knee joint. J Bone Joint Surg 46B:307, 1964.

15. Girgis FE, Marshall JL, Al Monajem ARS: The cruciate ligaments of the knee joint: Anatomical, functional, and experimental analysis. Clin Orthop 106:216–231, 1975.

16. Grood ES, Stowers SF, Noyes FR: Limits of movement in the human knee. J Bone Joint Surg 70A:88, 1985.

17. Cross MJ, Powell JF: Long-term follow up of posterior cruciate ligament rupture: A study of 116 cases. Am J Sports Med 12:292, 1984.

18. Trickey EL: Injuries to the posterior cruciate ligament: Diagnosis and treatment of early injuries and reconstruction of late instability. Clin Orthop Rel Res 147:76, 1980.

19. Hughston JC, Andrews JR, Cross MJ, et al.: Classification of knee ligament instabilities. Part I. The medial compartment and cruciate ligaments. J Bone Joint Surg 58A:159, 1970.

20. Satku K, Chew CN, Seow H: Posterior cruciate ligament injuries. Acta Orthop Scand 55:26, 1984.

21. Hughston JC: The absent posterior drawer test in some acute posterior cruciate ligament tears of the knee. Am J Sports Med 16:39, 1988.

22. Daniel DM, Stone ML, Burnett P, Sachs R: Use of quadriceps active test to diagnose posterior cruciate ligament disruptions and measure posterior laxity of the knee. J Bone Joint Surg 70A:386, 1988.

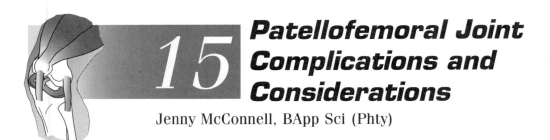

15 Patellofemoral Joint Complications and Considerations

Jenny McConnell, BApp Sci (Phty)

Patellofemoral pain syndrome is one of the most common conditions presenting to clinicians involved in the management of sports injuries.[1, 2] Twenty-five percent of the population will at some point in their lives suffer from patellofemoral symptoms. It is often the result of overuse, essentially because the patellofemoral joint is a soft tissue joint, and the position of the patella on the femur is very much reliant on the soft tissue structures. Management of patellofemoral problems is significantly enhanced if the therapist has a thorough understanding of the anatomy and biomechanics of the region.

This chapter examines the relevant anatomy and biomechanics of the patellofemoral joint; outlines the signs and symptoms of conditions of patellofemoral origin to assist in differential diagnosis; and provides assessment procedures and intervention strategies for the therapist.

ANATOMY

The patella is under the influence of the surrounding soft tissue structures for the first 20 degrees, where it is vulnerable and susceptible to problems. After 20 degrees of knee flexion, the bony architecture is increasingly responsible for controlling the position of the patella.

Soft Tissue Structures

The lateral side of the knee is made up of various fibrous layers, forming the superficial and deep lateral retinaculum. The anterior portion of the superficial layer of the lateral retinaculum consists of the fibrous expansion of vastus lateralis, running longitudinally along the lateral border and inserting into the patellar tendon.[3] Proceeding posteriorly, fibers from the iliotibial band interdigitate with fibers from the vastus lateralis and the patellar tendon to form the superficial oblique retinaculum.

The deep layer, or deep transverse retinaculum, consists of three major components: the epicondylopatellar band (lateral patellofemoral ligament), which provides superolateral static support for the patella; the midportion, which is the primary support structure for the lateral patella and courses directly from the iliotibial band to the patella; and the patellotibial band, which provides inferolateral stability for the patella.[2] Most of the lateral retinaculum arises from the iliotibial band, which provides both active, through the tensor fascia latae and gluteus maximus origins, and passive stabilization of the patella. If the iliotibial band is tight and the force is unopposed on the medial side, lateral displacement or lateral tilt and compression of the patella may arise. Passively, the structures are stronger on the lateral than on the medial side. The stability on the medial side is enhanced by the more muscular attachment of the medial quadriceps into the patella.

Medially, the capsule thickens to form a tough fibrous band, the medial patellofemoral ligament. This band inserts into the superior two thirds of the posterior part of the medial border of the patella. The stability on the medial side is further aided by the meniscopatellar ligament inferiorly, which inserts into the inferior third of the medial border of the patella, connecting the patella to the anterior part of the medial meniscus.[2–4] The passive and active stabilizers of the patellofemoral joint are inextricably linked. Most of the active stabilization of the patella is provided by the quadriceps muscle. The attachments of the individual heads of quadriceps into the patella are considered structurally in three components: superficial, intermediate, and deep.

The superficial plane contains the rectus femoris, which inserts into the superior pole and superior one third of the anterior surface. The intermediate plane consists of the vastus lateralis (VL) and vastus medialis (VM), which unite to form a solid aponeurosis that inserts into the base of the patella just posterior to the rectus femoris insertion. The remaining component, the deep plane, contains the vastus intermedius, which is the most efficient extensor. A 12 percent greater mean force is required by each of the other single long heads to complete the same motion.[5]

The VM and VL muscles are dynamically responsible for maintaining the position of the patella in a mediolateral direction. The VM is functionally divided, owing to the anatomic configuration of its fibers, into two parts: the longus, whose fibers are oriented 15 to 18 degrees medially to the frontal plane, and the obliquus, whose fibers are oriented 50 to 55 degrees medially in the frontal plane.[5] The vastus medialis longus acts with the rest of the quadriceps to extend the knee. Although the vastus medialis obliquus (VMO) does not extend the knee, it is active throughout knee extension to keep the patella centered in the trochlea of the femur.[5] The centered position of the patella, provided by the VMO, enhances the efficiency of the VL during knee extension.[5] The VMO arises from the tendon of the adductor magnus[6] and is supplied in most cases by a separate branch of the femoral nerve.[5]

On the lateral side, the VL is oriented 12 to 15 degrees laterally in the frontal plane, the obliquity of the distal fibers being greater. In a study by Hallisey et al.,[7] it was noted that an anatomically distinct group of VL fibers was separated from the main belly of the VL by a thin layer of fat. They found that this part interdigitated with the lateral intermuscular septum before inserting into the patella. Vastus lateralis obliquus provides a direct lateral pull on the patella because of its interdigitation with the lateral intermuscular septum.

If the attachment points of VMO and VL are changed anatomically, then the retropatellar surface area of contact can be dramatically changed.[8] This has significant implications for patients undergoing plication and realignment procedures for patellofemoral problems. It may explain why symptoms persist or recur in some of these patients. Symmetric displacement of the insertion points of the VMO and the VL tendons, either proximally or distally, results in greater changes at larger flexion angles (>60 degrees). If the insertion points are shifted in an asymmetric manner, then the effect is greater at low flexion angles (<60 degrees). At lower flexion angles, the effect of a lateral imbalance manifests itself as a rotation of the patella in the coronal plane, whereas at higher flexion angles, the imbalance is more likely to produce a tilt of the patella in the sagittal plane.

The location and the orientation of the pressure zone on the retropatellar surface are particularly sensitive to the magnitude and direction of tension in the VMO.[9] A 50 percent decrease in tension in the VMO may result in a 5-mm lateral displacement of the patella. If the VMO is deactivated or the tension in the VL is twice that of the VMO, then the pressure zone is almost entirely on the lateral facet. Pressure on the lateral facet will adversely affect the nutrition of the articular cartilage in the central and medial zones of the patella. Degenerative change will occur more readily in these areas. Therefore, one of the aims of management of patellofemoral problems is to facilitate a balance between medial and lateral structures, so the load through the joint is distributed as evenly as possible.

FUNCTIONS OF THE PATELLA

The patella links the divergent quadriceps muscle to a common tendon. Its major function is to increase the extensor moment of the quadriceps muscle. The patella also protects the tendon from compressive stress and minimizes the concentration of stress by transmitting forces evenly to the underlying bone.[2, 10–12]

The patella is like a balance beam, adjusting the length, direction, and force of each of its arms—the quadriceps tendon and the patella tendon—at different degrees of flexion.[10, 13, 14] With increasing flexion, the patellofemoral contact area moves from distal to proximal on the patella surface so that the quadriceps muscle has an increased, then a decreased, mechanical advantage. It means that terminal knee extension can occur with little increase in quadriceps demand, because the quadriceps is functioning with a longer lever in extension.

Patellar Excursion

The total proximal to distal excursion of the patella in the sagittal plane during knee flexion is between 5 and 7 cm.[15] In the frontal plane when the patella is relaxed, there is a mean displacement of the patella of approximately 22 mm, 12 mm in the medial direction and 10 mm in the lateral direction.[16]

At full extension, the patella sits lateral to the trochlea and rests on the supratrochlear fat pad. The fat pad is one of the most pain-sensitive structures in knee.[17] Not only is the fat pad responsible for contributing to symptoms around the knee, but the mechanoreceptors in the fat pad, as well as the cruciate ligaments, joint capsule, collateral ligaments, and skin, provide feedback to the muscles around the knee. Failure of any of these structures can result in atrophy of the quadriceps.[18]

Between 10 and 20 degrees, the articular surface of the patella comes into contact with the lateral femur through a small band of contact on the inferior patellar surface.[11, 19] In this position, the patellofemoral joint is relatively unstable, as the tibia has derotated, allowing the patella to move medially to be in contact with the trochlea. Thus, with increasing knee flexion, there is increasing stability of the joint. From 30 to 60 degrees, the middle surface of the patella comes into contact with the middle third of the trochlea, with a broader band of contact.[11, 19] By 60 to 90 degrees, the upper third of the patella has a broad band of contact deep within the trochlea and is firmly in position by the trochlear facets.[11, 19] By 90 degrees of flexion, the patella moves laterally again so that the contact areas split into two smaller areas medially and laterally on the upper patellar surface, corresponding to areas of contact on the medial and lateral condyles of the femur.[11] Although the patellofemoral contact area has diminished by this stage, there is extensive contact of the posterior surface of the quadriceps tendon with the trochlea.[19] It is not until 135 degrees of flexion that the odd facet of the patella makes contact with the trochlea. So, at full flexion, the lateral femoral condyle is completely covered by the patella, and the medial condyle, except for the lateral border, is completely exposed.[11, 19]

BIOMECHANICAL CONSIDERATIONS

The patellofemoral joint reaction force (PFJRF) is equal and opposite to the resultant force of the quadriceps tendon tension and the patellar tendon tension and acts perpendicular to the articular surfaces. The PFJRF increases with increasing flexion because the angle between the patellar tendon and the quadriceps becomes more acute.

The PFJRF changes from one-half times body weight during level walking, to three to four times body weight during stair ascending and descending, seven to eight times body weight during squatting, and 20 times body weight during jumping.[2, 20] Ericsson and Nissell[21] found a PFJFRF of 1.3 times body weight with ergonometric cycling, which further increased with increased workload and decreased seat height. The increase of PFJRF with flexion offers an explanation for the aggravation of patellofemoral symptoms experienced by individuals during bent knee activities. It is also the basis for the rationale of the management of patellofemoral pain, which emphasizes short arc quadriceps activity and straight leg raising maneuvers, thus avoiding weight-bearing and bent knee activities. However, joints are designed to handle compressive stress by maximizing the surface area of contact. The therapist's objective should be to optimize the area of contact to maximize the area of pressure distribution.

FACTORS PREDISPOSING TO PATELLOFEMORAL PAIN

Individuals with patellofemoral pain tend to demonstrate a failure of the intricate balance of the soft tissue structures around the joint, such that there may be an alteration of the pressure distribution from the patella to the femur. It has also been suggested that when the patellofemoral joint is outside its envelope of function and not in balanced homeostasis, the system breaks down and the patient presents with symptoms.[22]

Many different causes of patellofemoral

pain have been cited in the literature. The mechanism of pain production is not fully understood. There are many pain-sensitive structures in the knee. Patellofemoral pain is most likely due to either tension or compression of the soft tissue structures. Patellofemoral pain may therefore be classified by area of pain, as the site of pain usually indicates the compromised structure and the possible mechanism for the compromise. For example, lateral pain is indicative of adaptive shortening of the lateral retinaculum. Individuals presenting with lateral pain will have chronically tilted patellae (excessive lateral pressure syndrome), and there is often evidence of small nerve injury in the lateral retinaculum when the retinaculum is sectioned histologically.[2] If the patient presents with inferior patellar pain, the target irritated tissue in this instance is the infrapatellar fat pad. The infrapatellar fat pad has been found to be one of the most pain-sensitive structures in the knee.[22] A differential diagnosis of fat pad irritation and patellar tendonitis is outlined later in the chapter. A patient with a recurrently subluxing patella often presents with medial patellofemoral pain because the medial retinaculum is chronically overstretched. It is unusual for this type of patient to have tight lateral structures, as the patella is generally mobile in all directions and the VMO is poorly developed, often with a high attachment point into the patella.

It is postulated that in the individuals who complain of a deep ache in the knee, the articular cartilage has failed such that the load is now borne on the richly innervated underlying subchondral bone.[2] These patients often have the classic chondromalacia patellae, in which softening and fissuring are present on the undersurface of the patella.

Biomechanical Faults

Although a direct blow or a traumatic dislocation of the patella may precipitate patellofemoral pain, increasingly, suboptimal mechanics of the patella from biomechanical faults is thought to be the major contributory factor.[2, 23–26] The biomechanical faults can be divided into structural and nonstructural. Structural causes of malalignment can be divided into intrinsic and extrinsic causes and may be quite subtle. The extrinsic fac-

tors are more common and magnify the effect of the nonstructural faults.

Intrinsic structural factors relate to dysplasia of the patella or femoral trochlea and the position of the patella relative to the trochlea. Although uncommon, developmental abnormalities such as patella or trochlea dysplasia will create patellofemoral incongruence with resultant instability of the patella.[23, 24] Extrinsic structural faults are reported to cause a lateral tracking of the patella.[25–27] The extrinsic factors include increased Q angle, hamstrings, and gastrocnemius muscle tightness.

The Q angle has been used to estimate the angle of pull of the quadriceps muscle group.[2, 23, 26] The Q angle is formed by the bisection of a line from the anterosuperior iliac spine to the mid-pole of the patella with a line from the tibial tubercle to the mid-pole of the patella. It forms a valgus vector particularly in extension. The outer limit for Q angle for females is 15 degrees and for males 12 degrees.[26, 27] The explanation of the higher Q angle in females is the shape of the female pelvis. The Q angle varies dynamically, decreasing with knee flexion and increasing with knee extension owing to the external rotation of the tibia, which occurs during the screw-home mechanism to allow full extension to occur.[2, 27, 28] Increased femoral anteversion, external tibial torsion, or a lateral displacement of the tibial tubercle can cause an increase in Q angle.[29] Often, individuals with an increased Q angle have "squinting" patellae. These individuals usually present with an anteversion of the femur.[29]

Soft Tissue Tightness

A decrease in the flexibility of the soft tissue structures that surround the patella is a significant contributory factor in the etiology of patellofemoral pain. Soft tissue tightness is particularly prevalent during the adolescent growth spurt, in which the long bones are growing faster than the surrounding soft tissues.[30] This leads not only to problems with lack of flexibility and alteration of stress through joints but also to muscle control problems in which the motor program is no longer able to appropriately control the limb. A decrease in extensibility of the lateral retinaculum and a reduction in the flexibility of the tensor fasciae latae, hamstrings, gastrocnemius, or rectus femoris will adversely affect the tracking of the patella.

When the knee flexes, a shortened lateral retinaculum will come under excessive stress as the patella is drawn into the trochlea and the iliotibial band pulls posteriorly on the already shortened lateral retinaculum.[2, 31] This will cause a lateral tracking and tilting of the patella and often a weakness of the medial retinaculum.[31] Additionally, a tight tensor fasciae latae, through its attachment into the iliotibial band, will cause a lateral tracking of the patella, particularly at 20 degrees of knee flexion when the band is at its shortest.

Hamstrings and gastrocnemius tightness also cause a lateral tracking of the patella, by increasing the dynamic Q angle.[32-34] If an individual with tight hamstrings goes running, increased knee flexion occurs when the foot lands. Because the knee cannot straighten, an increased amount of dorsiflexion is required to position the body over the planted foot. If the range of full dorsiflexion has already occurred at the talocrural joint, further range is achieved by pronating the foot, particularly at the subtalar joint. This causes an increase in the valgus vector force and hence increases the dynamic Q angle.[32]

Muscle Imbalance

It would seem that the control and timing of the muscles of the lower limb are critical to the smooth functioning of the patellofemoral joint. However, the issue of muscle imbalance and timing is yet to be established in the literature. There is an assumption that a person with patellofemoral symptoms was, at one time when not symptomatic, like an asymptomatic person, much as we can say that apples and oranges are round pieces of fruit, yet we know that that is where the similarity ends. Thus with a patellofemoral sufferer, the factors that cause the patellofemoral symptoms have always been present, but the condition may not yet have manifested itself. The issue of VMO and VL timing is still controversial. Voight and Weider[35] found that the reflex response time of the VMO was earlier than that of the VL in an asymptomatic group, but in a symptomatic patellofemoral group, there was a

reversal of the pattern. These findings were recently confirmed by Witvrouw et al.,[36] but curiously these investigators found that there was a shorter reflex response time in the patellofemoral group relative to the control group. Dynamically, this issue has been supported by the work of Grabiner et al.,[37] who examined isokinetic knee extension at 250 degrees per second, following hamstrings preactivation. They found that the VMO activated 5.6 ms earlier than the VL. Even though this finding was statistically significant, these authors questioned the functional relevance.

These findings are at odds, however, with the findings of other investigators[38-40] who found that the VMO did not fire earlier than the VL in the asymptomatic group and that the firing of the VMO was not delayed in the symptomatic group. Because of this lack of change in the firing pattern, some of the investigators have concluded that general quadriceps strengthening only is required in the rehabilitation of patellofemoral pain. However, it has been found that taping the patella of patellofemoral pain sufferers causes an earlier activation of the VMO and a delayed activation of the VL, particularly on stair descent.[40] Perhaps it could be surmised that the VMO of the patellofemoral pain sufferer needs to fire earlier to overcome the abnormal tracking forces. Perhaps the ability to selectively fire the VMO is a learned skill rather than an innate ability, much as one would train the abductor hallucis or, for that matter, individually isolate one frontalis to elevate one eyebrow and not the other. Training should therefore further enhance this ability.

Although the early literature suggested that there was a difference in the ratio of the VMO and the VL activity, with the VL activity being greater than the VMO activity,[41] recent literature has not supported this contention. The early literature did not normalize the electromyelographic data. Normalization involves obtaining a ratio of the recorded muscle activity and muscle activity from the maximal voluntary contraction (MVC), which then enables a comparison to be made between the ratio of the activity of one muscle and another muscle. For example, if the recorded activity of the VMO is 20 μV and the maximum is 100 μV and the measured VL is 40 μV and the max is 200 μV, then the ratio of VMO to VL is 1:1. There has been some discussion that normalization is affected by the presence of pain, which will mask differences, as there may be error in the MVC, which may appear in the error of the recorded electromyelogram (EMG).[42]

Some debate exists about the reliability of the maximal contraction, throwing some concern on the normalization process. Howard and Enoka[43] found that there was considerable variation in the MVC of the VL EMG, even though the force exerted by the leg remained constant. Yang and Winter[44] found that the averaged rectified EMG data had a coefficient of variation (SD/mean) of 9.1 percent in one day and 16.4 percent between days. Where this leaves the clinician and what the best method is of facilitating recovery in a patient with patellofemoral pain are addressed in the section concerned with muscle training.

Altered Foot Biomechanics

Altered foot biomechanics such as excessive, prolonged, or late pronation will alter the tibial rotation at varying times through its range of motion, thus having an effect on patellofemoral joint mechanics.[32, 34] It is essential for the therapist to realize that the foot may be mobile or stiff, and that if a foot problem is discovered the only course of action is not necessarily orthotics, particularly if the foot is stiff. Movement is required in the foot for shock absorption and a rigid orthotic device deprives the foot even further of movement.

EXAMINATION

History

Obtaining a detailed history from the patient provides the clinician with the differential diagnosis, which is later confirmed or modified by the physical findings. The clinician needs to elicit the following from the history:
- area, behavior, and onset of the pain
- symptom-provoking activities
- presence of other symptoms such as clicking, giving-way, or swelling

This information provides an indication of the structure involved and the likely diagnosis. For example, if the patient was complaining of a "knife-like" lateral knee pain that was precipitated by running, the clinician would suspect an iliotibial friction syndrome.

SYMPTOMS OF PATELLOFEMORAL PAIN

The patient usually complains of a diffuse ache in the anterior knee, which is exacerbated by stair climbing and sitting with the knee flexed—the movie sign.[1, 2] Mild swelling, crepitus, and locking are among the other complaints. The crepitus is mostly due to tight deep lateral retinacular structures and can be improved with treatment. A mild effusion can have the effect of causing an asymmetric wasting of the quadriceps muscle.[45] Spencer et al.[45] found that after 20 mL of normal saline was injected into the knees of healthy college students, there was a diminution of the H reflex of the VM, whereas it took 50 to 60 mL of saline to diminish the H reflexes of the rectus femoris and the VL. The implication of this study is that anyone with a small low-grade effusion after an intra-articular pathologic lesion can end up with patellofemoral symptoms. The medial quadriceps may be inhibited before the lateral, which has the potential to set up an imbalance of the soft tissue forces and cause a consequent lateral tracking of the patella. So an athlete, who has primary intra-articular problems, such as a meniscal or ligamentous injury, may have great difficulty resolving the subsequent secondary patellofemoral symptoms, particularly if they are not identified.

Some patients may experience "giving-way" or a buckling sensation of their knee. This occurs during walking or stair climbing and is a reflex inhibition of the quadriceps muscle. It must be differentiated from the giving-way experienced when turning, which is indicative of an anterior cruciate–deficient knee. Locking is another symptom that must be differentiated from intra-articular pathology. Patellofemoral locking is usually only a catching sensation in which the patient can actively unlock the knee, unlike loose body or meniscal locking, in which the patient is either unable to unlock or can only passively unlock the knee.[1, 2]

When considering the possible differential diagnoses, the clinician must remember that the lumbar spine and the hip can refer symptoms to the knee. For example, the prepubescent male with a slipped femoral epiphysis may present with a limp and anterior knee pain that can initially be misdiagnosed as patellofemoral pain.[1, 2] Neural and fascial tissue can also be a source of symptoms around the patellofemoral joint. Lack of mobility of the L5 and S1 nerve roots and their derivatives can give rise to posterior or lateral thigh pain. Symptoms from neural tissue can be fairly easily differentiated from patellofemoral symptoms because the pain will be exacerbated in a sitting position, particularly when the leg is straight rather than in the classic movie sign position of a flexed knee. A positive response to the "slump" sitting test will quickly verify the neural tissue as being a source of the pain. Similarly, symptoms from a peripheral nerve, which may have become entrapped or stretched during arthroscopic surgery, may be reproduced by placing that particular nerve on stretch. The most common example is the infrapatellar branch of the saphenous nerve. Symptoms are sharp pain inferomedially with or without slightly altered sensation laterally. The symptoms are reproduced on deep bend and jumping, so they are frequently confused with patellar tendonitis symptoms because of the proximity to the tendon. Pain is reproduced with the patient prone, flexing the knee and externally rotating the tibia.

Differential Diagnosis

PATELLOFEMORAL INSTABILITY

Patellofemoral instability or recurrent patellofemoral subluxation is a variant of patellofemoral pain syndrome, in which there is actual subluxation of the patella. It is more common in females and tends to be associated with patella alta, a Q angle greater than 20 degrees and dysplasias of the trochlea and patella.[1, 46] Patients with instability will complain of a sensation of giving way on certain movements. This usually occurs when the femur internally rotates on a fixed externally rotated tibia.[46] This injury must be differentiated from the acute anterior cruciate ligament rupture, as the mechanism of injury is similar. It is important to take radiographs of all acute knee problems to ensure that the knee joint is intact and there is no bony involvement—that is, that there has been no disruption to the lateral femoral condyle, resulting in a loose body in the joint.

Patients with patellofemoral instability exhibit apprehension and sometimes pain on lateral movement of the patella. The apprehension sign confirms the diagnosis. Treatment is based on the same principles as those for patellofemoral pain management, since the predisposing factors are the same as for patellofemoral pain syndrome.

PATELLAR TENDONITIS

Patellar tendonitis is common in jumping sports. Some authors believe that because there appear to be signs of degeneration rather than signs of inflammation in the patellar tendon, the condition should be referred to as tendonosis of the patella. As many as 90 percent of professional volleyball and basketball players demonstrate degeneration of the patellar tendon on magnetic resonance imaging, yet only a small percentage of these individuals actually have symptoms. The clinician may question the validity of these degenerative changes being the source of all inferior patellar symptoms in jumping athletes. A recent study of college athletes over a 6-month period found that 78 percent of those diagnosed with patellar tendonitis showed an increased uptake in the fat pad on a T2-weighted magnetic resonance image, which is suggestive of inflammation of the fat pad.[47] It appears that the fat pad, rather than the patellar tendon, may be the source of the primary pathologic condition of many jumping athletes with patellar tendonitis diagnoses or that a combination of the two conditions may exist.

The patient's history helps differentiate patellar tendonitis with typical fat pad irritation. The patient with patellar tendonitis must have a history of eccentric loading of the quadriceps muscle, such as jumping or running downhill, whereas a patient with a fat pad irritation presents after a forceful extension maneuver, such as forceful kicking in swimming or locking of the knees in power walking. Both patient groups have inferior patella pain. With patellar tendonitis, the pain is exacerbated by squatting and jumping. The Q angle is generally straighter, less than 15 degrees in females and less than 12 degrees in males. With acute fat pad irritation, the pain is exacerbated by extension maneuvers such as straight leg raises and prolonged standing. The inferior pole of the patella is displaced posteriorly and the fat pad is puffy.[48]

ILIOTIBIAL BAND FRICTION SYNDROME

Iliotibial friction syndrome is a complaint of pain over the lateral femoral condyle. It is seen in distance runners who have changed footwear, increased the mileage, or altered the training terrain.[1-3, 49] These patients will have a tight iliotibial band, as confirmed on a modified Ober's test performed in side-lying position with the pelvis in a stable position. The hip is extended, adducted, and slightly externally rotated while the knee is flexed and extended to elicit pain or click-ing.[49] Correction of training errors as well as the correction of any faulty biomechanics must be addressed in treatment.

PLICA SYNDROME

Anterior knee pain, particularly along the medial edge of the patella, may be due to an inflamed synovial plica.[1, 2, 50, 51] The synovial plica is a redundant fold in the synovial lin-ing of the knee joint, extending from the fat pad medially under the quadriceps tendon, superiorly to the lateral retinaculum. Pain from an inflamed plica is usually worse in sustained flexed positions of the knee, and progressively improves with increased activ-ity. Some patients may be aware of a signifi-cant pop or snap as they flex and extend their knee. On examination, the plica is sometimes palpable as a thickened band, but the plica should be considered as the primary cause of the symptoms only if the patient fails to respond to the appropriate management of patellofemoral syndrome. An inflamed plica is usually only an indicator of a more complex problem involving abnormal patellofemoral mechanics.[1, 2, 51]

APOPHYSITIS IN THE ADOLESCENT KNEE PAIN SUFFERER

The tibial tubercle or the inferior pole of the patella may be tender to palpation in the active, rapidly growing, usually male, adoles-cent, indicating that there is an excessive traction on the soft tissue apophysis at the proximal or distal attachment of the patellar tendon.[52] If pain is elicited on palpation of the tibial tubercle, the patient is diagnosed as having Osgood-Schlatter disease, which is a more common condition than inferior

pole apophysitis (Sinding-Larsen-Johanssen syndrome). The diagnosis is a clinical one, so a radiograph is usually not necessary. However, a radiograph may be indicated to exclude bony tumor, particularly in cases in which the anterior knee pain is severe and there is a large amount of associated swell-ing. Bone tumors are rare, but in the 10- to 30-year-old age group, the knee is the site of osteogenic sarcoma.[1]

OSTEOCHONDRITIS DISSICANS IN THE ADOLESCENT KNEE PAIN SUFFERER

The patient with osteochondritis dissi-cans usually presents with intermittent pain and swelling of gradual onset. It must be differentiated from juvenile rheumatoid ar-thritis (Still's disease) and a partial discoid meniscus. In the acute situation, the patient with osteochondritis dissicans may have an extremely painful, locked, swollen knee. The swelling is a hemarthrosis and the locking is due to a loose body from a defect at the lateral aspect of the medial femoral con-dyle.[1] This is confirmed on radiograph and the patient requires an immediate orthope-dic referral for either fixation of the loos-ened fragment or removal of the detached fragment.[1, 52]

Radiologic Evaluation of the Patellofemoral Joint

To further aid in the diagnosis and man-agement of patellofemoral pain sufferers, dif-ferent radiologic procedures have been sug-gested. However, in the past, wide variability in the radiographic findings of patients with patellofemoral dysfunction, and the diffi-culty in demonstrating radiographic abnor-malities consistent with clinical findings, have contributed to the confusion in the diagnosis and classification of patellofem-oral pain disorders.[53, 54]

The patellofemoral joint is best visualized on an axial or tangential view. The "axial" view describes the parallel relationship of the x-ray beam with respect to the axis of the anterior tibia, while the "tangential" view describes the perpendicular relation-ship of the x-ray beam to the joint surfaces.[53, 54] Both methods provide cross-sectional information about the relationship of the patella to the trochlear groove.

CLINICAL EXAMINATION

The clinical examination confirms the diagnosis and helps determine the underlying causative factors of the patient's symptoms so that the appropriate treatment can be implemented. By examining the patient's standing position, the therapist has a fair indication of how the patient will move. The therapist can start at the feet and move up the lower limb or at the pelvis and move down the limb. From the front, the therapist can observe the femoral position, which is easier to see when the patient has the feet together. A position of internal rotation of the femur is a common finding with patients with patellofemoral pain. The internal femoral rotation often causes a squinting of the patellae. The internal rotation of the femur is usually associated with a tight iliotibial band and poor functioning of the posterior gluteus medius muscle. This gives rise to instability of the pelvis, causing an increase in the dynamic Q angle and increasing the potential for patellofemoral pain.

Moving down the leg to the knee, the therapist can observe the bulk of the different heads of the quadriceps muscle, the tightness of the iliotibial band attachment and any swelling or puffiness about the knee. An enlarged fat pad, for example, is indicative that the patient is standing in hyperextension or a "locked back" position of the knees. From this the clinician can infer that the quadriceps control, particularly eccentric control, in the inner range (0–20 degrees of flexion) will be poor. The position of the tibia relative to the femur (valgus/varus) is noted and the presence or absence of torsion of the tibia is determined, as these bony malalignments can affect the way the foot hits the ground as well as the patellofemoral position.

The clinician needs to palpate the talus on the medial and lateral sides to check for symmetry of position. In the relaxed standing position, there should be equal amounts of talus palpable on both the medial and lateral sides. This is the midposition of the subtalar joint. If the talus is more prominent medially, then the patient's subtalar joint is pronated. The position of the talus from the front is correlated with the position of the calcaneum from behind. If the talus is prominent medially, the calcaneum should be sitting everted. If the calcaneum is sitting straight or inverted, then the clinician can infer that the patient has a stiff subtalar joint and will pronate not at heel strike but at mid-stance, thus exhibiting a mid-foot collapse. The great toe and first metatarsal are examined for callus formation as well as position. If the patient has callus on the medial aspect of the first metatarsal or the great toe, or has a hallux valgus, then the therapist should expect the patient to have an unstable push-off in gait. When examined prone, this patient will have a forefoot deformity.

From the side, the clinician can check pelvic and lumbar spine position to determine whether the pelvis has an anterior or a posterior tilt or whether the patient has a "sway-back" posture. A sway-back posture is one in which the pelvis is displaced forward of the shoulders. The amount of extension of the knees, confirming the presence of hyperextension or a "locked back" position, can also be seen from the side.

From behind, the level of the posterosuperior iliac spine is checked to determine any leg length discrepancies, gluteal bulk is assessed, and the position of the calcaneum is observed. The clinician can therefore have a reasonable idea of the dynamic picture from a person's static alignment, so it should be possible to anticipate how the patient will move. Any deviations from the anticipated give a great deal of information about the muscle control of the activity.

Dynamic Examination

The aim of the dynamic examination is primarily to reproduce the patient's symptoms so that the clinician has an objective reassessment activity to evaluate the effectiveness of the treatment. Additionally, the effect of muscle action on the limb mechanics can be evaluated. The first dynamic activity examined is walking. For example, if an individual stands in hyperextension of the knees, the quadriceps will not function well in inner range due to lack of practice, so the initial shock absorption at heel strike will be minimal. Initial shock absorption occurs with knee flexion of 10 to 15 degrees, because the foot is supinated when the heel first strikes the ground. As soon as the heel hits the ground, the foot rapidly pronates, so if that same individual has a stiff subtalar joint, shock absorption must come from higher up in the body, in this case the pelvis. This patient will demonstrate a pelvic instability, which, depending on the tilt of the pelvis, will cause either an increase in pelvic and ultimately trunk rotation or lateral tilt. If the pelvis is anteriorly tilted, then the patient will exhibit an increase in pelvic rotation when walking, because that individual has a lack of hip extension and external rotation. If the pelvis is posteriorly tilted, the patient will present with a Trendelenburg gait, indicating weak gluteal musculature. The individual with a sway back posture walks with a combination of increased tilt and rotation. The optimal amount of pelvic movement is reported to be 10 degrees for rotation, 4 degrees for lateral tilt, and 7 degrees for anteroposterior tilt.[55]

The initial response, when evaluating a patient with abnormal pelvic motion, is to give that patient pelvic stability work to control the excessive motion. If this is the case, however, the patient, who is not shock-absorbing at the knee or the foot and now no longer shock-absorbing at the pelvis, must shock-absorb even higher up, perhaps at the cervical spine. This may be a potential cause of whiplash. If stabilization work is given to a patient, the therapist must make sure the patient has some scope for movement elsewhere, so asking the patient to walk with the knees slightly flexed will improve the shock absorption and decrease the need for the excessive movement at the pelvis.

If the patient's symptoms have not been provoked in walking, then evaluation of more stressful activities, such as stair-climbing, are performed. If symptoms are still not provoked, then squat and one-leg squat can be examined and used as a reassessment activity. With athletes, however, these clinical tests are not strenuous enough to reproduce their symptoms, as longer duration activities, such as running 15 km, provoke symptoms. In this situation, the clinician can evaluate the control of the one-leg squat to determine the effect of treatment outcome.

Supine Lying Examination

With the patient in the supine position, the clinician gains an appreciation of the soft tissue structures and begins to confirm the diagnosis. Gentle but careful palpation should be performed on the soft tissue structures around the patella. If pain is elicited in the infrapatellar region on palpation, the clinician should shorten the fat pad by lifting it toward the patella. If, on further palpation, the pain is gone, then the clinician can be relatively certain that the patient has a fat pad irritation. If the pain remains, then the patient has a patellar tendonitis. The knee is passively flexed and extended with overpressure applied, so the clinician has an appreciation of the quality of the endfeel. If any of these maneuvers reproduce pain, they can be used as a reassessment sign; for example, the symptoms of fat pad irritation are often reproduced with an extension overpressure maneuver.[48]

The flexibility of the hamstring, iliopsoas, rectus femoris, tensor fascia latae, gastrocnemius, and soleus muscles is determined. Tightness of any of these muscles has an adverse effect on patellofemoral joint mechanics and will have to be addressed in treatment. The iliopsoas, rectus femoris, and tensor fascia latae muscles can be tested using the Thomas test. To perform the Thomas test, the patient stands at the edge of the plinth. One leg is pulled up to the chest, to flatten the lumbar lordosis. The patient lies on the plinth, keeping the flexed leg close to the chest. The other leg should be resting such that the hip is in a neutral position (ie, on the plinth, at the same width as the pelvis) and the knee is flexed to 90 degrees. If the hip is in neutral position, but the knee is straight, the rectus femoris is tight. If the hip is flexed, but lying in the plane of the body, the iliopsoas is tight. If the hip remains flexed and abducted, the tensor fascia latae is tight. Lack of flexibility of the tensor fascia latae can be further confirmed in side-lying position by performing Ober's test.[56] The therapist needs to evaluate the flexibility of the muscles in each leg. Hamstrings flexibility can be examined by a passive straight leg raise maneuver, once the lumbar spine is flattened on the plinth and the pelvis is stable.[57] Normal hamstrings length should allow 80 to 85 degrees of hip flexion, when the knee is extended and the lumbar spine is flattened.[57]

With the patient in the supine position, the therapist can examine the orientation of the patella. Examination of orientation of the patella as an isolated procedure has been found to be unreliable, but determining the position of the patella relative to the femur is just part of the examination procedure and should be used to guide the treatment choice.[58] Unfortunately, determination of joint position and manual palpation in general is unreliable.[59–63] The position of the patella with respect to the femur needs to be considered not with respect to the normal, but with respect to the optimal, because the norm of the population is probably suboptimal. An optimal patellar position is one in which the patella is parallel to the femur in the frontal and the sagittal planes, and the patella is midway between the two condyles when the knee is flexed to 20 degrees.[64, 65] The position of the patella is determined by examining four discrete components: glide, lateral tilt, anteroposterior tilt, and rotation, in a static and a dynamic manner.

GLIDE COMPONENT

Determination of the glide component involves measuring the distance from the middle of the patella to the medial and lateral femoral epicondyles. The patella should be sitting equidistant ($+/-$ 5 mm) from each epicondyle when the knee is flexed 20 degrees. A 5-mm lateral displacement of the patella causes a 50 percent decrease in VMO tension.[14] In some cases, the patella may sit equidistant to the condyles, but as soon as the quadriceps contracts, the patella moves lateral, rather than in the line with the femur, indicating a dynamic problem. The dynamic glide demonstrates both the effect of the quadriceps contraction on patellar position and the timing of the activity of the different heads of quadriceps. The VMO should be activated simultaneously with, or even slightly earlier than, the VL if the patella is to remain centered in the trochlea.

TILT COMPONENT

If the passive lateral structures—the lateral retinaculum and the iliotibial band—are too tight, the patella will tilt so that the medial border of the patella will be higher than the lateral border and the posterior edge of the lateral border will be difficult to palpate. This is a lateral tilt, and, if severe, it can lead to excessive lateral pressure syndrome.[2] When the patella is passively moved in a medial direction, it should initially remain parallel to the femur. If the medial border quickly rides anteriorly, the patella has a dynamic tilt problem. This action of the patella is indicative of tight deep lateral retinacular fibers, which become taut at 20 degrees of knee flexion, affecting the seating of the patella in the trochlea.

ANTEROPOSTERIOR TILT

An optimal position also involves the patella being parallel to the femur in the sagittal plane. A most common finding is a posterior displacement of the inferior pole of the patella. This will result in fat pad irritation and often manifests itself as inferior patella pain, which is exacerbated by extension maneuvers of the knee.[65] A patient with a posterior displacement of the inferior pole of the patella will often have a dimple in the fat pad. When an active contraction of the quadriceps is performed, the foot usually comes off the plinth, so the proximal end of the tibia is moved posteriorly, pulling the inferior pole of the patella into the fat pad. This test examines the dynamic patellar posterior tilt.

ROTATION

To complete the ideal position, the long axis of the patella should be parallel to the long axis of the femur. In other words, if a line is drawn between the medial and lateral aspects of the patella, this line should be perpendicular to the long axis of the femur. If the inferior pole is sitting lateral to the long axis of the femur, the patient has an externally rotated patella. If the inferior pole is sitting medial to the long axis of the femur, then the patient has an internally rotated patella. The presence of a rotation component indicates that a particular part of the retinaculum is tight. Tightness in the retinacular tissue compromises the tissue and can be a potent source of the symptoms.

Side-Lying Examination

The side-lying position is used to assess the flexibility of the lateral structures—the lateral retinaculum, superficial and deep fibers, as well as the iliotibial band. To test the superficial retinacular structures, the knee is flexed to 20 degrees, where the therapist passively glides the patella in a medial direction. The therapist should be able to expose the lateral femoral condyle. The superficial retinacular fibers are tight if the lateral femoral condyle is not readily exposed. The deep fibers are tested with the patient in the same position. The therapist places his or her hand on the middle of the patella, takes up the slack of the glide in a medial direction, and applies an anteroposterior pressure on the medial border of the patella. The lateral border should move freely away from the femur. On palpation, the tension in the retinacular fibers should be similar. This test can also be used as a treatment technique. Iliotibial band tightness can be confirmed further by Ober's test,[56] which involves flexion of the underneath hip and knee to stabilize the pelvis. The knee of the upper leg is flexed to 90 degrees, while the hip is abducted, externally rotated, and slightly extended. If the iliotibial band is of normal length, the thigh should be resting on the plinth. However, if the band is shortened, the thigh remains abducted or flexes when the leg is released.[56]

Prone Lying Examination

Examination of some of the contributory factors to the patellofemoral problem is best performed in the prone position. Here, the therapist can examine foot position and anterior hip flexibility, and, if necessary, palpate the lumbar spine and sacroiliac joints. Primary foot deformities are determined by placing the foot in subtalar joint neutral position and determining the position of the forefoot relative to the rear foot and the position of the rear foot relative to the tibia. Additionally, the therapist can evaluate the amount of subtalar and first metatarsal joint movement. The contribution of the foot deformity to the patient's patellofemoral symptoms needs to be assessed, so the appropriate course of action, depending on the type and size of the foot deformity, can be taken. This may involve either prescription of orthotics or taping and specific muscle training.

With the patient in the prone position, the clinician is also able to evaluate the flexibility of the anterior hip structures by examining the patient in a figure-of-four position, with the underneath foot at the level of the tibial tubercle (Fig. 15–1). This position tests the available hip extension and external rotation, which is often limited because of chronic adaptive shortening of the anterior structures as a result of the underlying femoral anteversion. The distance of the ASIS from the plinth is measured, so the clinician has an objective measure of change. A lumbar spine and sacroiliac palpation can be performed at this stage of the examination, if the clinician feels that the knee symptoms have been referred from a primary pathologic condition of that region. Once the patellofemoral joint has been thoroughly examined and the primary problems have been identified, the patient is ready for treatment.

TREATMENT

Conservative

Most patellofemoral conditions are successfully managed with physical therapy. The aims of the treatment are twofold: first, to unload abnormally stressed soft tissue around the patellofemoral joint by optimizing the patellar position, and second, to improve the lower limb mechanics, which, if executed well, will significantly decrease the patient's symptoms.

Stretching the tight lateral structures and changing the activation pattern of the VMO may decrease the tendency for the patella to track laterally and should enhance the position of the patella. Stretching the tight lateral structures can be facilitated pas-

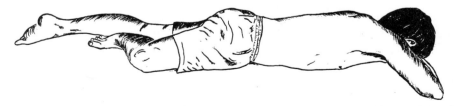

Figure 15–1. Assessment of anterior hip joint structure tightness. Patient in prone position flexes the knee and abducts and externally rotates one hip while the other leg rests on top of the flexed leg. The distance from the anterosuperior iliac spine to the plinth is measured. Ideally, the hip should be flat on the table.

sively, by the therapist's mobilizing and massaging the lateral retinaculum and the iliotibial band, as well as the patient's performing a self-stretch on the retinacular tissue (Fig. 15–2). However, the most effective stretch to the adaptively shortened retinacular tissue may be obtained by a sustained low load, using tape, to facilitate a permanent elongation of the tissues. This utilizes the creep phenomenon, which occurs in viscoelastic material when a constant low load is applied. It has been widely documented that the length of soft tissues can be increased with sustained stretching.[66–70] The magnitude of the increase in displacement is dependent on the duration of the applied stretch; that is, if the stretch is applied for long periods, the increase in displacement is large, hence the term "time-dependent."[69, 70] If the tape can be maintained for a prolonged period of time, then this, plus training of the VMO to actively change the patellar position, should have a significant effect on patellofemoral mechanics.

There is some debate, however, as to whether tape actually changes the position of the patella. Some investigators have found that tape changes patellofemoral angle and lateral patellar displacement but not congruence angle.[71] Others have concurred, finding no change in congruence angle when the patella is taped, but congruence angle is measured at 45 degree knee flexion, so subtle changes in patellar position may have occurred before this.[72] A recent study of asymptomatic subjects found that medial glide tape was effective in moving the patella medially (P = .003) but ineffective in maintaining the position after vigorous exercise (P<.001). But tape seems to prevent the lateral shift of the patella that occurred with exercise (P = .016).[73] The issue for a therapist, however, is not whether the tape changes the patellar position on the radiograph but whether the therapist can decrease the patient's symptoms by at least 50 percent so that the patient can exercise and train in a pain-free manner.

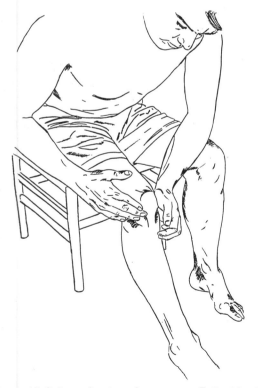

Figure 15–2. Lateral retinacular massage. Patient in sitting position presses the thenar eminence of one hand on the medial border of the patella. The other hand massages the lateral retinaculum.

PATELLAR TAPING

Patellar taping is unique to each patient, as the component is corrected, the order of correction and the tension of the tape are tailored for each individual, based on the assessment of the patellar position. The worst component is always corrected first and the effect of each piece of tape on the patient's symptoms should be evaluated by reassessing the painful activity. It may be necessary to correct more than one component. After each piece of tape is applied, the symptom-producing activity should be reassessed. The tape should always improve a patient's symptoms immediately. If it does not, then the order in which the tape has been applied or the components corrected should be re-examined.

If a posterior tilt problem has been ascertained on assessment, it must be corrected first, as taping over the inferior pole of the patella will aggravate the fat pad and exacerbate the patient's pain. The posterior component is corrected together with a glide or a lateral tilt, with the non-stretch tape being placed on the superior aspect of the patella, either on the lateral border to correct lateral glide or in the middle of the patella to correct lateral tilt. This positioning of the tape will lift the inferior pole out of the fat pad and prevent irritation of the fat pad.

If there is no posterior tilt problem, the glide can be corrected by placing tape from the lateral patellar border to the medial femoral condyle. At the same time, the soft tissue on the medial aspect of the knee is lifted toward the patella to create a tuck or fold in the skin. The skin lift helps anchor the tape more effectively and minimizes the friction rub (friction between the tape and the skin), which can occur when a patient has extremely tight lateral structures. In most cases, hypoallergenic tape is placed underneath the rigid sports tape to provide a protective layer for the skin, and if there seem to be additional skin problems, a plastic coating, either a spray or a roll-on, may be applied to the skin prior to the tape application.

The mediolateral tilt component is corrected by placing a piece of tape firmly from the middle of the patella to the medial femoral condyle. The object is to shift the lateral border away from the femur so that the patella becomes parallel with the femur in the frontal plane. Again, the soft tissue on the medial aspect of the knee is lifted toward the patella.

External rotation is the most common rotation problem, and to correct this, the tape is positioned at the inferior pole and pulled upward and medially toward the opposite shoulder while the superior pole is rotated laterally. Care must be taken so that the inferior pole is not displaced into the fat pad. Internal rotation, on the other hand, is corrected by taping from the superior pole downward and medially.

The patient must be taught how to position the tape on himself or herself. The patient should be in long sitting position with the leg out straight and the quadriceps relaxed (Fig. 15–3). The clinician is aiming for at least a 50 percent decrease in symptoms. If this has not been achieved, further correction may be necessary, with ongoing evaluation of patellar position, as correction of one component may change the other components.

If the tape cannot change the patient's symptoms or even worsens the symptoms, then one of the following must be considered:

- Patient requires tape to unload the soft tissues.
- Tape was poorly applied.

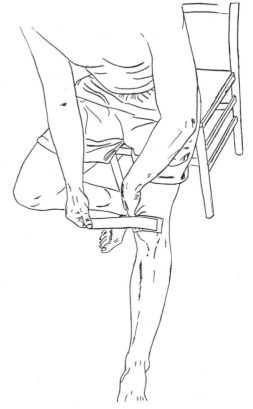

Figure 15–3. Taping the patella, the patient is sitting on the edge of the chair, leg relaxed, knee straight.

- Assessment of patellar position was inadequate.
- Patient has an intra-articular primary pathologic condition that is inappropriate for taping.

Unloading

The principle of unloading is based on the premise that inflamed soft tissue does not respond well to stretch. For example, if a patient presents with a sprained medial collateral ligament, applying a valgus stress to the knee will aggravate the condition, whereas a varus stress will decrease the symptoms. The same principle applies for patients with an inflamed fat pad, an irritated iliotibial band, or a pes anserinus bursitis. The inflamed tissue needs to be shortened or unloaded. To unload an inflamed fat pad, for example, a V tape is placed below the fat pad, with the point of the V at the tibial tubercle coming wide to the medial and lateral joint lines. As the tape is being pulled toward the joint line, the skin is lifted toward the patella, thus shortening the fat pad (Fig. 15–4). The same type of V tape can be used to unload the distal end of the iliotibial band when treating iliotibial friction syndrome. The point of the V is at the lateral joint line with the tape coming out wide to the anterior aspect of the femur above and the anterior aspect of the tibia below (Fig. 15–5).

It has been fairly well established that taping the patella relieves pain,[39, 40, 72, 74] but the mechanism of the effect is still being debated in the literature. It has been found that taping the patella of symptomatic individuals such that the pain is decreased by 50 percent results in an earlier activation of the VMO relative to the VL on both step-up and step-down. Stepping down in particular caused an 8.3 degree differential between the VMO and VL, as not only was the VMO activating earlier than in the pre-taped condition, but the VL was significantly delayed in the taped condition.[40] In a study by

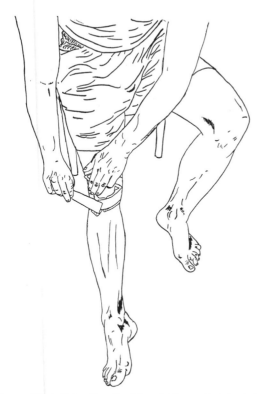

Figure 15–4. Unloading the fat pad. The patient is sitting on the edge of the chair, and the unload tape is started at the tibial tubercle and lifted out to the joint line. The soft tissue is lifted up to the patella.

Cerny,[74] however, in which all subjects had a medial tilt and internal rotation of the inferior pole taping, there was no change in activation pattern of the VMO and VL when the subjects were taped. But patellar taping has been associated with increases in loading response knee flexion as well as increases in quadriceps muscle torque. When the quadriceps torque of symptomatic army personnel was evaluated in taped, braced, and control conditions, it was found that the taping group generated higher concentric and eccentric torque than both the control and braced groups. The braced group did perform better than the control group in the eccentric situation. This increase in muscle torque did not correlate with pain reduction.[72]

Even in an osteoarthritic group, taping the patellofemoral joint in a medial direction has a significant effect on pain. Fourteen patients with a mean age of 70 years and radiographic evidence of tibiofemoral and patellofemoral osteoarthritis participated in a single-blind, blind-observer, randomized crossover trial of three different forms of taping: neutral, lateral, and medial. Patients were not told which tape was thought likely to be effective. The knee pain was recorded with a 10-cm visual analog scale before and 1 hour after tape application. Tape was kept on for 4 days and overall pain on each of the 4 days was recorded in a diary. After 4 days, the patients removed the tape and were asked to score the change in symptoms in the treated knee compared with before taping. After a 3-day interval, the procedure was repeated for the second tape position, and following a further 4 days of tape application and 3-day interval, the subjects entered the final arm of the study. At the end of the study, the assessor recorded which week of treatment each patient had preferred. Medial patellar taping was significantly better than lateral or neutral tape for pain scores, symptom change, and patient preference. In this elderly osteoarthritic group, medial patellar taping resulted in a 25 percent reduction in knee pain.[75]

Principles of Using Tape to Correct the Patella

The tape is kept on all day everyday until the patient has learned how to activate his or her VMO at the right time; that is, the

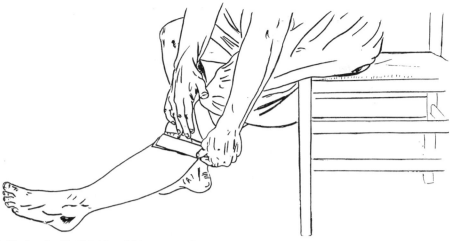

Figure 15–5. Taping for iliotibial band friction syndrome. The unload tape is a V around the lateral joint line.

tape is like training wheels on a bicycle and can be discontinued once the skill is established. The tape is removed with care in the evening, allowing the skin time to recover. The tape can cause a breakdown in the skin either through a friction rub or as a consequence of an allergic reaction. Preparation of the skin and skin care advice is essential.

The patient should never train with or through pain or effusion, as it has been shown quite conclusively in the literature that effusion has an inhibitory effect on muscle activity.[45, 76, 77] If the patient experiences a return of the pain, then the patient should readjust the tape. If the activity is still painful, the patient must cease the activity immediately. The tape will loosen quickly if the lateral structures are extremely tight or the patient's job or sport requires extreme amounts of knee flexion.

Muscle Training

The current debate when rehabilitating the patellofemoral joint is over the type of strengthening of the quadriceps muscle. Powers et al.[39] concludes that, because there is no difference in the activation pattern of the VMO and VL in symptomatic individuals and the ratio of the two muscles is the same, generalized quadriceps strengthening is all that is required when rehabilitating patients with patellofemoral pain. This seems at odds with clinical findings and other research, however, in which electrical stimulation of the VMO and electromyelographic biofeed-

back training have demonstrated similar positional changes on radiograph.[37]

To determine the effect of quadriceps training on the patellar position of asymptomatic college students, Ingersoll and Knight[78] conducted a 3-week training program. The students were randomly assigned to one of three groups—a control group, a group that trained with an electromyelographic biofeedback on the VMO to improve its activity, and a group that performed progressive resisted strengthening to the whole quadriceps.[78] The congruence angle of the patella was measured before and after training for each group. The position of the patella did not change in the control group. The electromyelographic biofeedback group demonstrated a medial glide of the patella and the patella was more centered in the trochlea, whereas the resisted strengthening group demonstrated a lateral displacement of the patella, even though there was a 170 percent increase in quadriceps strength in this group. This study indicates that it is possible to selectively train the VMO to have an effect on the patellar position. What types of exercises are most appropriate in training? From the current evidence available, it seems that closed chain exercise, that is, when the foot is on the ground, is the preferred method of training, not only because closed kinetic training has been shown to improve patellar congruence, but also because muscle training has been found to be specific to limb position.[79] In a group of patients with lateral patellar compression syndrome, it was found that open chain exercise with isometric quadriceps sets at 10-degree intervals with a 3-kg weight resulted in more lateral patellar tilt and glide from 0 to 20 degrees on computed tomographic scan. Closed chain exercise by pushing a foot-plate with resistance cords attached to provide 18 kg resistance demonstrated improved congruence from 0 to 20 degrees.[80] This study supported the findings of Koh et al.,[37] who found that stimulation of the VMO at full extension produced medial patellar rotation, tilt, and glide, whereas isometric quadriceps contraction produced lateral patellar rotation, tilt, and glide.

SPECIFICITY OF TRAINING

Before examining the issue of exercise prescription for the patellofemoral patient, some discussion on the different philosophies of strength training is required. The traditional strengthening view holds that strength gained in nonspecific muscle training can be harnessed for use in performance, that is, the engine (muscles) is built in the strength training room; learning how to turn the engine on (neural control) is acquired on the field.[81] Strength is therefore increased by utilizing the overload principle, meaning exercising at least 60 percent of maximal.[82] However, the muscles around the patellofemoral joint are stabilizing muscles and need to be endurance-trained, so working at 20 to 30 percent of maximal is more appropriate. A more recent interpretation of how to facilitate strength is based on the premise that the engine (muscles) and how it is turned on (neural control) should both be built in the strength training room.[81] Training should therefore simulate movement in terms of anatomic movement pattern, velocity, type, and force of contraction. Thus, with training, the neuromuscular system will tend to become better at generating tension for actions that resemble the muscle actions employed in training, but not necessarily for actions that are dissimilar to those used in training.

If the desired outcome of treatment is for the patient to be pain-free on weight-bearing activities, then the therapist must give the patient appropriate weight-bearing training. At no stage should the patient's recovery be compromised by training into pain.

A useful starting exercise is small-range knee flexion and extension movements (the first 30 degrees) with the patient in the

stance position, where the feet are facing forward and positioned at the width of the pelvis (Fig. 15–6). It is preferable that the patient has a dual channel biofeedback with electrodes on the VMO and the VL so that the patient can monitor the timing of the contraction and the amount of activity. The patient is instructed to squeeze the gluteals and slowly flex the knees to 30 degrees and slowly return to full extension without locking the knees back. The patient is aiming for the VMO to be activated before the VL and remain more than the VL during the activity. This clinical interpretation of the use of electromyelographic biofeedback is at odds with the research application, insofar as the activity of the VMO and the VL has not been normalized.

Progression of training involves simulation of the knee during the stance phase of walking, so the patient is in a walk stance

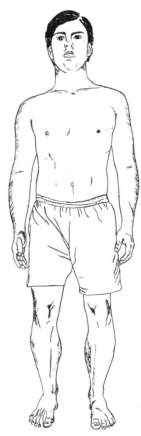

Figure 15–6. Training the vastus medialis obliquus and quadriceps muscles. Patient is in walk stance position, squeezes gluteals, and flexes knees to 30 degrees and comes back up slowly, not locking the knees back.

position (Fig. 15–7). In this position, VMO recruitment is usually poor and the seating of the patella in the trochlea is critical. Again, small amplitude movements need to be practiced. Emphasis should be given to the timing and intensity of the VMO contraction relative to the VL. For a patient who is having difficulty contracting the VMO, muscle stimulation may be used to facilitate the contraction. Further progression of treatment can be implemented by introducing step training. The patients need to practice stepping down from a small height initially. This should be performed slowly, in front of a mirror, so that changes in limb alignment can be observed and deviations can be corrected. Specific work on the hip musculature may be necessary to improve the limb alignment. Some patients may be able to do only one repetition before the leg deviates. This is sufficient for them to start with, as inappropriate practice can be detrimental to learning. The number of repetitions should be increased as the skill level improves. It

is therefore preferable for the therapist to emphasize quality not quantity. Initially, small numbers of exercises should be performed frequently throughout the day. The aim is to achieve a carry-over from functional exercises to functional activities. Later, the patient can move to a larger step, initially decreasing the number of contractions and slowly increasing them again. As the control improves, patients can alter the speed of their stepping activity and vary the place on descent where the stepping action is stopped. Weights can be introduced in the hands or in a backpack. Again, the number of repetitions and the speed of the movement should be decreased initially and built back up again.

Training should be applicable to the patient's activities or sport, so a jumping athlete, for example, should have jumping incorporated into his or her program. Figure-of-eight running, bounding, jumping off boxes, jumping and turning, and other plyometric routines are particularly appropriate for the high-performance athlete. However, the patient's VMO needs to be monitored at all times for timing and level of contraction relative to the VL. The number of repetitions performed by the patient at a training session will depend on the onset of muscle fatigue. The aim would be to increase the number of repetitions before the onset of fatigue. Patients should be taught to recognize muscle fatigue or quivering, so that they do not train through the fatigue and risk exacerbating their symptoms.

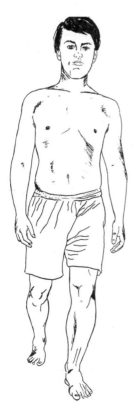

Figure 15–7. Training the vastus medialis obliquus progression. Patient is in walk stance position with heel of back foot off the floor. Patient slowly flexes and extends.

IMPROVING LOWER LIMB MECHANICS

A stable pelvis will minimize unnecessary stress on the knee. Training of the gluteus medius (posterior fibers) to decrease hip internal rotation and the consequent valgus vector force that occurs at the knee is necessary to improve pelvic stability. The posterior gluteus medius can be trained in weight-bearing with the patient standing side-on to a wall. The leg closest to the wall is flexed at the knee so the foot is off the ground. The hip is in line with the standing hip. The patient should have all the weight back through the heel of the standing leg, which is slightly flexed. The patient externally rotates the standing leg without turning the foot, the pelvis, or the shoulders. The patient should sustain the contraction for 20 seconds, so a burning can be felt in the gluteus medius region (Fig. 15–8).

Common errors include the following (Fig. 15–9):

- patient flexing too far forward with the hips so the tension is felt in the iliotibial band
- patient flexing the knee too much so the quadriceps bears the brunt of the exercise
- patient rotating the hips so tension is felt in the back
- weight too far forward on the toes, so the gastrocnemius feels tension

The training can be progressed to standing on one leg, where the pelvis is kept level and the lower abdominals and the glutei are worked together while the other leg is swinging back and forward, simulating the activity of the stance phase of gait (Fig. 15–10).

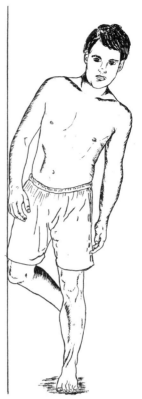

Figure 15–9. Some common problems with the gluteal training exercise.

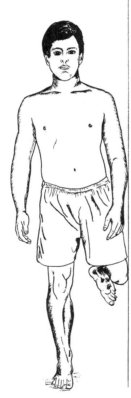

Figure 15–8. Gluteus medius posterior training, patient standing side-on to a wall. The leg closest to the wall is flexed at the knee so the foot is off the ground. The hip is in line with the standing hip. The patient should have all his or her weight back through the heel of the standing leg, which is slightly flexed. The patient externally rotates the standing leg without turning the foot, the pelvis, or the shoulders.

If the patient has marked internal femoral rotation, stretching of the anterior hip structures to increase the available external rotation may be required. The patient lies prone with the hip to be stretched in an abducted, externally rotated, and extended position. The other leg is extended and lies on top of the bent leg. The malleolus of the underneath leg is at the level of the tibial tubercle. The patient attempts to flatten the abducted and rotated hip by pushing along the length of the thigh and holding the stretch for 5 seconds (Fig. 15–11). This action activates the gluteals in inner range. Although it is not functional, it may facilitate gluteus medius activity in someone who is finding it difficult to activate the muscle in weight-bearing. If the patient can flatten the hip on the plinth, a further progression is to ask the patient to lift the knee off the plinth, keeping the hip and foot on the plinth. This can be attempted only if the patient can flatten the hip onto the plinth. It is a measure of the

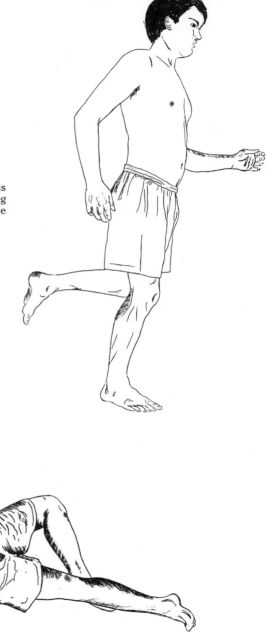

Figure 15–10. Progression of gluteal training. The patient is standing on one leg with the pelvis level while the other leg is swinging back and forward, simulating the activity of the stance phase of gait.

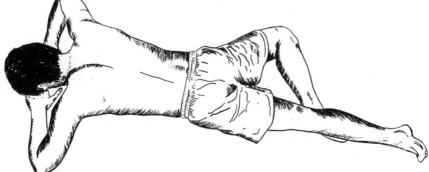

Figure 15–11. To stretch the anterior hip structures, the patient is prone with the hip to be stretched in an abducted, externally rotated, and extended position. The other leg is extended and lies on top of the bent leg. The malleolus of the underneath leg is at the level of the tibial tubercle. The patient pushes along the length of the thigh.

patient's ability to separate hip movement from spine movement and will minimize excessive pelvic rotation in gait.

Muscle Stretching

Appropriate flexibility exercises must be included in the treatment regime. The involved muscles may include hamstrings, gastrocnemius, rectus femoris, and tensor fascia latae/iliotibial band. One of the better methods for stretching the distal part of the iliotibial band is to have the patient in the long sitting position, maintaining the lumbar lordosis, while externally rotating and adducting the hip maximally before extending the knee. This stretch position should be maintained for 20 seconds (Fig. 15–12). If a hamstrings stretch is required, the hip remains straight while the knee is extended, and if the foot is dorsiflexed, the gastrocnemius also will be stretched. A tight gastrocnemius will increase the amount of subtalar joint pronation exhibited in the mid-stance phase of gait, so after the stretching, appropriate foot muscle training will be required.

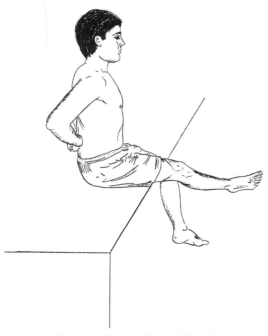

Figure 15–12. To stretch the iliotibial band, the patient is long sitting, maintaining the lumbar lordosis, while externally rotating and adducting the hip maximally before extending the knee.

CONSIDERATION OF FOOT PROBLEMS

The supinators of the foot, specifically tibialis posterior, should be trained if the patient demonstrates prolonged pronation during the mid-stance in gait. With the foot supinated, the base of the first metatarsal is higher than the cuboid, which will allow the peroneus longus to work more efficiently to increase the stability of the first metatarsal complex for push off. The therapist can train this action to improve the efficiency of push off. The position of training is in mid-stance, the patient is instructed to lift the arch while keeping the first metatarsal head on the floor, and then pushing the first metatarsal and great toe into the floor. If the patient is unable to keep the first metatarsophalangeal joint on the ground when the arch is lifted, then the foot deformity is too large to correct with training alone and orthotics will be necessary to control the excessive pronation.

SUMMARY

Management of patellofemoral pain is no longer a conundrum if the therapist can determine the underlying causative factors and address those factors in treatment. It is imperative that the patient's symptoms be significantly reduced. This is often achieved by taping the patella, which not only decreases the pain, but also promotes an earlier activation of the VMO and increases quadriceps torque. Management will need to include specific VMO training, gluteal control work, stretching tight lateral structures, and appropriate advice regarding the foot, be it orthotics, training, or taping.

References

1. Brukner P, Khan K. Clinical Sports Medicine. McGraw-Hill, 1993.
2. Fulkerson J, Hungerford D: Disorders of the Patello-femoral Joint, 2nd ed. Baltimore, Williams & Wilkins, 1990.
3. Reider B, Marshall J, Koslin B, et al.: The anterior aspect of the knee. J Bone Joint Surg 63A(3):351–356, 1981.
4. Fiske-Warren L, Marshall J: The supporting structures and layers on the medial side of the knee. J Bone Joint Surg 61A(1):61, 1979.
5. Lieb F, Perry J: Quadriceps function. J Bone Joint Surg 50A(8):1535–1548, 1968.
6. Bose K, Kanagasuntherum R, Osman M: Vastus me-

dialis oblique: An anatomical and physiologic study. Orthopaedics 3:880–883, 1980.

7. Hallisey M, Doughty N, Bennett W, Fulkerson J: Anatomy of the junction of the vastus lateralis tendon and the patella. J Bone Joint Surg 69A(4):545, 1987.

8. Ahmed AM, Burke DL, Yu A: In-vitro measurement of static pressure distribution in synovial joints: Part II. Retropatellar surface. J Biomed Engineering 105:226–236, 1983.

9. Amed A, Shi S, Hyder A, Chan K: The effect of quadriceps tension characteristics on the patellar tracking pattern. In Transactions of the 34th Orthopaedic Research Society, Atlanta, 1988, p. 280.

10. Buff H, Jones LC, Hungerford DS: Experimental determination of forces transmitted through the patellofemoral joint. J Biomechanic 21(1):17–23, 1988.

11. Hungerford DS, Barry M: Biomechanics of the patello-femoral joint. Clin Orthop Rel Res (144):9–15, 1979.

12. Reilly D, Martens M: Experimental analyses of the quadriceps muscle force and patellofemoral joint reaction force for various activities. Acta Orthop Scand 43:126–137, 1972.

13. van Eijden TMG, Kouwenhoven E, Verburg J, Weijs WA: A mathematical model of the patellofemoral joint. J Biomechanic 19(3):219–229, 1986.

14. Ahmed AM, Burke DL, Hyder A: Force analysis of the patellar mechanism. J Orthop Res 5:69–85, 1987.

15. Carson W, James S, Larson R, et al.: Patello-femoral disorders: Parts I and II. Clin Orthop Rel Res (185):165–174, 1984.

16. Burgess R: Patellofemoral joint transverse displacement and tibial rotation. Graduate Diploma Project Report, Manipulative Therapy, Southern Australia Institute of Technology, Adelaide, South Australia, 1985.

17. Dye S, Vaupel G, Dye C, et al.: Conscious neurosensory mapping of the internal structures of the human knee without intra-articular anaesthesia. Am J Sports Med 26(6):773–777, 1998.

18. Nyland J, Brosky T, Currier D, et al.: Review of the afferent neural system of the knee and its contribution to motor learning. J Orthop Sports Phys Ther 19(1)2–11, 1994.

19. Goodfellow J, Hungerford D, Zindel M: Patellofemoral joint mechanics and pathology. 1 & 2. J Bone Joint Surg 58B(3):287–299, 1976.

20. Matthews L, Sonstegard D, Henke J: Load bearing characteristics of the patellofemoral joint. Acta Orthop Scand (48):511–516, 1977.

21. Ericsson M, Nissell R: Patellofemoral forces during ergometric cycling. Phys Ther 67(9):1365–1368, 1987.

22. Dye S: The knee as a biologic transmission with an envelope of function. Clin Orthop Rel Res 325:10–18, 1996.

23. Radin E: A rational approach to treatment of patellofemoral pain. Clin Orthop Rel Res 144:107–109, 1979.

24. Townsend PR, Rose RM: The biomechanics of the human patella and its implications for chondromalacia. J Biomechan 10:403–407, 1977.

25. Insall J: Chondromalacia patellae: Patellar malalignment syndrome. Orthop Clin North Am 10:117–125, 1979.

26. Lyon L, Benzl L, Johnson K, et al.: Q angle: A factor—peak torque occurrence in isokinetic knee extension. J Orthop Sports Phys Ther 9(7):250–253, 1988.

27. Kramer P: Patella malalignment syndrome: Rationale to reduce excessive lateral pressure. J Orthop Sports Phys Ther 8(6):301–308, 1986.

28. Draganich L, Andriacchi T, Andersson G: Interaction between intrinsic knee mechanics and the knee extensor mechanism. J Orthop Res 5:539–547, 1987.

29. Malek M, Mangine R: Patellofemoral pain syndromes: A comprehensive and conservative approach. J Orthop Sports Phys Ther 2(3):108–116, 1981.

30. Micheli L, Slater J, Woods E, Gerbino P: Patella alta and the adolescent growth spurt. Clin Orthop Rel Res (213):159–162, 1986.

31. Fulkerson JP: Awareness of the retinaculum in evaluating patellofemoral pain. Am J Sports Med 10(3):147–149, 1982.

32. Subotnik S: The foot and sports medicine. J Orthop Sports Phys Ther 2(2):53–54, 1980.

33. Buchbinder R, Naparo N, Bizzo E: The relationship of abnormal pronation to chondromalacia patellae in distance runners. J Am Podiatr Assoc 69(2):159–161, 1979.

34. Root M, Orien W, Weed J: Clinical Biomechanics, Vol. II. Los Angeles, Clinical Biomechanics Corp, 1977.

35. Voight M, Weider D: Comparative reflex response times of the vastus medialis and the vastus lateralis in normal subjects and subjects with extensor mechanism dysfunction. Am J Sports Med 10:131–137, 1991.

36. Witvrouw E, Sneyers C, Lysens R, et al.: Comparative reflex response times of vastus medialis obliquus and vastus lateralis in normal subjects and subjects with patellofemoral pain syndrome. J Orthop Sports Phys Ther 24(3):160–166, 1996.

37. Koh T, Grabiner M, DeSwart R: In vivo tracking of the human patella. J Biomech 25(6):637–643, 1991.

38. Karst G, Willett G: Onset timing of electromyographic activity in the vastus medialis oblique and vastus lateralis muscles in subjects with and without patellofemoral pain syndrome. Phys Ther 75(9):813–822, 1995.

39. Powers C, Landel R, Sosnick T, et al.: The effects of patellar taping on stride characteristics and joint motion in subjects with patellofemoral pain. J Orthop Sports Phys Ther 26(6):286–291, 1997.

40. Gilleard W, McConnell J, Parsons D: The effect of patellar taping on the onset of vastus medialis obliquus and vastus lateralis muscle activity in persons with patellofemoral pain. Phys Ther 78(1):25–32, 1998.

41. Mariani P, Caruso I: An electromyographic investigation of subluxation of the patella. J Bone Joint Surg 61:169–171, 1979.

42. Souza D, Gross M: Comparison of vastus medialis obliquus: Vastus lateralis muscle integrated electromyographic ratios between healthy subjects and patients with patellofemoral pain. Phys Ther 71:310–320, 1991.

43. Howard J, Enoka R: Maximum bilateral contractions are modified by neurally mediated interlimb effects. J Appl Physiol 70:306–316, 1991.

44. Yang J, Winter D: Electromyography reliability in maximal contractions and submaximal isometric contractions. Arch Phys Med Rehabil 64:417–420, 1983.

45. Spencer J, Hayes K, Alexander I: Knee joint effusion and quadriceps reflex inhibition in man. Arch Phys Med 65:171–177, 1984.

46. Hughston J: Patellar subluxation: A recent history. Clin Sports Med 8(2):153–162, 1989.
47. Brukner P, McConnell J, Bergman A, Matheson G: Infrapatellar fat pad impingement: Correlation between clinical and MR findings. Am J Sports Med (In press).
48. McConnell J: Fat pad irritation: A mistaken patellar tendonitis. Sport Health 9(4):7–9, 1991.
49. Cross MJ, Crichton KJ: Clinical Examination of the Injured Knee. London, Harper & Row, 1987.
50. Jackson R, Marshall D, Fujisawa Y: The pathological medial shelf. Orthop Clin North Am 13(2):307, 1982.
51. Broom MJ, Fulkerson JP: The plica syndrome: A new perspective. Orthop Clin North Am 17(2):279–281, 1986.
52. O'Neill D, Micheli L: Overuse injuries in the young athlete. Clin Sports Med 7(3):591–610, 1989.
53. Merchant A, Mercer R, Jacobsen R, Cool C: Roentgenographic analysis of patellofemoral congruence. J Bone Joint Surg 56A:1391–1396, 1974.
54. Laurin C, Levesque H, Dussault S, et al.: The abnormal lateral patellofemoral angle. J Bone Joint Surg 60A(1):55–63, 1978.
55. Perry J: Gait Analysis. Thorofare, NJ, Slack, 1992.
56. Hoppenfeld S: Physical Examination of the Spine and Extremities. New York, Appleton-Century-Crofts, 1976.
57. Kendall F, McCreary L: Muscle Testing and Functioning. Baltimore, Williams & Wilkins, 1983.
58. Fitzgerald G, McClure P: Reliability of measurements obtained with four tests for patellofemoral alignment. Phys Ther 75(2):84–92, 1995.
59. Potter N, Rothstein J: Intertester reliability of selected clinical tests of the sacroiliac joint. Phys Ther 65(11):1671–1675, 1985.
60. Gonella C, Paris S, Kutner M: Reliability in evaluating passive intervertebral motion. Phys Ther 62(4):436–444, 1982.
61. Matyas T, Bach T: The reliability of selected techniques in clinical arthrometrics. Austr J Physiother 31:175–199, 1985.
62. Hardy D, Napier J: Inter and intratherapist reliability of passive accessory movement technique. N Z J Physiother X:22–24, 1991.
63. Maher C, Latimer J: Pain or resistance: The manual therapists' dilemma. Austr J Physiother 38(4):257–260, 1992.
64. McConnell J: The management of chondromalacia patellae: A long term solution. Austr J Physiother 32(4):215–223, 1986.
65. McConnell J: Training the vastus medialis oblique in the management of patellofemoral pain. In Proceedings of Tenth Congress of the World Confederation for Physical Therapy, Sydney, May 1987.
66. Frankel VH, Nordin M: Basic Biomechanics of the Skeletal System. Philadelphia, Lea & Febiger, 1980.
67. Herbert R: Preventing and treating stiff joints. In Crosbie J, McConnell J (eds): Key Issues in Musculoskeletal Physiotherapy. Oxford, Butterworth-Heinemann, 1993.
68. Hooley C, McCrum N, Cohen R: The visco-elastic deformation of the tendon. J Biomech 13:521, 1980.
69. Taylor D, Dalton J, Seaber A: Visco-elastic properties of muscle-tendon units. The biomechanical effect of stretching. Am J Sports Med 18:300, 1990.
70. Mckay-Lyons M: Low-load, prolonged stretch in treatment of elbow flexion contractures secondary to head trauma: A case report. Phys Ther 69:292, 1989.
71. Roberts JM: The effect of taping on patellofemoral alignment: A radiological pilot study. In Proceedings of the Sixth Biennial Conference of the Manipulative Therapists Association of Australia, Adelaide, 1989, pp. 146–151.
72. Conway A, Malone T, Conway P: Patellar alignment tracking alteration: Effect on force output and perceived pain. Isokinetics Exerc Sci 2(1):9–17, 1992.
73. Bockrath K, Wooden C, Worrell T, et al.: Effects of patella taping on patella position and perceived pain. Med Sci Sports Exerc 25(9):989–992, 1993.
74. Cerny K: Vastus medialis oblique/vastus lateralis muscle activity ratios for selected exercises in persons with and without patellofemoral pain syndrome. Phys Ther 8(75):672–683, 1995.
75. Cushnaghan J, McCarthy R, Dieppe P: The effect of taping the patella on pain in the osteoarthritic patient. Br Med J 308:753–755, 1994.
76. Stokes M, Young A: Investigations of quadriceps inhibition: Implications for clinical practice. Physiotherapy 70(11):425–428, 1984.
77. de Andrade J, Grant C, Dixon A: Joint distension and reflex muscle inhibition in the knee. J Bone Joint Surg 47A:313, 1965.
78. Ingersoll C, Knight K: Patellar location changes following EMG biofeedback or progressive resistive exercises. Med Sci Sports Exerc 23(10):1122–1127, 1991.
79. Powers CM: Rehabilitation of patellofemoral joint disorders: A critical review. J Orthop Sports Phys Ther 28(5):345–354, 1998.
80. Doucette S, Child D: The effect of open and closed chain exercise and knee joint position on patellar tracking in lateral patellar compression syndrome. J Orthop Sports Phys Ther 23(2):104–110, 1996.
81. Sale D, MacDougall D: Specificity of strength training: A review for coach & athlete. Can J Appl Sports Sci 6(2):87–92, 1981.
82. Grabiner M, Koh T, Dragnich L: Neuromechanics of the patellofemoral joint. Med Sci Sports Ex 1(26):10–21, 1994.

16 Optimizing Treatment of Joint Contracture Following Reconstruction

Bryan C. Heiderscheit, MS, PT, CSCS

A common goal of rehabilitation protocols following knee surgery is unrestricted range of motion (ROM). The effects of not achieving this goal can be disastrous for patients. The development of arthrofibrosis and joint contractures following knee ligament reconstruction has been reported to be as high as 35 percent,[1] with loss of knee motion being the primary complication following anterior cruciate ligament (ACL) reconstruction.[2-7] Abnormalities in function can result, such as inability to achieve full knee extension during gait or difficulty squatting down to lift an object. In addition, the risk of the patient's re-injuring the knee or developing degenerative joint disease is increased. This debilitating situation can often be avoided through appropriate surgical techniques and advanced rehabilitation protocols.[4, 6, 8]

REVIEW OF KNEE FUNCTIONAL ANATOMY

A detailed discussion of the functional anatomy of the knee is given in an earlier chapter, so only a brief overview is given here. The knee joint is a condyloid joint with two degrees of freedom, flexion-extension and rotation.[9] It is made up of three articulations: the tibiofemoral joint, the patellofemoral joint, and the superior tibiofibular joint. Each has its unique role in allowing effective joint function.

The tibiofemoral joint is often considered the primary articulation of the knee joint. The major ligaments of the knee support this joint, including the anterior and posterior cruciate ligaments and the medial and lateral collateral ligaments. In addition fibrocartilagenous menisci are present between the tibia and femur to increase joint stability, provide shock absorption, and provide joint lubrication. Therefore, the de-

rangements that occur to these ligaments and menisci will affect the ability of the tibiofemoral joint to function.

The patellofemoral joint consists of the articulation of the patella and the femur. The patella is a sesamoid bone enclosed in the distal tendon of the quadriceps femoris muscles whose primary function is to increase the mechanical advantage of the quadriceps femoris. Thus, compressive forces are present between the patella and femur.

Although the tibiofibular joint is the smallest of the three knee articulations, it should not be overlooked when describing mechanics of the knee joint. Proper kinematics, including anteroposterior glide, superoinferior glide, and rotation, are necessary to allow for effective knee function.

Additional soft tissue structures should be mentioned as well. The articulations of the knee are enclosed in a single articular capsule composed of both a fibrous outer layer and an inner synovial membrane. Friction-reducing structures such as bursae and fat pads are located throughout the knee complex, including between the infrapatellar tendon and the underlying tibiofemoral joint.

ETIOLOGY AND EPIDEMIOLOGY

Based on the degrees of freedom at the knee joint, contractures can develop to limit flexion-extension and rotation. Most classifications involving the contracture of the knee joint focus on flexion and extension limitations, as the rotational component will be secondarily compromised. Arthrofibrosis has frequently been associated with the development of motion loss.[10-12] Specifically, arthrofibrosis refers to the process of periarticular and intra-articular fibrous tissue formation related to trauma, thereby leading to flexion and extension limitation.[2, 3, 10] The terms *arthrofibrosis*, *contracture*, and *ankylo-*

sis are used interchangeably in the literature.

Etiologic factors involved with ROM loss are multifactorial. Possibilities include intercondylar notch scarring,[2] infrapatellar contracture syndrome,[3] postoperative immobilization, reflex sympathetic dystrophy,[4] and repair of structures in addition to the ACL.[4, 13] Gender has been addressed as a possible factor, with males being more susceptible.[13] Acute reconstruction has also been indicated as a primary risk factor for ROM loss. The occurrence of ROM loss was significantly greater in those patients undergoing reconstruction soon after the initial injury.[13] Delaying reconstructive surgery 3 weeks from the time of initial injury has been shown to significantly decrease the incidence of arthrofibrosis.[14, 15] Majors and Woodfin,[16] however, contradicted this finding by showing that the use of early or delayed reconstructive surgery had no influence on the incidence of ROM loss.

A flexion contracture maintains the knee in flexion, thereby preventing full knee extension. Limitations to knee flexion prevent the knee from achieving full flexion, disabling the individual from squatting. The incidence of motion loss associated with ACL reconstruction has been documented from 4 to 15 percent.[3–5, 17] Noyes et al.[6] reported the incidence of arthrofibrosis among patients who underwent ACL reconstruction with medial collateral ligament repair to be as high as 23 percent. Even with the advances in surgical and rehabilitation techniques, motion loss remains the most common complication following ligament surgery.[7]

Loss of knee motion following ACL reconstruction has been identified as the most frequent limitation.[2–5, 7] The majority of investigations into the causes of motion loss have usually focused on limitations in flexion.[18–20] Although flexion contractures can result in functional limitations, the relative disability associated with loss of extension is greater.[3, 10] Symptoms associated with extension loss include anterior knee pain, stiffness and crepitus, loss of strength, altered gait, and functional limitation.[3, 10]

HISTOLOGIC CHANGES

The histologic changes associated with arthrofibrosis are well documented. Enneking and Horowitz[21] investigated the intra-articular and histologic changes associated with immobilization of the human knee. Prolonged immobilization of unopposed surfaces led to the proliferation of the infrapatellar fat pad, suprapatellar pouch, and posterior fibro-fatty tissue into the joint cavity. This tissue eventually enclosed the cruciate ligaments and became continuous with the peripheral layers of the articular cartilage. A gradual resorption of the cartilage ensued, with the fibrous tissue eventually reaching the marrow. A similar process is found within directly opposing articular surfaces with the exception of additional cystic defects in the cartilagenous layers and eventual joint fusion.[21]

Limitation of flexion is thought to exist as a result of the fibrous tissue found in the anterior aspect of the knee. Capsular and patellofemoral adhesions along with invasion of the fibro-fatty tissue into the joint cavity result in flexion loss.[3, 11, 21] The presence of fibrotic tissue in the anterior region of the knee may lead to increased compressive forces at the patellofemoral joint, thereby limiting the flexion capabilities.

Lack of knee extension appears to result from the enclosure of the cruciate ligaments[2, 11, 21] in the fibro-fatty tissue and fibrosclerotic changes in the infrapatellar fat pad.[3] The enclosure of the cruciate ligaments in the fibrous tissue is often preceded by the presence of a fibrous nodule in the femoral notch located adjacent to the tibial attachment of the cruciate graft. This nodule, termed a cyclops lesion, results in a mechanical block to full extension (Fig. 16–1).[2] A similar obstruction has been described in the infrapatellar fat pad.[3] The fibrosclerotic changes that occur in the fat pad prevent the tibiofemoral opposition necessary to achieve full extension because of the fat pad's anatomic connection to the menisci. Paulos et al.[3] termed this condition infrapatellar contracture syndrome. This condition is discussed in greater detail later in this chapter.

Woo et al.[22] proposed a mechanism for the development of joint contractures and ROM deficits. Prolonged immobilization, which may follow knee ligament reconstruction, results in a loss of glycosaminoglycans and water from the connective tissues of the joint. This loss allows for the formation of new cross-links between molecules of the

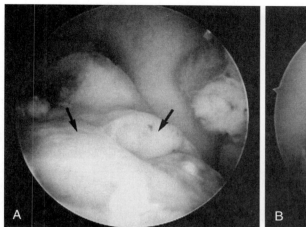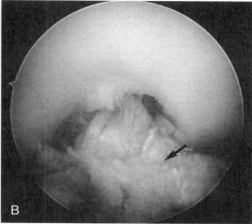

Figure 16–1. *A*, Arthroscopic view of intercondylar notch revealing a cyclops lesion. *B*, Same view with knee in extension after resection of cyclops. (From Fisher SE, Shelbourne KD: Arthroscopic treatment of symptomatic extension block complicating anterior cruciate ligament reconstruction. *Am J Sports Med* 21:558, 1993.)

periarticular connective tissue, ultimately limiting the extensibility of the tissue.

In addition to the connective tissue structures of the knee joint, the surrounding muscles undergo adaptive shortening when immobilized in a shortened position. Both the contractile and noncontractile components of muscle are structurally altered. A decrease in the number of sarcomeres occurs relative to the shortened position.[23] The noncontractile components of the muscle adaptively shorten, thus limiting the available ROM of the joint.[24]

CLASSIFICATION OF KNEE CONTRACTURE

Typically, a specified amount of ROM loss must occur before it is considered a contracture. Investigations traditionally have identified knee contractures based on a loss of knee extension of 10 degrees or more and total knee flexion less than 125 degrees.[3, 13, 15] It was thought that these criteria would result in functional limitations, such as gait deviations, difficulty climbing stairs, and inability to run.

Shelbourne et al.[11] stated that the traditional definition of a loss of 10 degrees or more of knee extension and knee flexion less than 125 degrees was appropriate for severe cases of arthrofibrosis but did not address the less severe cases. They redefined arthrofibrosis as any symptomatic limitation in motion relative to the contralateral knee.

They also proposed a clinical classification system for knee arthrofibrosis (Table 16–1). Classification is dependent on the direction and magnitude of the ROM limitation as well as patellar mobility.

Infrapatellar Contracture Syndrome

Paulos et al.[3] first described infrapatellar contracture syndrome (IPCS) in 1987 as a "little recognized cause of postoperative knee morbidity." Since then, this syndrome has been frequently cited in the literature. As stated earlier, IPCS involves the mechanical limitation of knee extension and flexion due to fibrosclerotic changes of the infrapatellar fat pads. The patients complain of knee stiffness and pain. Chronic swelling and flexed knee gait are also seen in these patients. Surgical observations made by Paulos et al.[3] regarding the anatomic changes resulting from IPCS included a fibrotic fat pad occupying the entire anterior joint space. The fat pad would become adherent to the patella, thereby entrapping it and limiting the knee's motion.

Three stages of IPCS have been described: the prodromal stage, the active stage, and the residual stage (Fig. 16–2).[3] The prodromal stage is one that every patient undergoing knee surgery enters, as it is a normal part of the healing process. The presence of IPCS during this stage will become apparent during the initial 2 to 8 weeks following sur-

Table 16–1. Clinical Classification System for Knee Arthrofibrosis

Type	Direction	Limitation Magnitude (degrees)	Patellar Motion	Patellar Infera
I	extension	<10	normal	none
	flexion	normal		
II	extension	>10	normal	none
	flexion	normal		
III	extension	>10	↓ medial/lateral	none
	flexion	>25		
IV	extension	>10	↓ medial/lateral	present
	flexion	>30		

Data from Shelbourne KD, Patel DV, Martini DJ: Classification and management of arthrofibrosis of the knee after anterior cruciate ligament reconstruction. Am J Sports Med 24:857, 1996.

gery. Extension limitations, diffuse edema in the infrapatellar tendon and fat pad, painful active ROM, and restricted patellar motion indicate the presence of IPCS. If these signs and symptoms go unrecognized, the syndrome can progress to the next stage.

The active stage often presents 6 to 20 weeks after the patient enters the prodromal stage. Marked loss of patellar mobility, primarily superior glide, and the presence of a "shelf sign" are frequently observed. The shelf sign appears as a result of the fibrous tissue infiltrating the infrapatellar tendon to its attachment at the tibial tuberosity, thereby creating an abrupt step-off or shelf.[3] Quadriceps atrophy and patellar crepitus

are found in addition to limitations in extension and flexion. Additional surgery or manipulations are often used in an unsatisfactory attempt to correct the limitations.

The final stage, the residual stage, presents 8 to 12 months after the IPCS onset. Restricted flexion and extension may remain with significant patellofemoral arthrosis. Although many of the overt physical signs of IPCS may have resolved, a residual patella infera is usually present.

OBJECTIVE MEASUREMENT

To quantify the extent of the contracture, a simple goniometric measure is often

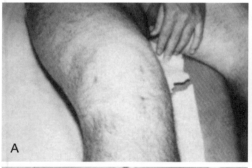
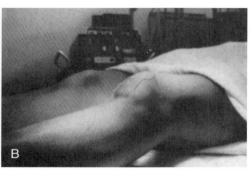
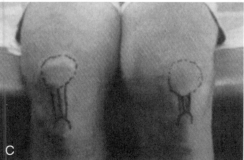

Figure 16–2. Stages of developing infrapatellar contracture syndrome (IPCS). *A*, Stage I: painful range of motion with limited patellar mobility. Marked by failure to progress with rehabilitation. *B*, Stage II: presence of shelf sign with continued loss of motion. *C*, Stage III: decrease in swelling with an increase in patellar mobility; however, patella infera is often present. (From Paulos LE, Rosenberg TD, Drawbert J, et al.: Infrapatellar contrature syndrome: An unrecognized cause of knee stiffness with patella entrapment and patella infera. *Am J Sports Med* 15:331, 1987.)

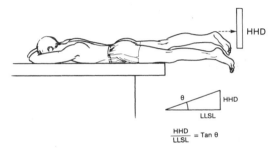

Figure 16–3. Alternative method for determining knee flexion contracture. The ratio of the heel height difference (HHD) to the lower limb segment length (LLSL) equals the tangent of the knee angle (θ). The knee flexion contracture therefore is equal to the arc tangent of the ratio; θ = arc tan (HHD/LLSL). (From Sachs RA, Daniel DM, Stone ML, et al.: Patellofemoral problems after anterior cruciate ligament reconstruction. *Am J Sports Med* 17:760, 1989.)

enough. The goniometer allows for the quick and easy measurement of extension or flexion deficits in both active and passive ROM. Standard goniometric technique involves the placement of the goniometer's axis at the lateral femoral epicondyle with the stationary arm aligned along the lateral femur to the greater trochanter.[25] The moveable arm is aligned along the lateral border of the fibula with the lateral malleolus as the reference.

The extension loss can also be measured at the heels. By placing the patient prone with the legs off the table, a knee flexion contracture will result in one heel being higher than the other. An objective measure can then be obtained by measuring the length of the leg from the knee to the sole of the foot, dividing by the heel height difference, and finally taking the arctangent of the result (Fig. 16–3). Sachs et al.[7] suggested that 1 cm heel height difference is comparable to 1 degree of flexion contracture. This, however, is a rough estimation, as it is based on individuals 72 cm in height.

Although these techniques are frequently used, they provide information only about the contracture at the end ROM. Further, a goniometric measure is a static measure from which minimal inference can be made regarding functional limitations. It has been demonstrated that various static measures are poor predictors of dynamic dysfunction.[26, 27] These findings suggest the need for a more comprehensive measurement of contracture or general knee stiffness.

In addition to the passive methods of quantifying knee stiffness,[28] Li, Heiderscheit, Caldwell, and Hamill (unpublished paper presented at the American Physical Therapy Association Combined Sections Meeting, Boston, MA, 1998) have proposed a rotational spring model from which knee joint stiffness can be measured throughout the stance phase of running. The mechanical model consists of a block and a rotational spring (Fig. 16–4). Changes in the joint angle and angular velocity of the spring will be reflected in alterations of the calculated stiffness. Based on a derivation of Hook's law, stiffness is estimated from knee angular velocity squared as a function of the knee angle squared (Fig. 16–4). A stiffness value is determined for each linear portion of the plot, providing a value of knee stiffness at different intervals of stance. This rotational spring model therefore represents the knee and the stiffness changes that occur during the support phase of running.

The sensitivity of the model to functional differences of subjects suggests its use as a discriminative measure between individuals. Although this model may not be clinically helpful for the patient with an acute post-surgical contracture, it can offer benefits in evaluating the patient with chronic knee stiffness. Distinct differences in knee stiffness values between healthy subjects and those with patellofemoral pain have been demonstrated, suggesting a potential diagnostic application. For example, as the maximum knee flexion angle during stance was approached, the subjects with patellofemoral pain consistently displayed higher knee stiffness values across a variety of running velocities.

Fisher and Shelbourne[10] utilized a stiffness score based on the patient's subjective evaluation of the symptomatic knee (Table 16–2). It does not provide an objective measure of stiffness, but it does incorporate the patient's perception of the limitation. An assessment of this type should not be overlooked during an evaluation, as the information gained can be beneficial to the clinician.

PREVENTION AND TREATMENT

Considering the characteristic progressive histologic changes that accompany contractures, prevention may be the best form of treatment. Forethought should be taken

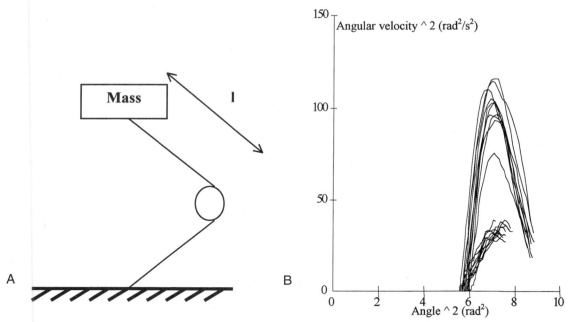

Figure 16–4. *A,* Rotational spring model of knee joint. The mass of the block (m) represents the body mass of the subject. The length (l) from the center of the mass to the center of rotation represents the distance between the joint centers of the hip and knee. *B,* Sample data from five running trials of one subject. The slope of the lines indicates the knee stiffness at various phases of support.

when deciding the appropriate time for ligament reconstruction. Based on the work of Shelbourne et al.,[19] reconstructive surgery should occur a minimum of 3 weeks follow-

Table 16–2. Patient Subjective Stiffness Score

Points	Stiffness Score
10	I have no stiffness in my knee. I can straighten it out completely without any conscious effort and at any given time.
8	I have occasional stiffness in my knee after certain activities. However, I can usually get it completely straight with little or no effort.
5	My knee often feels stiff, especially in the morning when I get out of bed, after sitting for 1 hour or more, or in cold weather. I can get it completely straight but only if I work at it.
2	My knee feels stiff every day. It is worse in the morning, after sitting, or in cold weather. I can straighten it out nearly completely with much effort.
0	My knee feels stiff all of the time and I am unable to straighten it compared to my other knee.

Modified from Fisher SE, Shelbourne KD: Arthroscopic treatment of symptomatic extension block complicating anterior cruciate ligament reconstruction. Am J Sports Med 21:558, 1993.

ing the injury. This post-injury delay allows for a reduction in the knee joint swelling and a return of full active ROM and strength, thus minimizing the risk for arthrofibrosis. Psychological benefits have also been noted with delaying of surgery that have resulted in a more positive attitude toward the impending reconstruction and rehabilitation.

Procedures accompanying the main reconstruction must also be considered in preventing ROM deficits. Several investigations have identified accompanying repair of the medial collateral ligament or meniscus with reconstruction of the ACL to be a prominent risk factor in arthrofibrosis development.[4, 13] This stands to reason, as post-surgical ROM restrictions are often more conservative when a medial collateral ligament or meniscal repair is performed in addition to the ACL reconstruction. Furthermore, attention must be paid to the use of a notchplasty in preventing impingement between the graft and femoral notch, as well as an isometric placement of the graft.[13]

Postoperatively, steps can be taken to minimize arthrofibrosis development. Traditional rehabilitation protocols sacrifice joint motion to maintain graft stability.[10] As the reliability of the graft has improved, however, early passive motion has been encouraged in postoperative rehabilitation. Emphasis should be placed on achieving extension equal to that of the contralateral knee within the first week following surgery. Shelbourne et al.[11] suggest that any delay in achieving this goal should be accompanied by the use of an extension board or extension casting. This shift to early passive motion has not resulted in graft instability but has reduced the occurrence of flexion contractures.[6, 8]

In addition to early passive motion, weight-bearing should be initiated at an early point in the rehabilitation program. This is continuous with the accelerated program proposed by Shelbourne and Nitz.[8] An accelerated program emphasizes full passive extension, early muscle control, early motion, cryotherapy, and immediate weight-bearing versus the slower progressions of conventional programs (Tables 16–3 and 16–4). The accelerated program has been shown to significantly reduce the development of arthrofibrosis.[14] Accelerated rehabil-

itation should be done with regard for the natural tissue healing process, however. Steps to minimize the inflammatory response and the accompanying pain and swelling should not be disregarded with the use of an accelerated program. An appropriate balance between the two goals must be maintained, based on the individual patient.

PHYSICAL THERAPY INTERVENTION

An accelerated rehabilitation program offers appropriate guidelines for the timeliness of achieving functional goals. Some additional information should be provided as to how these goals can be achieved.

The post-surgical patient should present weight-bearing as tolerated and often in a ROM-limiting brace. Such a brace allows for protective movement in the patient's avail-

Table 16–3. Conventional Rehabilitation Protocol Following Anterior Cruciate Ligament Reconstruction

Time after Surgery	Treatment
2–3 days	Continuous passive motion Passive range of motion (ROM) 0–60 degrees Partial weight-bearing with crutches and ROM-limiting brace
4 days	Discharge from hospital
1–2 weeks	ROM 0–90 degrees Wall slides, heel slides, straight leg raises Step-ups, calf raises Partial weight-bearing
3–4 weeks	ROM 0–100 degrees Prone hangs for terminal extension Full weight-bearing Unilateral knee bends, step-ups, calf raises Partial squats, bicycling (no tension)
5–6 weeks	ROM—terminal extension to 120 degrees Prone hangs Partial squats, leg press, calf raises Bicycling, swimming
10–12 weeks	ROM—terminal extension to 130 degrees Isokinetic evaluation with 20-degree block at 180 and 240 degrees per second Partial squats, leg press, bicycling with moderate resistance Jump rope
4 months	Full ROM Isokinetic evaluation at 60, 180, 240 degrees per second Continue strengthening, bicycling, swimming Functional progression if strength >70%
6 months	Isokinetic evaluation KT-1000 Increase agility workouts

Modified from Shelbourne KD, Wilckens JH, Mollabashy A, et al.: Arthrofibrosis in acute anterior cruciate ligament reconstruction: The effect of timing of reconstruction and rehabilitation. Am J Sports Med 19:332, 1991.

●━━ Table 16-4. Accelerated Rehabilitation Protocol Following Anterior Cruciate Ligament Reconstruction

Time after Surgery	Treatment
2-3 days	Continuous passive motion Passive range of motion (ROM) exercises for terminal extension and 90 degrees of flexion Weight-bearing as tolerated
3-4 days	Discharge from hospital
7-10 days	ROM—terminal extension Prone hangs and towel extensions Wall slides, heel slides, active-assisted flexion Strengthening—knee bends, step-ups, calf raises Partial to full weight-bearing
2-3 weeks	ROM—terminal extension to 110 degrees Unilateral knee bends, step-ups, calf raises Weight room activities—leg press, quarter squats, and calf raises in the squat rack Bicycling, swimming
5-6 weeks	ROM—terminal extension to 130 degrees Isokinetic evaluation with 20-degree block at 180 and 240 degrees per second If isokinetic score >70%, start lateral shuffles, cariocas, and jumping rope Continue weight room activities Continue bicycling and swimming
12 weeks	Full ROM Isokinetic evaluation at 60, 180, 240 degrees per second KT-1000 Increase agility workouts
16 weeks	Isokinetic evaluation KT-1000 Increase agility workouts

Modified from Shelbourne KD, Wilckens JH, Mollabashy A, et al.: Arthrofibrosis in acute anterior cruciate ligament reconstruction: The effect of timing of reconstruction and rehabilitation. Am J Sports Med 19:332, 1991.

able ROM. Depending on the surgical procedure performed, the brace allowing full extension immediately following surgery has been shown to reduce the risk of arthrofibrosis. Full extension allows the graft to locate in the intercondylar notch of the femur to prevent excessive hemorrhage and scar tissue formation.[13]

Cosgarea et al.[15] compared the incidence of arthrofibrosis in patient groups with varying ROM guidelines following ACL reconstruction.[15] Patients were either splinted in 45 degrees of flexion with passive ROM started 7 days postoperatively, splinted in 45 degrees of flexion with passive ROM started 2 days postoperatively or splinted in full extension with passive ROM started the first day. The patient group placed in full extension and allowed immediate passive ROM displayed a significant reduction in the incidence of arthrofibrosis, with only 2.7 percent of the patients developing it. The groups splinted in 45 degrees of flexion with passive motion initiated on day 7 or day 2 were at a much greater risk for developing arthrofibrosis, as 23.4 percent and 10.2 percent did, respectively.

Full passive knee extension is a priority following knee ligament reconstruction. Full hyperextension that is easily achieved should occur 2 weeks following surgery. Additional methods, such as extension casting and prone hangs, can be used to obtain extension equal to that of the contralateral knee. The clinician can measure achievement of this goal by blocking the thigh motion with one hand and passively raising the patient's heel with the other (Fig. 16-5).

Patellar mobilizations should be initiated immediately. These should consist of glides in the medial and lateral as well as superior and inferior directions. Caution must be taken, however, in regard to the healing surgical incision and arthroscopic portals, as well as the patient's tolerance. The patient should be instructed in this technique and asked to perform it frequently throughout the day. The importance of this technique

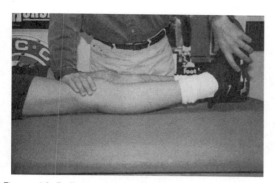

Figure 16–5. Determining whether the knee motion is equal to the contralateral limb is easy if the examiner places one hand on the distal thigh to stabilize the femur while the other hand raises the foot. (From Shelbourne KD, Patel DV, Martini DJ: Classification and management of arthrofibrosis of the knee after anterior cruciate ligament reconstruction. *Am J Sports Med* 24:857, 1996.)

has been noted in preventing IPCS.[3] Once the sutures are removed, scar mobilization techniques should be performed and taught to the patient to prevent adherence between the cutaneous and subcutaneous tissues. Anteroposterior glides to the superior tibiofibular joint should also be included to maintain the accessory joint motion.

Inflammation should be controlled in the early stages, as capsular effusion may induce ROM limitations. Anti-inflammatory medication has been shown to be helpful in controlling post-surgical inflammation.[3] Cold and compression have been shown to be beneficial in reducing swelling, as well as in controlling pain.

Early quadriceps contraction should be stressed in a postreconstruction rehabilitation program. Isometric contraction of the quadriceps with the knee in full extension allows for active motion of the patella and the periarticular tissues, thereby further reducing the risk of developing IPCS.[3] The return of strength in the quadriceps is also important in preventing flexion contractures, as it is the primary knee extensor. The progression to straight leg raises should be questioned if a quadriceps lag is present. Active knee extensions should also be performed in a closed chain position (standing) as the articular surfaces are approximated with the graft engaging the intercondylar notch. Neuromuscular stimulators may also prove to be beneficial in initiating early quadriceps activity.

Casting and splinting have been frequently

recommended in preventing and treating loss of knee joint motion.[3, 11, 29, 30] An extension cast is recommended if the patient is having difficulty passively achieving full extension (Fig. 16–6). The cast can be worn at various intervals throughout the day, as well as through the night. Care should be taken with forceful extension measures, as an acceleration of chondral lesions can occur.[3] Paulos et al.[3] recommend the use of extension casts for only 3 to 5 days, at which time, if this treatment is unsuccessful, surgery is recommended. Following operative correction of the ROM loss, an extension cast is recommended.[11]

In addition to all the steps taken to ensure early full extension, full flexion is also required. This, however, is not stressed until week 3 or 4 of the rehabilitation program. The inclusion of patellar mobilizations early allows for easier return of full flexion. Exercises can be incorporated such as wall slides, heel slides, and stationary bicycling with no tension in addition to flexion mobilizations performed by the clinician and patient.[11]

SURGICAL INTERVENTION

If preventative methods and aggressive physical therapy fail to restore extension equal to that of the contralateral knee, a surgical approach may be indicated. This often consists of a closed manipulation using anesthesia or an arthroscopic débridement of the scar tissue.

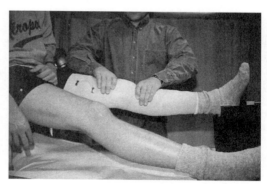

Figure 16–6. Application of a knee extension cast may be useful if difficulty is encountered achieving full extension. This cast is frequently used following debridement. (From Shelbourne KD, Patel DV, Martini DJ: Classification and management of arthrofibrosis of the knee after anterior cruciate ligament reconstruction. *Am J Sports Med* 24:857, 1996.)

Closed Manipulation Under Anesthesia

Following knee ligament reconstruction and appropriate physical therapy, a resultant ROM loss can be treated by manipulating the knee. This consists of the patient being given a general or spinal anesthetic agent prior to the procedure to provide complete muscle relaxation. The patient's lower extremity is placed into 90 degrees of hip flexion with the tibia firmly grasped. The surgeon then begins to bend the knee to achieve full flexion, stopping when no further adhesions separate.[17] To achieve extension, the knee is straightened with the ankle placed atop a bolster while a posterior force is applied at the knee. In general, the contralateral knee's motion is used as a guide for the total motion imposed on the involved knee.[17] This procedure is usually not attempted until 2 to 3 months following surgery or when no ROM improvement is noted. Although this procedure is not invasive, additional injuries can result, such as supracondylar fractures of the femur, avulsions of the patellar tendon, and myositis ossificans.[17, 31, 32]

Few investigations have been performed to determine the efficacy of closed manipulations. Dodds et al.[17] examined the results of knee manipulation following ACL reconstruction of 42 knees. They showed an increase in ROM from 95 degrees of flexion before manipulation to 127 degrees after, and 11 degrees of extension loss before manipulation to 4 degrees of extension loss after. Following the manipulation, the patients returned to physical therapy for continued rehabilitation. The investigators did not find any increased graft laxity following the procedure. In addition, the length of time from the ACL reconstruction to the manipulation did not affect the ROM outcome. It should be noted, however, that 16 of the 42 knees required additional manipulations or arthroscopic débridement to achieve the desired ROM.

Arthroscopic Debridement

Debridement of the involved scar tissue is achieved using an arthroscopic procedure. Tissue that is preventing flexion and extension must be excised or resected to enable full ROM. Extension is typically regained by excising a cyclops lesion found at the tibial attachment site of the ACL graft.[11, 12] An additional femoral notchplasty may be performed to prevent further impingement between the graft and femoral notch (Fig. 16–7).[11] Flexion is usually regained with a release of scar tissue found on the anterior aspect of the knee and graft. Retropatellar tendon and anterior tibial scar tissue is resected with excision of any fibrotic capsule to allow unrestricted patellar mobility.[11]

Postsurgical Rehabilitation

Once full ROM is achieved through either closed manipulation or arthroscopic débridement, it must be maintained. An aggressive physical therapy regimen is resumed, with the priority being full ROM. Because of the functional importance of full extension, attempts may be made to maintain full extension while potentially sacrificing flexion ROM. Attempts at serial casting in extension may be utilized, especially following arthroscopic débridement. Shelbourne et al.[11] recommended casting the patient's knee into full extension immediately following débridement accompanied by forced-extension casting until full extension is achieved. The authors based achieving full extension on the extension of the contralateral knee. Physical therapy sessions were recommended twice

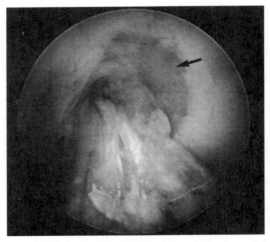

Figure 16–7. Arthroscopic view of knee following notchplasty. (From Fisher SE, Shelbourne KD. Arthroscopic treatment of symptomatic extension block complicating anterior cruciate ligament reconstruction. *Am J Sports Med* 21:558, 1993.)

daily for ROM management with flexion exercises initiated after the patient easily achieved full extension.[11]

SUMMARY

Arthrofibrosis and ROM loss remain the primary complication following knee ligament reconstruction.[2-7] Although invasive and noninvasive procedures exist to treat this dilemma, given its progressive nature, it is often unavoidable once begun. Knowledge of the risk factors and steps taken to avoid them can decrease the incidence. The combination of appropriate surgical techniques and the use of an accelerated rehabilitation protocol have proved beneficial in minimizing the occurrence of arthrofibrosis.

References

1. Strum GM, Friedman MJ, Fox JM, et al.: Acute anterior cruciate ligament reconstruction. Clin Orthop 253:184, 1990.
2. Jackson DW, Schaefer RK: Cyclops syndrome: Loss of extension following intra-articular anterior cruciate ligament reconstruction. Arthroscopy 6:171, 1970.
3. Paulos LE, Rosenberg TD, Drawbert J, et al.: Infrapatellar contracture syndrome: An unrecognized cause of knee stiffness with patella entrapment and patella infera. Am J Sports Med 15:331, 1987.
4. Graf B, Uhr F: Complications of intra-articular anterior cruciate reconstruction. Clin Sports Med 7:835, 1988.
5. Mohtadi NGH, Webster-Bogaert S, Fowler PJ: Limitation of motion following anterior cruciate reconstruction: A case control study. Am J Sports Med 19:620, 1991.
6. Noyes FR, Mangine RE, Barber S: Early motion after open and arthroscopic anterior cruciate ligament reconstruction. Am J Sports Med 15:149, 1987.
7. Sachs RA, Daniel DM, Stone ML, et al.: Patellofemoral problems after anterior cruciate ligament reconstruction. Am J Sports Med 17:760, 1989.
8. Shelbourne KD, Nitz P: Accelerated rehabilitation after anterior cruciate ligament reconstruction. Am J Sports Med 18:292, 1990.
9. Segal P, Jacob M: The Knee. Chicago, Year Book Medical Publishers, 1973.
10. Fisher SE, Shelbourne KD: Arthroscopic treatment of symptomatic extension block complicating anterior cruciate ligament reconstruction. Am J Sports Med 21:558, 1993.
11. Shelbourne KD, Patel DV, Martini DJ: Classification and management of arthrofibrosis of the knee after anterior cruciate ligament reconstruction. Am J Sports Med 24:857, 1996.
12. Cosgarea AJ, DeHaven KE, Lovelock JE: The surgical treatment of arthrofibrosis of the knee. Am J Sports Med 22:184, 1994.
13. Harner CD, Irrgang JJ, Paul J, et al.: Loss of motion after anterior cruciate ligament reconstruction. Am J Sports Med 20:499, 1992.
14. Shelbourne KD, Wilckens JH, Mollabashy A, et al.: Arthrofibrosis in acute anterior cruciate ligament reconstruction: The effect of timing of reconstruction and rehabilitation. Am J Sports Med 19:332, 1991.
15. Cosgarea AJ, Sebastianelli WJ, DeHaven KE: Prevention of arthrofibrosis after anterior cruciate ligament reconstruction using the central third patellar tendon autograft. Am J Sports Med 23:87, 1995.
16. Majors RA, Woodfin, B: Achieving full range of motion after anterior cruciate ligament reconstruction. Am J Sports Med 24:350, 1996.
17. Dodds JA, Keene JS, Graf BK, et al.: Results of knee manipulations after anterior cruciate ligament reconstruction. Am J Sports Med 19:283, 1991.
18. Benum P: Operative mobilization of stiff knees after surgical treatment of knee injuries and post-traumatic conditions. Acta Orthop Scand 53:625, 1976.
19. Sprague N, O'Connor R, Fox J: Arthroscopic treatment of postoperative knee arthrofibrosis. Clin Orthop 166:165, 1982.
20. Thompson TC: Quadricepsplasty to improve knee function. J Bone Joint Surg 26:366, 1944.
21. Enneking WF, Horowitz M: The intra-articular effects of immobilization on the human knee. J Bone Joint Surg 54:973, 1972.
22. Woo SL-Y, Matthews JV, Akeson WH, et al.: Connective tissue response to immobility: Correlative study of biomechanical and biochemical measurements of normal and immobilized rabbit knees. Arthritis Rheum 18:257, 1975.
23. Williams PE, Goldspink G: Changes in sarcomere length and physiological properties in immobilized muscle. J Anat 127:459, 1978.
24. Williams PE, Goldspink G: Connective tissue changes in immobilized muscle. J Anat 138:343, 1984.
25. Norkin CC, White DJ: Measurement of Joint Motion: A Guide to Goniometry. Philadelphia, F.A. Davis, 1985.
26. Hamill J, Bates BT, Knutzen KM, et al.: Relationship between selected static and dynamic lower extremity measures. Clin Biomech 4:217, 1989.
27. McPoil TG, Cornwall MW: The relationship between static lower extremity measurements and rearfoot motion during walking. J Orthop Sports Phys Ther 24:309, 1996.
28. Oatis C: The use of a mechanical model to describe the stiffness and damping characteristics of the knee joint in healthy adults. Phys Ther 73:740, 1993.
29. Jansen CM, Windau JE, Bonutti PM, et al.: Treatment of a knee contracture using a knee orthosis incorporating stress-relaxation techniques. Phys Ther 76:182, 1996.
30. McClure PW, Blackburn LG, Dusold C: The use of splints in the treatment of joint stiffness: Biologic rationale and an algorithm for making clinical decisions. Phys Ther 74:1101, 1994.
31. Friedman MJ, Blevins F: Slipped distal femoral epiphyseal plate following closed manipulation of the knee. Am J Sports Med 13:201, 1985.
32. Ivey M: Myositis ossifications of the thigh following manipulation of the knee. Clin Orthop 98:102, 1985.

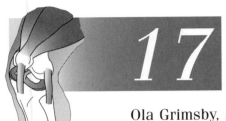

17 Manual Therapy Approach to Knee Ligament Rehabilitation

Ola Grimsby, PT, MOMT, MNSMT, FAA OMPT,
and Brian Power, PT, MOMT

HISTORY

Manual therapy has a rich history dating back as far as Hippocrates in his work called *Corpus Hippocrateum*, circa 400 BC. In 1916, Dr. James Mennell published his concept of "joint play" and how to influence the joints through manipulation. Dr. James Cyriax continued the works of Dr. Mennell and developed a diagnostic approach to differential diagnosis that is still used by physical therapists and osteopathic physicians. Currently, there are many approaches to manual therapy and numerous schools of thought throughout the world.[1a, 1b]

DEFINITION

Manual therapy is the application of one's knowledge of anatomy, histology, physiology, and kinesiology to provide the optimal stimulus of regeneration for the specific tissues in lesion. It demands a thorough evaluation of musculoskeletal and systemic functions to diagnose the specific tissue and identify contraindications to treatment.[1c]

The evaluation procedural flow is an imperative aspect of the treatment process and as such needs to be defined. An evaluation flow that is used by the Ola Grimsby Institute is a clinically applied approach combining various scientific research findings to diagnose the tissue in lesion (Table 17–1). This flow of procedures is used with the diagnostic pyramid to selectively rule out tissue that is not part of the dysfunction (Table 17–2). The clinician is then left with the involved tissue and can then determine the appropriate treatment program.

There are basically five tissues in the human body that physical therapists work with: collagen, bone, cartilage, disc, and muscle. Each of these tissues has a specific optimal stimulus for regeneration and needs to be given that stimulus to regenerate the desired tissue. This stimulus for regeneration depends on the tension that is given to the tissue. Free-floating undifferentiated mesenchymal cells are responsible for producing various types of tissue. The product of this cell is dependent on the applied biomechanical energy. The human cell has the ability to change the nature of its product;[2] therefore, the clinician needs to identify the tissue that is to be treated so that the optimal biomechanical energy is given and unwanted results do not occur, such as osteophytic formation and the creation of a pseudoarthrosis at a fracture site.

This chapter deals with ligamentous structures, and the optimal stimulus for regeneration for that specific tissue is modified tension in the line of stress. We cannot, however, ignore the fact that along with the ligaments, motion also occurs at the joints. Cartilage is therefore affected as a result of the injury as well as the techniques and

---

Table 17–1. Examination

1. Initial observation
2. History/interview
3. Structural inspection
4. Active movements
5. Passive movements
6. Resisted movements × 3
7. Palpation
8. Specific mobility tests and positional faults
9. Neurologic evaluation
10. Specific regional tests
11. Additional information (radiograph, magnetic resonance image, computed tomographic scan, electromyograph, laboratory tests)
12. Correlation
13. Treatment plan
14. Prognosis

Courtesy of the Ola Grimsby Institute, San Diego, CA.

■ Table 17-2. The Diagnostic Pyramid

	Metabolism	Vascular	Bone	Disc	Nerve	Joint Entrapment	Joint Cartilage	Bursa	Joint Capsule	Muscle Tendon	Ligament Fascia	Subcutaneous	Skin
Radiograph/Lab tests	144 ——	145 ——	146 ——	147 ——	148 ——	149 ——	150 ——	151 ——	152 ——	153 ——	154 ——	155 ——	156 ——
MRI/CT/EMG													
Segmental Play	131 ——	132 ——	133 ——	134 ——	135 ——	136 ——	137 ——	138 ——	139 ——	140 ——	141 ——	142 ——	143 ——
Joint Play	118 ——	119 ——	120 ——	121 ——	122 ——	123 ——	124 ——	125 ——	126 ——	127 ——	128 ——	129 ——	130 ——
Special Tests	105 ——	106 ——	107 ——	108 ——	109 ——	110 ——	111 ——	112 ——	113 ——	114 ——	115 ——	116 ——	117 ——
Neurologic Tests	92 ——	93 ——	94 ——	95 ——	96 ——	97 ——	98 ——	99 ——	100 ——	101 ——	102 ——	103 ——	104 ——
Palpation	79 ——	80 ——	81 ——	82 ——	83 ——	84 ——	85 ——	86 ——	87 ——	88 ——	89 ——	90 ——	91 ——
Resisted Motion	66 ——	67 ——	68 ——	69 ——	70 ——	71 ——	72 ——	73 ——	74 ——	75 ——	76 ——	77 ——	78 ——
Passive Motion	53 ——	54 ——	55 ——	56 ——	57 ——	58 ——	59 ——	60 ——	61 ——	62 ——	63 ——	64 ——	65 ——
Active Motion	40 ——	41 ——	42 ——	43 ——	44 ——	45 ——	46 ——	47 ——	48 ——	49 ——	50 ——	51 ——	52 ——
Structural Inspection	27 ——	28 ——	29 ——	30 ——	31 ——	32 ——	33 ——	34 ——	35 ——	36 ——	37 ——	38 ——	39 ——
History-Interview	14 ——	15 ——	16 ——	17 ——	18 ——	19 ——	20 ——	21 ——	22 ——	23 ——	24 ——	25 ——	26 ——
Initial Observation	1 ——	2 ——	3 ——	4 ——	5 ——	6 ——	7 ——	8 ——	9 ——	10 ——	11 ——	12 ——	13 ——

These numbers indicate the steps in the evaluation process. A total of 156 steps are considered for a complete evaluation to determine the tissue lesion.
+ = Positive   ? = Questionable   x = Eliminated   [Blank] = Not applicable/Cannot test
Courtesy of the Ola Grimsby Institute, San Diego, CA.

concepts described. The optimal stimulus for regeneration of cartilage is compression-decompression with gliding. It is not within the scope of this chapter to explain the reasons for these stimuli for regeneration. The techniques that follow are to be seen not only as methods to inhibit pain and improve arthrokinematic motion but also to apply biomechanical energy to the collagen and cartilage that has been traumatized. It is only through a complete evaluation of the biomechanical and physiologic models to identify specific tissues in lesion that a clinician should consider a treatment program. Without such, we as a profession do not have a rationale for the approach that we have chosen.

TECHNIQUES

Flexion-Extension

The tibiofemoral joint is a modified saddle joint in the coronal plane and a hinge joint in the sagittal plane. Because of the difference between the two planes, one needs to be aware of which plane is being affected by the different techniques. If one looks first at the sagittal plane, the hinge joint is such that the concave tibial plateau articulates with the convex femoral condyle (Fig. 17–1). The axis of motion for this plane is within the femoral condyle and changes with various degrees of motion.[3] According to the osteopathic paradigm, structure governs function.[4] The joint play allows the structures to move appropriately, and the soft tissue guides and limits the available motion.

According to the rules of concavities and convexities, if a concavity moves on a convexity, arthrokinematic and osteokinematic motion occur in the same direction. If a convexity moves on a concavity, arthrokinematic and osteokinematic motion occur in opposite directions. Because the knee is functionally a weight-bearing joint, the convex-on-concave rule applies when the knee is in a closed kinetic chain. If one moves the concave tibial plateau in a posterior direction or rolls or glides the convex femoral condyle in an anterior direction, the structures that primarily limit the motion will be the posterior cruciate ligament and, to a lesser degree, the collateral ligaments (Fig. 17–2).

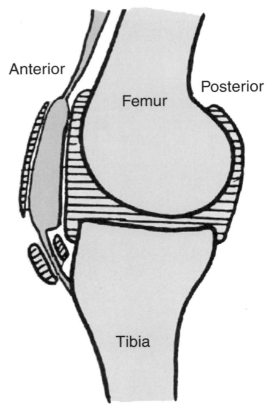

Figure 17–1. Tibiofemoral joint: sagittal view. (Courtesy of the Ola Grimsby Institute, San Diego, CA.)

With this knowledge, one can influence the arthrokinematics to improve knee flexion. To influence extension, the application is reversed and the primary tissue influenced is the anterior cruciate ligament and secondarily the collateral ligaments (Fig. 17–3).

Ligaments are made up of primarily type I collagen, which is histologically competent to resist shearing forces.[5] The main components of collagen are fibroblasts and glycosaminoglycans. These two components are directly linked to each other in terms of viability. Tension is the biomechanical energy that stimulates fibroblastic activity as well as the production of glycosaminoglycans. Glycosaminoglycans provide nutrition to the fibroblasts and lubrication for the newly synthesized fiber. Without tension, there is no regenerative stimulus for the collagen, which will reduce the amount of fibroblastic activity and production of glycosaminoglycans.

Tension also allows the practitioner to

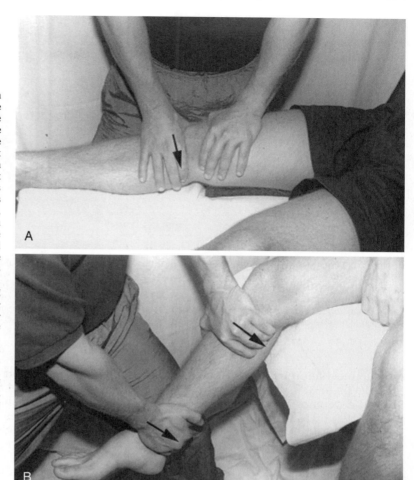

Figure 17–2. This technique can be used to test or mobilize the posterior glide of the tibia on the femur. The indication would be limited motion in flexion of the tibia on the femur. *A,* The patient is lying supine on the table with a firm pad under the distal part of the femur. The operator is standing lateral to the patient's leg, facing the patient's knee. *B,* An alternative technique with the patient sitting with the knee off the edge of the table. The end of the tibia is supported by one hand and the other hand moves the tibia in a posterior direction. The operator's one hand is fixing the distal end of the patient's femur against the pad and the table. The other hand is as close to the joint space as possible, holding around the anterior part of the patient's proximal tibia. The operator moves the tibia in a posterior direction. The size of the pad under the patient's femur is decided by the amount of contracture in the joint.

work with receptors to either facilitate or inhibit muscle tone. Wyke[30] has identified various receptors that are prevalent in areas that are predominantly tonic or phasic. The areas that have the capacities of both have more equal numbers of either receptor in that area. Knowledge of these receptors can aid the clinician to be more effective in the treatment. Type I mechanoreceptors are found in all joints. They are prevalent in the tonic joints such as the neck, hip, and shoulder and are located in the superficial layers of the joint capsule between the collagen fibers. Their importance lies in the fact that they give postural and kinesthetic awareness. These are the receptors that allow us to know where our body is in relation to the environment. They also enable us to begin recruiting stabilizing muscles prior to motion to ensure proper arthrokinematic movements of the joints. They have inhibitory function in that they are slow-adapting and respond to the beginning and end range of tension. They are, in essence, our inhibitory stretch receptors.

Type II mechanoreceptors are located in the deep layers of the joint capsule. They allow for inhibitory effects in the lumbar, foot, hand, and jaw. The elbow and the knee have equal concentrations of type I and type II mechanoreceptors. Type II mechanoreceptors allow us to know when our joints are moving in that they are the phasic receptors. They are fast-adapting and therefore do not respond to tension. These receptors work well with oscillations of a rate of one per second.

As stated earlier, the knee has an equal concentration of both receptors. The clinician can therefore utilize either type I or

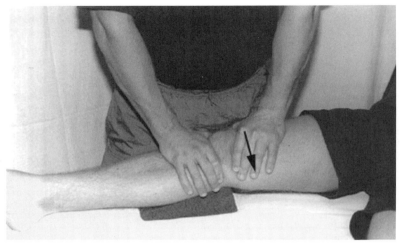

Figure 17–3. This technique is used to test or mobilize posterior glide of the femur on the tibia. Indication for this technique is limited motion in extension. The patient is lying supine on the table with a firm pad under the proximal part of the tibia. The operator is standing lateral to the patient's leg, facing the patient's knee. The operator's one hand is fixing the proximal end of the tibia against the pad and the table. The other hand is as close to the joint space as possible, holding around the anterior part of the patient's femur. The operator moves femur in a posterior direction. The size of the pad under the patient's femur is decided by the amount of contracture in the joint.

type II mechanoreceptors to facilitate the quadriceps or hamstrings, depending on the desired outcome. This was shown in a 1996 dissertation by Natalie K. Howard and Penny P. Tussing for their Master's thesis at Grand Valley State University in Allendale, Michigan. Their study showed that during a closed chain isometric squat with an anterior tibial force, there was an average of a 14 percent increase in quadriceps recruitment.

Raunest et al.[6] discuss the electromyographic activity of quadriceps and hamstrings when the fascicle bundles of the cruciate ligaments are exposed to tension with the knee joint in various ranges of motion. Their study showed that when the anteromedial fascicle group of the anterior cruciate ligament was loaded, there was a significant increase in the electromyographic activity of the ipsilateral hamstrings. The quadriceps were silent during the period of ligament loading. Mechanical loading of the posterolateral fascicles in the anterior cruciate ligament induced agonistic excitation of the quadriceps. When a load was placed in the anterior or posterior fascicles of the posterior cruciate ligament, there was an increase in the electromyographic activity of the ipsilateral hamstrings and an inhibition of the quadriceps. These studies show the importance of the receptor input for facilita-

tion or inhibition of muscular activity to induce the desired outcome of the treatment.

Figure 17–4 shows the set-up of weight-bearing exercises that utilizes the mechanoreceptors to facilitate the desired muscle group. The same exercise can be applied as a self-mobilization technique to improve flexion or extension, depending on the direction of the pulley forces.

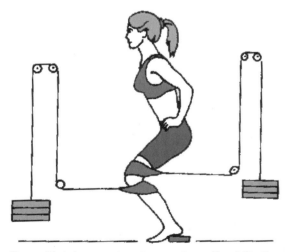

Figure 17–4. Lower extremity exercise: self-mobilization for extension. (Courtesy of the Ola Grimsby Institute, San Diego, CA.)

Medial-Lateral Glide

When looking at the tibiofemoral joint in the coronal plane, we see that it is a modified sellar joint because of the intercondylar notch (Fig. 17–5). This suggests that there is both concavities moving on convexities and convexities moving on concavities. Figure 17–6 shows articulation techniques to restore the medial and lateral glide components of the tibiofemoral joint. These motions are often overlooked and can be the limiting factor for full extension or flexion.

Medial and lateral glides place tension on the collateral ligaments, applying the optimal stimulus of regeneration to these structures. The applied tension also influences the mechanoreceptors in the area. There is equal distribution of type I and type II mechanoreceptors in the collateral ligaments, meaning that either oscillatory or stretch techniques can be performed to obtain the desired response. No research has been done to determine the facilitation function of these ligaments on the thigh musculature, as has been done for the cruciate ligaments.

Adjunct and Conjunct Rotation

Adjunct rotation is described as the amount of rotation available in a joint complex that can be voluntarily influenced. An example of this in the knee is the availability of tibial rotation when the knee is flexed to 90 degrees. This rotation is due to the differing length of the femoral condyles, the shape of the meniscus, and the influence of the collateral ligaments and muscular contractions. Conjunct rotation is the amount of rotation a joint complex has that is not under voluntary control. This type of rotation is seen with the "screw-home" mechanism in the knee where the tibia, in an open chain, undergoes an external rotation in the final degrees of knee extension. In a closed chain system, the tibia is "fixed"; therefore, the rotation would be relatively internal to the femur. Figure 17–7 shows techniques that can affect the ability of the knee to allow the proper amount of conjunct rotation during functional activities. This type of rotation is often overlooked by clinicians as they try to achieve full range of motion.

Proximal and Distal Tibiofibular Joints

The proximal and distal tibiofemoral joints have an important link to the optimal function of the tibiofemoral complex. The proximal tibiofibular joint is an almost plane joint with a slight convexity on the oval tibial facet and a slight concavity of the fibular head. The tibial facet faces laterally, posteriorly, and inferiorly. The tendon of the biceps femoris muscle attaches to the fibular head. Because of this attachment, the fibular head moves in a posterior direction with knee flexion following the concave-on-convex rule. Because of this interaction, a decrease in posterior glide of the fibular head can restrict full flexion of the tibiofemoral joint. Likewise, when the knee travels into extension, the fibular head must glide in an anterior direction. Figure 17–8 demonstrates the technique for posterior and anterior glide of the proximal fibula on the tibia.

The distal tibiofibular joint consists of a concave tibial surface and a convex or plane surface on the medial distal end of the fibula. There is no voluntary movement in the proximal or distal tibiofibular joints. The

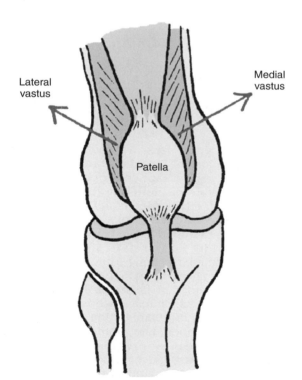

Figure 17–5. Tibiofemoral joint: coronal view. (Courtesy of the Ola Grimsby Institute, San Diego, CA.)

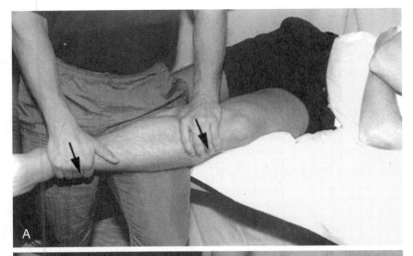

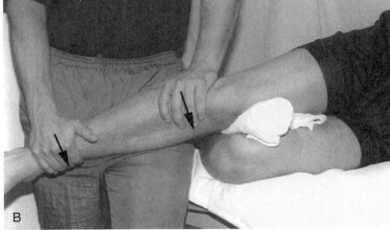

Figure 17–6. These techniques can be used to test or mobilize lateral or medial glide of the tibia against the femur. They are indicated for a limitation of motion in flexion and extension. *A*, The patient is side-lying with a slightly flexed knee and the leg extending over the edge of the table. The opposite leg is flexed. The operator is standing, facing the dorsal side of the patient's leg. The operator supports the patient's leg against his body with one hand. The operator's other hand is placed on the proximal part of the tibia's medial side and his forearm is 90 degrees to the leg. The operator moves the leg in a lateral direction, parallel to the joint plane in the knee, with a simultaneous motion of both hands. *B*, For a medial glide, the lowest leg in a flexed position can be a fulcrum against the distal part of the femur. Use a towel between the patient's knees. The mobilization procedure is the same as in the lateral glide.

movements that do occur are primarily a result of the ankle's influence. An evaluation of talocrural motion provides the following results. With supination of the foot, the head of the fibula glides distally and posteriorly. Plantar flexion of the foot produces a distal glide with a slight medial rotation of the fibula. Dorsiflexion of the ankle yields a proximal glide. The fibula rotates externally around its longitudinal axis. Pronation gives a proximal and anterior glide with an external rotation of the fibula.

Because of the interaction between the proximal and distal tibiofibular joints with the knee and the ankle function, the clinician should always evaluate the functional mobility of both these complexes when treating one or the other. Figure 17–9 shows a technique for testing and improving anterior mobility of the distal tibiofibular joint. Figure 17–10 demonstrates the technique for posterior glide of the distal tibiofibular joint.

Nutritional Components

We have been discussing modified tension as being important for regeneration of collagen. Another important consideration is the nutritional state of the tissue that has been traumatized, either mechanically or surgically. As physical therapists, we traditionally have been excluded from providing nutritional support for our patients; however, this is beginning to change. Interest in alternative medical therapies is beginning to increase and nutrition is at the forefront of this approach. As clinicians who are the primary providers of rehabilitation to individuals who have undergone trauma, we are natural candidates to provide nutritional support. We must not overlook the causes of these potential nutritional deficits, either. With trauma, there is a certain degree of inflammation. We must consider the foods or

Figure 17–7. *A* and *B*, Distraction of the tibia from the femur during internal and external rotation of the knee joint. These techniques are indicated to improve limitation of motion in rotation. The patient is sitting on the table with the leg positioned over the edge. The operator is sitting on a chair with the patient's leg between his flexed knees, his legs crossed at the ankle, and a foam pad between his knees and the patient's leg. The operator's knees fix the patient's leg and his hands hold the proximal part of the tibia from the lateral and medial side. The patient's femur is stable, resting on the table. The operator gives distraction to the knee joint by extending his own knees and maintains the distraction while he rotates the tibia in a medial or lateral direction. Anterior glide/external rotation increases extension, posterior glide/internal rotation increases mobility in flexion. The operator obtains less distraction during the medial rotation because the cruciate ligaments now are coiled around each other and thus prevent separation of the joint surfaces. Distraction can also be performed with a fixation belt around the patient's ankle and the operator's foot.

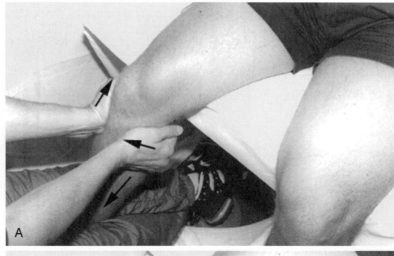

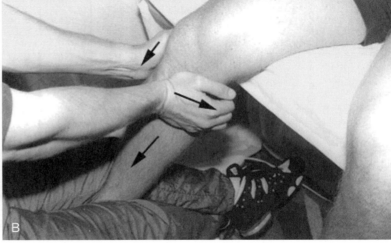

medications that will affect the inflammatory process. Nonsteroidal anti-inflammatory drugs block the cyclooxygenase and lipoxygenase pathways of the omega-6 polyunsaturated fatty acid synthesis. They have also been shown to decrease the mucous lining of the stomach,[7] which prevents the full digestion of proteins and allows for an increase in cell wall permeability. Owing to the decrease in this enzymatic activity and the increase in cell wall permeability, larger protein molecules are absorbed by the gastrointestinal system. This activity produces an autoimmune response as the body reacts to the foreign matter. This response creates an inflammatory response similar to a viral infection. "The leaky gut syndrome" is the result of this process and is described in detail by Rooney et al.[8]

Food allergies can cause a similar reaction that will add to the inflammatory response and decrease the healing process. There are also a variety of foods that have a high content of arachidonic acid, which is a type of prostaglandin known to have inflammatory effects. Prostaglandins are a type of eicosanoid. Eicosanoids are produced from omega-6 and omega-3 polyunsaturated fatty acids present in the cell membrane phospholipids. Omega-3 polyunsaturated fatty acids have an anti-inflammatory response. They are best found in flax seed oil and cold-water fish oils. Omega-6 polyunsaturated fatty acids have more pro-inflammatory influence, as arachidonic acid is a by-product of the synthesis. Foods that have omega-6 polyunsaturated fatty acids, including canola, corn, and sunflower oils, should be avoided. The consumption of meat contributes to a considerable amount of arachidonic acid. The

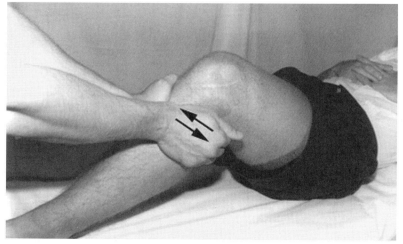

Figure 17–8. This technique shows testing and mobilization of anteroposterior glide of the proximal fibula against the tibia. It is indicated to test or improve motion of the head of the fibula. The patient is lying supine with the hip and the knee flexed and the foot resting on the table. The operator is sitting on the table at the patient's foot, facing the anterior part of the patient's leg. The operator stabilizes the patient's tibia from the medial side. The operator's other hand holds around the head of the fibula with the thenar and the index finger. The operator moves the head of fibula in an anterolateral or posteromedial direction. The operator should mold the fingers around the head of the fibula as gently as possible to avoid irritation of the peroneal nerve.

dietary ratio of omega-6 to omega-3 fatty acids in the United States has been estimated to range between 20:1 and 25:1. A more healthful ratio may be closer to 5:1 to 10:1.[9, 10]

Bioflavonoids, which are a group of naturally occurring substances displaying effects similar to vitamin B, can inhibit the cyclooxygenase and lipoxygenase pathways. Bioflavonoids can be found in citrus fruits, tea, and wine (D. Sopler, personal communication, 1997).

Once the inflammatory process is controlled, we need to look at the nutritional aspects of wound healing. Chondrocytes are responsive to mechanical, biochemical, and micro-environmental stimuli.[11] Ressel[12] shows clinical and experimental evidence that cartilage may heal with identical tissue or a mixture of fibrocartilage and hyaline cartilage.

Damage to connective tissue was believed to be irreparable, although there is now evidence that supports the contrary.[11] The basic structural unit of a collagen fiber is a long protein chain assembled from amino

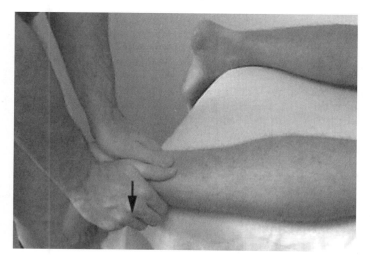

Figure 17–9. This technique shows testing or mobilization of anterior glide of the distal part of the fibula at the distal tibiafibular joint. It is indicated to improve limited motion in eversion of the foot. The patient is lying prone on the table with the leg on the table, but as close to the edge as possible. The foot is extending over the end of the table with a pad between the ankle and the table. The operator stands at the end of the table facing the plantar side of the patient's foot. The operator holds one hand around the medial and anterior part of the ankle, thus fixing the tibia against the table. The operator holds the heel of the other hand on the posterior part of the lateral malleolus. The operator moves the lateral malleolus anteriorly by moving his body weight over his extended elbow.

Figure 17–10. This technique demonstrates testing or mobilization of posterior glide of the distal part of the fibula at the distal tibia-fibular joint. It is indicated to improve limited motion in inversion of the foot. The patient is lying supine on the table with the leg and the calcaneus on the table, but as close to the edge as possible. The lateral malleolus is thus extending over the edge of the table. The operator stands at the end of the table facing the plantar side of the patient's foot. The operator holds one hand around the dorsal part of the calcaneus from the medial side with the hand between the calcaneus and the table. The operator holds the heel of the other hand on the anterior part of the lateral malleolus. The operator moves the lateral malleolus posteriorly by moving his body weight over his extended elbow.

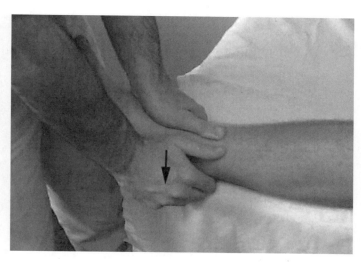

acids.[13] Collagen fibers give connective tissue its tensile strength. A load of at least 10 kg is needed to break a collagen fiber 1 mm in diameter.[14]

Proteoglycans are a key component of the ground substance that makes up connective tissue. Glucosamine sulfate is the stimulus for proteoglycan synthesis. Some studies have shown glucosamine sulfate to normalize cartilage metabolism and decrease pain and inflammation in arthritic patients.[15, 16] Other nutritional components to tissue healing include D-glucuronic acid, which is part of the make-up of hyaluronic acid. Hyaluronic acid is a mucopolysaccharide that is the primary component of proteoglycans and synovial fluid. Vitamin E is a major antioxidant and reduces free radicals, which may damage connective tissue and cause chronic inflammation. There is evidence that a reduction in free radicals will benefit wound healing and connective tissue repair.[17] Vitamin C is required for collagen fiber synthesis and therefore aids in tissue repair. It also functions as an antioxidant by regenerating other antioxidants, especially vitamin E. Copper maximizes vitamin C synthesis. Bioflavonoids activate an enzymatic process necessary for collagen cross-linking.[18] They bind to elastin and prevent degradation by elastases, which are released as a result of inflammation.[19]

Patellofemoral Joint

The patellofemoral joint has two types of tissue of concern: The first is collagen, which provides stability and function. The other is cartilage, which articulates with the femur.

The medial aspect of the posterior surface of the patella is covered with thick cartilage, which develops in response to the increase in pressures in this area with functional activities such as descending stairs and rising from a full squat. On either side of the median ridge are two biconcave facets, one medial and one lateral. As the patella moves vertically during flexion, it comes into contact with the trochlea on its inferior aspect in full extension, on its central aspect at about 30 degrees of flexion, and on its superior and superomedial aspects in full flexion.[20] The patella must have the mobility to travel approximately twice its length in flexion. Figures 17–11 and 17–12 demonstrate techniques for improving patellar mobility in all planes to achieve proper arthrokinematic motion. These techniques not only affect the collagen of the patellar tendon but also apply regenerative forces through the patella with compression and decompression added to the glides.

Compression and Distraction

Compression and distraction can be powerful techniques to inhibit pain and muscle guarding as well as to modify the tension on the injured tissue. A small amount of distraction is always applied to any treatment technique as it places tension on the receptors and gives a decompressive force through the joint. Figure 17–13 shows a tech-

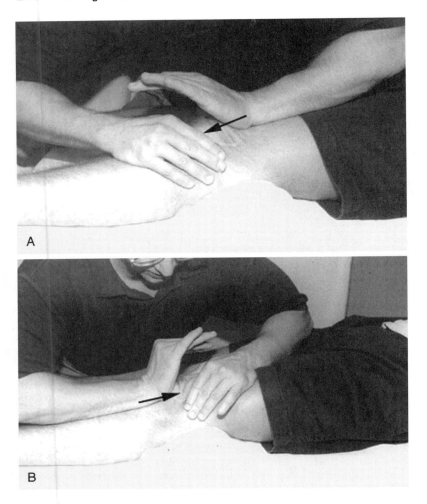

Figure 17–11. These techniques demonstrate testing or mobilization of the patella in a distoproximal direction. It is indicated to test or to improve motion of the patella. The patient is lying supine on the table with the knee in slight flexion on top of a towel roll. *A*, The operator's right hand is held inferior to the patella, preventing patellar compression. The operator moves the patella parallel to the anterior femoral condyles in a distal direction, using the palm of his left hand. *B*, Hand placement for patellar mobilization in a proximal direction.

nique for decompression of the tibiofemoral joint by applying a distraction force.

The techniques described are used to inhibit pain and muscle tone. They can also be used to gain "joint play" as described by Mennell. All tissue has elastic and plastic properties. The clinician determines whether the goal is to gain elasticity or plasticity. If the joint has been immobilized, either through bracing or muscle guarding, one of the first components to be lost is glycosaminoglycan.[21] According to Akeson et al.,[21] constituents of glycosaminoglycan begin to degrade in approximately 1.7 to 7 days. This loss is responsible for the sensation one experiences after immobilization. The muscles have to generate more force to overcome the loss of elasticity and the sensation is stiffness. Once the limb is actively moved, the tension stimulates the pro-

duction of fibroblasts, which produce fiber and glycosaminoglycans. The more glycosaminoglycan that is produced, the more lubrication between the collagen fibers and the less resistance the muscles have to overcome. Since the limb may have been immobilized for an extended amount of time, there may not be any elasticity available. In this case, the clinician must first improve plasticity in the tissue to restore some of the joint play. This is accomplished by taking the tissue to its end range of tension and applying a 10-second to 1.5-minute static stretch. Approximately 80 percent of the available deformation will occur with a 10-second hold. It is important that the clinician not apply so much tension that pain is perceived by the patient. Pain, remember, results from abnormal stresses and is a direct response to trauma.

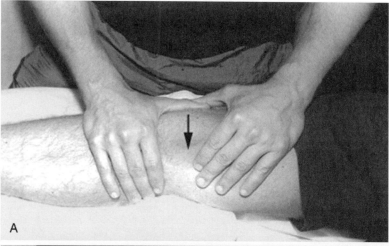

Figure 17–12. These techniques demonstrate testing or mobilization of the patella in a mediolateral direction. They are indicated to test or to improve patella mobility. The patient lies supine on the table with the knee in slight flexion, with a small towel roll under the knee. The operator stands on the side of the knee opposite to the direction of movement. The operator's left thenar web space is superior and the right thenar web space is inferior to the patella. *A*, The operator's thumb moves the patella in a medial direction. *B*, Mobilizing the patella in a lateral direction.

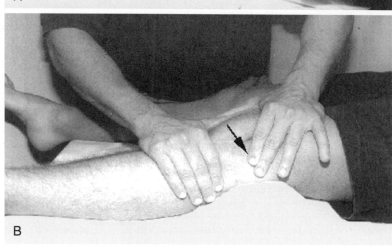

Collagen has the capacity to deform 20 percent of its length before rupture occurs. It can only deform some 3 percent before evidence of micro-trauma is present. To gain plasticity, the clinician must only apply tension up to 3 percent of the collagen's available range. Pain will be the response if one exceeds the collagen's ability to tolerate the tension being applied.

Once the clinician has maintained the tension, plasticity is acheived, allowing an increase in motion. Actively moving the limb and applying modified tension through the collagen stimulates fibroblasts, which produce fiber and glycosaminoglycans. The glycosaminoglycans will improve the lubrication and nutrition of the collagen, whereas the fiber will improve the collagen's ability to tolerate the stresses that will be a part of the rehabilitation program.

Dosing Tension

No matter what techniques we use to gain range of motion or to inhibit pain, we must improve the tissue's tolerance to tension. This is the key concept of rehabilitation. Clinicians must make sure that the tissue in lesion has the capacity to tolerate the various stresses that are placed on it. The main goal of any rehabilitation program is to regain optimal function of the system that is in lesion. Optimal function is the ability to move around a physiologic axis with full mobility and stability. That means that for every 1 degree of motion that we improve in a joint, we must dynamically stabilize that degree both concentrically and eccentrically. In the extremities, 1 degree does not seem like much motion, but in the spine when the total amount of motion is 3 de-

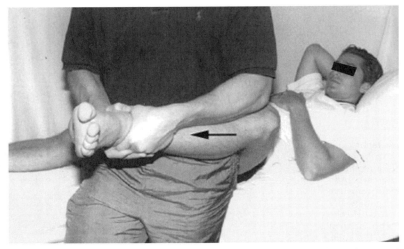

Figure 17–13. This technique shows distraction of the tibia from the femur. The indication is to improve any limitation of motion. The patient is lying supine on the table with the hip flexed, externally rotated, and abducted with flexion in the knee joint. The operator is sitting on the table with his back against the patient, medial to the patient's leg. The patient's femur is fixed against the operator's back and the operator holds both hands distal to the malleolus from the anterior and posterior side. The operator's forearm is parallel to the patient's leg. The operator moves the leg in a distal direction, thus separating the tibia from the femur. These techniques are most beneficial when the patient is unable to flex the knee joint more than approximately 30 degrees.

grees, that 1 degree of motion represents one third of the total motion available.

Ligaments are relatively avascular and as such do not obtain significant nutrition from direct circulation. Of greater importance to this tissue is modified tension placed on the tissue to stimulate the fibroblast to produce fiber and glycosaminoglycans. Whatever exercise we choose, it must be of modified tension in the line of stress with many repetitions. In the line of stress would be functional exercises that reproduce the stress of daily activities.

The initial stage of exercise is concerned with increasing circulation to the tonic system, preventing atrophy, increasing protein synthesis, and reducing the level of metabolites. The functional quality we aim to influence is endurance as well as coordination.[22] For endurance work to take place, the amount of energy expanded must be equal to the amount of energy supplied. This occurs after some 5 to 6 minutes of exercise at a constant intensity level and is called *steady state.* The question is how do we decide the dosage with specific reference to each particular patient's exercise ability. In this phase, we are not primarily concerned with qualities like range of motion and strength. We do, however, need a formula for the number of repetitions, resistance, and speed the

patient can perform in a pain-free synergy. As the number of repetitions is determined by the resistance, we need to find a percentage of maximal resistance the patient can overcome enough times to develop endurance and therefore coordination. In 1948, De-Lorme defined the term *resistance maximal.*[23] It was introduced as the resistance a group of muscles can overcome once, and this factor was then used as a measure of strength.

In 1953, Hettinger and Mueller published work on isometric strength training. They showed that a 6-second hold of 75 percent of maximal resistance was sufficient to increase strength.[24, 25] At the same time, East German scientists and sports trainers developed the relationship between the percentage of resistance maximum (RM) and the number of repetitions that an exercise can be performed with a certain weight. Various functional qualities were defined by that relationship. In Norway, Holten and Faugli[26] developed a curve to that effect (Fig. 17–14).

In patients, we are rarely able to test 100 percent of a RM because of pain and the danger of overloading the tissue in lesion. In practical terms, we choose a resistance from experience that we think the patient will be able to use to perform the number of repetitions we need to achieve the desired functional quality. According to the Holten

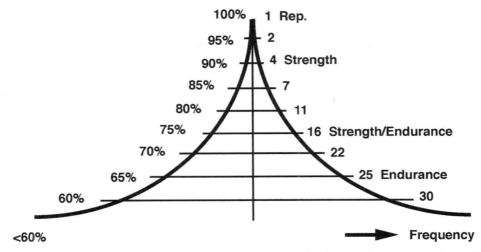

Figure 17–14. Male female concentric curve. (Courtesy of the Ola Grimsby Institute, San Diego, CA.)

curve, endurance is acheived at approximately 75 to 60 percent of 1 RM when 20 to 30 repetitions are performed.

At times, the patient's own weight may be too much and may exceed 1 RM. The person can either lose weight quickly, be placed in gravity-controlled room, or more simply be "de-weighted". This can be done with counter-weights. For the knee, the use of a lat bar with weight on the weight stack will be sufficient to decrease the patient's body weight to allow functional exercises to be performed.

In most functional exercises based on concentric work, fatigue is a consequence and must be considered when doing exercises so that the patient's tolerance is not exceeded. The exercise is performed with slow speed around physiologic axes in a pain-free range until fatigue. Fatigue may also occur as a lack of coordination observed by the clinician but not perceived by the patient. To acheive an increase in the total number of repetitions while maintaining a tolerable dosage, we must increase the sets. To go from one set to three sets, the patient must reduce either the amount of repetitions per set or the resistance. If one reduces the resistance, there may be a change in the functional quality. To avoid this, we reduce the number of repetitions by 10 to 20 percent.

The rest period between sets is determined by the time the individual needs to return to the steady state respiratory rate. As the respiratory rate reaches steady state, the oxygen debt created by the exercise is decreasing.

An important component of exercise is to utilize tension specificity to recruit and facilitate muscle fibers. According to Blix's Length/Tension curve (Fig. 17–15), the greatest amount of tension the muscle can achieve is a 20 percent increase in fiber length measured from the resting length.[27] This is partly because of the structural interaction between the muscle fibers and collagen as well as the mechanical advantage of the muscle and the receptors in the collagen

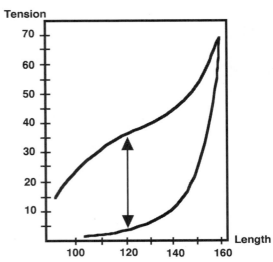

Figure 17–15. The diagram shows the relationship between "passive tension" and "total tension." When the passive curve is deducted from the total, the actual active tension is achieved. Greatest tension can be achieved at 20 percent increase in fiber length measured from resting position. (Courtesy of the Ola Grimsby Institute, San Diego, CA.)

of the associated joint capsule, recruiting both tonic and phasic muscle fibers when the collagen is in the beginning range of tension (resting position of the joint).[28-30] The clinical implications are that the patient can tolerate less resistance in the beginning of range and the end of range of contraction and can overcome more resistance 20 percent beyond resting contraction. The patient will accelerate toward the maximal length/tension range of motion and decelerate away from it. Acceleration and deceleration are the most important components of all activities (Fig. 17–16). Since all exercises are task-specific, the variables of speed and resistance throughout the range of contraction are of greatest importance for fiber recruitment and physiologic coordination.[31]

GENERAL PROGRESSION OF KNEE REHABILITATION

First, a thorough examination is carried out to identify the tissue in lesion. Secondly, soft tissue techniques are performed to reduce tonic guarding of the vastus medialis oblique muscle. Next exercises are performed to coordinate the vastus medialis oblique muscle and to improve the vascularity. This is done with concentric exercises using modified tension, which initially may be non-weight-bearing. Functional qualities are to be decided such as coordination, strength, and so forth. Once the weight-bearing status has progressed, closed chain exercises are initiated. These exercises are performed with modified tension, possibly with de-weighting. The exercises are performed according to the Holten Curve and are dosed to gain the functional quality that is lacking. Eccentric exercises and plyometrics are incorporated, emphasizing lateral and diagonal movements in functional patterns. This overview of course is simplified, but the clinician should have the understanding that the exercise program is individualized to the patient's needs. No one protocol is sufficient to properly rehabilitate all patients with the variety of needs and stages of healing that are seen in our clinics.

SUMMARY

However one decides on a rehabilitation program, functional exercises for the knee should include variables of speed with acceleration and deceleration, concentric and eccentric movement and weight-bearing. They should closely mimic the range and planes of motion that the knee needs to be able

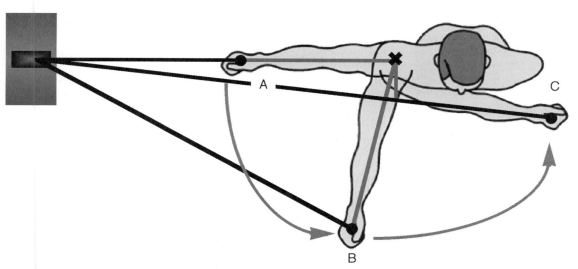

Figure 17–16. Pulley resistance. Variable resistance (ability to overcome inertia) in various ranges of motion during concentric work is determined by the length of the lever arm. The patient is initiating a concentric contraction from the starting position A. Acceleration occurs to position B, where the force arm is the longest and the length/tension is maximal. Observe how the force arm (distance from the line of resistance to the axis of motion) becomes reduced as the patient contracts toward the inner range, where the muscle can develop less tension in position C. (Courtesy of the Ola Grimsby Institute, San Diego, CA.)

to tolerate, keeping in mind, "you get what you train."

Note: The information in this chapter is an overview only of the concepts of manual therapy. For detailed information and residency programs regarding manual therapy, contact the American Academy of Orthopedic Manual Physical Therapists.

References

1a. Cyriax J: Textbook of Orthopaedic Medicine, 8th ed. London, Balliere Tindall, 1978.
1b. Mennell J: The role of manipulation in therapeutics. Lancet 400:1932.
1c. The Ola Grimsby Institute. San Diego, CA.
2. Wolff J: Gesetz der Transformation der Knocken. Berlin, A. Hirschwald, 1884.
3. Kapandji IA: The Physiology of the Joints, Vol. 2. New York, Churchill Livingstone, 1987.
4. Stoddard A: Manual of Osteopathic Practice. London, Hutchinson Medical Publications, 1969.
5. White A, Panjabi M: Clinical Anatomy of the Lumbar Spine. Philadelphia, J.B. Lippincott, 1990.
6. Raunest J, Sager M, Burgener E: Proprioceptive mechanisms in the cruciate ligaments: An electromyographic study on reflex activity in the thigh muscles. J Trauma. 41:488–493, 1996.
7. Russo PJ: NSAID-induced gastroenteropathy: A biochemical dissection. Hosp. Pract. Dec.:123–132, 1992.
8. Rooney PJ, Jenkins RT, Buchanan WW: A short review of the relationship between intestinal permeability and inflammatory joint disease. Clin Exp Rheum 8:75–83, 1990.
9. Simopoulos AP: Omega-3 fatty acids in health and disease and in growth and development. Am J Clin Nutr 54:438–463, 1991.
10. Erasmus U: Fats That Heal, Fats That Kill, 2nd ed. Burnaby, Canada: Alive Books, 1993.
11. Bland JH, Cooper SM: Osteoarthritis: A review of the cell biology involved and evidence for reversibility, management rationally related to known genesis and pathophysiology. Semin Arthritis Rheum 14(2):106, 1984.
12. Ressel OJ: Disk regeneration: Reversibility is possible in spinal osteoarthritis. ICA Int Rev Chiropract. Mar/April: 39–61, 1989.
13. Percival M: Nutritional support for connective tissue repair and wound healing. Nutritional Pearls 26:1–4, 1996.
14. Stryer L: Biochemistry, 2nd ed. San Francisco, W.H. Freeman, 1975.
15. Setniker I: Antireactive properties of chondroprotective drugs. Int J Tissue React 14(5):253–261, 1992.
16. Vaz AL: Double-blind clinical evaluation of the relative efficacy of glucosamine sulfate in the management of osteoarthritis of the knee in out-patients. Curr Med Res Opin 8:145–149, 1982.
17. Bucci LR: Nutrition Applied to Injury Rehabilitation and Sports Medicine. Boca Raton, FV, CRC Press, 1995.
18. Havsteen B: Flavinoids, a class of natural products of high pharmacological potency. Biochem Pharmacol 32(7):1141–1148, 1983.
19. Tixier JM, Godeau G, Robert AM, Hornebeck W: Evidence by in vivo and in vitro studies that binding of pycnogenols to elastin affects its rate of degradation by elastases. Biochem Pharm 33(24):3933–3939, 1984.
20. Kapandji IA: The Physiology of the Joints, Vol. 2. New York, Churchill Livingstone, 1987.
21. Akeson W, Woo S, Amiel D, Coutts R, Daniel D: The connective tissue response to imobility: Biomechanical changes in periarticular connective tissue of the immobilized rabbit knee. Clin Orthop Rel Res 93:356–361, 1973.
22. Shepard R, Astrand P: Endurance in Sport. Oxford, England, Blackwell Scientific Publications, 1992.
23. DeLorme T, Watkins a: Progressive Resistance Exercise. New York, Appleton Century, 1951.
24. Hettinger T: Isometrisches Muskeltraining. Stuttgart, Germany, 1964.
25. Mueller K: Statische und Dynamische Muskelkraft. Frankfurt, Germany, M. Thun, 1987.
26. Holten O, Faugli H: Medisinsk Treningsterapi. Universitetsforlaget, 0608 Oslo, Norway, 1993.
27. Blix M: Length and tension. Scand Arch Physiol 93–94, 1892.
28. Dean E: Physiology and therapeutic implications of negative work. Phys Ther 68:233–237, 1988.
29. Frankel V, Nordin M: Basic Biomechanics of the Skeletal System. Philadelphia, Lea & Febiger, 1980.
30. Wyke B, Polacek P: Articular neurology: The present position. J Bone Joint Surg 57(B):40, 1975.
31. Grimby G, Thomee R: Principles of rehabilitation after injuries. *In* Dirix A, Knuttgen HG, Tittel K (eds): The Olympic Book of Sports Medicine, Vol. 1. Oxford, England, Blackwell Scientific Publications, 1984.

18 Bracing: Science or Psychology?

Patrick W. Cawley, OPA, RT, CRA

HISTORY

It is often assumed by those in the orthopedic sports medicine community that functional bracing of the knee is a relatively modern phenomenon. However, in the fourth century BC, Hippocrates alluded to the practice of splinting and bracing of the lower extremity following soft tissue and joint injuries that resulted in instability.[1] In the first century AD, noted Greek physician Galen discussed bracing methods to permit mobility following destabilizing injuries of the joints of the lower extremity.[2] Despite an apparent understanding of the potential biomechanical benefits of functional knee bracing by some physicians, it is clear that bracing was neither commonly used nor widely accepted during these periods. In intervening centuries, there are few references that specifically address functional bracing of instabilities of the knee until the writings of Bonnet in 1845.[3] Not only do his writings reveal an intimate understanding of the biomechanical result of the disruption of the knee ligaments, but he also provides detailed drawings of an articulated knee brace to address these deficits.

Lower extremity bracing was widely employed in the 19th century for a variety of conditions, particularly for congenital and acquired neuromuscular disorders. It was not until the late 1960s that functional knee bracing came into common use for knee ligament instability with the introduction of the Lenox Hill Derotation Brace. Despite surgical reconstruction, many athletes continued to experience episodes of instability during this period. From the beginning of the 1970s through the decade of the 1980s, functional knee bracing gained wide acceptance, particularly for athletes, and companies that made knee braces proliferated. Many of these companies were started by orthopedic surgeons. The rise in the popularity of functional knee bracing can be correlated with the dramatic rise in professional athlete's salaries and television exposure, and the inability of the surgical procedures of the day to restore complete functional stability to the knee.

The 1990s witnessed a dramatic evolution in both surgical and rehabilitation technologies, owing primarily to an improved understanding of the biomechanical, neuromuscular, and neurosensory mechanisms governing knee function. Minimally invasive surgical techniques and more biomechanically accurate reconstructive procedures can restore nearly normal mechanical stability in the knee. Perhaps more important to the ultimate outcome of knee ligament injuries have been new rehabilitation strategies that focus not only on restoration of strength and range of motion but also on restoration of neurosensory and kinematic function. As a result of these improvements, many clinicians now question whether knee bracing serves a necessary purpose, particularly following knee ligament reconstruction. Current attitudes regarding functional knee bracing are based in many cases on limited qualitative or anecdotal evidence. The lack of validated long-term outcome data, particularly data on cost-versus-benefit analyses, makes any conclusion problematic. Complicating this picture are the changes in reimbursement policies. Fee capitation and declining incomes have also had an impact on the use of ancillary modalities such as bracing and rehabilitation following surgical reconstruction of the knee.

CURRENT LITERATURE

Brace Mechanical Function

One of the impediments the clinician faces in attempting to validate the decision to employ a functional knee brace, particularly in

252

a primarily prophylactic application following ligament reconstruction, is the lack of good long-term outcome data. Though a substantial body of research literature on knee bracing is available, this literature is diverse, sometimes difficult to find, and generally very narrow in focus. The majority of research available on the effects of functional knee bracing has focused on the control of tibial translation and rotation.[4-13] The clear conclusion from these investigations is that functional knee braces do provide increased mechanical stability to the knee under low, subphysiologic loading conditions. Many clinicians claim that these same effects would not be seen under true physiologic loading conditions. In 1995, Soma et al.[14] addressed these concerns in a study using an instrumented mechanical surrogate. These investigators found that functional knee braces do provide increased mechanical stability to the knee under high physiologic loads and that this function is dependent on rate of loading, brace design, and material properties.

Several investigations have shown that functional bracing may increase energy expenditure and reduce functional performance.[15-20] While this finding would seem to contraindicate the use of a functional brace, particularly during the rehabilitation process, other work indicates that patients may quickly adapt to this increased demand.[15, 21] In fact, these authors speculate that this increased demand enhances the return of strength and may constitute a form of resistive exercise, which is beneficial to long-term outcome. They also note that over 90 percent of subjects report a significant functional and performance improvement when using a functional knee brace. A number of investigations have demonstrated that functional knee bracing may have beneficial effects on restoration of both kinematics and functional performance.[22-26] It is generally accepted that, despite surgical reconstruction of the anterior cruciate ligament, some significant physiologic deficits remain after surgery.[25, 26] The referenced studies have demonstrated that the use of a functional knee brace can restore force and torque generation to near-normal levels and can restore near-normal kinematic patterns in both anterior cruciate ligament (ACL)–deficient and reconstructed knees. This restoration of near-normal kinematics to the knee may have significant implications for the long-term outcome, particularly acceleration of

articular cartilage degeneration, following both conservative and surgical treatment of knee ligament injuries.

An aggressive surgical approach to treatment of anterior cruciate ligament tears is frequently justified by the claim that reconstruction is necessary to restore normal knee kinematics to ameliorate long-term degenerative change in the joint.[27, 28] A number of investigators have demonstrated that replacement of the ACL with a graft, regardless of technique, does not restore normal kinematic patterns to the knee.[29-31] Rather, the graft functions more as a "check-rein" against large excursions in the frontal plane. Based on these findings, we must conclude that reconstruction does not mitigate the incidence of degenerative processes resulting from abnormal motion patterns. A recent study from Daniel et al.[32] tends to confirm this conclusion. Greater degrees of degenerative change were noted in the reconstructed subjects than were seen in conservatively treated subjects in this long-term prospective investigation. In a recent study, Wojtys et al.[33] investigated muscle firing patterns and anterior tibial translation in response to induced anteriorly directed forces at the tibia in partially weight-bearing subjects. While demonstrating a reduction in anterior tibial displacement ranging from 15 to 30 percent with muscles relaxed and 60 to 80 percent with muscles contracted, the authors identified what they termed a "latency," or delay, in hamstring firing when the limb was braced. Interestingly, the longest latency for hamstring firing was associated with braces that produced the greatest reduction in anterior tibial translation. These authors concluded that functional bracing interferes with normal hamstring function. Another reasonable conclusion based on these same data is that functional knee bracing, particularly by braces that provide the best anterior stability, reduced the need for coactivation of the hamstrings for knee stabilization.

BIOMECHANICAL, PHYSIOLOGIC, AND PSYCHOLOGICAL PERSPECTIVES ON POTENTIAL KNEE BRACE EFFECTS

Post-Surgical Ligament Remodeling

There is little controversy surrounding functional knee bracing in the chronically unstable knee or in the conservative treatment of knee ligament injuries. It is not surprising in light of the recent surgical revolution that many surgeons now question the necessity of functional knee bracing following ligament reconstruction. In the decades of the 1970s and 1980s, most postoperative failures were related to failure of graft fixation. This phenomenon has all but disappeared in the 1990s. The result of this has been a more aggressive approach to rehabilitation involving both early weight-bearing and early resistive exercise. Although short-term results with these techniques have been excellent, an understanding of the graft remodeling process suggests that small and insidious changes, possibly not evident for 5 to 10 years, may occur without some consideration for mechanical protection of the remodeling graft.

Postoperative remodeling of the ligament graft has been extensively studied.[34–37] This process is characterized by four stages: (1) time zero (i.e., immediately following implantation of the graft) avascularity and necrosis, (2) revascularization, (3) cellular repopulation, and (4) structural remodeling. As can be seen in Figure 18–1, graft remodeling is a staged process. Almost immediately following implantation, the avascular graft undergoes a necrotic phase in which collagen fragmentation occurs. Up to two-thirds of the graft's mass may be resorbed by the body during this phase. The ultimate strength of the graft drops quickly with this fragmentation and disorganization of the collagen matrix. Whereas a 10-mm patellar tendon graft may have constituted 170 percent the strength of the original ACL, by the fourth postoperative week, this graft may be as little as 10 percent of the strength of the original ACL.[34–37]

As shown in Figure 18–1, cellular repopulation and revascularization of the graft require up to 24 weeks before these processes are complete. Reorganization of the collagen

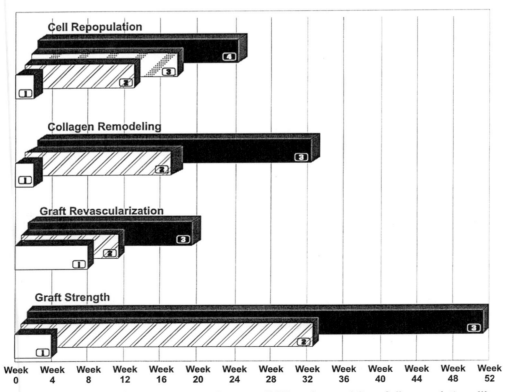

Figure 18–1. Natural history of anterior cruciate ligament (ACL) graft remodeling. Cell repopulation: (1) complete acellularity; (2) cell repopulation begins; (3) generalized cellular proliferation; (4) cellular repopulation complete. Collagen remodeling: (1) collagen fragmentation/resorbtion; (2) generalized cross-linking of collagen evident; (3) collagen reorganization resembles native ACL. Graft revascularization: (1) graft synovialization begins; (2) intrinsic vascularization begins; (3) vascularization complete. Graft strength: (1) graft strength 10 percent of normal ACL; (2) graft strength 20 to 30 percent of normal ACL; (3) graft strength 40 to 60 percent of normal ACL.

into a structure roughly resembling a ligament can take as long as 32 weeks. During this interval, collagen strands are disorganized and not aligned along the lines of stress and have a reduced capability to resist tensile stresses. This process is somewhat analogous to construction of a bridge. Until all of the mechanical components are in place, the bridge is not really a mechanically functional structure. Excessive loads during early phases of construction would result in collapse of the bridge. Likewise, it is necessary that all of the components of functional remodeling be in place for a graft to be structurally functional. Our best evidence indicates that at 12 months following surgery, the graft possess only 40 to 60 percent of the original ultimate strength of the normal ACL. Our best evidence indicates that although the tendon graft remodels into a structure roughly resembling a ligament, neither its biochemical or material properties ever match those of the native ACL.[38] In particular, tendon grafts exhibit significantly higher material stiffness than do normal ligaments and are thus at greater risk of loading, which might result in plastic or permanent deformation. Accordingly, mechanical protection of the graft from deforming loads seems to be indicated, at least during the early stages of rehabilitation.

Modern rehabilitation protocols conscientiously avoid activities that might overstress a graft, such as high-resistance open-chain exercises. It is also clear, however, that low-load cyclic stresses can also influence this remodeling process.[39–42] Cyclic stresses can result in long-term deformation of the graft, which affects both knee stability and joint kinematics and, consequently, acceleration of degenerative changes within the knee. These changes would be subtle and would not be apparent on physical examination, particularly while the patient is able to use compensatory muscular strategies to compensate for minor kinematic and stability deficiencies. As was discussed earlier, bracing may play an important role not only in protecting the graft from low-level cyclic stresses, but also in kinematic guidance of the remodeling graft.[22–26]

There is evidence in the literature suggesting that functional knee bracing does provide mechanical stress protection to the remodeling graft. In 1992, Beynnon et al.[43] found that some functional braces reduced ACL strain under some conditions during open-chain testing in vivo. In a 1997 follow-up,[44] these same investigators found that functional bracing had a significant strain-protective effect on the ACL in both weight-bearing and non-weight-bearing conditions during in vivo testing. However, our ability to assess the efficacy of bracing in protecting the remodeling graft is compounded by our inability to characterize these small and insidious changes in stability or kinematics in vivo as well as the traditional clinical focus on short-term results and lack of good long-term outcome data.

Neurosensory Effects of Functional Knee Bracing

One of the most perplexing issues in the controversy over functional knee brace efficacy is an apparent paradox in the quantitative results versus the subjective responses in regard to brace efficacy. Despite the fact that a number of investigators have been unable to demonstrate significant mechanical efficacy for functional knee braces, subjective response regarding both functional and performance efficacy is overwhelmingly favorable.[21] A potential explanation for this discrepancy might be an enhancement of neurosensory function associated with brace use. Several investigators using electromyographic analysis of muscular function during dynamic activity have stated that, based on electromyographic results, functional knee bracing has little or no effect on proprioception in the lower extremity.[25, 26, 33] It should be noted that these studies addressed only efferent components of the motor control loop and can tell us very little about either proprioception or kinesthesia.

In 1996, I and coinvestigators[45] reported on the results of neurosensory testing in a group of chronically ACL-deficient subjects following a period of 1 month of functional knee bracing using a similar group of subjects for control subjects. Using an instrumented system to characterize motor control performance, these authors performed an index evaluation on all subjects. Half of the subjects were then fitted with functional knee braces and instructed to use them during athletic activities; otherwise, all subjects were instructed not to alter normal daily activities during the 1-month evaluation period. All subjects returned after 1 month and motor control tests were re-administered. Results of this study are shown in Figure 18–2. As can be seen with the exception of single-limb tests on the non-injured limb, all braced subjects demonstrated significant motor control improvement for both static and dynamic tests. No significant changes were shown for non-braced controls. Although a neurosensory benefit was demonstrated in this study, the mechanism behind this improvement is not understood. It is hypothesized that this result is a combination of increased mechanical stability of the joint combined with enhanced afferent output elicited from both musculotendinous and cutaneous mechanoreceptors in the limb. We are pursuing further investigation in this area.

Psychological Aspects of Functional Knee Bracing

A review of the literature will produce only a limited discussion of the potential psychological effects of functional knee bracing.[21, 46, 47] In an unpublished 1984 investigation, Cawley[48] reported on some of the psychological aspects of functional knee bracing in a group of 73 subjects who had undergone ACL reconstruction. Using clinical interviews and patient diaries, this investigator reported that patients were more aggressive in their approach to physical therapy when their knee was braced, were more compliant with physical therapy prescriptions, and reported that they felt more confident in performing resistive exercise when their knees were braced. The author reported that a functional knee brace may also function as a tactile "reminder," which may induce protective adaptations in gait and functional activities that result in avoidance of potentially dangerous loading conditions to the knee.

Two potential undesirable side effects were identified associated with knee brace use. The first was termed "risk-taking" behavior and was found to be a trait associated predominantly with male patients involved in contact sports. In this behavior, patients whose knees were braced tended to take risks with the braced knee under the assumption that the brace protected them from injury. The second of these effects was termed "dependence" behavior and was

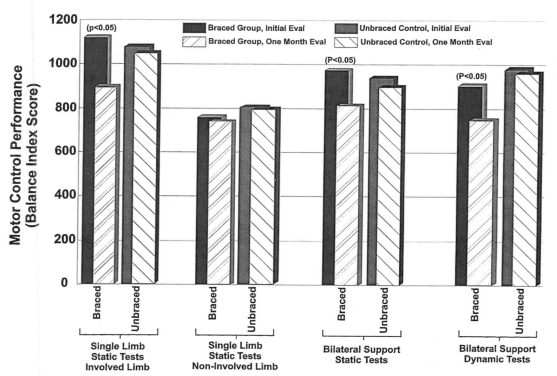

Figure 18–2. Motor control test scores in braced subjects after 1 month of bracing as compared with nonbraced subjects. A lower score indicates a better performance.

most commonly seen in females with a more sedentary lifestyle. These patients tended to become reliant on the brace for stability and tended to use the brace for all activities, including those for which the therapist had recommended the brace be removed. Typically, these patients failed to progress as rapidly as other patients and took significantly longer to recover muscular strength. The author points out that these potential problems are actually patient communication issues. All patients must be apprised of both the benefits and limitations of functional knee brace use. If the patient is included in treatment decisions and fully understands the function of all treatment modalities, problems resulting from misunderstandings can be reduced or eliminated.

Mechanical and Material Factors Affecting Brace Function

Soft tissue is the principal mechanical interface between the brace and the limb. Since the axial soft tissues of the limb have little resistance to tangential loading, functional knee braces provide little or no control of rotation about the long axis of the lower extremity under physiologic loading conditions, despite the claims to the contrary of a number of brace manufacturers. A good analogy for this phenomenon is to grasp the wrist at the level of the ulnar styloid very tightly. Despite a good anatomical interface, you can still rotate the hand on the wrist you are grasping. This phenomenon is exaggerated on the large muscle masses of the lower extremity. The only advantage available to the brace designer is that the lower limb is composed of the two longest lever arms in the body, the femur and tibia. Using these two lever arms, the brace can address translations and rotations in the frontal and saggital planes. Accordingly, all functional knee braces work essentially the same way—leverage. An example of the optimal leverage points to control anteroposterior translation at the knee is shown in Figure 18–3A, while an example of the optimal leverage points to control varus-valgus rotation of the knee is shown in Figure 18–3B. Using the same leverage systems, brace manufacturers address control of translations and rotations in a variety of different ways. It is the clinician's responsibil-

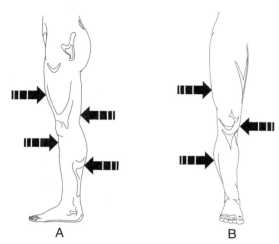

Figure 18–3. Arrows represent examples of the optimal leverage points to control anteroposterior translation at the knee *(A)* and the optimal leverage points to control varus-valgus rotation of the knee *(B)*.

ity to determine whether the design elements of a given brace correctly address the pathologic conditions present when a brace is prescribed, or to determine whether the brace utilizes leverage systems appropriate to a specific patient's needs. It can be truthfully said that no one brace design is appropriate for all patient needs.

A particular area of contention concerns hinge design on functional knee braces. A number of manufacturers claim to have hinges that duplicate the normal kinematics of the knee. If this were true, medial and lateral hinges on the braces would be of different designs, reflecting differences in motion between medial and lateral compartments of the knee, and the brace hinges would also be required to accommodate normal automatic rotation of the lower extremity during gait. No currently marketed functional knee brace incorporates such a hinge design. Due primarily to the soft tissue interface between brace and limb, it has been conclusively demonstrated that hinge design has little or no effect on knee kinematics.[49–52] Rather, the function of the brace hinge is to provide range-of-motion control when desired and to facilitate leverage by transferring loads between femoral and tibial levers of the brace. Whether the hinge design is monocentric (a single center of rotation) or polycentric (multiple or changing centers of rotation) is of little importance as long as the design provides an effective load transfer mechanism. For polycentric hinges, gearing is generally required to accomplish this load transfer effectively.

It is common to hear clinicians state that they prefer custom-made functional knee braces over so-called off-the-shelf designs because they get a better fit. This statement is true when significant geometric or anatomic variation is present. However, most off-the-shelf designs offer the flexibility of in-office reforming should interval girth or contour changes occur during the treatment period, and each off-the-shelf orthosis is generally "custom" fit to the patient at the initial application. The greatest difference between custom-made and off-the-shelf braces is usually in the materials and manufacturing methods employed. Custom-made braces generally employ materials such as advanced composites that can only be formed using special manufacturing techniques. Once formed, these braces generally cannot be changed if some interval change in the limb occurs. An advantage of these advanced materials is a significant strength-versus-weight ratio and enhanced stiffness or durability, particularly for high loading environments such as football. Special materials and manufacturing processes also result in higher unit costs for custom-made knee braces.

A complete understanding of knee brace function requires that the clinician understand the influence of brace material properties on ultimate effect. As Soma et al.[14] point out, knee brace performance is dependent on brace design (how leverage is applied), brace materials properties, and how the brace is loaded. Upon first inspection, many will pick up a knee brace and bend or twist the structure to characterize its material properties. Frequently, if the brace bends or twists too much, it will be discarded as not having enough material strength. However, when a brace is applied to the limb, a "composite" structure is formed that has a "composite" material response. Although the brace is intended to provide mechanical support to the limb, the limb likewise may also add mechanical support to the brace. Accordingly, testing of functional knee braces, whether in vitro or in vivo, must be conducted on a limb or an accurate surrogate thereof. Some manufacturers have begun to take advantage of this fact in designs that are lighter in weight and more compli-

ant but still provide superior control of rotations and translations about the joint.

The ultimate response of most materials and structures is "rate-dependent" in nature, or the response of the structure to load is dependent on how fast the loading is applied. This is especially true of the composite structure of the braced knee. This is significantly influenced by the material stiffness of the knee/brace composite structure. For example, it is assumed that a very mechanically stiff brace is needed under high-rate impact loads to provide protection to the joint. In actuality, it has been shown that impacts to very stiff braces might result in acceleration of the knee within the brace, resulting in joint injury.[53] In this loading situation, it is desirable that some deformation of the brace occur to change the rate of loading, to absorb some of the energy, and to distribute some of the energy to be absorbed in the soft tissues. Conversely, high brace stiffness is an important factor when external forces create bending moments along the axis of the limb, such as an external rotation-valgus injury in skiing. Obviously, tissue compliance factors exert a significant influence on this behavior. The mechanical interface of a brace is significantly better on limbs with well-toned musculature and control of rotations and translations is enhanced. In limbs with much more compliant tissues, significant displacement of the mechanical structure of the brace can occur while interfaced with the limb, thus reducing brace effectiveness.

Brace Selection and Application Notes

The decision regarding whether to use a functional knee brace must remain a purely clinical one based on the best evidence available. If the decision is made to use a functional knee brace, a number of factors should be taken into consideration in choosing a particular brace:

1. Define the principal role for the brace as well as the planes of instability. If the application is to be used for a chronically unstable knee, the main role of the brace is to provide mechanical control in one or more planes. Usually, the brace must enhance antero-posterior stability of the knee and,

secondarily, should also increase resistance to varus-valgus rotation of the knee. Thirdly, prevention of hyperextension may be desired. If the brace is primarily prophylactic in nature, such as protection of a remodeling ACL graft, prevention of excessive valgus or varus rotation at the knee would be the primary requirement. Secondarily, the brace should prevent hyperextension on the limb. Although it is not clear in the literature, a functional knee brace can also serve to protect a remodeling graft from small cyclic displacements that might result in permanent deformation over time, so increased anteroposterior stiffness may be beneficial as well. Once the plane or planes of instability are defined, pick the brace whose leverage points match the intended application.

2. If addressing chronic instability, define the nature of the instability. A *mechanical instability* is the direct result of disruption of one or more of the soft tissue stabilizers about the joint and is usually measurable either through manual or instrumented techniques. This type of instability responds well to external mechanical stabilization in the form of bracing. A *functional instability* is most often the result of either a neurosensory or neuromuscular deficit and is generally not measurable in a traditional sense. Rather, a functional instability is determined from patient history. Although both functional and mechanical instabilities frequently coexist, a predominantly functional instability should be addressed through rehabilitation, as it will not respond well to functional bracing.

3. Define any special morphologic or physiologic requirements. Substantial deformity of the limbs dictates that a custom-made brace be used to accommodate any morphologic variations. Neurovascular conditions such as diabetes may dictate a brace design with a larger surface area to avoid point pressures that could result in ischemic damage to the tissues. Tissue compliance, particularly in elderly individuals, is a special concern. Care must be taken that pressure points on the brace do not produce tissue abrasion or maceration.

4. Define the patient expectations and intended application of the brace. A young athletic individual involved in contact sports or a sport in which the brace may be subject to both high loading and repetitive abrasion will usually dictate a custom-made orthosis. Although light in weight, a custom-made brace of advanced composite material can withstand the expected rigors of the sport. Alternatively, a recreational athlete engaged in the same sport at a lower level may do very well in an off-the-shelf orthosis. More sedentary individuals who require some support for walking and jogging may do well with a hinged neoprene orthosis.

Above all, it is incumbent upon the clinician to involve the patient in the treatment process through adequate communication. The patient must understand that there are many activities for which the brace should not be used, such as controlled closed chain resistive exercises, jogging on well-groomed surfaces, or riding a bicycle. The brace should be used for activities involving high shearing or rotational moments across the joint. Based on the data presented earlier, I recommend that a functional brace be used for at least 6 months following ACL reconstruction. Most critically, the patient must understand not only the potential benefits of a functional knee brace but also the inherent limitations of a functional knee brace. If the patient is told nothing else, he or she should be told not to depend on the functional knee brace to provide protection in unusual loading situations.

SUMMARY

The answer to the question "Is knee bracing science or psychology?" actually is quite simple; the efficacy of knee bracing is based both on science and on psychology. Although it has not been extensively studied, clinicians understand intuitively that there is a strong psychological component associated with all aspects of the treatment of significant knee joint injuries. Concerns over the outcome of both surgical and conservative treatment protocols can influence a patient's perspective, his or her approach to recovery, and his or her quality of life. The overwhelmingly favorable subjective response in the literature would indicate that the patients themselves feel that bracing serves an important function in their recovery. Not only do patients report an enhanced sense of security when using functional knee braces, but the majority also report a subjective sense of improved functional performance when a brace is used. The subjective feeling that braces serve an important function is supported by the finding that the majority of patients continue to use knee braces, even long beyond the period recommended by the therapist or physician. As in other areas of traditional medicine, the psychological aspects of injury and treatment deserve further study.

Nowhere in the published literature has it been reported that functional knee bracing causes harm. And a rather substantial body of evidence tends to support the scientific efficacy of functional knee bracing. Enhanced mechanical stability, restoration of kinematics, potential strain protection of the remodeling graft, and enhanced neurosensory function have all been reported. Despite this, many clinicians question the validity of the data presented and instead rely on primarily anecdotal evidence in the decision process. A number of factors may be responsible for this attitude. With few exceptions, the scientific study of functional knee braces has been the exclusive province of clinicians. Brace manufacturers have not taken the lead in validation of their products, resulting in suspicion of manufacturer claims of brace efficacy. More importantly, there are no rigorously controlled prospective outcome data available to support the use of functional knee bracing. Traditionally, all that was required to sell a specific brand of brace was to apply the orthosis to a prominent athlete. To resolve remaining questions about the scientific efficacy of functional knee braces, manufacturers must take a more active role in the validation of their products. Likewise, clinicians must work more closely with manufacturers in this regard to produce rigorously controlled, long-term outcome studies that address not only mechanical issues but also psychological and cost issues.

References

1. Adams FR: The Genuine Works of Hippocrates. Translated from Greek, with preliminary discourse and annotations. New York, William Wood, 1891.
2. Galen: On The Usefulness of the Parts of the Body, 2 Vols. Translated, with introduction and commentary by MT May. Ithaca, Cornell University Press, 1968.
3. Paessler HH: The history of the cruciate ligaments: Some forgotten (or unknown) facts from Europe. Knee Surg Sports Traumatl Arthroscopy 1:13, 1993.
4. Baker BE, Van Hanswiyk E, Bogosian S, et al. A biomechanical study of the static stabilizing effect of knee braces on medial stability. Am J Sports Med 15:566, 1987.
5. Bassett GS, Fleming BW: The Lenox Hill brace in anterolateral rotatory instability. Am J Sports Med 11:345, 1989.
6. Beck C, Drez D Jr, Young J, et al. Instrumented testing of functional knee braces. Am J Sports Med 14:253, 1986.
7. Branch TP, Hunter R, Reynolds P: Controlling anterior tibial displacement under static load: A comparison of two braces. Orthopedics 11:1249, 1988.
8. Colville MR, Lee CL, Cuillo JV: The Lenox Hill brace: An evaluation of effectiveness in treating knee instability. Am J Sports Med 14:257, 1986.
9. Coughlin L, Oliver J, Barretta G: Knee bracing and anterolateral rotatory instability. Am J Sports Med 11:161, 1983.
10. Mishra DK, Daniel DM, Stone ML: The use of functional knee braces in control of pathologic anterior knee laxity. Clin Orthop Rel Res 241:213, 1989.
11. Mortenson WW, Foreman K, Daniel, DM, et al. An in vivo study of functional knee orthoses in the ACL disrupted knee. Orthop Res 13:520, 1988.
12. Wojtys EM, Goldstein SA, Redfern M, et al. A biomechanical evaluation of the Lenox Hill knee brace. Clin Orthop Rel Res 220:179, 1983.
13. Zogby RG, Baker BE, Seymour RJ, et al. A biomechanical evaluation of the effect of functional knee braces on anterior cruciate ligament instability using the Genucom Knee Analysis System. Trans Orthop Res Soc 14:212, 1989.
14. Soma CA, Vangsness CT, Cawley PW, Liu SH: Functional knee braces: The effects of rate of force application on anterior tibial translation in custom fit versus premanufactured braces. Presented at the 62nd Annual Meeting, American Academy of Orthopedic Surgeons, Orlando, FL, 17 May, 1995.
15. Branch TP, Hunter RE: Functional analysis of anterior cruciate ligament braces. Clin Sports Med 9(4):771, 1990.
16. Houston ME, Goemans PH: Leg muscle performance of athletes with and without knee support braces. Arch Phys Med Rehab 63:431, 1982.
17. Inglehart TK: Strength and Muscular Performance as Affected by the Carbon Titanium Knee Brace in Normal Healthy Males. Irvine, CA, Innovation Sports, 1985.
18. Tegner Y, Lysholm J: Derotation brace and knee function in patients with anterior cruciate ligament tears. Arthroscopy 1:264, 1985.
19. Tegner Y, Pettersson G, Lysholm J, et al. The effect of derotation braces on knee motion. Acta Orthop Scand 59:284, 1988.
20. Zetterlund AE, Serfass RC, Hunter RE: The effect of wearing the complete Lenox Hill Derotation brace on energy expenditure during horizontal treadmill running at 161 meters per minute. Am J Sports Med 14:73, 1986.
21. Cawley PW, France EP, Paulos LE: The current state of functional knee brace research. Am J Sports Med 19(3):226, 1991.

22. Knutzen KM, Bates BT, Hamill J: Electromyography of post-surgical knee bracing in running. Am J Phys Med 62:172, 1983.
23. Knutzen KM, Bates BT, Schot P, et al. A biomechanical investigation of two functional knee braces. Med Sci Sport Exerc 19:303, 1987.
24. Cook FF, Tibone JE, Redfern FC: A dynamic analysis of a functional brace for anterior cruciate ligament insufficiency. Am J Sports Med 17:519, 1989.
25. Branch TP, Hunter R, Donath M: Dynamic EMG analysis of anterior cruciate deficient knees with and without bracing during cutting. Am J Sports Med 17:35, 1989.
26. Branch TP, Indelicato PA, Riley S, Miller G: Kinematic analysis of anterior cruciate deficient subjects during side-step cutting with and without a functional knee brace. Clin J Sports Med 3:86, 1993.
27. Noyes FR, Mooar PA, Mathews Ds, et al. The symptomatic anterior cruciate deficient knee: Part 1: The long-term functional disability in athletically active individuals. J Bone Joint Surg 65A:154, 1983.
28. Hirshman HP, Daniel DM, Miyasaka K: The fate of unoperated knee ligament injuries. In Daniel DM, Akeson WH, O'Connor JJ (eds): Knee Ligaments: Structure, Function, Injury, and Repair. New York, Raven Press, 1991, p.481.
29. Fuss FK: Optimal replacement of the cruciate ligaments from the functional-anatomical point of view. Acta Anat 140:260, 1991.
30. Hefzy MS, Grood ES: Sensitivity of insertion locations on length patterns of anterior cruciate ligament fibers. J Biomech Eng 108:73, 1986.
31. Lewis JL, Lew WD, Hill JA, et al. Knee joint motion and ligament forces before and after ACL reconstruction. J Biomech Eng 111:97, 1989.
32. Daniel DM, Stone ML, Dobson BE, et al. Fate of the ACL injured patient: A prospective outcome study. Am J Sports Med 22:632, 1994.
33. Wojtys EM, Kothari SU, Huston LJ: Anterior cruciate ligament functional brace use in sports. Am J Sports Med 24(4):539, 1996.
34. Amiel D, Kleiner JB, et al. The phenomenon of "ligamentization": Anterior cruciate ligament reconstruction with autogenous patellar tendon. J Orthop Res 4:162, 1986.
35. Arnoczky SP, Warren RF, Ashock MA: Replacement of the anterior cruciate ligament using patellar tendon autograft. J Bone Joint Surg 68A(3):176, 1986.
36. Kleiner JB, Amiel D, et al: Early histologic, metabolic, and vascular assessment of anterior cruciate ligament autografts. J Orthop Res 7:235, 1989.
37. Ballock RT, Woo SL-Y, et al. Use of patellar tendon autograft for anterior cruciate ligament reconstruction in the rabbit: Long-term histological and biomechanical study. J Orthop Res 7:184, 1987.
38. Woo SL-Y, Ohland KJ, McMahon PJ: Biology, healing, and repair of ligaments. In Finerman GAM, Noyes FR (eds): Biology and Biomechanics of the Traumatized Synovial Joint: The Knee as a Model. Rosemont, IL, American Academy of Orthopedic Surgeons, 1992, p. 241.
39. Shino K, Inoue M, et al. Maturation of allograft tendons transplanted into the knee: An arthroscopic and histologic study. J Bone Joint Surg 70B:556, 1988.
40. Weisman G, Pope MH, Johnson RJ: The effect of cyclic loading on knee ligaments. Trans Orthop Res Soc 4:24, 1979.
41. Viidik A: Structure and function of normal healing tendons and ligaments. In Abstracts of the First World Congress of Biomechanics, La Jolla, CA, 1991.
42. Clayton ML, Weir GJ Jr: Experimental investigations of ligamentous healing. Am J Surg 98:373, 1959.
43. Beynnon BD, Pope MH, et al. The effect of functional knee braces on anterior cruciate ligament strain in vivo. J Bone Joint Surg 74(9):1298, 1992.
44. Beynnon BD, Johnson RJ, et al. The effect of functional knee bracing on the anterior cruciate ligament in the weightbearing and nonweightbearing knee. Am J Sports Md 25(3):353, 1997.
45. Losse GM, Howard ME, Cawley PW: Effect of functional knee bracing on neurosensory function in the lower extremity in a group of anterior cruciate deficient knees. Presented to the American Academy of Orthopedic Surgeons, 63rd Annual Meeting, Atlanta, GA, Feb 24, 1996.
46. Cawley PW: Functional knee bracing for skiing. A review of factors affecting brace choice. Top Acute Care Trauma Rehab 3:73, 1988.
47. France EP, Cawley PW, Paulos LE: Choosing functional knee braces. Clin Sports Med 9(4):743, 1990.
48. Cawley PW: Some psychological aspects associated with bracing of the knee following reconstructive surgery. Presented at the Staff Sports Medicine Symposium, Mission Bay Hospital, San Diego, CA, May 19, 1984.
49. Walker PS, Emerson R, et al. The kinematic rotating hinge: Biomechanical and clinical application. Orthop Clin North Am 31(1):187, 1982.
50. Rovick JS, Reuben JD, et al. An experimental study of knee kinematics in vitro. Presented at the RESNA 8th Annual Conference, Memphis, TN 1985.
51. Walker PS, Kurosawa H, Rovick JS, Zimmerman BS: External knee joint design based or normal knee motion. J Rehab Res Dev 22(1):9, 1985.
52. Regalbuto MA, Rovick JS, et al. The forces in a knee brace as a function of hinge design and placement. Am J Sports Med 17(4):535, 1989.
53. France EP, Paulos LE: In vitro assessment of prophylactic knee brace function. Clin Sports Med 9(4):823, 1990.

19 Anterior Cruciate Ligament Injury in the Female Athlete

Lori Thein Brody, MS, PT, SCS, ATC

*T*he movement of women off the bench and onto the playing field is a relatively recent phenomenon. Although the young female athlete of today presumes sports participation to be a normal aspect of any girl's life, it has not always been so. Kathy Switzer's 1967 Boston Marathon run, the 1973 Billie Jean King vs. Bobby Riggs tennis match, and the 1986 entry of girls into high school football are milestone events in women's sporting history. It was not until 1983 that the first all-woman's triathlon was held, and in 1986 an athletic shoe company opened the first women's division.[1] The pivotal event in current women's sporting history is the passage of the Higher Education Act of 1972 with its Title IX provision. Title IX requires equal treatment of men and women in sport, as it states, "no person in the U.S. shall, on the basis of sex be excluded from participation in, or denied the benefits of, or be subjected to discrimination under any educational program or activity receiving federal aid." This provision required that schools receiving federal funds provide athletic opportunities for men and women in equal proportion to the enrollment in the general student body.[2]

Since that time, sports participation by girls of all ages has exploded. The number of girls in interscholastic sports programs increased by 600 percent between 1970 and 1979.[3] In 1989, an estimated 333,149 girls were playing high school basketball, compared with 380,783 boys.[4] Overall, intercollegiate opportunities for female athletes continues to increase, with basketball, volleyball, tennis, cross country, and softball the five most popular sports.[5] However, disparity still exists at many levels. An estimated 1.85 million girls participate annually in interscholastic sports, compared with 3.5 million boys. At the collegiate level, there are 186,045 males and 96,467 females on NCAA teams.[2] Male college athletes receive roughly $179 million more per year in athletic scholarships than female college athletes.[2] Only 28.9 percent of the 1992 Barcelona Olympics participants were female.[1, 6]

Although the female's increased sports participation has been praised by most, a concern has arisen over the consequences of this participation. One possible consequence is an increase in injuries among female athletes, and particularly injuries to the anterior cruciate ligament (ACL). The purpose of this chapter is to investigate the relationship between ACL injuries and the female athlete as well as possible contributors to this relationship.

EPIDEMIOLOGY OF INJURY

Does a difference in the incidence of ACL injuries between male and female athletes exist, or are female's injuries simply a reflection of increased participation? Epidemiologic studies generally express the injury rate as the number of injuries per 1000 exposures. An *exposure* implies participation in one practice or game where an injury might occur. A *reportable injury* is one that requires medical attention and results in restriction from play for 1 or more days. The number of ACL injuries encountered in various athletic and clinical settings has been documented. In a prospective study of 902 high school athletes, the risk of ACL injury was 1 in 39 for the males and 1 in 25 for the females. Overall the incidence of ACL injury was 1.6/100 players/year, a rate 1000 times that of the nonathletic population.[7] The National Athletic Trainers Association found that 22.8 percent of the high school girls and 22.1 percent of the high school boys sustained an injury during basketball.[4] However, the girls sustained more moderate and major injuries while the boys sustained more minor injuries. Of the basketball injuries, the girls injured their knee 18 percent of the time, compared with 10 percent for the boys. Moreover, more of the girls went on to surgery (3.4 percent) than the boys (2.5 percent). Whieldon and Cerny[6] found conflicting results in their prospective study at four high schools. Varsity boys in contact sports had significantly higher total injuries per 100 athletes and per 1000 exposures than varsity girls in contact sports.

Gray et al.[8] studied female basketball player's injuries and found the knee to be injured 72 percent of the time, with the ACL accounting for 25 percent of knee injuries. A total of 19 ACL ruptures were found in women compared with four in men. The incidence of adolescent female ACL injuries was five times that of their male counterparts, with the mean age of injury of 17 ± 1.5 years. The mechanism of injury was landing from a jump 58 percent of the time, pivoting 38 percent of the time, and being knocked down in 4 percent of cases. Zillmer et al.[9] studied injury patterns in 2392 female and 2683 male high school varsity basketball players over two seasons. During that time, 734 injuries occurred involving 536 players, of which 14 percent in females and 8 percent in males involved the knee. The females had more severe knee injuries, and 21 percent of the females went on to surgery compared with 18 percent of the males. Of the major injuries sustained by girls, 58 percent involved the knee.

The National Collegiate Athletic Association (NCAA) has been keeping statistics on injuries since 1982 as part of its *Injury Surveillance System*. Injury data are collected on a sample of representative institutions. Comparing ACL injury rates in women versus men showed a women-to-men ratio of 3.17 in gymnastics (0.52:0.17), 2.30 in soccer (0.31:0.13), 3.72 in basketball (0.23:0.06), and 0.76 in lacrosse (0.15:0.19). The only male sport with ACL injury rates approaching those found in sports where women participated was spring football, with an injury rate of 0.23 per 1000 exposures.[10]

Similar statistics were found in another collegiate study. Twenty-nine institutions representing the Atlantic Coast, Big Ten, and Pacific Ten conferences of the NCAA were surveyed for ACL injuries and the total number of participants over a 5-year period.[11] Data were obtained from the NCAA *Injury Surveillance Report*. The prevalence of ACL injuries was 2.1 percent in the males and 19.3 percent in the females. This produced

an odds ratio of 8.38, or an eight times greater likelihood of ACL injury in the female. Arendt and Dick[12] also studied injury patterns among collegiate basketball players over a 5-year period. Knee injuries constituted 19 percent of all women's injuries and 12 percent of all men's injuries. The knee injury rate (per 1000 exposures) was 0.70 for men's basketball and 1.0 for women's. When looking at specific structures within the knee, an interesting pattern was found. The rate of injury to the ACL and meniscus were significantly higher in the women, whereas all other injury patterns were remarkably similar (Table 19–1). The likelihood of ACL injury was four times greater in females than in males. Additionally, a greater percentage of women's injuries were noncontact.

Similar collegiate level studies were also conducted on soccer players over a 5-year period. Data were collected on 461 men's teams and 278 women's teams. Again, more knee injuries occurred in the female athletes, with a knee injury rate per 1000 exposures of 1.6 for women and 1.3 for men. Knee injuries constituted 19 percent of all women's soccer injuries and 16 percent of all men's soccer injuries. The ACL injury rate in women was more than double that of men, with similar disparity in the meniscal tear rate (0.34 in women vs. 0.19 in men)

◑━ Table 19–1. Knee Injury Rates for Men's and Women's Basketball from 1989 to 1993

Injured Structure	Men's Basketball		Women's Basketball		P†
	Number	Rate*	Number	Rate*	
Collateral ligament	158	0.21	181	0.28	.01
Torn cartilage (meniscus)	100	0.13	189	0.29	.00
Patella or patellar tendon	196	0.26	158	0.24	—
Anterior cruciate ligament	49	0.07	189	0.29	.00
Posterior cruciate ligament	5	0.01	9	0.01	—

*Rate based on injuries per 1000 athlete-exposures. Athlete-exposures: men's, 626,223; women's, 308,748.
†Probability based on χ^2 tables
From Arendt E, Dick R: Knee injury patterns among men and women in collegiate basketball and soccer. NCAA data and review of the literature. Am J Sports Med 23(6):694–701, 1995.

Table 19–2. Knee Injury Rates for Men's and Women's Soccer from 1989 to 1993

Injured Structure	Men's Soccer		Women's Soccer		
	Number	*Rate**	*Number*	*Rate**	*P†*
Collateral ligament	316	0.51	192	0.62	.02
Torn cartilage (meniscus)	119	0.19	105	0.34	.00
Patella or patellar tendon	130	0.21	92	0.30	.01
Anterior cruciate ligament	81	0.13	97	0.31	.00
Posterior cruciate ligament	22	0.04	12	0.04	—

*Rate based on injuries per 1000 athlete-exposures. Athlete-exposures: men's, 626,223; women's, 308,748.
†Probability based on χ^2 tables
From Arendt E, Dick R: Knee injury patterns among men and women in collegiate basketball and soccer. NCAA data and review of the literature. Am J Sports Med 23(6):694–701, 1995.

(Table 19–2). Again, a greater percentage of women's ACL injuries were noncontact.[12]

At the national level, a study of U.S. Olympic Basketball trial participants found females to sustain more knee injuries and to require more surgery than their male counterparts.[11] Eleven of 80 male participants sustained knee injuries, 3 of which were ACL injuries. In contrast, 34 of 64 females sustained knee injuries, 13 of which were ACL injuries. A sample of 52 volleyball players participating at various levels in the Italian National Championship was studied to determine factors related to ACL injury.[13] Of the 52 ACL-injured players, 42 were women and 10 were men. The initial injury occurred during game play in 32 of 52 cases, and during a phase of jumping in 48 of 52 injuries. Of these, the injuries occurred during "smashing" in 38 and while blocking in 10. Only two players were hurt as the result of contact with another player. This finding is consistent with other studies suggesting jumping activities as a major source of ACL injuries in female athletes.

Clearly a disparity in the incidence of ACL injuries between male and female athletes exists. The likelihood of an ACL injury in a female athlete ranges from 3 to 10 times higher than in a male in the same sport. Although more females are now participating in sports, the total numbers of females is still less than of males. Despite the lower numbers, the number of injuries per exposure is still greater in women. Some possible causes and potential solutions will be explored.

CONTRIBUTING FACTORS

A number of factors have been suggested as potential causes or contributing factors to the high rate of ACL injuries in females. Delineating interrelated factors is difficult with current measurement techniques. For example, physiologic laxity, hamstring flexibility, and proprioception are potential contributors that may be related. Determining primary and secondary causes and avenues for successful preventative intervention are difficult at this time. However, some research studies have shed light on these issues. They will be roughly categorized as intrinsic or extrinsic factors (Table 19–3). Some factors have both intrinsic and extrinsic components (eg, flexibility, posture).

Extrinsic Factors

TRAINING AND CONDITIONING
Differences in the training and conditioning between male and female athletes may underlie the ACL injury disparity. An unintended consequence of Title IX may have been an explosion in the number of inexperienced participants. Prior to the implementation of Title IX, those girls with natural athletic ability were drawn to sports, whereas other girls self-selected other activities. The increase in sports availability may have produced a larger pool of less skilled players, resulting in an increased ACL injury rate.

Table 19–3. Factors Associated with Anterior Cruciate Ligament Injuries in Female Athletes

Extrinsic Factors
1. Training and conditioning
2. Coaching
3. Position

Intrinsic Factors
1. Hamstring flexibility
2. Physiologic laxity
3. Hormonal effects
4. Posture
5. Notch size

That is, compared with boys who participate in sports from a very young age, girls initially entered sports at an older preteen or teen age. If this is the case, the number of ACL injuries in females should approach that of the males in the coming years as females begin participation at an earlier age. This is yet to be seen.

A cohort of male and female basketball players were studied to determine force production characteristics of leg extensor and trunk flexor and extensor muscles.[14] As expected, the absolute values for strength and vertical jumping height were greater for the males. However, the time needed to produce the same relative torque was greater in the female. Additionally, the females produced less force relative to body weight than the males. These results suggest that torque production deficits are not fully accounted for by body weight differences, and that a difference in the type or volume or preparatory training may exist.

In contrast, the high number of ACL injuries in women at the intercollegiate, Olympic, and professional levels would suggest that training and conditioning are not factors. One would certainly believe that the female athlete at this level of competition would be well-trained and conditioned. Despite this, a high injury rate persists in this population. However, the issue of training and conditioning may not be one of volume or specific drills, but *how* those drills are done. A study by Hewett et al.[15] evaluated the impact of a jump-training program on the landing mechanics and lower extremity strength in female athletes involved in jumping sports. A group of 11 female high school volleyball players and a group of 9 males matched to height and weight were studied throughout a 6-week jump-training program. A key component of their training was learning the neuromuscular control of landing, or *how* to land correctly, rather than simple plyometric drilling. The four basic techniques taught were (1) correct posture and body alignment throughout the jump, (2) straight vertical jumping without antero-posterior or lateral sway, (3) soft landing with flexed knees and toe-to-heel rocking, and (4) instant recoil in preparation for the next jump. These skills were taught in the first, or technique, phase (phase I). This was followed by the fundamentals phase (phase II) and the performance phase (phase III). Post-training testing showed a 22 percent decrease in the

peak landing forces and a 50 percent reduction in knee adduction and abduction moments. Hamstring muscle power increased 44 percent on the dominant side and 21 percent on the nondominant side, and vertical jump height increased 10 percent. These findings support a focus on *how training is carried out*, not just the overall drill choice (Table 19–4). Improved control and efficiency of movement were altered by coaching in technique, not sports skills. This factor is a critical component of the training and conditioning and coaching programs.

COACHING

Related to training and conditioning is the issue of coaching. Another unintended consequence of Title IX was the loss of women's head coaching and administrative positions to men. In 1972, prior to the enactment of Title IX, 90 percent of women's collegiate athletic programs were administrated by women. In 1992, that proportion was 16.8 percent.[2] The number of women heading a merged men's and women's athletic department were 2 in 107, 3 in 88, and 3 in 103 in Division IA, IAA, and IAAA, respectively.[16] Before 1972, more than 90 percent of women's teams were coached by women; that number has since diminished to approximately 48 percent. Although the number of women holding these positions increased by 181 from 1982 to 1992, men still hold 631 more of these positions than women.[2] Moreover, coaches of women's sports are paid less than coaches of male sports, and within women's sports, the female coaches are paid less than the male coaches.[2]

The questions of whether women need to be coached differently from men and the relationship of coaching to ACL injury are still unanswered. However, some data exist suggesting that coaching and training techniques may influence *how* a female plays. It is possible that females need a different coaching emphasis than males at some levels. Perhaps more emphasis at a younger age should be placed on fundamentals of starting, stopping, acceleration, deceleration, jumping and so on, rather than on specific sports skills. The Hewett et al.[15] study referred to in the previous section supports neuromuscular training techniques to improve these fundamental skills.

Griffis et al.[17] implemented a program of improved fundamental player techniques in

● **Table 19-4. Sample Jump-Training Program***†

Exercise	Repetitions or Time	
Phase I: Technique	**Week 1**	**Week 2**
1. Wall jumps	20 sec	25 sec
2. Tuck jumps‡	20 sec	25 sec
3. Broad jumps stick land	5 reps	10 reps
4. Squat jumps‡	10 sec	15 sec
5. Double-leg cone jumps‡	30 sec/30 sec	30 sec/30 sec (side-to-side & back-to-front)
6. 180-degree jumps	20 sec	25 sec
7. Bounding in place	20 sec	25 sec
Phase II: Fundamentals	**Week 3**	**Week 4**
1. Wall jumps	30 sec	30 sec
2. Tuck jumps‡	30 sec	30 sec
3. Jump, jump, jump, vertical jump	5 reps	8 reps
4. Squat jumps‡	20 sec	20 sec
5. Bounding for distance	1 run	2 runs
6. Double leg cone jumps‡	30 sec/30 sec	30 sec/30 sec (side-to-side & back-to-front)
7. Scissor jump	30 sec	30 sec
8. Hop, hop, stick land‡	5 reps/leg	5 reps/leg
Phase III: Performance	**Week 5**	**Week 6**
1. Wall jumps	30 sec	30 sec
2. Step, jump up, down, vertical	5 reps	10 reps
3. Mattress jumps	30 sec/30 sec	30 sec/30 sec (side-to-side & back-to-front)
4. Single-legged jumps distance‡	5 reps/leg	5 reps/leg
5. Squat jumps‡	25 sec	25 wec
6. Jump into bounding‡	3 runs	4 runs
7. Single-legged hop, hop stick	5 reps/leg	5 reps/leg

*Emphasis was on quality of jumping rather than simply performing plyometric exercises.
†Before jumping exercises, subjects did stretching (15–20 minutes), skipping (2 laps), and side shuffle (2 laps). After training, subjects did a cool-down walk (2 minutes) and stretching (5 minutes). Each jump exercise was followed by 30-second rest period.
‡These jumps performed on mats.
From Hewett TE, Stroupe AL, Nance TA, Noyes FR: Plyometric training in female athletes. Am J Sports Med 24(6):765–773, 1996.

a junior college women's basketball program over the course of two seasons. The three fundamental movement patterns of focus were (1) plant and cut, (2) straight knee landings, and (3) one-step stop. In their experience, planting and cutting accounted for 29 percent of all ACL injuries, whereas straight knee landings and deceleration accounted for 28 percent and 26 percent of ACL injuries, respectively. Rather than a plant and cut to change directions, the athletes were taught an accelerated rounded turn technique. This prevents sudden deceleration and allows the athlete to continue accelerating through the turn rather than abruptly stopping and changing direction. The straight knee landings were improved by teaching a bent-knee landing. This prevents the hyperextension injury frequently seen on landings. Finally, the players were taught to take a three-step stop when decelerating rather than the single step stop commonly used. This prevents the sudden deceleration with a straight knee, a common cause of ACL injuries. After implementation of this program, the incidence of ACL injuries decreased by 89 percent.[18]

POSITION

An athlete's position may have an impact on ACL injuries. This factor is closely related to specific skill training. In their study of basketball players, Gray et al.[8] examined player position relative to the mechanism of injury. Of the nine centers injured, six were injured while landing from a jump, two from pivoting, and one from being knocked down. In contrast, those playing guard were injured as a result of pivoting 78 percent of the time. The center spends more time jumping, whereas the guards twist and pivot more often, and these positional differences are reflected in the respective mechanisms of injury.

Zillmer et al.[9] looked at body characteristics as contributing factors to injuries in high school varsity basketball players. They found a significant relationship between knee injury and player sex and height. Short girls (66 inches or less) were more likely to sustain a knee injury than their teammates. The shorter girls may be more at risk because their height may better suit a guard position, which requires more twisting and pivoting. As such, the training, conditioning, and preventative measures should address the specific position within a sport.

Intrinsic Factors

HAMSTRING FLEXIBILITY

The role of the hamstring muscles in providing stability to the knee is clear both theoretically and clinically. It is theorized that because males tend to have shorter hamstring muscles, they maintain a more flexed knee posture, decreasing the chances of hyperextension. The relationship between hamstring flexibility and ACL injuries is yet to be clarified. Harner et al.[19] examined hamstring flexibility in 31 patients with bilateral noncontact ACL injuries and 23 control subjects. Hamstring flexibility was measured via a sit-and-reach test. No significant differences between the patients and control subjects were found. However, there was a significant difference in hamstring muscle tightness between men and women in the control group, with the women reaching farther than men. Loudon et al.[20] studied several factors related to static posture in a group of ACL-injured athletes and a control group. Hamstring length was measured via the hip flexion angle when the knee was placed in a neutral position. No differences were found between the ACL-injured group and the control group. However, within gender, the ACL-injured females had tighter hamstring muscles than the uninjured, whereas the opposite was true for the males.

PHYSIOLOGIC LAXITY

A greater inherent physiologic joint laxity in females over males has been considered as a factor in ACL injuries. A predisposition toward greater laxity, whether due to genetics or to hormonal differences, could differentially affect females versus males. Individuals possessing hypermobile joints are identified by at least three of the following findings: (1) hyperextension of the elbows, (2) hyperextension of the knees, (3) 90-degree hyperextension of the metacarpopha-

langeal joints, (4) ability to bring the thumb down to the volar surface of the forearm, and (5) ability to touch the palms of the hands on the floor with the knees extended.[21]

Hypermobile joints are associated with numerous problems such as patellar instability, shoulder instability, and rotator cuff injury.[22] In a study of male soldiers, those individuals with excessive laxity had significantly more musculoligamentous injuries than those with less laxity, particularly at the knee and ankle. When applied to ACL injuries, a knee with this type of laxity is called a *cruciate-dependent knee*.[10, 23] The cruciate-dependent knee relies more heavily on static ligamentous structures for stability than a more inherently stable joint.[10] The hyperextended posture common in females suggests posterior capsule laxity and, when combined with a reduced muscle mass, may result in greater dependence on the ACL for stability. The individual with this knee profile may be more likely to fail conservative treatment and to require surgery.[10] Additionally, this inherent hypermobility may increase the chances that the ACL graft may stretch, and rehabilitation may need to be modified accordingly.[24] This concept is particularly relevant in autograft ACL reconstructions, where the individual's own tissue is used to create a new ACL. The same collagen make-up of the graft tissue may predispose the graft to the same failure as the original ACL.

Questioning the supposition of greater physiologic laxity in female athletes, Brannan et al.[25] studied the anterior knee laxity in 30 intercollegiate gymnasts and in nongymnasts. All subjects were without a history of knee injury, and the control subjects were taken from physical education activity classes at a Division I university. The KT-1000 (MEDmetric Corporation, San Diego, CA) testing was performed and showed no difference between the gymnasts and the nongymnasts. However, no male population was used for comparison purposes, narrowing the application of results.

HORMONAL EFFECTS

Females may be more prone to hypermobility or to frank ACL injuries due to levels of hormones such as estrogen, progesterone, and relaxin.[10, 26] Estrogen has many effects on connective tissue, including increasing a tissue's sensitivity to relaxin. Relaxin subsequently produces laxity in the target tissue by decreasing the density and organization of collagen and increasing the ground substance. Progesterone also affects the collagenous make-up of musculoskeletal tissues. Estrogen and progesterone receptors are a prerequisite for the respective hormone action in a tissue. Both estrogen and progesterone target cells have been identified in the human ACL.[26] However, the mere presence of these receptors does not ensure specific action targeted to the ACL. In fact, estrogen and progesterone target cells were found in both male and female specimens.

Subsequently, the effects of 17β-estradiol on the cellular proliferation and collagen synthesis of fibroblasts derived from rabbit ACLs were studied.[27] The presence of these receptors in the rabbit was confirmed, a primary cell culture established, and the fibroblasts exposed to various concentrations of estrogen. The estrogen was increased in near log concentrations, ensuring levels consistent with those of the normal menstruating female (0.025–0.3 ng/mL).[27] Results showed declining collagen synthesis first noted at a 17β-estradiol level of 0.025 ng/mL. At estradiol concentrations between 0.025 and 0.25 ng/mL, collagen synthesis was reduced by more than 40 percent compared with control subjects. These findings suggest that fluctuation in serum estrogen levels throughout the menstrual cycle may affect collagen metabolism in the ACL. Whether these changes are significant enough to produce a change in the mechanical properties of the ACL is yet to be determined.

POSTURE

Related to hamstring flexibility and hypermobility is the issue of resting posture. Females have a wider pelvis, increased femoral anteversion, a greater knee valgus angulation, increased genu recurvatum, and greater external tibial torsion and foot pronation.[23] This static posture combined with poor dynamic muscular control (e.g., weak hip external rotators) can predispose the female athlete to multiple injuries, including ACL injuries. The increased anterior pelvic tilt associated with this posture makes a neutral knee position difficult. The default position associated with anterior pelvic tilt is knee hyperextension and excessive prona-

tion. This hyperextended position may impinge the ACL and, when combined with excessive rotation from pronation, may excessively load the ACL.

Loudon et al.[20] studied the relationship between several measures of static posture and ACL injury. They found genu recurvatum, the navicular drop test, and excessive subtalar joint pronation to be discriminators for those with ACL injuries. Similar findings were noted in a study of male and female interscholastic and intercollegiate athletes.[28] Athletes with ACL injuries had greater measures of navicular drop, suggesting that pronation was associated with ACL injury. Regression analysis indicated that the navicular drop test predicts injury status for 87.5 percent of the females and 70.5 percent of all cases. In contrast, Smith et al.[29] found no relationship between navicular drop test and ACL injuries. Using regression analysis, the authors were unable to predict group membership by navicular drop measurements.

NOTCH SIZE

The trochanteric notch size has gained attention as a potential predisposing factor to ACL injury. Noncontact ACL injuries are suggested to occur more frequently in those individuals with intercondylar notch stenosis. It is unclear whether the stenosis itself underlies the ACL injuries, or if the stenosis is a sign of a congenitally smaller ACL, with a smaller load to failure. Defining stenosis is the first step in determining this relationship.

Notch morphology measurement has focused on the anterior and posterior openings of the intercondylar notch and the total condylar width. Some authors have measured the actual size of the openings,[30, 31] whereas others have compared a ratio of the opening to the total condylar width.[7, 32–34] Houseworth et al.[35] compared three ratios from notch view radiographs in 50 individuals with acute ACL injuries and in 50 control subjects. Ratios were determined using a computer graphics station. Anterior, posterior, and total area were determined and ratios calculated. The authors found a significantly smaller posterior-to-total ratio in those with acute ACL injuries.

Most authors have focused on measurement of the anterior notch opening.[7, 30, 31, 33, 34] Good et al.[30] measured the widest portion of the anterior outlet of the intercondylar notch in 93 patients with chronic ACL-deficient knees, in 62 patients with acute ACL injuries, and in 38 cadaver knees. Significant differences were found between all groups, with the chronic ACL group having the smallest opening (16.1)mm, followed by the acutely injured group (18.1 mm) and the cadaveric group (20.4 mm). Lund-Hanssen et al.[31] used notch view radiographs to determine the notch width index (NWI), defined as the ratio of the anterior notch width to total condylar width. A ratio was used to eliminate problems due to individual size and magnification. Measurements were taken in a group of 20 female handball players with unilateral ACL injuries and in 26 control subjects. The NWI of 0.224 in the injured players was significantly smaller than the 0.243 in the control subjects. In athletes with an anterior notch opening of 17 mm or less, the risk of ACL injury was seven times higher. The same trend of increasing injury risk with decreasing NWI was seen.

LaPrade and Burnett[36] performed a 2-year prospective study of 213 Division I intercollegiate athletes. Bilateral intercondylar notch view radiographs were taken on all athletes. The average NWI was 0.244 ± 0.036 for males and 0.238 ± 0.037 for females. Seven athletes with an average NWI of 0.193 ± 0.013 (0.188 ± 0.013 for males and 0.200 ± 0.010 for females) tore their ACL. Six of those injuries occurred during cutting or planting and one by direct contact. When defining a stenotic knee as one with an NWI of 0.20 or less, the odds of an ACL tear in a stenotic knee was 66 times higher than in a nonstenotic knee. An NWI of 0.20 is outside the range of 1 standard deviation (SD) of the mean. This is in agreement with Souryal et al.[7] in a study of 783 ACL-injured patients. The NWI of those sustaining noncontact ACL injuries averaged 0.189 (0.165 for females and 0.214 for males), whereas the NWI in contact injuries was 0.233. They defined "critical stenois" as 0.20 in males and 0.18 in females. Those greater than 1 SD from the threshold were 26 times more likely to tear their ACL.

Notch stenosis is suggested to be a factor in nonsimultaneous bilateral ACL injuries.[34, 37] Studies of bilateral nonsimultaneous ACL injuries found an incidence range from 2 to 9.6 percent.[33, 37] Souryal et al.[34] found no difference in NWI between normal subjects and those with acute ACL injuries, whereas those with bilateral injuries had a significantly smaller NWI. Using computed tomography, Anderson found patients with unilateral and bilateral ACL injuries to have a smaller maximum notch width to condylar width ratio.

The relationship between ACL injury and the NWI has been challenged by some. Herzog et al.[32] validated imaging techniques using radiology, magnetic resonance imaging, and direct cadaveric dissection. The plain film measurements were significantly different from the direct measurements, whereas the magnetic resonance imaging measurements were not different from the direct measurements. All radiographic measurements were greater than the direct or magnetic resonance imaging measurements. In the second part of the study, 20 asymptomatic athletes with chronic ACL insufficiency were compared with 20 matched control subjects. No difference was found for notch measurements on magnetic resonance images or radiographs. Tietz et al.[38] studied the symmetry of the femoral notch width index in 40 male and 40 female patients, half of whom had noncontact ACL injuries. The authors found that the notch width indexes of right and left knees were symmetrical regardless of sex or injury status, and that there was no difference in notch width index between patients with and without ACL injuries.

Although some conflicting evidence exists, some relationship between ACL injuries and notch stenosis is present. It is unknown whether notch size itself is the issue or whether notch size is a marker for some other factor. Currently, most ACL reconstructions include notchplasty as a routine procedure. How findings of notch stenosis prior to ACL injury will interplay with prevention measures is yet to be determined.

PREVENTION

Prevention of ACL injuries in female athletes must focus on factors over which we have control. Routinely performing a notchplasty during ACL reconstruction may prevent a reinjury but does not prevent the initial injury. Aspects of prevention that may be instituted prior to ACL injury focus on coaching, coordination, and fundamental skill development. Fundamental skill development should be carried out at the youngest possible age, without interfering with the "play" aspects of sport in the very young. These skills include jumping, landing, direction changes, starting, and stopping. Basic balance and coordination exercises can also be included and tend to be challenging yet fun for young athletes. Part of the training program should focus on postural education and body awareness. Training in these areas provides the foundation for movement patterns that minimize the risk of injury. Performing basketball skill drills will not prevent ACL injuries if the athlete's posture of choice is knee hyperextension.

Rationale for Training the Nervous System

Neurologic control of the knee is commonly emphasized in knee rehabilitation programs following injury or surgery, but is rarely addressed in prevention programs. Closed chain, balance, and proprioception exercises are examples of activities used to train the nervous system. Several factors support the importance of this type of training. Poorer joint position sense was found in a group of patients with ACL-deficient knees when compared to age-matched control subjects.[39] A poor correlation exists between clinical ligament testing and proprioception, whereas accuracy of proprioception and functional outcome are correlated with patient satisfaction. In a separate study, a significant correlation between differential hamstring latency and the frequency of "giving way" existed.[40]

The muscle and muscle spindle system along with the afferent system at the joint play an important role in joint stability. Because joint afferents are activated throughout the range of motion, they play a major role in muscle stiffness regulation, rather than simply serving as "limit detectors."[41, 42] Pope et al.[43] demonstrated that the pain response produced from valgus stress on the medial collateral ligament does not travel quickly enough to initiate muscular reaction to prevent an injury. Even when the same situation was analyzed using knee joint afferent fibers (which are faster than pain fibers), time was still inadequate to prevent injury. Muscle stiffness, a result of training

and regulated to some extent by joint afferents, represents the first line of defense against pertubations. Muscle contraction causes a significant increase in the stiffness of the knee joint, whereas simultaneous co-contraction of agonists and antagonists further increases the joint stability.[42]

The relationship between muscle stiffness in joint stability highlights the importance of muscle firing patterns during exercise. Closed chain exercise presumes muscle co-contraction about a joint. However, the hamstrings are not always fully active during closed chain exercise, and this finding may provide a clue to why some athletes get injured.[44, 45] Differences in the muscle activation patterns during the same activity may predispose some individuals to injury. Therefore, training procedures should focus on active conscious muscle activation during specific activities.

Learning a skill, whether a simple skill such as jumping, or a complex task such as a gymnastics routine, follows a learning path. The activity is initially *cognitive* and requires attention to the task. Gross motor strategies to deal with the problem are developed. In this phase, the athlete must provide conscious attention to body position and muscle activation. Appropriate coaching can lead to postures and muscle activation patterns that minimize injury. The next phase is the *associative*, in which strategies are further refined and movement patterns become more efficient. The final stage is the *autonomous*, in which little cognitive processing is necessary. The goal of an effective training program is to get the athlete to the autonomous phase, choosing postures and muscle activation patterns that minimize the risk of injury.

POSTURAL TRAINING

Postural retraining exercises may improve lower extremity posture. The key posture in the prevention of ACL injuries is the maintenance of a slightly flexed knee posture. However, knee posture is intricately linked with lumbopelvic posture, and this must be addressed simultaneously. Maintenance of a neutral spine posture minimizes the hyperextended knee posture commonly associated with an exaggerated lumbar lordosis. Teaching the athlete to keep the knees slightly flexed is difficult in the presence of excessive lumbar lordosis, and, as such, the closed chain relationships in the lower extremity joints must be addressed. Training the proprioceptive system so that the slightly flexed knee position is the "neutral" position may prevent the female athlete from seeking hyperextension as the "default" or position of comfort (Fig. 19–1). This posture should be reinforced during all other skill training activities.

BALANCE AND COORDINATION TRAINING

Balance and coordination training should include both open and closed chain exercise. It is prudent to recall that many of the ACL injuries incurred by female athletes are the result of landing from a jump. If the incorrect motor program is selected mid-air (in an open chain), closing the chain on landing will not prevent the injury. At that point, the afferent input to the system does not travel rapidly enough to prevent an injury. Thus, the athlete must preactivate the appropriate muscles and choose the optimal

posture to ensure a safe landing. This choice occurs in an open chain. Open chain active repositioning exercises with or without resistance can be used for open chain training. An isokinetic device with a very narrow torque range (5 to 10 ft-lb between upper and lower limit) can be used to train an athlete to activate her quadricep or hamstring muscles at a certain level. Combination open and closed chain exercises such as jumping or hopping can be used, with emphasis on presetting appropriate muscle activity and posture prior to landing.

Closed chain exercises using a variety of foam rollers, balance board, or balance beams may be a routine part of physical education classes or team practices. These exercises should emphasize proper posture throughout the legs, spine, and shoulders, with a focus on quality rather than quantity. The issue is not whether the athlete performs the exercise, but *how* she carries out the exercise. Based on motor learning techniques, early training requires feedback and information about posture and muscle acti-

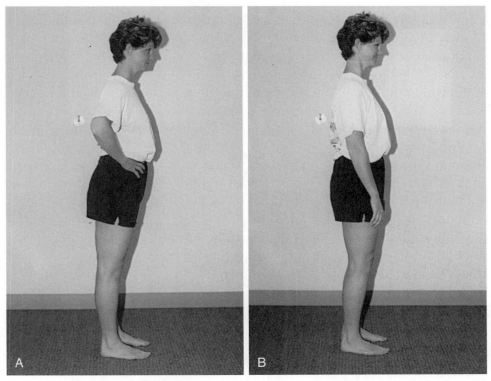

Figure 19–1. *A*, Standing in an extended lumbopelvic posture results in hyperextension at the knee joint. *B*, Correction of the lumbopelvic posture by finding neutral spine allows the knees to maintain a neutral or slightly flexed position. Neuromuscular retraining is now necessary to ensure maintenance of this posture as the "default" posture.

vation. As proficiency improves, the exercise difficulty should be progressively increased. Exercises progress from double support to single leg balance and may incorporate movement patterns specific to the athlete's sport or implements routinely used. Equipment can be used in a variety of ways to achieve this progressive difficulty (Fig. 19–2).

The pool may be used for balance and coordination exercises. The hydrodynamics of water provide tremendous balance challenges. Single-leg balance, postural training, and simple plyometric exercises in shallow water can teach fundamental skills. Additionally, open chain positional awareness drills in deep water prove particularly challenging. In this situation, no joint compres-

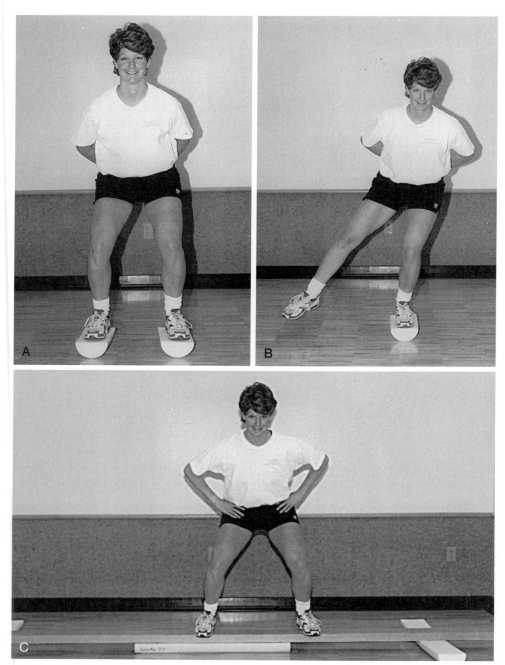

Figure 19–2 *See legend on opposite page*

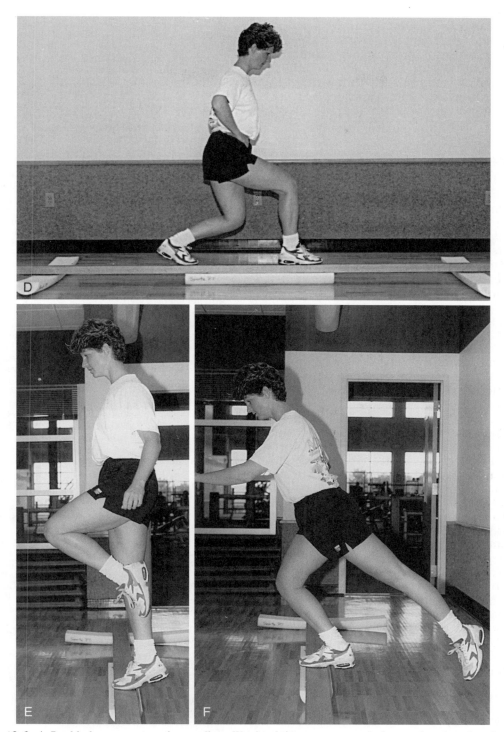

Figure 19–2. *A*, Double leg support on foam rollers. Weight shifting, eyes open and eyes closed, and various ball-handling skills can be performed in this position. *B*, Progression to single-leg balance on foam roller. Similar skills can be performed on a single leg. *C*, A balance beam can be placed on foam rollers to increase the challenge. Activities should be initiated in double stance, with frontal plane movements less challenging than sagittal. *D*, Sagittal plane movements performed on a balance beam on foam rollers. *E*, A toe-raise position increases the balance challenge. *F*, Positions that challenge postural mechanisms throughout the entire kinetic chain can enhance stability in awkward positions.

sive forces from weight-bearing are available to provide joint position information. The athlete must rely on muscle receptors to provide position input. Training the athlete in unfamiliar patterns such as backward bicycling in the deep water is particularly useful.

SUMMARY

A difference in ACL injuries in males versus females exists. The contributions to this finding are multifactorial and include both intrinsic and extrinsic factors. The relative weights of each of these factors in the ACL injury equation are yet to be delineated. Future research must focus on the interrelationships among these factors to devise effective strategies to prevent these injuries. In the meantime, prevention approaches must focus on factors that are amenable to intervention. Changes in coaching, training, and conditioning to include postural awareness, balance, and coordination training and fundamental technique (eg, jumping) training should be implemented at a young age. Training and conditioning must extend beyond mere strength and endurance training, just as coaching must reach beyond sports drills. These changes are not difficult and can be incorporated into traditional athletic programs with success.[18]

Finally, these differences in ACL and other injuries between females and males should be used to understand differences between male and female athletes, not to disqualify or discourage women from sports participation. The benefits of regular exercise continue to far outweigh the potential for injury. These benefits extend beyond the physical and reach to the emotional, psychological, and social as well. A better understanding of the differences between male and female athletes will improve the sporting experience for all.

References

1. Jaffe R: History of women in sport. *In* Agostini R (ed): Medical and Orthopedic Issues of Active and Athletic Women. St. Louis, MO, Hanley and Belfus, 1994, pp. 1–6.
2. Lopiano DA: Gender equity in sports. *In* Agostini R (ed): Medical and Orthopedic Issues of Active and Athletic Women. St. Louis, MO, Hanley and Belfus, 1994, pp. 13–27.
3. Boutilier MA, SanGiovanni L: The Sporting Woman. Champaign, IL, Human Kinetics Publishers, 1983.
4. Powell J: Injury toll in prep estimated at 1.3 million. J Athl Training 24(4):360–373, 1989.
5. Acosta RV, Carpenter LJ: Women in Intercollegiate Sport: A Longitudinal Study—a 19-Year Update 1997–1996. Brooklyn, NY, Brooklyn College, 1996.
6. Whieldon TJ, Cerny FJ: Incidence and severity of high school athletic injuries. J Athl Training 25(4):344–350, 1990.
7. Souryal TO, Freeman TR: Intercondylar notch size and anterior cruciate ligament injuries in athletes: A prospective study. Am J Sports Med 21(4):535–539, 1993.
8. Gray J, Taunton JE, McKenzie DC, Clement DB, McConkey JP, Davidson RG: A survey of injuries to the anterior cruciate ligament of the knee in female basketball players. Int J Sports Med 6:314–316, 1985.
9. Zillmer DA, Powell JW, Albright JP: Gender-specific injury patterns in high school varsity basketball. J Women's Health 1(1):69–76, 1992.
10. Hutchinson MR, Ireland ML: Knee injuries in female athletes. Sports Med 19(4):222–236, 1995.
11. Malone TR, Hardaker WT, Garrett WE, Feagin JA, Bassett FH: Relationship of gender to anterior cruciate ligament injuries in intercollegiate basketball players. J South Orth Assoc 2(1):36–39, 1993.
12. Arendt E, Dick R: Knee injury patterns among men and women in collegiate basketball and soccer. NCAA data and review of the literature. Am J Sports Med 23(6):694–701, 1995.
13. Ferretti A, Papandrea P, Conteduca F, Mariani PP: Knee ligament injuries in volleyball players. Am J Sports Med 20(2):203–207, 1992.
14. Hakkinen K: Force production characteristics of leg extensor, trunk flexor and extensor muscles in male and female basketball players. J Sports Med Phys Fitness 31(3):325–331, 1991.
15. Hewett TE, Stroupe AL, Nance TA, Noyes FR: Plyometric training in female athletes. Am J Sports Med 24(6):765–773, 1996.
16. 1992–1993 NCAA Directory. Overland Park, KS, National Collegiate Athletic Association, 1992.
17. Griffis ND, Vequist SW, Yearout KM: Injury prevention of the anterior cruciate ligament [abstract]. *In* American Orthopaedic Society for Sports Medicine: Meeting Abstracts, Symposia and Instructional Courses, 15th Annual Meeting Traverse City, MI, 1989.
18. Yearout K: Prevention of ACL injuries using improved player techniques. Presented at: Sports Physical Therapy Section Team Concept Meeting, Kona, Hawaii, 1988.
19. Harner CD, Paulos LE, Greenwald AE, Rosenberg TD, Cooley VC: Detailed analysis of patients with bilateral anterior cruciate ligament injureis. Am J Sports Med 22(1):37–43, 1994.
20. Loudon JK, Jenkins W, Loudon KL: The relationship between static posture and ACL injury in female athletes. J Orthop Sports Phys Ther 24(2):91–97, 1996.
21. Dubs L, Gschwend N: General joint laxity: Quantification and clinical relevance. Arch Orthop Trauma Surg 107:65–72, 1988.
22. Diaz MA, Estevez EC, Guijo PS: Joint hyperlaxity and musculoligamentous lesions: Study of a population of homogenous age, sex and physical exertion. Br J Rheumatol 2:112–120, 1993.

23. Ireland ML, Gaudette M, Crook S: ACL injuries in the female athlete. J Sport Rehab 6:97–110, 1997.
24. Hardin JA, Voight ML, Blackburn TA, Canner GC, Soffer SR: The effects of a "decelerated" rehabilitation following anterior cruciate ligament reconstruction on a hyperelastic female adolescent: A case study. J Orthop Sports Phys Ther 26(1):29–35, 1997.
25. Brannan TL, Schulthies SS, Myrer JW, Durrant E: A comparison of anterior knee laxity in female intercollegiate gymnasts to a normal population. J Athl Training 30(4):298–303, 1995.
26. Liu SH, Al-Shaikh R, Panossian V, Yang RS, Nelson SD, Soleiman N, et al: Primary immunolocalization of estrogen and progesterone target cells in the human anterior cruciate ligament. J Orthop Res 14:526–533, 1996.
27. Liu SH, Al-Shaikh R, Panossian V, Finerman GAM, Lane JM: Estrogen affects the cellular metabolism of the anterior cruciate ligament: A potential explanation for female athletic injury. Am J Sports Med 25(5):704–709, 1997.
28. Woodford-Rogers B, Cyphert L, Denegar CR: Risk factors for anterior cruciate ligament injury in high school and college athletes. J Athl Training 29(4):343–349, 1994.
29. Smith J, Szczerba JE, Arnold BL, Martin DE, Perrin DH: Role of hyperpronation as a possible risk factor for anterior cruciate ligament injuries. J Athl Training 32(1):25–29, 1997.
30. Good L, Odensten M, Gillquist J: Intercondylar notch measurements with special reference to anterior cruciate ligament surgery. Clin Orthop 263:185–189, 1991.
31. Lund-Hanssen H, Gannon J, Engebretsen L, Holen KJ, Anda S, Vatten L: Intercondylar notch width and the risk for anterior cruciate ligament rupture. Acta Orthop Scand 65(5):529–532, 1994.
32. Herzog RJ, Silliman JF, Hutton K, Rodkey WG, Steadman JR: Measurements of the intercondylar notch by plain film radiography and magnetic resonance imaging. Am J Sports Med 22(2):204–210, 1994.
33. Schickendantz MS, Weiker GG: The predictive value of radiographs in the evaluation of unilateral and bilateral anterior cruciate ligament injuries. Am J Sports Med 21(1):110–113, 1993.
34. Souryal TO, Moore HA, Evans JP: Bilaterality in anterior cruciate ligament injuries: Associated intercondylar notch stenosis. Am J Sports Med 16(5):449–454, 1988.
35. Houseworth SW, Mauro VJ, Mellon BA, Kiefer DA: The intercondylar notch in acute tears of the anterior cruciate ligament: A computer graphics study. Am J Sports Med 15(3):221–225, 1987.
36. LaPrade RF, Burnett QM: Femoral intercondylar notch stenosis and correlation to anterior cruciate ligament injuries. Am J Sports Med 22(2):198–203, 1994.
37. Anderson AF, Lipscomb AB, Liudahl KJ, Addlesonte RB: Analysis of the intercondylar notch by computed tomography. Am J Sports Med 15(6):547–552, 1987.
38. Tietz CC, Lind BK, Sacks BM: Symmetry of the femoral notch width index. Am J Sports Med 25(5):687–690, 1997.
39. Barrett DS: Proprioception and function after anterior cruciate reconstruction. J Bone Joint Surg 73B-5:833–837, 1991.
40. Beard DJ, Kyberd PJ, Fergusson CM, Dodd CA: Proprioception after rupture of the anterior cruciate ligament. J Bone Joint Surg 75B-2:311–315, 1993.
41. Hutton RS, Atwater SW: Acute and chronic adaptations of muscle proprioceptors in response to increased use. Sports Med 14(6):406–421, 1992.
42. Johansson H, Sjolander P, Solka P: A sensory role for cruciate ligaments. Clin Orthop 268:161–178, 1991.
43. Pope MH, Johnson RJ, Brown DW, Tighe C: The role of the musculature in injuries to the medial collateral ligament. J Bone Joint Surg 61A:398, 1979.
44. Brask B, Lueke R, Soderberg G: Electromyographic analysis of selected muscle during the lateral step-up exercise. Phys Ther 64:324–329, 1984.
45. Graham VL, Gehlsen GM, Edwards JA: EMG evaluation of closed and open kinetic chain knee rehabilitation exercises. J Athl Training 28(1):23, 1993.

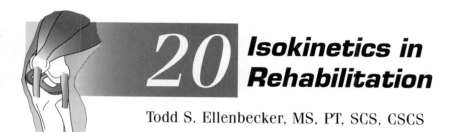

20 Isokinetics in Rehabilitation

Todd S. Ellenbecker, MS, PT, SCS, CSCS

Since the introduction of the first isokinetic dynamometer by J.J. Perrine in the late 1960s, the use of isokinetic dynamometers for musculoskeletal rehabilitation and performance enhancement has dramatically increased.[1] Despite the trend away from isokinetic open kinetic chain exercise toward what is referred to as more "functional" closed kinetic chain exercise, isokinetic dynamometers continue to provide a reliable resource for testing and training the musculature of the extremities and trunk.

Indications and rationale for the inclusion of isokinetic training and testing in rehabilitation of the patient following knee ligament injury are the primary focus of this chapter. One example is commonly used that clearly highlights the rationale for application of isokinetics based on research. In 1981, Wyatt and Edwards[2] published research showing that the human knee joint articulated at approximately 233 degrees per second during a normal gait pattern. Scientifically based research has been applied to rehabilitation with isokinetics, which has led to the use and inclusion of exercise that attempts to mimic the joint speeds and concentric and eccentric muscular activation demands inherent in functional activities. The use of 240 degrees per second as a testing and training speed has been advocated and included in rehabilitation programs for many years, based on this research finding and specificity principle.[3] The reader is also referred to Chapter 4 by Paine and Johnson for additional isokinetic testing information including standardized patient testing applications, and dynamometer specifications.

BASIC PRINCIPLES OF ISOKINETIC EXERCISE

The definition of isokinetic or constant "speed" exercise includes a fixed velocity that is preset and dependent on technology (currently 1 to 600 degrees per second), which produces a resistance to the limb or segment that is accommodating in nature.[3, 4] Because of changes in musculoskeletal leverage and the length-tension curve, the resistance level incurred by the limb or segment with isokinetic exercise accommodates to the individual at each point in the range of motion during exercise or testing.[3, 4]

Force-Velocity Relationship

Because of the objectivity of isokinetics incurred with testing and data collection, several physiologic principles are demonstrated in isokinetic research. The force-velocity curve has been reproduced with isokinetic testing through a velocity spectrum in intact human skeletal muscle (Fig. 20–1).[5, 6] The force-velocity curve demonstrates that as the velocity of shortening of the skeletal muscle or joint increases, the force, or torque, generated by the musculature decreases in nearly a linear fashion.[3, 5, 6] Figure 20–2 shows the force-velocity relationship for concentric and eccentric muscular contractions. Eccentric isokinetic testing has confirmed the force-velocity curve found in previous research using other methods regarding the presence of in-

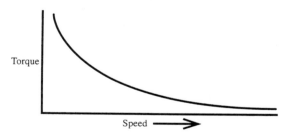

Figure 20–1. Force velocity curve. (From Davies GJ, George J. A Compendium of Isokinetics in Clinical Usage, 4th ed. Onalaska, WI, S & S Publishers, 1992.)

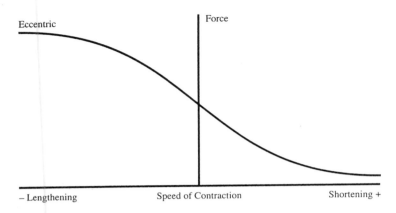

Eccentric

Force

– Lengthening   Speed of Contraction   Shortening +

Figure 20–2. Force velocity curve for concentric and eccentric muscular contractions. (From Davies GJ, George J. A Compendium of Isokinetics in Clinical Usage, 4th ed., Onalaska, WI, S & S Publishers, 1992.)

creased muscular force or torque generation as the velocity of lengthening increased with eccentric muscular work.[3, 7–9] Eccentric isokinetic testing, however, has identified a plateau in the force-velocity curve at approximately 100 degrees per second.[7] At testing or training speeds of 100 degrees per second or higher, no further increase in force generation from the muscle tendon unit is measured in vivo.[7]

These findings have clinical implications for the application of isokinetic exercise to patients following knee ligament rehabilitation. The presence of lower force outputs at higher, more functional contractile velocities may enhance patient tolerance to strengthening at these speeds.[2] According to Bernoulli's principle, compressive forces between two surfaces articulating in a fluid environment are inversely proportional to velocity. High-velocity isokinetic exercise has demonstrated favorable results in experimental studies. Bell et al.[10] conducted a 5-week training study of isokinetic knee extension-flexion exercise at 180 degrees per second. Pre- and post-testing revealed significant strength improvements at all testing speeds ranging between 90 and 240 degrees per second, as well as increases in muscle cross-sectional area and myofibrillar ATPase activity. Their findings show that even short-term high-velocity isokinetic training improves strength and in vivo force-velocity relationships. The use of faster isokinetic training speeds when applied in vivo to the patient following knee ligament injury are indicated, therefore, for functional, biomechanical, and physiologic reasons.

Patterns of Fiber Recruitment

Of additional interest to the clinician rehabilitating patients with moderate or exten-

sive muscular weakness following knee ligament injury is recruitment of muscle fibers. The recruitment pattern of the two major types of muscle fiber in human muscle has been shown to be dependent on the metabolic cost and effort of the exercise or activity being performed.[11] According to Henneman and Olson,[12] recruitment patterns follow the size principle, which states that recruitment of a motor neuron is inversely proportional to its size; smaller type I fibers are generally the first to be recruited, followed by the larger type II fibers as the metabolic cost and intensity of the exercise increases. The clinical application of this information lies in the use of submaximal isokinetic exercise training during the progression of rehabilitative exercise following knee ligament injury. Edstrom[13] and Haggmark et al.[14] have demonstrated selective atrophy of slow twitch (type I) muscle fibers following anterior cruciate ligament (ACL) injury. The use of submaximal isokinetic exercise is then indicated as a means to objectively ensure the submaximal nature of the exercise and provide an accommodating submaximal resistance level to address the selective atrophy and musculotendinous adaptations following injury.

INTEGRATION OF ISOKINETIC EXERCISE IN KNEE LIGAMENT REHABILITATION

Isokinetic exercise for the patient following knee ligament injury has traditionally followed a pattern or progression that allows or ensures patient readiness and tolerance to the isokinetic mode of resistance. Figure 20–3 contains Davies resistive exercise pro-

STAGES:

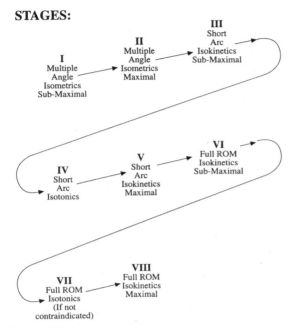

Figure 20–3. Davies resistive exercise progression. ROM = range of motion. (From Davies, George J. A Compendium of Isokinetics in Clinical Usage, 4th ed., Onalaska, WI, S & S Publishers, 1992.)

gression for musculoskeletal rehabilitation.[3] This figure details the sequence beginning with multiple-angle isometrics, progressing to isotonic and subsequently isokinetic forms of resistance. In each of the three resistive exercise categories, the patient is progressed from a submaximal to a more maximal level of intensity. This progression is followed and recommended by this author, whose guidelines for advancement to isokinetic resistance exercise are listed in Table 20–1.

⊙▬ Table 20–1. **Precursors to Isokinetic Exercise Introduction**

* Full weight-bearing
* Non-antalgic gait pattern
* No joint effusion
* Range of motion greater than testing or training motion on dynamometer
* Knee ligament laxity <3 mm compared with contralateral knee with arthrometer testing
* Ability to perform straight-leg raises with 8 lbs or more
* Ability to perform open kinetic chain extension with 20 lbs or more
* Closed kinetic chain squat or leg press with body weight or more

These precursors must be tolerated pain-free.

Timing of Isokinetic Exercise Introduction

Although individual differences must be accounted for in all aspects of human rehabilitation, application of isokinetic exercise following knee ligament reconstruction follows some typical guidelines. Shelbourne et al.[15] perform isokinetic testing as early as 4 to 6 weeks following autogenous ACL reconstruction. Others report isokinetic testing and training occurring after 8 to 12 weeks.[3, 16, 17] Research testing the effects of maximal-effort isokinetic knee extension on knee ligamentous laxity was published by Maitland et al.[18] They found that the performance of a maximal-effort knee extension isokinetic test did not increase tibial translation 6 months following autogenous ACL reconstructions. A resistance exercise progression as well as a knowledge of physiologic healing times of the graft, based on animal research,[19, 20] helps guide clinicians in placement of stress onto the healing graft following surgery. Although full revascularization and remodeling of the graft does not occur for up to 1 year following reconstruction, careful progression of resistive exercise and use of isokinetic testing and training can be a safe and integral part of the rehabilitation process.

Range of Motion Utilized in Knee Ligament Rehabilitation

The range of motion during isokinetic testing and training of the patient following knee ligament rehabilitation has significant clinical implications. Wilk and Andrews[21] studied tibial translation during isokinetic knee extension using an instrumented knee laxity device. Results of their research demonstrated greater tibial translation during knee extension beyond 30 degrees with peak values for anterior tibial translation being found between 30 and 15 degrees of knee extension range of motion. This finding is consistent with similar research performed with quadricep isometric and isotonic exercise using radiography,[22] cadaveric limbs,[23, 24] and in vivo testing.[25]

Introduction of the patient following ACL injury or reconstruction to the isokinetic dynamometer is performed using a range of motion from 90 degrees of knee flexion to approximately 30 degrees of knee flexion. The last 30 degrees in the range of motion is not used initially because of the consistent finding[21, 25] of increased tibial translation with resistive exercise in this movement arc. Upon progression in resistive exercise and dynamic stabilization provided by the surrounding musculature in rehabilitation, the patient is gradually introduced to isokinetic exercise using a full range of excursion between 90 degrees flexion and near complete extension. Care is taken with isokinetic as well as isotonic knee extension exercise to prevent full terminal extension or hyperextension because of the biomechanical implications of the screw-home mechanism on the ligamentous structures,[26] as well as stress to the posterior capsular structures. Terminal resisted extension therefore can stress structures other than the ACL and can be potentially deleterious following medial collateral ligament injury or disruption secondary to the rotation of tibia.[3]

Additional Factors Limiting Anterior Tibial Translation

Several additional factors can be employed by the clinician when integrating isokinetic exercise in patients following knee ligament injury. These include angular velocity selection and pad placement.

Research has demonstrated that anterior tibial translation decreases as angular velocity of testing or training increases. Wilk and Andrews[21] identified a linear decrease in anterior tibial translation between isokinetic testing speeds of 60 to 360 degrees per second. Clinical recommendation for faster isokinetic training speeds based on these findings is warranted to decrease anterior shear forces, which produce anterior tibial translation secondary to quadriceps contraction.

Pad placement during isokinetic knee extension and flexion training is typically just proximal to the medial and lateral malleolus.[3] This allows for full, unrestricted ankle dorsiflexion range of motion and optimizes the musculoskeletal leverage by lengthening the perpendicular distance from the dynamometer input shaft to the point of resistance application. Several authors have suggested utilizing a more proximal pad placement with patients following ACL re-

construction or injury.[3, 27, 28] Johnson[29] introduced an "anti-shear device," which has both a proximal and a distal pad to prevent excessive anterior tibial translation during isokinetic exercise. The application of a posteriorly directed force by the proximal pad to the proximal tibia by the dual pad device was found to decrease anterior tibial translocation in an experimental condition.[30]

Wilk and Andrews[21] experimentally compared a distal (2.5 cm proximal to medial malleolus) with a more proximal (7.5 cm proximal to medial malleolus) pad placement and the effect on anterior tibial translation (Fig. 20–4). Placement of the pad proximally significantly decreased the torque generated by the subjects at all three angular velocities. Anterior tibial translation was also significantly reduced with a proximal pad placement. Use of a more proximal pad placement (7.5 cm proximal to medial malleoli) is indicated for patients who need special protection against anterior tibial translation during isokinetic training. In nearly all cases, special care must be taken to ensure consistency of pad placement during testing, since differences of as little as 5 cm do significantly affect torque production and hence could jeopardize reliability.[21, 31]

Intensity of Isokinetic Exercise Progression

Consistent with the Davies resistive exercise progression,[3] a submaximal intensity is initially employed with all patients when utilizing isokinetic dynamometers. Owing to the presence of accommodating resistance and the potential for maximal physiologic loading throughout the range of motion with isokinetic resistance, submaximal exercise intensities for one to two trial treatments are recommended. Progression to more maximal exertion levels following the submaximal trial treatments is recommended and followed based on patient signs and symptoms.

Isokinetic Angular Velocity Selection

As stated, faster isokinetic training speeds are typically recommended because of the fast joint speeds inherent in functional activities such as walking and running.[2, 3] Table

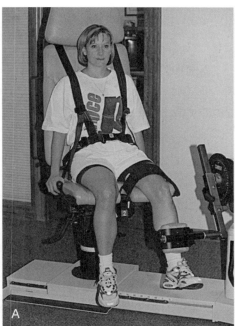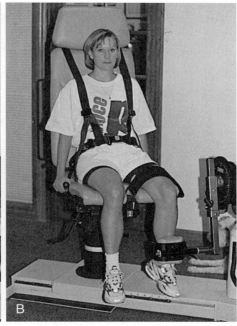

Figure 20–4. Isokinetic knee extension/flexion set-up with proximal *(A)* and distal *(B)* pad placement on the Cybex NORM Isokinetic dynamometer system.

20–2 displays the typical classification of angular velocities. Training velocities typically range from 180 degrees per second to 360 degrees per second. Velocities above 360 degrees per second are typically not used because of the difficulty for the patient in catching the pre-set angular velocity during the exercising range of motion.

Selection of isokinetic training speeds is an important decision for the clinician. Angular velocities that are too slow can produce increased joint compressive forces and invoke patellofemoral pain.[3] Training speeds that are too fast may result in only a small portion of the range of motion being truly isokinetic. Figure 20–5 shows the three portions of a typical isokinetic torque curve. The three portions are termed acceleration, load range, and deceleration.[3, 32] Acceleration occurs upon initiation of limb move-

ment and involves what is termed "free limb acceleration," where the limb does not encounter any extrinsic loading other than the weight of the lever arm and gravitational forces.[3] Load range is the portion of the range of motion at which the limb is exercised at a constant velocity. Deceleration occurs as the limb is brought to end range of motion and involves eccentric activation of the antagonistic musculature prior to reaching the range of motion stop and reversing directions. Optical isokinetic angular velocity selection involves maximizing the load range portion of the curve while utilizing the fastest, most functionally indicated angular velocities specifically indicated for that patient's activity or sport-related demands.

One additional factor relevant in the application of isokinetics to patients with knee ligament injury is the relationship between co-activation and angular velocity. A study of the co-activation of the quadricep and hamstring musculature using electromyography was done by Hagood et al.[33] They found a significant increase in both hamstring and quadriceps antagonistic co-activation during the final 40 degrees in the range of motion with isokinetic loading in healthy knees. These authors conclude that as limb velocity increased under isokinetic loading, there

⊙▬ Table 20–2. Isokinetic Angular Velocity Classification

Speed (degrees/sec)	Classification
0–60	Slow
60–180	Intermediate
180–300	Fast
300–600	Functional

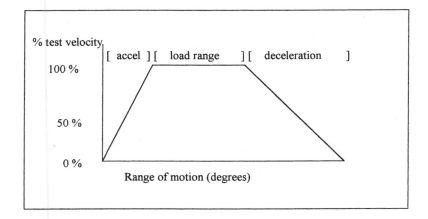

Figure 20–5. Isokinetic velocity graph depicting the portions of the exercise range of motion designated as acceleration, load range, and deceleration.

is a substantial, reflexive increase contribution of the antagonistic musculature, which increases joint stiffness and reduces laxity. Therefore, faster speeds may be of additional importance because of the inherent physiologic muscular recruitment issues discussed in this research.

Isokinetic Training Volume and Rest Issues

Many different protocols have been used regarding exercise volume and rest periods. One of the most widely published isokinetic training workout protocols is Davies' VSRP, or velocity spectrum rehabilitation protocol.[3, 34] The VSRP consists of 10 sets of 10 repetitions of exercise through a velocity spectrum. Typical velocity spectrums used by this author range between 180 and 300 degrees per second with angular velocity increases every 30 degrees per second.[34] The number of repetitions per set of exercise is typically formatted to address both strength and improvement of local muscular endurance.[35] To address this goal, 10 to 20 repetitions per set is commonly used.[34]

Rest intervals with isokinetic exercise represent another important clinical decision that requires both practical and scientific consideration. Following an acute bout of maximal-effort muscular performance, a rest period of 20 seconds will allow 50 percent of muscular adenosine triphosphate and creatine phosphate to be restored.[36] Rest periods of 40 and 60 seconds result in 75 and 87 percent, respectively, of phosphagen repayment.[36] Knowledge of this repayment schedule allows clinicians to make scientifically

based decisions on the amount of rest needed or desired following muscular work. Rest periods of up to 90 seconds between speeds[37] and up to 3 minutes between velocity spectrum rehabilitation programs[38] have been deemed optimal for recovery but are not always clinically practical. Altering rest periods based on sport or activity specificity is also recommended. An example of this would be 25-second rest periods for tennis players, since 25-second rest periods are allowed between points in a tennis match.

ISOKINETIC TESTING

To enhance the reliability of the data acquisition, a standardized approach to the isokinetic evaluation of any patient or joint should be followed[3, 39] The reader is referred to Chapter 4 for a detailed description of the factors inherent in a standardized testing protocol as well as the works by Davies,[3] Wilk et al.,[39] and Sapeaga.[40] One additional concept important to enhance the reliability of data acquisition when using an isokinetic device is order of angular velocity during testing. Wilhite et al.[41] varied the testing order of angular velocities during isokinetic knee extension testing over multiple occasions. Their findings indicated a significant difference in test-retest reliability based on testing speed sequence. Significantly greater test-retest reliability was garnered when researchers followed a sequence of testing from slower angular velocities to faster angular velocities. Starting with faster testing velocities compromised the reliability of the data acquisition, as did a random speed sequence. Clinically, this author begins all isokinetic testing using the slowest speed in the testing sequence and progressing via the velocity spectrum from slowest speed to fastest speed to enhance reliability.

The importance of isokinetic testing in knee ligament rehabilitation can be highlighted by the results of a study by Wilk et al.[42] Manual muscle testing of the quadriceps and hamstrings was carried out by two physical therapists and one orthopedist who all were experienced in the use of manual muscle testing. Upon determination of the patient as having bilaterally symmetrical 5/5 or normal grade manual muscle testing strength, the patient underwent a bilateral isokinetic knee extension flexion test. Results of the testing on 176 post-arthroscopy patients demonstrated differences in muscular strength between extremities ranging between 23 to 31 percent.[42] Isokinetic testing is particularly useful in determining subtle differences in strength between extremities, even in patients who have 5/5 (normal grade) manual muscle testing results.

Interpretation of Isokinetic Test Data

Again the reader is referred to Chapter 4 as well as to the reports by Davies,[3] Davies et al.,[4] and Davies and Ellenbecker[34] for a complete description and discussion of isokinetic data parameters and test interpretation. Interpretation of isokinetic test data by this author is primarily carried out in three main areas: bilateral comparison, unilateral strength ratios, and normative data.

BILATERAL COMPARISON

Comparison of the injured or postoperative limb to the contralateral limb forms one of the basic premises of orthopedic strength assessment. Several authors have recommended that a bilateral comparison of 85 to 90 percent be achieved prior to the patient being discharged from formal strengthening exercises and a unilateral emphasis on training.[3, 4, 34, 43] Most reports on lower extremity isokinetic normative data profiles on normal, healthy populations[44, 45] as well in certain populations of athletes[46] show no significant dominance effect between extremities. Bilateral symmetry of lower extremity muscular function is therefore typically assumed un-

less excessive ergonomic or unilateral athletic musculoskeletal demands are encountered.

The parameters of peak torque and single repetition work have been utilized by many clinicians and are the primary variables or parameters referenced in the interpretation by this author. Peak torque represents the highest point on the torque curve, regardless of where in the range of motion it occurs, and is known as a "point" measurement since it only indicates strength at one point in the range of motion.[3, 4, 34] Single repetition work represents the area under the torque curve and is indicative of the individual's ability to produce force through a range of motion.[3, 4, 34, 47] Single repetition work, total work, and power are all known as "whole curve" measures, since they are indicative of muscular strength throughout the range of motion. Since these measures are whole curve measures, it is imperative that data acquisition occur through identical ranges of motion. Discrepancies in the range of motion between testing limbs can falsely lower or raise the whole curve isokinetic parameters and cause an error in interpretation.

Isokinetic dynamometers are also used to assess muscular endurance or fatigue resistance.[3, 4, 34] Isokinetic strength data are typically sampled using five testing repetitions because most individuals demonstrate both peak torques and maximum work effort during the second and third test repetition.[48] Testing for muscular endurance or fatigue resistance is typically performed using as few as 15 and up to 50 or more test repetitions.[3, 4, 49] Absolute endurance parameters have been reported,[3, 49] such as the work over the total number of testing repetitions or work in the last five repetitions of the testing set, as well as relative endurance test parameters such as the fatigue ratio, which is normally determined as the work in the second half of the testing repetitions divided by the work in the first half of the test repetitions multiplied by 100.[47] Another example of relative endurance testing is counting the number of repetitions until a certain percentage of initial torque production is achieved.[49] Relative muscular fatigue indexes and blood lactate concentrations were found to correlate significantly in an experimental investigation by Douris.[50] Douris also found that the relative muscular fatigue index and blood lactate concentration increased as angular velocity of testing increased from 30 to 300 degrees per second using 1-minute maximal effort work bouts.

In a 7-week training study examining the efficacy of absolute and relative isokinetic endurance tests, Kannus et al.[49] found the relative fatigue index to be unchanged because of the equal improvements in the amount of muscular performance in the beginning and end of the 25 testing repetitions. They conclude that relative endurance tests should be used to establish and determine muscular endurance, but cannot document improvement longitudinally because of equal increases in function with training, which keep the fatigue ratio relatively constant.[49] Absolute measures of endurance are recommended to document and assess improvements in muscular endurance following periods of training.

UNILATERAL STRENGTH RATIOS

Unilateral strength ratios are used to assess strength balance between agonist and antagonist musculature.[3, 4, 34] The hamstring-to-quadricep ratio is calculated and has been shown to be velocity-dependent[3, 4, 51] owing to the different fiber type orientation of the hamstrings and quadriceps. Table 20–3 lists quadricep and hamstring ratios that are used as general guidelines. These ratios show increased hamstring performance as the angular velocity of testing increases. Alterations of this hamstring-to-quadricep ratio exist among athletic populations[52] as well as in the presence of ACL deficiency.[51, 53] Research attempting to demonstrate a statistical relationship between thigh muscular imbalance and injury (H:Q ratio) did not identify this empirically based notion.[54] Despite a lack of direct scientific correlation, unilateral strength ratios are an important parameter to evaluate when interpreting test data from patients with knee ligament injury.

NORMATIVE DATA COMPARISON

When rehabilitating a patient from a distinct, specific population, such as an elite junior tennis player, normative data comparison becomes an additional avenue for interpretation with isokinetic testing. Normalized data, such as peak torque and single-repetition work–to–body-weight ratios, allow scientists and clinicians to compare individual performances in subjects or patients with results from established descriptive or normative data studies.

Table 20–3 shows an example of a normative data sample from elite junior tennis players who are uninjured.[46] No significant difference was found between extremities in quadriceps or hamstring strength, indicating limb symmetry among normal tennis players. Data concerning normalized body weight ratios and unilateral strength ratios can be compared with data from subjects of similar age, sex, and athletic background.[3, 4] Additional articles are published using athletes from soccer,[55, 56] football,[57] racquet sports, and track and field.[52] Caution must be taken when applying normative data profiles, since isokinetic data have been shown to be both population- and apparatus-specific.[58]

OBJECTIVE CHARACTERISTICS INHERENT IN PATIENTS FOLLOWING KNEE LIGAMENT INJURY AND RECONSTRUCTION

Isokinetic testing has been utilized to quantify muscular strength following ACL reconstruction. Several important concepts have been identified regarding the return of muscular strength following reconstruction based on objective strength measurement.

Effects of Immobilization

The effect of complete immobilization of patients following ACL reconstruction was discussed in research by Feiring et al.[59] Two groups of patients following ACL reconstruction underwent identical rehabilitation, except that one group of patients (n = 28), were immobilized in a brace and had a delayed period of immobilization time, resulting in a longer period of time before isokinetic training and testing could take place and the other group (n = 28) underwent immediate rehabilitation and no brace immobilization time. Bilateral comparisons in each group showed differences in the return of quadriceps knee extension strength. The group that underwent brace immobilization had bilateral comparison results of 70 percent slow-speed function and 78 percent fast-speed function at 36 weeks following re-

Table 20–3. **Isokinetic Normative Knee Extension-Flexion Data from Elite Junior Tennis Players Generated on the Cybex 6000 Dynamometer (Age 14–17)**

Knee extension/flexion data for peak torque and single repetition work-to-body-weight ratios for elite junior male tennis players*

Parameter/Speed	Left		Right		*t*-Value	Sig
	Mean	*SD*	*Mean*	*SD*		
Knee extension:						
Torque/BW 180	60.2	21.7	60.5	22.5	0.30	0.766
Torque/BW 300	53.8	6.8	54.0	8.8	0.22	0.827
Work/BW 180	61.4	23.5	62.1	24.5	0.47	0.644
Work/BW 300	54.1	12.7	52.8	12.6	1.72	0.090
Knee flexion:						
Torque/BW 180	36.6	13.5	36.0	13.5	1.04	0.305
Torque/BW 300	33.7	5.9	32.6	5.9	1.41	0.168
Work/BW 180	35.2	13.6	35.2	14.3	0.03	0.973
Work/BW 300	29.5	8.1	29.5	7.7	0.06	0.954

Knee extension/flexion data for peak torque and single repetition work-to-body-weight ratios for elite junior female tennis players*

Parameter/Speed	Left		Right		*t*-Value	Sig
	Mean	*SD*	*Mean*	*SD*		
Knee extension:						
Torque/BW 300	44.4	5.5	47.4	6.7	2.31	0.049
Work/BW 300	43.3	7.6	42.6	7.2	0.60	0.554
Knee flexion:						
Torque/BW 300	30.7	6.1	31.3	4.9	0.57	0.584
Work/BW 300	27.2	7.0	26.5	5.9	0.96	0.348

Hamstring/quadricep peak torque and single repetition work ratios for elite male and female junior tennis players†

Parameter	Left		Right	
	Torque	*Work*	*Torque*	*Work*
Males:				
H/Q 180	61%	58%	59%	58%
H/Q 300	63%	55%	62%	56%
Females:				
H/Q 300	69%	64%	66%	63%

*All values expressed in foot pounds relative to body weight in pounds.
†All values expressed as percent hamstring strength relative to quadricep strength.
   From Ellenbecker TS, Roetert EP: Concentric quadricep and hamstring strength in elite junior tennis players. Isok Exerc Sci 5(1):3–6, 1995.

construction. The intra-articular ACL reconstruction group that did not have any immobilization had bilateral (injured/uninjured) comparisons of 82 and 87 percent at the slow and fast speed, respectively, at only 25 weeks postoperatively. Results from this study show that immediate rehabilitation and earlier strengthening result in a faster return of both slow- and fast-speed isokinetically documented quadricep strength. The immobilization group showed significantly greater slow-speed deficits, which is consistent with the finding of greater atrophy of type I muscle fibers following injury and immobilization.[13, 14]

Intra-articular Versus Extra-articular Anterior Cruciate Ligament Reconstruction

An objective isokinetic muscular function study of intra-articular and extra-articular ACL reconstructions was performed by Feiring et al.[60] Results of this study showed no significant difference in isokinetic knee extension-flexion bilateral work comparisons between a group of patients with 89 extra-articular ACL reconstructions and 44 intra-articular reconstructions using accelerated rehabilitation programs. This finding is in contrast to research by Oni and Crowder,[61] who found greater deficits in both quadriceps and hamstring strength measured with isokinetic testing in intra-articular ACL reconstructions in a prospective randomized clinical trial.

Patellar Tendon Versus Hamstring Autogenous Reconstruction

Isokinetic testing of patients following autogenous ACL reconstruction using both the patellar tendon and semitendonosis muscle has been done to determine whether specific graft-dependent strength deficits exist following harvesting. Harter et al.[62] compared isokinetic knee extension-flexion bilateral comparisons among a group of 30 patients with patellar tendon autografts with 16 patients who had ACL reconstruction using the semitendonosis at a mean of 48 months postoperatively. Results showed no significant difference among quadriceps and hamstring strength regardless of the type of graft used. The authors conclude that even at 48 months following autogenous ACL reconstruction, bilateral deficits in both open chain knee flexion and extension strength are present. Findings of quadriceps and hamstring strength deficits 8 years following knee ligament injury have been consistently reported in the literature.[63, 64] Carter[65] also reported no significant difference between quadriceps and hamstring bilateral deficits among three groups of patients following autogenous ACL reconstruction with either the patellar tendon, semitendinosis, or semitendinosis/gracilis grafts. Carter's findings did demonstrate significant bilateral strength deficits at 6 months following reconstruction in all three reconstruction groups. Collectively, these authors[62–65] recommend increased patient education and emphasis on long-term strengthening for the patient after ACL reconstruction because of the consistent finding of long-term isolated strength deficiencies in objectively oriented outcomes research.

Open Versus Closed Chain Isokinetic Testing

Feiring and Ellenbecker[66] tested 23 patients 15 weeks following an autogenous ACL reconstruction. Subjects underwent an accelerated rehabilitation program with both open and closed chain rehabilitation methods. Subjects were tested using a traditional open kinetic chain knee extension test as well as a supine leg press type closed chain extension test using a concentric Cybex isokinetic dynamometer. Results showed that the closed chain isokinetic leg press–type testing produced peak torque and single repetition work bilateral comparisons of 92 to 95 percent. Open kinetic chain knee extension testing revealed 71 to 75 percent quadriceps knee extension strength relative to the uninjured extremity. The results of this study show significant differences between open and closed chain isokinetic tests of muscular performance in patients following ACL reconstruction. The addition of muscular substitution and compensation present with closed kinetic chain testing due to the interconnecting segments of the lower extremity kinetic chain may explain the apparent return of leg extension strength measured with closed chain testing as compared with the more isolated knee extension strength deficits identified in these patients 15 weeks following ACL reconstruction.

RELATIONSHIP BETWEEN ISOKINETIC TESTING AND FUNCTIONAL PERFORMANCE IN THE LOWER EXTREMITY

One of the potential arguments against isokinetic testing is that the inherent open kinetic chain knee extension-flexion pattern is not "functional." Several studies have indeed tested the relationship between open chain knee extension-flexion testing and various functional performance measures in an attempt to demonstrate a relationship between an isolated test of muscular function and functional performance measures.

Wilk et al.[67] tested 50 patients 25 weeks following ACL reconstruction using three commonly applied functional tests as well as isokinetic knee extension-flexion testing. A statistically significant and positive correlation was found between a hop for time and distance, cross-over triple hop, and isokinetic knee extension strength at 180 and 300 degrees per second. No positive correlations were found for knee flexion testing and the functional performance measures.

Wilson and Murphy[68] tested subjects isokinetically, isometrically, and with a vertical jump to determine the relationship between these test results and cycling performance. They found a significant relationship between isokinetic knee extension at 60, 180, and 300 degrees per second and cycling performance. The isokinetic testing and vertical jump were also able to discriminate among cyclists of different levels of ability. The isometric rate of force development test also utilized by these authors did not have any correlation with functional performance. In a similar comparison between cycling performance and isokinetic knee extension strength, Mannion et al.[69] found significant strength improvements following 16 weeks of isokinetic knee extension in two groups, one training at 60 degrees per second and the other at 240 degrees per second. These strength improvements also produced significantly greater peak pedal velocity and peak power outputs during cycle ergometry tests.

The relationship between isokinetic testing and functional performance is not limited to cycling. Westblad et al.[70] tested elite middle distance runners using a 100-repetition maximal effort concentric and 100-repetition maximal effort eccentric endurance test and compared isokinetic muscular performance of the quadriceps with submaximal and maximal treadmill running capacities. Significant correlations were found for both concentric and eccentric endurance of the quadriceps as well as blood lactate levels. Feltner et al.[71] also studied isokinetic training effects on running. Subjects trained the inverter and everter musculature of the ankle isokinetically and found a decrease in the pronation and supination angles at heel strike and a change in rearfoot motion from isokinetic training.

Not all studies examining the relationship between lower extremity performance measures and isokinetic performance have revealed a significant correlation. Anderson et al.[72] and others[73–75] found no statistical relationship between lower extremity functional tests and isokinetic open chain knee extension. Further research is clearly needed to better understand the relationship between objectively measured isolated muscular strength and functional performance.

ECCENTRIC ISOKINETICS: APPLICATION IN KNEE LIGAMENT REHABILITATION

Comparing the research base of concentric isokinetics with that of eccentric isokinetics identifies a huge discrepancy in the amount of published, clinically applicable research in the area of eccentric isokinetics. Despite this research void, eccentric isokinetics are used in clinical practice for the patient with a knee ligament injury.

Initiation of Eccentric Isokinetics

Following the Davies resistive exercise continuum, eccentric isokinetics are progressed from submaximal levels initially to maximal effort levels based on patient signs and symptoms. Eccentric isokinetics are only recommended following the initiation and tolerance of maximal effort concentric isokinetic exercise.[3, 4, 76] One of the primary benefits garnered with the addition of an eccentric isokinetic component is isolation. With the addition of an eccentric phase, isolation of a particular muscle group is possible by combining the eccentric muscle activation with a concentric activation of the same muscle group. Hence, in knee ligament rehabilitation, in which substantial deficits are traditionally found in the quadriceps,[63–66] eccentric and concentric activation of the quadriceps can be performed, thereby negating the hamstring muscle work that would normally take place during reciprocal isokinetic training. The added benefit of isolation to the obvious advantage of contraction mode specificity make eccentric isokinetic exercise, particularly in end-stage rehabilitation, an attractive option.

The inherent principles of eccentric isokinetics also create cause for caution with respect to application to human subjects during rehabilitation. The internal muscle tension generated with an eccentric muscular contraction is the highest relative to concentric and isometric muscular contractions (Elftman Principle).[8] The additive benefit afforded by the noncontractile tissue that produces this increased tissue tension with eccentric isokinetics can lead to delayed-onset muscle soreness or exercise-induced muscle damage and often produce greater subjective muscular soreness following workouts.[76] Use of an exercise progression from submaximal to maximal intensities, as well as careful monitoring of patient signs and symptoms and patient education regarding delayed-onset muscle soreness and exercise-induced muscle damage will assist the clinician and patient in applying eccentric isokinetics during rehabilitation of a knee ligament injury.

Further research is needed to determine the optimal number of exercise sets, repetitions, and rest cycles for eccentric exercise. Preliminary research by Yanagi et al. (unpublished paper, 1990) found 15 training repetitions per set to be optimal with eccentric isokinetics. Additionally, Helbing et al.[77] found three to five sets of 15 repetitions to be superior to one set of 15 repitions but found no difference between three and five sets with eccentric isokinetic training. As the eccentric isokinetic research base grows, further guidance and clinical application will be available for the clinician to better utilize this modality.

SUMMARY

Isokinetic testing and training provide an objective source that can assist the clinician in the rehabilitation of the patient with knee ligament injury. The knowledge base provided by extensive research allows a scientific platform for optimal assessment and training of the lower extremity, both for performance enhancement and, especially, rehabilitation. Knowledge of the basic physiologic, biomechanical, and clinical principles inherent with isokinetics will allow the clinician to safely utilize this important rehabilitation tool in knee ligament rehabilitation. Isokinetic dynamometers provide a reliable[78–85] instrument for the assessment of muscular strength and endurance and can be an integral part of both rehabilitation and objective outcomes research in knee ligament rehabilitation.

References

1. Perrine JJ: The biophysics of maximal muscle power outputs: Methods and problems of measurement. *In* Jones NL, McCartney N, McComas AJ (eds): Human Muscle Power. Champaign, IL, Human Kinetics Publishers, 1986.
2. Wyatt MP, Edwards AM: Comparison of quadriceps and hamstring torque values during isokinetic exercise. J Orthop Sports Phys Ther 3:48–56, 1981.
3. Davies GJ: A Compendium of Isokinetics in Clinical Usage, 4th ed. LaCrosse, WI, S & S Publishers, 1992.
4. Davies GJ, Wilk KE, Ellenbecker TS: Assessment of Strength. *In* Malone TR, McPoil T, Nitz AJ (eds): Orthopaedic and Sports Physical Therapy, 3rd ed. St. Louis, Mosby, 1997.
5. Thorstensson A, Grimby G, Karlsson J: Force velocity relations and fiber composition in human knee extensor muscles. J Applied Physiology 40(1):12–16, 1976.
6. Hansen TI, Kristensen JH: Force velocity relationships in the human quadriceps muscles. Scand J Rehab Med 11:85–89, 1979.
7. Hanten W, Wieding D: Isokinetic measurements of the force velocity relationship of concentric and eccentric contractions. Phys Ther 68:801, 1988.
8. Elftman H: Biomechanics of muscle. J Bone Joint Surgery 48:363, 1966.
9. Ellenbecker TS, Davies GJ, Rowinski MJ: Concentric versus eccentric isokinetic strengthening of the rotator cuff: Objective data versus functional test. Am J Sports Med 16:64–68, 1988.
10. Bell GJ, Peterson SR, Maclean DC, Quinney HA: Effect of high velocity resistance training on peak torque cross sectional area and myofibrillar ATPase activity. J Sports Med Phys Fitness 32:10–18, 1992.
11. Ahlquist LE, Bassett DR, Sufit R, Nagle FJ, Thomas DP: The effect of pedalling frequency on glycogen depletion rates in type I and type II quadriceps muscle fibers during submaximal cycling exercise. Eur J Appl Physiol 65:360–364, 1992.
12. Henneman E, Olson CB: Relations between structure and function in the design of skeletal muscles. J Neurophysiol 28:581–589, 1965.
13. Edstrom L: Selective atrophy of red muscle fiber in the quadriceps in long standing knee joint dysfunctions: Injuries to the anterior cruciate ligament. J Neurological Sci 11:551–558, 1970.
14. Haggmark T, Jansson E, Eriksson E: Fiber type area and metabolic potential of the thigh muscle in man after knee surgery and immobilization. Int J Sports Med 1(2):12–17, 1981.
15. Shelbourne KD, Klootwyk TE, DeCarlo MS: Update on accelerated rehabilitation after anterior cruciate ligament reconstruction. J Orthop Sports Phys Ther 15:303–308, 1992.
16. Mangine RE, Mangine ME: Isokinetic approach to selected knee pathologies. *In* Davies GJ (ed): A Compendium of Isokinetics in Clinical Usage, 4th ed. LaCrosse, WI, S&S Publishers, 1992.
17. Lai ETS, Ng GYF: A survey on the rehabilitative management of anterior cruciate ligament injuries in Hong Kong. Hong Kong Physiother J X:15–21, 1997.
18. Maitland ME, Lowe R, Stewart S, Fung T, Bell GD: Does Cybex testing increase knee laxity after anterior cruciate ligament reconstructions? Am J Sports Med 21(5):690–695, 1990.
19. Arnoczky SP, Tarvin GB, Marshall JL: Anterior cruciate ligament replacement using patellar tendon: An evaluation of graft revascularization in the dog. J Bone Joint Surg 64A:217–224, 1982.
20. Butler DL: Anterior cruciate ligament: Its normal

response and replacement. J Orthop Res 7:910–921, 1989.

21. Wilk KE, Andrews JR: The effects of pad placement and angular velocity on tibial displacement during isokinetic exercise. J Orthop Sports Phys Ther 17(1):24–30, 1993.

22. Yasuda K, Sasaki T: Exercise after anterior cruciate ligament reconstruction. The force exerted on the tibia by the separate isometric contractions of the quadriceps and hamstrings. Clin Orthop 220:275–283, 1987.

23. Arms SW, Pope MH, Johnson RJ, Fischer RA, Arvidsson I, Eriksson E: The biomechanics of anterior cruciate ligament rehabilitation and reconstruction. Am J Sports Mec 12:8–18, 1984.

24. Grood ES, Suntay WJ, Noyes FR, Butler DL: Biomechanics of the knee extension exercise. Effect of cutting the anterior cruciate ligament. J Bone Joint Surg 66A(5):725–734, 1984.

25. Henning CE, Lynch MA, Glick KR: An in-vivo strain gauge study of elongation of the anterior cruciate ligament. Am J Sports Med 13(1):22–26, 1985.

26. Canner GC: Biomechanics and biomaterials of the knee. *In* Engle RP (ed): Knee Ligament Rehabilitation. New York, Churchill Livingstone, 1991.

27. Wilk KE, Andrews JR: Current concepts in the treatment of anterior cruciate ligament disruption. J Orthop Sports Phys Ther 15(6):279–293, 1992.

28. Nisell R, Erickson MO, Nemeth G, Ekholm J: Tibiofemoral joint forces during isokinetic knee extension. Am J Sports Med 17:49–54, 1989.

29. Johnson D: Controlling anterior shear during isokinetic knee extension. J Orthop Sports Phys Ther 4:23–31, 1982.

30. Timm KE: Validation of the Johnson anti-shear accessory as an accurate and effective clinical isokinetic instrument. J Orthop Sports Phys Ther 7(6):298–303, 1986.

31. Taylor RL, Casey JJ: Quadriceps torque production on the Cybex II dynamometer as related to changes in lever arm length. J Orthop Sports Phys Ther 8:147–152, 1986.

32. Brown LE, Whitehurst M, Findley BW, Gilbert R, Buchalter DN: Isokinetic load range during shoulder rotational exercise in elite male junior tennis players. J Strength Conditioning Res 9(3):160–164, 1995.

33. Hagood S, Solomonow M, Baratta R, Zhou BH, D'Ambrosia R: The effect of joint velocity on the contribution of the antagonist musculature to knee stiffness and laxity. Am J Sports Med 18(2):182–187, 1990.

34. Davies GJ, Ellenbecker TS: Application of isokinetics in testing and rehabilitation. *In* Andrews JR, Harrelson GL, Wilk KE (eds). Physical Rehabilitation of the Injured Athlete, 2nd ed. Philadelphia, WB Saunders, 1998.

35. Fleck S, Kraemer W: Designing Resistance Training Programs. Champaign, IL, Human Kinetics Publishers, 1987.

36. Fleck S: Interval training: Physiological basis. J Strength Conditioning Res 5:4–7, 1983.

37. Ariki P, Davies GJ, Siewert M, et al.: Rest interval between isokinetic velocity spectrum training speeds. Phys Ther 65:735–736, 1985.

38. Ariki P, Davies GJ, Siewert M, et al.: Rest interval between isokinetic velocity spectrum training sets. Phys Ther 65:733–734, 1985.

39. Wilk KE, Arrigo CA, Andrews JR: Standardized isokinetic testing protocol for the throwing shoulder: The throwers series. Isok Exerc Sci 1:63–71, 1991.

40. Sapeaga AA: Muscle performance evaluation in orthopaedic practice. J Bone Joint Surgery 73-A(10)1562–1574, 1990.

41. Wilhite MR, Cohen ER, Wilhite SC: Reliability of concentric and eccentric measurements of quadriceps performance using the Kin Com dynamometer: The effect of testing order for three different speeds. J Orthop Sports Phys Ther 11:419–420 (Abstract), 1990.

42. Wilk KE, Arrigo CA, Andrews JR: A comparison of individuals exhibiting normal grade manual muscle test and isokinetic testing of the knee extension/flexion [abstract]. Phys Ther 72(6):71, 1992.

43. Malone TR, Blackburn TA, Wallace LA: Knee Rehabilitation. Phys Ther 60:1602, 1980.

44. Hageman PA, Gillaspie DM, Hill LD: Effects of speed and limb dominance on eccentric and concentric isokinetic testing of the knee. J Orthop Sports Phys Ther 10(2):59–65, 1988.

45. Lucca JA, Kline KK: Effects of upper and lower limb preference on torque production in the knee flexors and extensors. J Orthop Sports Phys Ther 11(5):202–207, 1989.

46. Ellenbecker TS, Roetert EP: Concentric quadricep and hamstring strength in elite junior tennis players. Isok Exerc Sci 5(1) 3–6, 1995.

47. Cybex Applications Manual. Hauppague, NY, Cybex Inc. A Division of Henley Health Care, 1998.

48. Wilk KE, Arrigo CA: Peak torque and maximum work repetition during isokinetic testing of the shoulder internal and external rotators. Isok Exerc Sci 4(4):171–175, 1994.

49. Kannus P, Cook L, Alosa D: Absolute and relative endurance parameters in isokinetic tests of muscular performance. J Sport Rehabil 1:2–12, 1992.

50. Douris PC: The effect of isokinetic exercise on the relationship between blood lactate and muscle fatigue. J Orthop Sports Phys Ther 17(1):31–35, 1993.

51. Murray SM, Warren RF, Otis JC, Kroll M, Wickiewicz TL: Torque velocity relationships of the knee extensor and flexor muscles in individuals sustaining injuries of the anterior cruciate ligament. Am J Sports Med 12(6):436–440, 1984.

52. Read MTF, Bellamy MJ: Comparison of hamstring/quadriceps isokinetic strength ratios and power in tennis, squash, and track athletes. Br J Sports Med 24(3):178–182, 1990.

53. Kannus P: Ratio of hamstring to quadriceps femoris muscles' strength in the anterior cruciate ligament insufficient knee: Relationship to long term recovery. Phys Ther 68(6):961–965, 1988.

54. Grace TG, Sweetser ER, Nelson MA, Ydens LR, Skipper BJ: Isokinetics muscle imbalance and knee-joint injuries: A prospective blind study. J Bone Joint Surg 66-A(5):734–740, 1984.

55. Mangine RE, Noyes FR, Mullen P, Barber SD: A physiological profile of the elite soccer athlete. J Orthop Sports Phys Ther 12(4):147–152, 1990.

56. Agre JC, Baxter TL: Musculoskeletal profile of collegiate soccer players. Arch Phys Med Rehabil 68:147–150, 1987.

57. Parker MG, Ruhling RO, Holt D, Bauman E, Drayna M: Descriptive analysis of quadriceps and hamstrings muscle torque in high school football players. J Orthop Sports Phys Ther 5(1):2–6, 1983.

58. Francis K, Hoobler T: Comparison of peak torque values of the knee flexor and extensor muscle groups using the Cybex II and Lido 2.0 isokinetic dynamometers. J Orthop Sports Phys Ther 8:480–483, 1987.

59. Feiring DC, Ellenbecker TS, Derscheid GL: Difference in isokinetic muscle function related to the post-surgical care of intra-articular ACL reconstructions [abstract]. Phys Ther 71(6):S32, 1991.

60. Feiring DC, Ellenbecker TS, Derscheid GL: Recovery time and isokinetic evaluation following ACL reconstruction: A 3 group comparative analysis [abstract]. Phys Ther 71(6):S33, 1991.

61. Oni OOA, Crowder E: A comparison of isokinetics and muscle strength ratios following intra-articular and extra-articular reconstructions of the anterior cruciate ligament. Injury 27(2):195–197, 1996.

62. Harter RA, Osternig LR, Standifer LW: Isokinetic evaluation of quadriceps and hamstrings symmetry following anterior cruciate ligament reconstruction. Arch Phys Med Rehabil 71:465–468, 1990.

63. Kannus P, Latvala K, Jarvinen M: Thigh muscle strengths in the anterior cruciate ligament deficient knee: Isokinetic and isometric long-term results. J Orthop Sports Phys Ther 9(6):223–227, 1987.

64. Kannus P, Jarvinen M: Thigh muscle function after partial tear of the medical ligament compartment of the knee. Med Sci Sports Exerc 23(1):4–9, 1991.

65. Carter TR, Edinger S: Isokinetic evaluation of anterior cruciate ligament reconstruction: Hamstring versus patellar tendon. J Arthro Rel Res 15:169–172, 1999.

66. Feiring DC, Ellenbecker TS: Single versus multiple joint isokinetic testing with ACL reconstructed patients. Isok Exerc Sci 6:109–115, 1996.

67. Wilk KE, Romaniello WT, Soscia SM, Arrigo CA, Andrews JR: The relationship between subjective knee scores, isokinetic testing, and functional testing in the ACL reconstructed knee. J Orthop Sports Phys Ther 20(2):60–73, 1994.

68. Wilson G, Murphy A: The efficacy of isokinetic, isometric and vertical jump tests in exercise science. Austr J Sci Med Sport 27(1):20–24, 1995.

69. Mannion AF, Jakeman PM, Willan PLT: Effects of isokinetic training of the knee extensors on isometric strength and peak power output during cycling. Eur J Appl Physiol 65:370–375, 1992.

70. Westblad P, Svendenhag J, Rolf C: The validity of isokinetic knee extensor endurance measurements with reference to treadmill running capacities. Int J Sports Med 17:134–139, 1996.

71. Feltner ME, Macrae HH, Macrae PG, Turner NS, Hartman CA, Summers ML, Welch MD: Strength training effects on rearfoot motion in running. Med Sci Sports Exerc 26(8):1021–1027, 1994.

72. Anderson MA, Gieck JH, Perrin D, Weltman A, Rutt R, Denegar C: The relationships among isometric, isotonic, and isokinetic concentric and eccentric quadriceps and hamstring force and three components of athletic performance. J Orthop Sports Phys Ther 14(3):114–120, 1991.

73. Noyes FR, Barber SD, Mangine RE: Abnormal lower limb symmetry determined by function hop tests after anterior cruciate ligament rupture. Am J Sports Med 19:513–518, 1991.

74. Swarup M, Irrgang JJ, Lephart S: Relationship of isokinetic quadriceps peak torque and work to one legged hop and vertical jump. Phys Ther 72:S88, 1992.

75. Delitto A, Irrgang JJ, Harner CD, et al. Relationship of isokinetic quadriceps peak torque and work to one legged hop and vertical jump in ACL reconstructed subjects. Phys Ther 73:S85, 1993.

76. Davies GJ, Ellenbecker TS: Eccentric isokinetics. Orthop Phys Ther Clin North Am 1(2):297–336, 1992.

77. Helbing AK, Fater DC, Anderson MA, Davies GJ: The optimal number of exercise sets for eccentric power gains of the quadriceps [abstract]. Wisconsin Physical Therapy Association State Meeting, 1991.

78. Wilson GJ, Walshe AD, Fisher MR: The development of an isokinetic squat device: reliability and relationship to functional performance. Eur J Appl Physiol 75:455–461, 1997.

79. Burdett RG, VanSwearingen J: Reliability of isokinetic muscle endurance tests. J Orthop Sports Phys Ther 8(10):484–488, 1987.

80. Pincivero DM, Lephart SM, Karunakara RA: Reliability and precision of isokinetic strength and muscular endurance for the quadriceps and hamstrings. Int J Sports Med 18:113-115, 1997.

81. Steiner LA, Harris BA, Krebs DE: Reliability of eccentric isokinetic knee flexion and extension measurements. Arch Phys Med Rehabil 74:1327–1335, 1993.

82. Bandy WD, McLaughlin S: Intramachine and intermachine reliability for selected dynamic muscle performance tests. J Orthop Sports Phys Ther 18(5):609–613, 1993.

83. Levene JA, Hart BA, Seeds RH, Fuhrman GA: Reliability of reciprocal isokinetic testing of the knee extensors and flexors. J Orthop Sports Phys Ther 14(3):121–127, 1991.

84. Timm KE, Genrich P, Burns R, Fyke D: The mechanical and physiological performance reliability of selected isokinetic dynamometers. Isok Exerc Sci 2(4):182–190, 1992.

85. Feiring DC, Ellenbecker TS, Derscheid GL: Test retest reliability of the Biodex isokinetic dynamometer. J Orthop Sports Phys Ther 11(7):298–300, 1990.

21 Open and Closed Kinetic Chain Rehabilitation

George J. Davies, MEd, PT, SCS, ATC, CSCS,
Bryan C. Heiderscheit, MS, PT, CSCS,
and Michael Clark, MS, PT, CSCS

*R*ehabilitation of patients with knee injuries or surgeries has gone through a series of interesting evolutions. The following observations can be made regarding the shifting between various rehabilitation paradigms:

1970s: open and closed kinetic chain and sports rehabilitation
1980s: open kinetic chain (OKC) rehabilitation with emphasis on isokinetics
1990s: closed kinetic chain (CKC) rehabilitation

Some of the trends regarding rehabilitation of various pathologic knee conditions involve almost exclusive use of CKC exercises. In contrast, few clinicians recognize the potential benefits offered with OKC exercises. Perhaps the philosophy that "if everyone is doing it, it must be okay" is prevailing. It is the purpose of this chapter to review the scientific and clinical literature regarding the use of OKC and CKC rehabilitation protocols for patients with knee injuries and to provide rationale for integrating the two protocols. It is our desire that the trend in knee rehabilitation return to an integrated design with an emphasis on functional tasks.

An OKC exercise can be considered an activity in which the distal component of the extremity is not fixed but is free in space. Further, it is commonly considered to be a non-weight-bearing activity. An example of such a movement would be performing a seated knee extension exercise. When the distal component of the extremity is fixed, often involving weight-bearing, the movement becomes a CKC activity. Examples of this would be squatting or a leg press exercise.

It is questionable whether most exercises can be considered purely OKC or CKC when many show characteristics of both. For example, during walking, both an OKC and a CKC position exist with swing and stance phase, respectively. Further, riding a bicycle requires the individual's foot to be fixed to the pedal (CKC), but the pedal and foot are still moving in space (OKC). These activities and those that are similar should not be considered entirely CKC or OKC but rather a succession of CKC and OKC activities.[1] As a remedy to the confusion of classifying an exercise as CKC or OKC, a classification system involving four distinct divisions has been proposed (Table 21–1).[1] For the purpose of this text, an OKC activity is operationally defined as non-weight-bearing with a free distal segment, whereas a CKC activity is weight-bearing with a fixed distal segment.

OPEN KINETIC CHAIN ASSESSMENT AND REHABILITATION

Characteristics

An example of the OKC pattern is moving the knee from flexion to extension or the reverse while sitting. This OKC pattern will serve as the model to demonstrate the following characteristics that are often used to describe OKC exercises:

- Distal end is free
- Isolated angular joint pattern
- Muscle recruitment limited to the single joint movers
- Stable joint axis during movement pattern
- Non-weight-bearing movement pattern
- Production of joint shear forces dependent on placement of resistance
- Usually limited to a single plane of movement
- Use of equipment provides artificial means of stabilization

◉━ Table 21-1. Exercise Classification Based on Kinetic Chain

Exercise	Definition	Example
Open kinetic chain	Terminal segment is free to move	Knee extension
Closed kinetic chain	Terminal segment is fixed	Squat, lunge, step-up
Partial kinetic chain	Terminal segment meets resistance but is not completely fixed or stationary	Slide board, skiing
Succession drills	Terminal segment repeatedly and rapidly converts between free and fixed	Running, plyometrics

Data from Wilk KE, Escamilla RF, Fleisig GS, Arrigo CA, Barrentine SW: Open and closed kinetic chain exercise for the lower extremity: Theory and clinical application. Athletic Train Sports Health Care Perspect 1:336, 1995.

Rationale

With the trend moving toward the use of CKC rehabilitation, advantages that may be gained by OKC tasks are often overlooked. In addition to the numerous investigations demonstrating the efficacy of OKC rehabilitation,[2–4] authors have demonstrated inadequate rehabilitation without the incorporation of OKC activities.[5, 6]

Snyder-Mackler et al.[6] conducted a prospective randomized clinical investigation into the effects of intensive CKC rehabilitation programs with different types of electrical stimulation on patients with ACL reconstruction. These researchers previously demonstrated the strength of the quadriceps femoris muscle to be well correlated with the function of the knee during the stance phase of gait. In the present study,[6] following an intensive CKC rehabilitation program, a residual weakness remained in the quadriceps that produced alterations in the normal gait function of these patients. The authors concluded that CKC exercise alone does not provide an adequate stimulus to the quadriceps femoris to permit more normal knee function in the stance phase of gait following ACL reconstruction. The authors recommend the application of OKC exercise for the quadriceps femoris muscle following ACL reconstruction to improve muscle strength and the functional outcome for the patients.

To recognize an individual muscle group deficit as described by Snyder-Mackler et al.[6] requires an OKC assessment. Because of compensations and substitutions that can occur, whole limb testing, as is the case with CKC exercise, may not be as sensitive. The weak link in the kinetic chain may not be identified unless specific isolated OKC testing is performed. If periodic OKC testing is not performed, an existing deficit can remain undetected. This can give both the patient and the clinician a false-positive finding in determining an appropriate discharge date.

Individual testing should not be limited to just the prime movers of the injured joint but should include accessory muscles and muscles of adjacent joints. Nichols et al.[7] demonstrated resultant weakness of the ipsilateral hip abductors and adductors in patients with ankle and foot problems. The authors concluded that injuries at distal joints, irrespective of severity, appear to produce the greatest amount of total limb weakness.

OKC tasks can often be initiated early in the rehabilitation. While restricted weight-bearing may prevent certain CKC exercises from being utilized, OKC tasks are not limited due to their non-weight-bearing nature. Further, the control offered the clinician during an OKC task allows its early utilization. The clinician can control such parameters as range of motion, speed of movement, translational stresses (by shin pad placement), and varus-valgus forces.

With the goal of every patient's rehabilitation being increased function, the protocol selected must ensure that this happens. The use of OKC tasks has been demonstrated to improve the functional performance of patients, including individuals following anterior cruciate ligament(ACL) reconstruction.[2, 3, 8–10]

Methods

To enable the sequential progression of a rehabilitation program, pre-established objective assessment techniques are required. The various clinical techniques used for OKC assessment can include strength testing (isometrics, isotonics, isokinetics) and proprioceptive testing.

ISOMETRICS

Isometric testing assesses muscle strength at a single point in the range of motion. The muscle being tested is neither shortening nor lengthening during the assessment. This method of testing is most commonly referred to as manual muscle testing (MMT). MMT (performed isometrically as "break tests") is used to assess the muscular weakness following disorders primarily involving the contractile muscle elements, the neuromuscular junction, and the lower motor neuron.[11] Careful observation and palpation are essential for effective testing. In addition, stabilization and correct positioning should be considered to minimize muscle substitution or compensation. In attempts to decrease the inherent subjectivity of MMT, hand-held dynamometers have become popular. While still relying on appropriate testing conditions, the hand-held dynamometer allows for greater objectivity in quantifying isometric MMT.

ISOTONICS

Isotonic testing allows for assessment of dynamic strength. Unlike isometric testing, isotonic testing measures strength throughout a range of motion. As demonstrated by a muscle length-tension curve, muscle force production varies throughout the range of motion. Therefore, testing at a single point in the motion may not provide the clinican with enough information to appropriately assess the patient.

ISOKINETICS

Isokinetic assessment allows the clinican to objectively assess muscle performance in a safe environment. While both isotonic and isokinetic testing are performed throughout the available range of motion, isokinetics also offer the advantage of controlling the speed of movement. Isokinetic testing has been demonstrated to be reliable and valid.[12-17] A standard orthopedic testing protocol should be followed during isokinetic testing. Davies[18] recommends the use of a velocity spectrum testing protocol. Velocity spectrum testing refers to testing at slow (1–60 degrees per second), intermediate (60–180 degrees per second), fast (180–300 degrees per second), and functional (300–1000 degrees per second) velocities. Three to five test repetitions at each speed are

suggested. If assessment of muscle endurance is the goal, 20 to 30 repetitions at a fast speed (240–300 degrees per second) may prove to be more appropriate than fewer repetitions at a slower speed. Isokinetic testing allows for a variety of testing protocols. It is beyond the scope of this chapter to discuss all the details, so the reader is referred to Davies[18] for a detailed description of the various options.

The same general principles described for each of the three strength assessments apply to these modes in training. The appropriateness of one versus the others is based on the patient's status. For example, a patient 1 week after ACL reconstruction should not be performing multiple sets of isokinetics, although the implementation of an isometric program may prove to be beneficial. Irrespective of the type of strength program used during the rehabilitation program, the basic principles of training should be followed. These include specificity, intensity, volume, rest periods, training frequency, and muscle balance.[19-21] The program should always be individualized to the patient's needs and deficits, keeping in mind the ultimate goal of both the clinician and patient.

PROPRIOCEPTIVE TESTING

The term *proprioception* was originally used by Sherrington[22] to describe vestibular, joint, and muscle receptor input to the nervous system. This afferent feedback mechanism includes both active and passive information. The active component, kinesthesia, refers to the sensations of joint motion, while the passive movement, joint position sense, is specific to the joint position.[23, 24] Kinesthesia was originally used to describe sensations related to both position and motion of the body.[25] Over the years, it appears that *kinesthesia* has been redefined as the active division of the more encompassing term *proprioception*. For the purpose of this chapter, *kinesthesia* is used in reference to joint motion, with *proprioception* encompassing both kinesthesia and joint position sense.

Tactile, visual, and vestibular input, as well as information from receptors located in the joints and muscles, controls proprioception. Joint receptors, however, may have primary control.[26-28] It has been demonstrated following injury that joint mechanoreceptors are damaged and subsequently do not function effectively.[29] Proprioceptive deficits have been noted with various joint injuries and disruptions,[29, 30–34] as well as following several surgical procedures.[35–37] It has even been suggested that kinesthetic deficits can predispose an individual to injury.[38] Various assessment methods, including joint movement description and joint angle replication, have been described and should be included.[39] Joint angle replication is a technique frequently used to assess joint proprioception. Joint angle replication measured with a goniometer or inclinometer can provide an objective assessment of joint proprioception.

CLOSED KINETIC CHAIN ASSESSMENT AND REHABILITATION

Characteristics

Examples of the CKC pattern include the standing squat, lunge, and step-up.[40–42] The standing squat will serve as the model to demonstrate the following characteristics frequently used to describe CKC exercises. As previously defined, a CKC exercise involves a fixed distal segment, most often in a weight-bearing position.
- Fixed distal end segment
- Motion at multiple joints
- Muscle recruitment at each moving joint
- Moving joint axis relative to external room coordinates
- Weight-bearing movement pattern
- Joint compression
- Multiple planes of movement

Rationale

Several authors have suggested that CKC exercises are safer than OKC exercises for patients with knee ligament injury secondary to the decreased shear forces present at the knee joint.[43–47] This becomes a significant factor when considering the effect of anterior tibial translation on a recent ACL reconstruction. Cadaveric studies have demonstrated that joint geometry in combination with axial loading will limit anterior tibial displacement even when the menisci, ACL, and medial collateral ligament (MCL) have been removed.[43, 48–51] This indicates that the increased knee joint compressive forces present during a CKC activity may reduce the stress on the healing ACL graft. In contrast, OKC knee extension exercises during initial flexion (0–60 degrees) generated shear forces that increased anterior tibial translation, thereby increasing the stress on the ACL.[51, 52–55]

The effects of OKC exercises on ACL strain have been investigated.[50, 52, 56, 57] Quadriceps contraction during an OKC activity increased ACL strain during initial knee flexion (0–45 degrees), whereas flexion beyond 75 degrees reduced the strain to the ACL. The use of a terminal knee extension program following ACL reconstruction may therefore be inappropriate, as the excessive strain may be placed on the healing graft. As anticipated, hamstring contraction during an OKC movement decreased ACL strain.[50, 53] This supports the use of a CKC exercise, as the co-contraction of the hamstrings can act to stabilize the tibia, preventing anterior translation.

Bynum et al.[58] performed the first prospective randomized study comparing OKC and CKC exercises. Patients who had recently undergone ACL reconstruction were the subject sample. Using a KT-1000 knee ligament arthrometer, the CKC group displayed significantly lower bilateral differences for ACL laxity than the OKC group. Further, the CKC group returned to activities of daily living sooner than expected. The authors concluded that a CKC exercise protocol should be exclusively used following ACL reconstruction.[58]

Differences in patellofemoral joint forces and contact stress may also exist between OKC and CKC activities. Reily and Martens[59] calculated that the peak patellofemoral joint reaction force during OKC knee extension occurred at 36 degrees of flexion. At this knee angle, a relatively small portion of the patella is in contact with the femur, suggesting that the large joint force is concentrated on a small articular surface. This results in a high patellofemoral contact stress per unit area. During a CKC activity, the patellofemoral contact stress is less than the OKC during initial knee flexion (0–45 degrees).[60] At knee angles greater than 50 degrees, the contact stress differences between OKC and CKC activities depend on the specific CKC activity performed. For example, CKC squat produces less contact stress than OKC knee extension,[61] whereas

CKC leg press produces more contact stress.[60] These observed differences between OKC and CKC activities indicate that the proper CKC exercise can reduce the articular stresses incurred by the patellofemoral joint during rehabilitation.

Previous investigations have been conducted to describe electromyographic (EMG) activity during controlled OKC and CKC exercises.[42] Results indicate that open and closed kinetic chain activity causes different muscular recruitment patterns throughout the range of motion. Low levels of quadriceps and hamstrings co-activation were demonstrated during OKC leg extensions, as evidenced by a 6:1 EMG ratio between quadriceps and hamstrings.[42] CKC exercises result in simultaneous movement of all segments in the kinetic chain in a predictable manner and require coordinated muscular effort involving co-contraction of antagonistic muscles and stabilizing muscles to control motion.[42] When compared with leg press and leg extensions, CKC vertical squats produced the most co-contraction during initial knee flexion.[42, 62] EMG ratios for quadriceps to hamstrings have been reported at 1.5:1 for vertical squats and 4:1 for leg press.[42, 62] Another widely used CKC exercise, lateral step-ups, elicits significantly greater quadriceps EMG activity as compared to squats, leg presses, or stair stepping.[63, 64] Contraction of the hamstrings appears to be insufficient to neutralize the shear forces produced during lateral step-ups.[63, 64] Further research is needed to determine which exercises are safe and in what ranges of motion they should be performed.

In addition to improved muscular co-contraction, CKC training may produce greater activation of the joint mechanoreceptors than OKC training, thereby improving joint proprioception.[40] Proprioception and kinesthesia are critical to athletic performance. After joint injury, proprioception and kinesthesia are diminished. It is therefore necessary to use functional exercises that will help restore normal neuromuscular control. Stimulation of joint mechanoreceptors during CKC exercises improves the coordinated neuromuscular controlling mechanism required for joint stability.[40, 41]

Methods

Enhancing the ability to function effectively should be the main objective of the rehabilitation process. A planned, systematic approach to rehabilitation can effectively and efficiently allow a patient to achieve a full functional recovery. A functional continuum should be utilized to progressively advance the clinical rehabilitation program. The appropriate design and implementation of a CKC rehabilitation program is necessary for restoring normal neuromuscular control. General guidelines for a CKC program design are as follows:

- Program should be planned, organized, and systematic
- Determine patient's current rehabilitation level
- Set realistic goals
- Perform sports-specific CKC exercises
- Use criterion-based progressions
- Achieve muscular balance
- Exercises should be proprioceptive dominant
- Re-evaluate on a regular basis

Exercises performed in a CKC appear to be more functional than OKC exercises. CKC exercise stimulates specific mechanoreceptors that improve postural control and kinesthetic awareness, thus improving neuromuscular control.[40, 42] Furthermore, using CKC exercises for rehabilitating patients with patellofemoral dysfunction and ACL reconstruction in the ranges from 0 to 45 degrees of knee flexion has been supported by current research.[19, 50, 65–68] However, utilizing CKC exercises exclusively may fail to provide an adequate stimulus to a weak link in the kinetic chain if compensations occur.[6, 41]

Muscle imbalances and joint restrictions in other related segments must be monitored during CKC exercises. For example, if a patient has patellofemoral pain and concomitant decreased ankle dorsiflexion, then compensatory subtalar joint pronation may occur during CKC exercises. This compensation mechanism may change the recruitment patterns of the surrounding musculature or alter the segment angles, potentially placing excessive stress on the knee. Restoring normal arthrokinematics will minimize the occurrence of abnormal compensation patterns with the use of CKC exercises.

Program design is critical to achieve a functional outcome. Clinical control is utilized to elicit the appropriate responses. Dynamic stability is achieved first to allow for controlled joint translation and appropriate patterns of muscular recruitment. Once dynamic stabilization has been achieved, the focus of the program should switch to restoring function during normal activities of daily living and sporting activities. Exercises should progress from simple to complex, slow to fast, well controlled to less controlled, and static to dynamic. For a sample set of CKC rehabilitation exercises, see Table 21–2.

INTEGRATED APPROACH WITH FUNCTIONAL REHABILITATION

Many theoretical and descriptive models have been defined regarding the use of certain exercise regimens; however, the outcome studies are lacking. A classic example is the increased use of CKC exercises almost exclusively in the patient with an ACL reconstruction. The apparent functional gains offered by a CKC-only rehabilitation program have resulted in the disregard of substantiated OKC exercises. Yet the scientific literature may not be able to support this shift. Crandall et al.[69] presented a review of the literature at the 1994 meeting of the American Orthopedic Society for Sports Medicine concerning ACL surgery and rehabilitation.

⊙▬ Table 21–2. **Sample Exercises to Be Used in the Design of a Closed Kinetic Chain Rehabilitation Program**

Goal	Exercise
Quadriceps dominant	Wall squats
	Leg press
	Lateral step-ups
Hamstrings dominant	Wide stance squats
	Retrograde stair stepping
	Multiple position lunges
	Single leg touchdowns
	Forward step-ups
	Straight leg deadlift
Quadriceps/hamstrings co-contraction	Fitter
	Slide board
	Vertical squat (0–45 degrees)
Proprioception dominant	Balance board
	Sport beam
	Mini-tramp
	BAPS board
Functional activities (sport-specific)	Speed drills
	Lateral speed and agility drills
	Plyometrics
	Medicine ball exercises
	Physioball exercises

BAPS = biomechanical ankle platform system.

The review indicated that only 5 of the 1167 papers published on this topic since 1975 met the criteria to be included in a meta-analysis. The majority of the papers on ACL surgery and rehabilitation are simply descriptive studies, with very few prospective, randomized, controlled clinical studies.

The advantages and disadvantages of both exercise regimens were discussed previously in this chapter. An integration of the OKC and CKC protocols provides the patient with the benefits of both while offsetting the negative aspects of each. Note that the disadvantages of one may be compensated for by the advantages of the other. A common complaint of OKC exercise is that it may not offer the functional motor pattern available with a CKC task. However, isolated muscle weakness may be present as compensations occur at other points in the kinetic chain. As previously stated, quadriceps muscle weakness has been demonstrated to exist among patients treated only with "aggressive CKC exercises" following ACL reconstruction.[6] The proposed use of an integrated program would provide the patient with the functional motor pattern gained through CKC activities, as well as the ability to address the quadriceps weakness with specific OKC training.

Further, investigations have demonstrated that testing the entire kinetic chain may not recognize isolated deficits.[7, 70, 71] Although these deficits exist, the results of the CKC testing are within normal limits in a bilateral comparison.[5, 72] Davies[5] performed bilateral muscle testing of over 300 patients with knee injuries or following knee surgery. All patients were tested with a Linea CKC computerized isokinetic testing system[73] and with a Cybex OKC computerized isokinetic testing system. The results demonstrated that while CKC testing produced similar bilateral scores, the OKC testing indicated the presence of bilateral deficits (Table 21–3).[74]

Simultaneous testing of multiple muscle groups with the development of a composite force output score appears to result in the weakened muscles being compensated for by the others. This compensation can result in the whole limb displaying a smaller deficit than what might actually exist. With bilateral symmetry frequently used as a discharge criterion, much importance is placed on this value. If a clinician were to deem a patient ready for discharge based on the CKC values without considering the presence of com-

⊙ Table 21–3. Comparison of Open and Closed Kinetic Chain Isokinetic Dynamometer Testing of 300 Patients with Various Pathologic Knee Conditions or After Surgery

	Cybex (Open)			Linea (Closed)		
Parameter (degrees/sec)	*Peak Torque* (ft-lb)*	*Bilateral Deficit† (%)*	*Parameter (inches/sec)*	*Force (lb)*	*Bilateral Deficit† (%)*	
60			10			
U	142		U	462		
I	101	29	I	420	9	
180			20			
U	99		U	374		
I	78	21	I	331	11	
300			30			
U	80		U	302		
I	64	20	I	253	16	

I = involved, U = uninvolved.
*Values for quadriceps muscle group only.
†Determined as ratio of involved to uninvolved.

Modified from Davies GJ, Ellenbecker TS: Application of isokinetics in testing and rehabilitation. *In* Andrews JR, Harrelson GL, Wilk KE (eds): Physical Rehabilitation of the Injured Athlete, 2nd ed. Philadelphia, WB Saunders, 1998, p. 219.

pensation, the likelihood of injury recurrence may increase.

These results were further supported by the findings of Feiring and Ellenbecker.[72] This study also demonstrated differences between OKC and CKC testing. A particular point noted with both studies[5, 72] is that if only CKC testing is performed, isolated

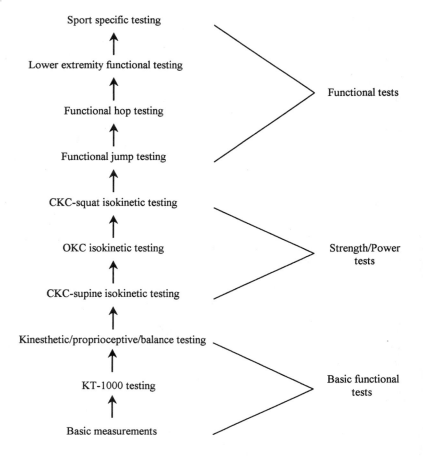

Figure 21–1. Functional testing algorithm (FTA) for the lower extremity. (Modified from Davies GJ, Wilk K, Ellenbecker TS: Assessment of strength. *In* Malone TR, McPoil T, Nitz AJ (eds.): Orthopedic and Sports Physical Therapy, 3rd ed. St. Louis, Mosby–Year Book, 1997.)

Sport specific testing
↑
Lower extremity functional testing
↑
Functional hop testing
↑
Functional jump testing
} Functional tests
↑
CKC-squat isokinetic testing
↑
OKC isokinetic testing
↑
CKC-supine isokinetic testing
} Strength/Power tests
↑
Kinesthetic/proprioceptive/balance testing
↑
KT-1000 testing
↑
Basic measurements
} Basic functional tests

deficits that exist in the lower extremity may be overlooked. It is only by testing each part of the kinetic chain that we can identify any existing deficits. The OKC component can address isolated muscle weakness that the CKC exercises cannot.[75]

The scientific validation of an integrated approach, however, needs to be addressed. A clinical project is currently being conducted by Davies to investigate the effects of two different rehabilitation protocols for patients following ACL reconstruction. One group of patients will undergo a purely CKC protocol, while the second group will receive an integrated OKC and CKC protocol. The results of such an investigation will either support or refute the use of an integrated rehabilitation program.

Functional Testing Algorithm

The integration of OKC and CKC protocols follows the functional testing algorithm (FTA) (Fig. 21–1).[76, 77] The reader is referred to Chapter 25 for complete details of this concept. Briefly, the patient is tested at an early level in the FTA. With successful completion, the patient is progressed and tested at the next level. If unable to complete the task at a minimal criterion, the patient remains at the same level. The focus of the rehabilitation program is then oriented to help the patient successfully complete the requirements to progress to the next FTA level. The FTA test results therefore provide the basis for an efficient, specific rehabilitation program involving both OKC and CKC tasks.

SUMMARY

This chapter reviews the literature regarding OKC and CKC rehabilitation protocols for individuals with knee injuries. Advantages and disadvantages of both methods have been defined. Rationale for the integration of the two rehabilitation techniques was provided. A program that uses both OKC and CKC exercises is functionally directed while recognizing and correcting isolated deficits.

References

1. Wilk KE, Escamilla RF, Fleisig GS, Arrigo CA, Barrentine SW: Open and closed kinetic chain exercise for the lower extremity: Theory and clinical application. Athletic Train Sports Health Care Perspect 1:336, 1995.
2. Timm KE: Post-surgical knee rehabilitation: A five year study of four methods and 5,381 patients. Am J Sports Med 16:463, 1988.
3. Wilk KE, Rominello BR, Soscia S, et al.: The relationship between subjective knee scores, isokinetic testing, and functional testing in ACL reconstructed knees. J Orthop Sports Phys Ther 20:60, 1994.
4. Blattner SE, Noble L: Relative effects of isokinetic and plyometric training on vertical jump performance. Res Q 50:583, 1979.
5. Davies GJ: Descriptive study comparing open kinetic chain and closed kinetic chain isokinetic testing of the lower extremity in 300 patients with selected knee pathologies, abstracted, p. 906. Proceedings of the 12th International Congress of the World Confederation for Physical Therapy, Washington, DC, June, 1995.
6. Snyder-Mackler L, Delitto A, Bailey SL, et al.: Strength of the quadriceps femoris muscle and functional recovery after reconstruction of the anterior cruciate ligament. J Bone Joint Surg 77(A):1166, 1995.
7. Nicholas JA, Strizak AM, Veras G: A study of thigh muscle weakness in different pathological states of the lower extremity. Am J Sports Med 4:241, 1976.
8. Greenberger HB, Paterno MV: Comparison of an isokinetic strength test and functional performance test in the assessment of lower extremity function, abstracted. J Orthop Sports Phys Ther 19:61, 1994.
9. Shaffer SW, Payne ED, Gabbard LR, et al.: Relationship between isokinetic and functional tests of the quadriceps, abstracted. J Orthop Sports Phys Ther 19:55, 1994.
10. Tegner Y, Lysholm J, Lysholm M, et al.: A performance test to monitor rehabilitation and evaluate anterior cruciate ligament injuries. Am J Sports Med 14:156, 1986.
11. Daniels L, Worthingham C: Muscle Testing: Techniques of Manual Examination, 3rd ed. Philadelphia, WB Saunders, 1986.
12. Barbee J, Landis D: Reliability of Cybex computer measures. Phys Ther 68:737, 1984.
13. Francis K, Hoobler T: Comparison of peak torque values of the knee flexor and extensor muscle groups using the Cybex II and Lido 2.0 isokinetic dynamometers. J Orthop Sports Phys Ther 8:480, 1987.
14. Mawdsley RH, Knapik JJ: Comparison of isokinetic measurements with test repetitions. Phys Ther 62:169, 1982.
15. Reitz CL, Rowinski M, Davies GJ: Comparison of Cybex II and Kin-Com reliability of the measures of peak torque: Work and power at three speeds, abstracted. Phys Ther 69:782, 1988.
16. Snow DJ, Johnson K: Reliability of two velocity controlled tests for the measurement of peak torque of the knee flexors during resisted muscle shortening and resisted muscle lengthening. Phys Ther 68:781, 1988.
17. Timm KE: Reliability of Cybex 340 and MERAC isokinetic measures of peak torque, total work, and average power at five test speeds. Phys Ther 69:782, 1988.
18. Davies GJ: A Compendium of Isokinetics in Clinical Usage and Rehabilitation Techniques, 4th ed. Onalaska, WI, S and S Publishers, 1992.

19. Solomonow M, Baratta R, Zhov BH, et al.: The synergistic action of the anterior cruciate ligament and thigh muscles in maintaining joint stability. Am J Sports Med 15:207, 1987.

20. Kisner C, Colby CA: Therapeutic Exercise: Foundations and Techniques, 2nd ed. Philadelphia, FA Davis, 1985.

21. Knight KL: Quadriceps strengthening with DAPRE technique: Case studies with neurological implications. Med Sci Sports Exerc 17:636, 1985.

22. Sherrington CS: On the proprioceptive system, especially in its reflex aspects. Brain 29:247, 1906.

23. Horch KW, Clark FJ, Burgess PR: Awareness of the knee joint. An anatomical and histological study in the cat. J Neurophysiol 38:1436, 1975.

24. Lephart SM, Pincivero DM, Giraldo J, Fu FH: The role of proprioception in the management and rehabilitation of athletic injuries. Am J Sports Med 25:130, 1997.

25. Bastian HC: The "muscular sense," its nature and corticol localisation. Brain 10:1, 1888.

26. Ferrel WR, Gandevia SC, McCloskey DI: The role of joint receptors in human kinesthesia when intramuscular receptors cannot contribute. J Physiol (Lond) 386:63, 1987.

27. Grigg P: Peripheral neural mechanisms in proprioception. J Sports Rehabil 3:2, 1994.

28. Grigg P, Greenspan BJ: Response of primate joint afferent neurons to mechanical stimulation of knee joint. J Neurophysiol 40:1, 1977.

29. Wyke B: The neurology of the joints. Ann R Coll Surg Engl 41:25, 1967.

30. Barrack RL, Skinner HB, Buckley SL: Proprioception in the anterior cruciate deficient knee. Am J Sports Med 17:1, 1989.

31. Barrack R, Bruckner J, Kneisl J, et al.: The outcome of non-operatively treated complete tears of the anterior cruciate ligament in active young adults. Clin Orthop 259:192, 1990.

32. Barrett DS, Cobb AG, Bentley G: Joint proprioception in normal, osteoarthritic, and replaced knees. J Bone Joint Surg 73(B):53, 1991.

33. Kennedy JC, Alexander IJ, Hayes KC: Nerve supply of the human knee and its functional importance. Am J Sports Med 10:329, 1982.

34. DeCarlo MS, Talbot RW: Evaluation of ankle joint proprioception following injection of the anterior talofibular ligament. J Orthop Sports Phys Ther 8:72, 1986.

35. Grigg P, Finerman GA, Riley LH: Joint position sense after total hip replacement. J Bone Joint Surg 55(A):1016, 1973.

36. Lephart SM, Kocher MS, Fu FH, et al.: Proprioception following anterior cruciate ligament reconstruction. J Sports Rehabil 1:188, 1992.

37. Smith R, Brunolli J: Shoulder kinesthesia after anterior glenohumeral dislocation. Phys Ther 69:106, 1989.

38. Allegrucci M, Whitney SL, Lephart SM, et al.: Shoulder kinesthesia in healthy unilateral athletes participating in upper extremity sports. J Orthop Sports Phys Ther 21:220, 1995.

39. Davies GJ, Hoffman SD: Neuromuscular testing and rehabilitation of the shoulder complex. J Orthop Sports Phys Ther 18:449, 1993.

40. Prentice WE: Closed kinetic chain exercise. In Rehabilitation Techniques in Sports Medicine, 2nd ed. St. Louis, Mosby, 1994.

41. Snyder-Mackler L: Scientific rationale and physiological basis for the use of closed kinetic chain exercise in the lower extremity. J Sport Rehab 5:2, 1996.

42. Wilk KE, Escamilla RF, Fleisig GS, et al.: The comparison of tibiofemoral joint forces and electromyography during open and closed kinetic chain exercises. Am J Sports Med 24:518, 1996.

43. Frndak PA, Berasi CC: Rehabilitation concerns following anterior cruciate ligament reconstruction. Sports Med 12:338, 1991.

44. Irrgang JJ: Modern trends in anterior cruciate ligament rehabilitation: Nonoperative and postoperative man. Sports Med 12:797, 1993.

45. Lutz GE, Stuart MJ, Sim FH: Rehabilitative techniques for athletes after reconstruction of the anterior cruciate ligament. Mayo Clin Proc 65:1322, 1990.

46. Shelbourne KD, Nitz P: Accelerated rehabilitation after anterior cruciate ligament reconstruction. Am J Sports Med 18:292, 1990.

47. Shelbourne KD, Klootwyk TE, DeCarlo MS: Update on accelerated rehabilitation after anterior cruciate ligament reconstruction. J Orthop Sports Phys 15:303, 1992.

48. Grood ES, Suntay WJ, Noyes FR: Biomechanics of knee extension exercise. J Bone Joint Surg 66A:725, 1984.

49. Henning CE, Lynch MA, Glick KR: An in vivo strain gauge study of elongation of the anterior cruciate ligament. Am J Sports Med 13:22, 1985.

50. Renstrom P, Arms SW, Stanwyck TS, et al.: Strain within the anterior cruciate ligament during hamstring and quadriceps activity. Am J Sports Med 14:83, 1986.

51. Shoemaker SC, Markolf KL: Effects of joint load on the stiffness and laxity of ligament deficient knees: An in vitro study of the anterior cruciate and medial collateral ligaments. J Bone Joint Surg 67A:136, 1985.

52. Arms SW, Pope MH, Johnson RJ, et al.: The biomechanics of anterior cruciate ligament rehabilitation and reconstruction. Am J Sports Med 12:8, 1984.

53. Johnson H, Karrholm J, Elmqvist LG: Kinematics of active knee extension after tear of the anterior cruciate ligament. Am J Sports Med 17:796, 1989.

54. Lutz GS, Palmitier RA, An KN, et al.: Comparison of tibiofemoral joint forces during open kinetic chain and closed kinetic chain exercise. J Bone Joint Surg 75A:732, 1993.

55. Wang C-J, Walker PS: Rotary laxity of the human knee joint. J Bone Joint Surg 56A:161, 1974.

56. Arms SW, Johnson RJ, Pope MH: Strain measurement of the human posterior cruciate ligament. Trans Orthop Res Soc 9:355, 1994.

57. Bennyon B, Howe JG, Pope MH, et al.: The measurement of anterior cruciate ligament strain in vivo. Int Orthop 16:1, 1992.

58. Bynum EB, Barrack RL, Alexander AH: Open versus closed kinetic chain exercises after cruciate ligament reconstruction: A prospective randomized study. Am J Sports Med 23:401, 1995.

59. Reiley DT, Martens M: Experimental analysis of the quadriceps muscle force and patellofemoral joint reaction force for various activities. Acta Orthop Scan 43:126, 1972.

60. Steinkamp LA, Dillingham MF, Markel MD, et al.: Biomechanical considerations in patellofemoral joint rehabilitation. Am J Sports Med 21:438, 1993.

61. Hungerford DS, Barry M: Biomechanics of the patellofemoral joint. Clin Orthop 144:9, 1979.
62. Escamilla RF: The effects of technique variations on tibiofemoral forces and muscle activity during the squat and leg press. Doctoral dissertation, Auburn University, 1995.
63. Brask B, Lueke R, Soderberg G: Electromyographic analysis of selected muscles during the lateral step-up exercise. Phys Ther 64:324, 1984.
64. Cook TM, Zimmerman CL, Lux KM, et al.: EMG comparison of lateral step-up and stepping machine exercise. J Orthop Sports Phys Ther 16:108, 1992.
65. Hsieh HH, Walker PS: Stabilizing mechanisms of the loaded and unloaded knee joint. J Bone Joint Surg 58:87, 1976.
66. Markolf KL, Bargar WL, Shoemaker SC, Amstutz HC: The role of joint load in knee stability. J Bone Joint Surg 63A:570, 1981.
67. Yack HJ, Collins CE, Whieldon TR: Closed kinetic chain exercise for the ACL deficient knee. Am J Sports Med 21:49, 1993.
68. Yack HJ, Riley LM, Whieldon TR: Anterior tibial translation during progressive loading of the ACL deficient knee during weight-bearing and non-weight-bearing isometric exercise. J Orthop Sports Phys Ther 20:247, 1994.
69. Crandall D, Richmond J, Lau J, et al.: A meta-analysis of the treatment of anterior cruciate ligament. Research paper presented at the American Orthopaedic Society for Sports Medicine, Palm Desert, CA, June, 1995.
70. Bolz S, Davies GJ: Leg length differences and correlation with total leg strength. J Orthop Sports Phys Ther 6:123, 1984.
71. Gleim GW, Nicholas JA, Webb JN: Isokinetic evaluation following leg injuries. Phys Sportsmed 6:74, 1978.
72. Feiring DC, Ellenbecker TS: Single versus multiple joint isokinetic testing with ACL reconstructed patients. Isok Exerc Sci 6:109, 1996.
73. Davies GJ, Heiderscheit BC: Reliability of the Lido Linea closed kinetic chain isokinetic dynamometer. J Orthop Sports Phys Ther 25:133, 1996.
74. Davies GJ, Ellenbecker TS: Application of isokinetics in testing and rehabilitation. *In* Andrews JR, Harrelson GL, Wilk KE (eds): Physical Rehabilitation of the Injured Athlete, 2nd ed. Philadelphia, WB Saunders, 1998, p. 219.
75. Davies GJ: The need for critical thinking in rehabilitation. J Sports Rehabil 4:1, 1995.
76. Davies GJ: Functional testing algorithm for patients with knee injuries, abstracted, p. 91. Proceedings of the 12th International Congress of the World Confederation for Physical Therapy, Washington, DC, June, 1995.
77. Davies GJ, Wilk K, Ellenbecker TS: Assessment of strength. *In* Malone TR, McPoil T, Nitz AJ (eds): Orthopedic and Sports Physical Therapy, 3rd ed. St. Louis, Mosby–Year Book, 1997, p. 231.

22 Kinetic Chain Concept

W. Ben Kibler, MD

*T*he goal of rehabilitation of knee ligament injuries is the return of knee function. This is often a complex goal because it deals not only with local knee function but also with the function of the knee in the context of specific types of athletic activity. To be able to return the knee to normal, the therapist and clinician must understand the functions that the knee performs in athletic activities. These functions should be analyzed in terms of both physiologic activities and biomechanical actions. The knee and its ligaments can be looked at as an isolated entity, but should also be looked at in the context of how the knee and the ligaments work in concert with the rest of the body to allow the athlete to function for the particular sport or activity that he or she is engaged in. This chapter is designed to explore some of the functional requirements of the knee and the ligaments and to describe them in the context of a kinetic chain of events.

The kinetic chain is a useful concept that may be used as a framework to describe the function of the entire limb and the athlete in athletic activity. It can help explain the functions of kicking, running, or jumping, in "lower body" activity and can help describe how the knee works in predominantly upper body sports in terms of contributing to efficient throwing, serving, and hitting of the ball in baseball or ground strokes in tennis. The kinetic chain can also be used to describe the dysfunctions that exist in the knee, knee ligaments, and entire body after injury or after treatment. This concept can provide a scientific basis for accelerated rehabilitation of the knee in the context of local function and sport-specific activities. It should also be used as a tool in helping to evaluate outcomes. Total limb function cannot be considered normal unless the kinetic chain is intact.

The kinetic chain refers to a sequential activation of the limb segments of the leg in an optimal fashion to allow for efficient generation of the force, stabilization of the leg, and transfer of the force to the distal end of the chain, whether it be the opposite foot or the arm. The activation sequence usually progresses from the base of support through each consecutive segment (ground → foot → leg → thigh → trunk). The activation sequence is sport- or activity-specific and is dependent on joint position and muscle support. In most sports, the activation starts at the ground with a ground reaction force. This occurs in all ground-based sports, including running, jumping, kicking, baseball, tennis, and soccer. The activation produces force, both from the ground and through muscle activation in the proximal segments. The activation also allows for load absorption and joint and segment stabilization to allow the more proximal segments of the chain to be a stable base for activation of the next segment. Through this combination of force generation and joint stabilization, the generated force is transferred from the ground through successive segments, with additional force and velocity being added through the activation of each segment. This activation terminates in a distal segment at which maximum force and velocity are applied.

The knee is a very important link in most kinetic chains of athletic activity. It is the central point of the leg, which is the force-generating unit for most activities. The knee requires stability to allow the large force-generating muscles to have an effective pull on the rest of the segments and to support the rest of the body weight on the legs. It also requires smooth motion to allow the movements of the knee to be harmonized with the movements of the other joints to allow for smooth motion of the entire limb. If the ligaments are injured or unstable, the kinetic chain is broken and force transfer and force regulation are compromised. This causes a problem in the more distal segments as decreased force is provided to the other segments or they have to provide a larger share of the force generation. In either case, total activity for athletic performance is compromised.

The kinetic chain concept has both a biomechanical and a physiologic basis. Understanding the biomechanical and physiologic bases of the kinetic chain allows a proper evaluation of knee ligament injuries, proper evaluation prior to rehabilitation, and smooth framework for rehabilitation.

BIOMECHANICAL BASIS FOR THE KINETIC CHAIN CONCEPT

The kinetic chain is based on the work of Hanavan,[1] who first modeled the body as a series of links. These links constituted a segment of the body, usually a bone and its adjoining joint. It was shown that the optimal activation of these links and stabilization of these links allow for efficient activity, whether it be in normal daily activities or in sports activities.[2]

The importance of proper sequential activation of the links was also demonstrated by the work of Putnam,[3] who demonstrated two methods of biomechanically accomplishing a complex activity involving several links. The first method was by the coordination of partial momenta.[4] In this construct, an athletic activity is accomplished by allowing the terminal ends of every segment of the link system to be moving at their optimal velocity at the exact same moment. This would result in a very long lever arm and rigid body, moving the terminal segment at a very rapid speed. An example of this type of activation would be trying to kick a ball with the leg extended and locked at the hip and knee, and dorsiflexed and locked at the ankle, and pivoting the entire leg around the plant leg hip. The major problem is that it is difficult to coordinate all of the segments into this exact pattern and the compliance of the tissues will not allow the body to be this rigidly stiff. The more proximal segments would have a huge stress placed on them because of the requirements of moving the more distal segments. In athletic practice, this does not occur except in rare situations.

Sequential activation, or summation of speed, however, has been shown to be very effective in allowing maximal velocity at the terminal segments.[5] In this situation, all of the terminal ends of the segments move in a coordinated sequence so that the purpose of the kinetic chain is realized. This is the more familiar pattern of kicking, in which the plant leg and hip act as a fulcrum to allow successive activation of hip flexion from extension, hip internal rotation from external rotation, knee extension from flexion, and ankle dorsiflexion from plantar flexion. This allows the terminal link, which is usually much smaller, to move at a maximum velocity and with the most range of motion to allow an effect similar to the end of a cracking whip. The larger proximal segments do not move as rapidly or go through large ranges of motion, but provide large torques. Most athletic activities are biomechanically made up of a sequential activation of the links of the segmented system. The knee should be looked at in this context and should be rehabilitated with proper activation of these segments in mind.

The forces that are seen at the knee are made up of several elements.[3, 6, 7] The first element is the moment that is experienced at the knee based on muscle activation around the knee joint. This element is the factor that has been most widely studied. Muscle activation studies, joint force analysis, and strength testing studies have focused almost exclusively on this area. Although important, because the knee is the source of the overt clinical symptoms and pathologic conditions, this is not the sole factor. The second contributor to the force at the knee is the position of the adjacent segments, the tibia and the femur, in terms of flexion, extension, or rotation. The third contributing factor to the force around the knee is the velocity as well as acceleration of the segments around the knee joint.

The position and motion of the segments are also determined by the articulations above and below the knee joint. Position plus motion of the hip joint is a major determinant of the forces at the knee. Muscle activation patterns about the knee, the varus-valgus angle of the knee, and compression loads on the knee can be varied by the position of the hip and pelvis. The more varus angulation that the hip is exposed to, the more internal rotation and valgus stress is placed on the knee. Gluteus medius and gluteus maximus activity decrease the load at the knee by allowing more valgus of the hip and a negative Trendelenburg position.

The more proximal segments of the kinetic chain of kicking are very influential in the forces at the knee. The most important muscles for causing maximum foot velocity in the kicking motion are the hip flexors.[6] After the hip flexors move the entire leg forward, the knee extensors are activated to counteract knee flexion and to help create knee extension.

The force seen at the knee of the swing leg in running is dependent on plant leg hip activation.[8] As the swing leg is raised higher, as in longer or faster strides, the plant leg hip faces larger internal-external rotation and varus-valgus moment, indicating rotation of the entire body about the hip in both the transverse and coronal planes. A slight valgus positioning of the plant leg hip, with slight elevation of the pelvis on the swing leg, allows better stabilization and power in push off on the plant leg, and more power and velocity in the knee in the swing leg.

Hip position, hip angle, and hip muscle strength are also important factors in facilitating rehabilitation after knee injury or surgery. DeVita[9] has evaluated hip and knee kinematics, kinetics, and energetics before ACL reconstruction and in early ACL reconstruction. Preoperatively, knee and hip kinematics, and energetics were markedly altered. In the postoperative phases, knee kinematics progressed in a significant trend toward normal, but knee energetics (loadbearing and stabilization characteristics) were not progressing. Both hip kinematics and energetics were significantly progressing toward normality. In fact, hip energetics 5 weeks postoperatively were better than pre-injury levels. It was thought that the clinical improvement in knee function was in large part attributable to increased function of the hip stabilizing muscles. This allowed optimal positioning of the body over the leg and loading of the knee so that the moments seen at the knee were appropriate for the level of healing at the knee.

These findings confirm the function of the knee as a link in the kinetic chain and emphasize the importance of the proximal and distal segments of the leg in modifying the loads on the knee, allowing the knee to function in a stable situation both in performance and injury. This study also emphasizes the need to look at the motions and positions of the proximal and distal links around the knee when evaluating and treating the knee itself.

PHYSIOLOGIC BASIS FOR THE KINETIC CHAIN CONCEPT

Motor activation for specific athletic activities is organized according to the architecture of the muscles, the position of the limb segments in space, and the specific activities.[10] These are learned patterns that are governed by spinal cord–mediated pattern generators, modulated by repetition, and controlled by reflex feedback through sensory mechanisms. There are two main patterns of motor organization that affect muscles in an athletic activity. They are the link-dependent and the force-dependent systems.

The link-dependent system is concerned with coordinating motor activity around one joint (Table 22–1). The major function of the link-dependent patterns is to control perturbations to the joint, conferring joint stability in concert with ligamentous activity. The major sensory organs that control the activation of the link-dependent system are the muscle spindle receptors. They work in real time to give a continuous feedback of joint position and muscle activity to the spinal cord. These muscle patterns are the ones that are usually documented by EMG evaluation of the muscles around the joint. This is the activation pattern that is produced on EMG evaluation of the gastrocnemius, hamstring, and quadriceps muscles in various jumping, running, and cutting activities. The predominant mode of muscle activation in this pattern is co-contraction force couple, which emphasizes stability of the joint rather than torque to the moving limb. These co-contractions are modulated in a pattern of reciprocal inhibition so that a relatively low level of muscle activation is adequate to provide optimal stiffness to the joint. The stiffness decreases abnormal motions owing to perturbations of the joint. Reciprocal inhibition is a neurologic pattern that allows modulation of the agonist and antagonist firing patterns so that there is

● ▬ Table 22–1. **Link-Dependent System**

- Coordinated activity at one joint
- Muscle spindle receptors: primary
- Predominant muscle contraction: co-contraction
- Motor activation increases joint stiffness

control of stiffness of the joint without maximal muscle contraction. By modulating the agonist pattern and by intensifying the antagonist pattern, a balance of muscle activity can be achieved at about 35 to 40 percent of maximum muscle firing capacity while still maintaining the stiffness of the joint. This is an organized pattern. It is not strictly based on reflexes, although modulation and improvement of the stiffness can be done through reflex activation by repetitive movements. It has been shown that in the ankle joint, ankle disc training causes a stabilization effect of muscle firing, not by increasing peroneal activation but by modulating peroneal and tibialis activation to allow for a stabilization of the joint.

Proprioceptive feedback from the ligaments around the joints also appears to have some influence on the link-dependent patterns but does not appear to have the major influence. Motor activation patterns can be returned to normal activation patterns in the absence of ligamentous constraints and ligamentous proprioceptive contributions.

The second organizational pattern for motor activation is the force-dependent pattern (Table 22–2). This pattern is responsible for generation of force throughout several link segments. It harmonizes the movements of the segments to allow for maximal velocity of the most distal segment of the chain. It also stiffens the entire limb and all the involved segments by coordinating the force-dependent and link-dependent patterns simultaneously. This activation pattern is more efficient at faster speeds of motion and is responsible for the quick reactions that can occur in athletic activities. It is modulated by Golgi tendon receptors and is very angle specific for the joints.

Motor firing patterns in the force-dependent pattern can be altered by changes of joint position as little as 15 degrees or joint velocity changes of 10 percent. The exact pattern of muscle activation in the force-dependent pattern is based on the position

and stability of the joints determined by the link-dependent pattern. Abnormal laxity of the joint or abnormal position of the joint causes an alteration and a decrease in efficiency of firing of the link-dependent pattern, thereby breaking the link system.

This organizational pattern is not as well investigated in the literature. There are few studies that demonstrate activation of the other segments of the leg in various running and jumping patterns. One such study did show that muscle activation around the hip and knee is dependent on whether the angle of cutting is at 45 degrees or 90 degrees and is different between male and female athletes. Motor activation patterns are also affected by the direction of the force vectors. Activation sequences are different when the leg is on the ground, as in a closed chain activity, versus when the leg is in the air, as in an open chain activity. Motor control theory based on this model of motor activation and on matching of activation patterns with sports or activity demands suggests that conditioning and rehabilitation be done by simulating normal force applications, joint loads, and motor activation patterns. With respect to knee rehabilitation, it is more important to have the foot in a closed chain activity pattern, as this is how the muscles work in normal athletic activities.

The muscle activity around the knee is a complex interaction of link-dependent and force-dependent patterns. Ligamentous instability or stiffness plays a role in the motor activation patterns. Once the ligaments have been restored, however, normalization of the muscle firing patterns needs to be accomplished to allow for biomechanical movements. It is insufficient to look only at the muscle firing patterns around the knee because the knee also works in the context of the force-dependent pattern; therefore, the firing patterns and activations of the hip and foot musculature also must be considered in knee rehabilitation. It is very probable that the major benefits that closed chain rehabilitation bring to knee ligament rehabilitation include not only that the muscles around the knee are allowed to work in a co-contraction fashion but also, more importantly, that the hips, knee, and foot are placed in a weight-bearing position, that the hip musculature is brought into play at the proper early time in rehabilitation to allow for normal load across the knee, and that this allows normal

---

○▬ Table 22–2. **Force-Dependent System**

- Generation of force through several joints
- Responsible for quick reaction-type movements
- Motor activation dependent on joint positions
- Golgi tendon organs, primary receptors involved

firing patterns to occur throughout the entire extremity.

CLINICAL APPLICATIONS OF THE KINETIC CHAIN CONCEPT

This review has emphasized the fact that the entire leg participates in athletic activity. The knee does not exist in isolation, either physiologically or biomechanically. Hip position is one of the major factors in allowing normal kinematics and energetics of the knee in normal function. The kinetic chain concept allows an understanding of all of the factors that go into normal function of the knee in athletic activities and emphasizes the importance of evaluation and rehabilitation of all of the segments of the kinetic chain in the rehabilitation sequence.

Before the patient begins knee rehabilitation, he or she should be checked for kinetic chain alterations. Lumbar flexion and extension and range of motion should be assessed along with "lumbopelvic rhythm," which is the composite motion that allows smooth coupling of lumbar spine motion and pelvic rotation. Hip range of motion should be evaluated in flexion-extension, abduction-adduction, and, especially, rotation. Rotation should be measured goniometrically. Hip abductor, flexor, and extensor strength should be specifically tested, in both the supine and the standing positions. Dynamic pelvic control should be tested in single-leg stance, straight ahead walking, pushing off with an exaggerated stride, climbing an 8- to 12-inch step, and when possible, a single-leg half-squat. A positive Trendelenburg sign, with pelvic tilt toward the non-stance leg and plant leg hip varus, indicates the need for proximal hip exercises. Ankle plantar and dorsiflexion strength and range of motion should also be tested.

In the early phases of rehabilitation, the hip strength and range of motion may be rehabilitated without compromising any of the knee ligament healing. Early weight-bearing with normal gait patterns, avoiding a Trendelenburg position of the hip and pelvis, and avoiding an excessive hip flexion and knee flexion should be emphasized to allow for the early return of the normal motor patterns. In skilled athletes, these patterns are very well developed but are very fragile and drop out somewhat quickly, to be replaced by substitute patterns of muscle activation and substitute patterns of biomechanics at the hip and the knee.

Early return to the more normal physiologic and biomechanical patterns can be accomplished and should be encouraged in order to restore the normal motor patterns. Closed chain exercises are an extremely efficient way to accomplish these purposes. Placing the foot on the ground and allowing a normal pattern of activation from the hip to the foot and from the foot to the hip through the knee allow the normal activation patterns to be re-established. By placing the knee, hip, and ankle in normal positions, the exercises allow the previously established length-dependent patterns to be reinstituted. By allowing joint loading through all of the links and segments of the leg, closed chain exercises also reinstitute the normal force-dependent patterns. Their activation increases stiffness of the entire limb to protect the healing ligament, allow normal patterns of load transfer from the foot through the knee to the hip, and allow normal patterns of load transfer from the plant to the swing leg. In all ground-based athletic activities, closed chain activation of the force-dependent pattern is the predominant mode of muscle organization. This pattern, which replicates the activities of running, jumping, walking, and kicking, and even is evident in upper body activities such as throwing,[11] should be reinstituted and re-emphasized all the way through the rehabilitation process. "Accelerated" rehabilitation, which appears to offer many advantages and few disadvantages, depends to a great extent on closed chain concepts of early weight-bearing, decreased external support, exercising in physiologic ranges with the foot on the ground, and emphasis on total leg control. The kinetic chain concept provides the physiologic and biomechanical supports for the institution of closed chain accelerated rehabilitation. This concept also accurately predicts that systems of rehabilitation that adhere to closed chain principles will have a high percentage of favorable outcomes.

The criteria for return to play should also be governed by the kinetic chain concept. It is not sufficient to have full range of motion and good anatomic stability of the knee itself, but also normal activation of all of the segments in the kinetic chain. Normal hip strength and motion, and normal ankle range of motion, should be present as well as normal knee motion and normal knee activation patterns. Special emphasis should be placed on specific patterns that are important for specific sports, such as push-offs in sprinters or kicks in soccer players, landing in basketball players, stabilization and twisting patterns in basketball players, and load-bearing in a backward peddling direction for down linemen or defensive backs in football. These patterns involve not only the knee musculature but also the leg, hip, and back musculature.

SUMMARY

The kinetic chain concept can be a very important concept to understand when rehabilitating patients who have suffered injuries to the ligaments about the knee. Alterations in the biomechanics and physiology of the normal functions of the knee, both locally and distantly, accompany knee ligament injuries, immobilization due to the injuries, and treatment or immobilization of the injury itself. Anatomic restoration of the ligaments, either by surgery or bracing, is not sufficient in and of itself to restore the normal kinetic chain activation. Both the physiology and the biomechanics suffer as a result of knee ligament injury and should be brought back to normal patterns as soon as possible to complete the rehabilitation of the knee. By knowing the normal functions of the knee, normal patterns of motor firing organization, and normal biomechanical demands on the knee, a therapist or clinician can then design appropriate rehabilitation protocols to restore the physiologic and bio-

mechanical functions of the knee in addition to the anatomic integrity of the knee. Closed chain rehabilitation patterns are the most efficient way of restoring the physiology and biomechanics of the knee and have shown great utility in accomplishing these results.

References

1. Hanavan EP: Mathematical Model of the Human Body. Wright-Patterson Air Force Base, Pub. No. AMRL-TR-64-102, 1964.
2. Marino M: Current concepts of rehabilitation in sports medicine. In Nicholas JA, Hershman EB (eds): The Lower Extremity and Spine in Sports Medicine. St. Louis, Mosby, 1986, pp. 117–195.
3. Putnam CA: Sequential motions of body segments in stroking and throwing skills: Descriptions and explanations. J Biomechanics 26:125–135, 1993.
4. Van Gheluwe B, Hebbelinck M: The kinematics of the serve movement in tennis. In Winter D (ed): Biomechanics IX-B. Champaign, IL, Human Kinetics, 1985, pp. 521–526.
5. Bunn JW: Scientific Principles of Coaching. Englewood Cliffs, NJ, Prentice Hall, 1972.
6. Putnam CA: A segment interaction analysis of proximal to distal sequential segment motion patterns. Med Sci Sports Exerc 23:130–144, 1991.
7. Zajac FE, Gordon ME: Determining muscle's force and action in multi-articular movement. Exerc Sports Sci Rev 17:187–230, 1989.
8. Chou LS, Draganich LF: Stepping over an obstacle increases the motions and moments of the joints of the trailing limb in young adults. J Biomechanics 30:331–337, 1997.
9. DeVita P, Hortobagyi T, Barrier J: Gait mechanics are not normal after ACL reconstruction and accelerated rehabilitation. Med Sci Sports Exerc 30:1481–1488, 1998.
10. Nichols TR: A biomechanical perspective on spinal mechanisms of coordinated muscular action: An architectural principle. Acta Anat 151:1–13, 1994.
11. Kibler WB: Biomechanical analysis of the shoulder during tennis activities. Clin Sports Med 14:79–86, 1995.

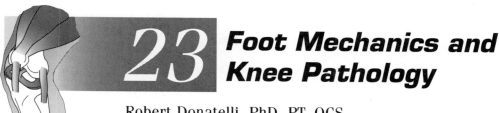

23 Foot Mechanics and Knee Pathology

Robert Donatelli, PhD, PT, OCS,
and Bruce Greenfield, PT, MMSc, OCS

Musculoskeletal injuries to the knees are commonly classified as either macrotrauma or microtrauma injuries.[1] Macrotrauma injuries usually result in a partial or complete ligamentous tear or bone fracture and occur in patients who often undergo surgical repair or reconstruction. Microtrauma injuries or overuse injuries result in microtear of tissue followed by inflammation and soft tissue healing.[2]

Although the etiology of knee macrotrauma injury resulting from a single, high-impact event is easily discerned with a proper history, the causes of microtrauma injuries to the knee that result from repetitive low-insult stress to tissue are often multifactorial and difficult to determine.[3, 4] The factors are divided into intrinsic and extrinsic (Table 23–1) predisposing causes.[5] Extrinsic factors include, but are not limited to, vocational stresses such as repetitive climbing on a ladder or walking on concrete surfaces, or avocational or sports stresses such as overtraining, incorrect training, or, in runners, incorrect running shoes.[6–8] Intrinsic factors of the lower extremity often include changes in normal alignment and mechanics of the foot and ankle.[9] The hip,

knees, and ankle joints compose the lower extremity kinetic chain as a series of interconnected joints that produce an interdependent movement pattern during specific activities.[10] Because the foot is the terminal segment in contact with the ground, changes in position and movement of the foot and ankle influence the position and movement of the knee. Several authors have described the kinetic chain movement of the lower extremity during gait and have documented correlation of foot and ankle problems with selective knee conditions.[11–13] The result is that many clinicians evaluate the position and movement of the foot and ankle as a predisposing intrinsic factor to overuse injury at the knee.

Application of appropriate treatment including correction of foot and ankle malalignment in the presence of knee overuse injuries are therefore predicated on knowledge of normal function. Positional changes in the normal anatomic alignment of the lower extremity resulting in either genu valgus or varus may place increased stress on the collateral and capsular ligaments, in addition to the anterior and posterior cruciate ligaments. Changes in stress patterns may influence the rate and quality of healing after injury or surgery. The purpose of this chapter is to review the normal and abnormal mechanics of the foot and ankle and relate the mechanics to changes in knee position, function, and injury.

Table 23–1. Overuse Injuries: Intrinsic and Extrinsic Factors

Factor Type	Examples
Predisposing (intrinsic)	Malalignment of the lower extremity, e.g., genu valgum, genu varum Leg length discrepancy Muscle imbalances
Precipitating (extrinsic)	Training errors Shoe wear Running surfaces Overstriding
Perpetuating (intrinsic and extrinsic)	Continued training without correction of predisposing or precipitating factors

ALIGNMENT OF THE LOWER EXTREMITY AND FOOT AND ANKLE

An understanding of normal alignment of the lower extremity is imperative to assess the effects of altered foot and ankle mechanics on the kinematics and kinetics of the knee. The following discussion of lower extremity alignment is extrapolated from Norkin and Levangie.[14] Because the femoral neck overhangs the femoral shaft (angle of inclination), the long axis of the femur is oblique, directed inferiorly and medially from its proximal to its distal end. The anatomic axis of the tibia is directed almost vertically. Consequently, the femoral and tibial longitudinal axes normally form an angle medially at the knee joint of 185 to 190 degrees (Fig. 23–1). That is, the femur is angled off vertically 5 to 10 degrees, creating a physiologic valgus angle at the knee. The result is that the mechanical axis or the weight-bearing forces directed from the ground to the femoral head at the hip courses equally between the medial and lateral compartments of the knee (Fig. 23–2). Weight-bearing stresses during bilateral stance are therefore equally distributed between the medial and lateral tibiofemoral articulations and the knee can function most efficiently and with the least amount of stress to the extra- and intra-articular soft tissues and muscles.

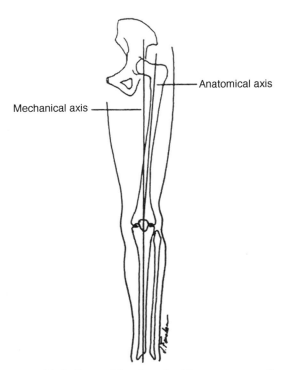

Figure 23–2. Femoral head at the hip courses equally between the medial and lateral compartments of the knee. (From Norkin CC, Levangie PK: Joint Structure and Function: A Comprehensive Analysis, 2nd ed. Philadelphia, F. A. Davis, 1992.)

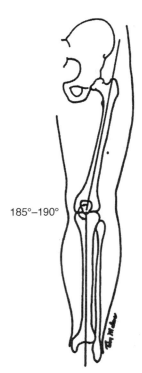

185°–190°

Figure 23–1. Femoral and tibial long axis normally form an angle medially at the knee joint of 185 to 190 degrees. (From Norkin CC, Levangie PK: Joint Structure and Function: A Comprehensive Analysis, 2nd ed. Philadelphia, F. A. Davis, 1992.)

If the medial tibiofemoral angle is greater than 10 degrees, an abnormal condition called genu valgum is produced (Fig. 23–3A). The result is that the mechanical axis of the lower extremity shifts toward the lateral compartment of the knee, resulting in increased compression, with increased tensile stress along the medial structures, including the tibial collateral ligament, coronary ligament, and, to some extent, the anterior cruciate ligament. A decrease in the physiologic valgus angle produces a condition called genu varum (Fig. 23–3B). The mechanical axis shifts medially, increasing compression through the medial tibiofemoral compartment, with increased tensile stress within the structures along the lateral knee, including the lateral collateral ligament, the distal iliotibial band, and the anterior cruciate ligament. Structures both proximal (at the hip) and distal (at the foot and ankle) can produce alterations from the normal anatomic axis at the knee. The changes from normal alignment and function of the foot and ankle are the primary focus of this chapter.

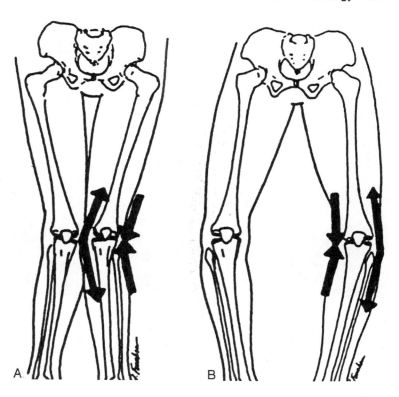

Figure 23–3. *A*, Genu valgum (tibio-femoral angle greater than 10 degrees). *B*, Genu varum. (From Norkin CC, Levangie PK: Joint Structure and Function: A Comprehensive Analysis, 2nd ed. Philadelphia, F. A. Davis, 1992.)

Normal and Abnormal Alignment of the Foot and Ankle

According to Root et al.,[15] the ideal posture of the foot and ankle from which normal function occurs is where the subtalar joint is neither excessively supinated nor pronated. Observation of the ideal posture of the foot and ankle is when the rearfoot is in line with the midline of the calf and the forefoot is perpendicular to the midline of the heel (Fig. 23–4). Root et al. define normal anatomic forefoot position as 0 degrees of varus or valgus relative to the rearfoot (heel) with the subtalar joint in neutral. Forefoot varus is defined as the inversion of the forefoot on the rearfoot with the subtalar joint in neutral (Fig. 23–5). Forefoot valgus is eversion of the forefoot with the subtalar joint in neutral (Fig. 23–6). Forefoot varus and valgus are the most common causes of foot and ankle abnormal pronation and supination, respectively. The ideal position is the position of the foot from which the normal amount of pronation and supination during gait and running occurs.

Theoretically, forefoot varus is a rigid de-

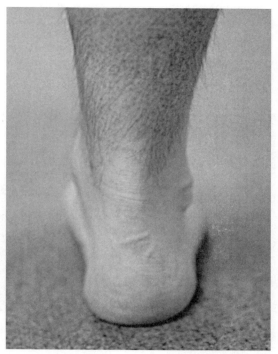

Figure 23–4. Ideal posture of the foot and ankle (midline of calf and forefoot is perpendicular to the midline of the heel).

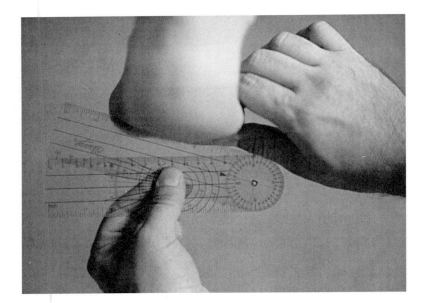

Figure 23–5. Forefoot varus.

formity that creates an abnormal gait pattern with weight-bearing under the lateral metatarsal heads during propulsion. The inverted position of the forefoot keeps the medial metatarsal heads off the weight-bearing surface during stance. A rigid forefoot varus deformity that is uncompensated during weight-bearing is rare; however, a compensated hypermobile forefoot varus is common. The definition of hypermobile forefoot varus for the purposes of this text is excessive inversion and limited eversion of the forefoot (Fig. 23–7). The hypermobile forefoot is secondary to instability of the midtarsal joints and collapse of the medial arch during weight-bearing activities. The excessive motion of the midtarsal joint area can cause an overpronation of the rearfoot.

Pathologic conditions seen clinically are most often related to the compensatory mechanisms that allow the forefoot to bear weight (Fig. 23–8). The most common compensatory mechanism during the gait cycle that allows the medial metatarsal's contact with the weight-bearing surface is subtalar joint pronation.

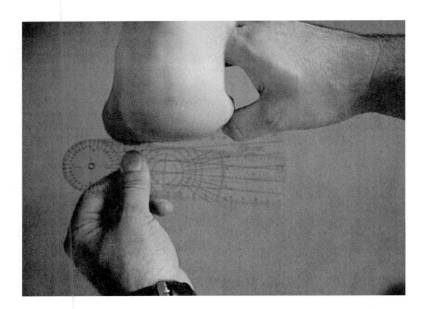

Figure 23–6. Forefoot valgus.

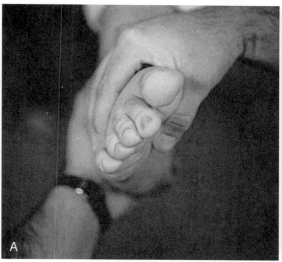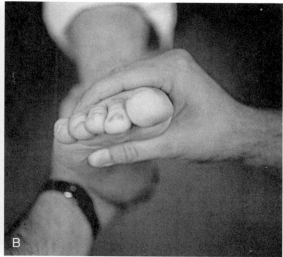

Figure 23-7. *A*, Excessive inversion of the forefoot while the rearfoot is stabilized. *B*, Limited eversion of the forefoot, unable to move the forefoot past midline.

Abnormal pronation of the foot has been implicated in many pathologic conditions of the foot, ankle, and knees.[16-20] Normally, subtalar joint pronation provides a mechanism for shock absorption and adaptation to uneven terrain early in the stance phase of

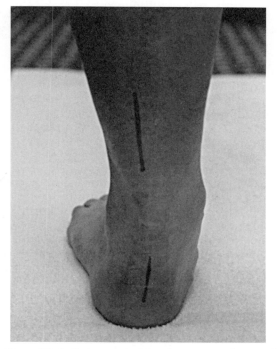

Figure 23-8. Compensated forefoot varus: abnormal alignment.

gait. The subtalar joint is in neutral or slight supination at heel strike. A normal amount of pronation occurs for two reasons. First, the center of gravity falls medial to the subtalar joint axis, resulting in calcaneal eversion. Second, the talus follows the action of the tibia in the transverse plane during weight-bearing movements. When the tibia internally rotates during initial stance, the talus adducts and the plantar flexes. Pronation during weight-bearing consists of these concurrent motions of calcaneal eversion, talar adduction, and talar-plantar flexion. Abnormal pronation continues beyond 20 to 35 percent of stance phase when supination normally occurs. Excessive pronation is pronation that is of greater magnitude than normal. Excessive pronation is difficult to define; a literature review reveals no study indicating the degree of subtalar joint pronation in a large number of normal subjects.

Most biomechanists and clinicians have found that the ideal position of the foot is not ubiquitous in the general population. Taunton et al.[13] define a mild forefoot varus deformity as 4 to 6 degrees in the general population. A related study, examining the forefoot position of 240 feet in 120 normal subjects, found an average of 8 degrees of forefoot varus.[21] A mild degree of forefoot varus is common and does not, in and of itself, result in significant pathomechanics of the foot and pathology. Muscle fatigue and the effects of extrinsic factors such as overtraining or improper footwear, superimposed on malalignment, may result in overuse injuries.

EFFECTS OF ABNORMAL FOOT MECHANICS ON THE KNEE

Abnormal mechanics of the foot and ankle has been identified as an intrinsic factor that can both predispose to and perpetuate an overuse injury at the knee. The following is a discussion of the pathomechanics of knee overuse injury resulting from abnormal foot and ankle pronation and supination.

Effect of Abnormal Pronation

Excessive and prolonged rearfoot pronation produces obligatory internal tibial rotation. The rearfoot normally pronates from heel strike until midstance, causing internal tibial rotation. External rotation of the tibia, femur, and pelvis normally occurs from the beginning of midstance to terminal stance (toe-off) in response to supination of the foot and ankle. Excessive pronation may prolong internal rotation of the tibia into stance phase. This relative internal rotation is translated up through the lower extremity and causes internal rotation that effectively forces the lateral portion of the femoral trochlear groove anteromedially against the lateral patellar facet during weight-bearing.[16]

PATELLAR COMPRESSION SYNDROME

Chronic irritation of the lateral patellar facet can result in lateral patellar compression syndrome with pathologic changes in the hyaline cartilage of the lateral patellar facet. Fulkerson[17, 18] also identified that irritation of a small sensory nerve along the lateral border of the patella may result from this condition. Histologic evidence of retinacular nerve injury is often associated with patellofemoral malalignment. If pronation of the involved extremity is greater than the patient's normal contralateral leg, the clinician should be suspicious that pronation is excessive and potentially aggravating to patellofemoral function. The prolonged, obligatory internal rotation of the tibia that occurs with excessive foot pronation through the

gait cycle applies a tensile force to the attachment site of the iliotibial band at Gerdy's tubercle that can tether the iliotibial band tightly against the lateral femoral epicondyle and result in irritation of the iliotibial band during running. The result is iliotibial band friction syndrome.[19]

FUNCTIONAL GENU VALGUM

Excessive or prolonged pronation may also result in a functional genu valgum, as well as an obligatory tibial internal rotation. As the calcaneus everts, the talus adducts, moving the tibia medial relative to the femur.[21] The effect is to increase opening along the medial tibiofemoral joint and tensile strain along the deep medial capsule and medial collateral ligament.

LIGAMENTOUS RESTRAINTS OF ANTEROPOSTERIOR DRAWER

The anterior cruciate ligament (ACL) primarily resists anterior tibial shear, but it has a secondary function of resisting tibial valgum and internal rotation.[22] The position of excessive tibial internal rotation and valgum may therefore with time overstress the ACL.[23] This is particularly relevant in the presence of a healing reconstructed ligament, or in the presence of a partial ACL tear.

CHANGE IN Q ANGLE

The Q angle of the knee represents the quadriceps angle of pull along the femur produced by the quadriceps muscle pull superiorly and the patellar tendon pull at the tibial tubercle inferiorly. The Q angle is measured by placing a goniometer over the center of the patella with the patient standing or supine. The stationary arm of the goniometer is aligned with the anterior superior iliac spine and the moveable arm is aligned with the tibial tubercle (Fig. 23–9). The normal Q angle measures approximately 10 degrees in men and 15 degrees in women and normally reflects the anatomic valgus angle of the lower extremity. Any biomechanical problem that increases the Q angle potentially results in an increase in lateral vector of the quadriceps muscle pull that can result in an increase in the amount of lateral patellar tracking. As the foot is pronating beyond the normal 4 to 6 degrees and

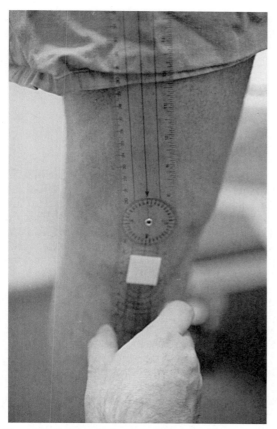

Figure 23–9. Q angle (anterosuperior iliac spine to tibial tubercle).

Effect of Abnormal Supination

Abnormal supination is the inability of the foot to pronate effectively during the stance phase of gait.[20] Pes cavus, or the high-arched foot, is commonly associated with abnormal supination. The foot type described is also associated with a rigid structure that is a poor shock absorber and is limited in the presence of terrain. Pes cavovarus is a specific foot type defined by a rigid plantar-flexed first ray or medial column. The plantar-flexed position of the medial column is often described as an everted position of the forefoot on the rearfoot.[21] During weight-bearing, the rigid plantar-flexed medial column is compensated for by the rearfoot moving into inversion, or supination (Fig. 23–10). Reduction in normal subtalar joint pronation decreases attenuation of forces at the foot and ankle and may increase forces up to the knee. The inability to absorb ground reaction forces at heel strike, especially during high-impact running, has been closely linked with pain and dysfunction in other joints.

A potential result of a compensated supinated foot is obligatory external tibial rotation. The external rotation of the tibia may also position the femur limb in a relative externally rotated posture. The abnormal posture of the lower limb may create a functional genu varum.[26] According to Noyes et al.,[27] a varus alignment at the knee increases

beyond 25 percent of stance phase, the tibia is carried into excessive and prolonged internal rotation. This causes the tibia to be in internal rotation at the same time in certain individuals that the pelvis is causing the femur to migrate into external rotation. The result is an increase in the Q angle and lateral pulling of the patella.

Eng and Pierrynowski[24] used foot orthoses to significantly alter the pain in lateral patellofemoral pain syndrome. The foot orthoses were designed to control overpronation of the rearfoot and midfoot during the stance phase of gait. In another study, Eng and Pierrynowski[25] demonstrated with three-dimensional lower limb kinematics that foot orthoses reduced the frontal and transverse plane movements of the talocrural and subtalar joint. In addition, the frontal plane motion at the knee during contact and midstance phases of running was also significantly reduced.

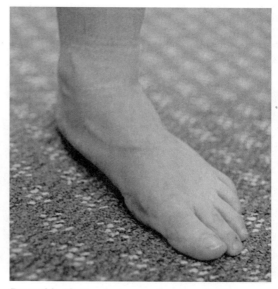

Figure 23–10. Rearfoot varus (compensated).

lateral tibiofemoral joint opening and increases stress along the lateral collateral ligament and the iliotibial band. The varus malalignment becomes significant in the presence of patients with an ACL-deficient knee with a positive lateral pivot shift or subluxation of the lateral tibiofemoral compartment of the knee. Chronic stress to the lateral structures of the knee in the presence of genu varum can result in potential overstretching of these secondary restraints to the ACL, resulting in dynamic instability.

Leg Length Difference

Excessive pronation or supination in one lower extremity can result in, or may be a compensatory mechanism of, leg length discrepancy. As pronation occurs with functional dropping of the medial aspect of the foot, a resulting functional shortening of the extremity occurs. The knee may be subjected to abnormal stress on both the long-limb and short-limb sides. If an individual attempts to compensate on the long-limb side by rearfoot pronation and internally rotating the lower extremity at the hip, an increased valgus force will be imparted to the knee joint, resulting in increase in compression forces within the lateral tibiofemoral joint, increase in stress along the medial knee ligaments, and predisposition to lateral patellofemoral compression syndrome. Conversely, supination in one lower extremity may produce a functional lengthening of that limb. The result may be a functional genu varus with increased compression stress and increased tensile stress along the medial and lateral aspects of the knee, respectively.

The long-limb side may also maintain a longer stance phase of gait, subjecting the limb to greater ground reaction forces.

EVALUATION

A static evaluation should be performed in the presence of knee orthopedic injuries based on the assumption that posture and alignment may reflect underlying impairments. The patient is observed anteriorly in relaxed standing to assess for genu valgus or varus, and increase or decrease in the normal anatomic valgus angle of the knee. The clinician should ask the patient to turn around and observe both feet for excessive pronation or supination and associated rearfoot valgus or varus, respectively (Fig. 23–11). In standing, the position of the calcaneus reflects the compensated subtalar joint position. Next, the clinician should observe the patient's gait to assess the mechanics of the subtalar joint during the phases of gait.

Static analysis of rearfoot neutral and rearfoot/forefoot relationships can be obtained to assess the amount of subtalar joint deviations from the neutral position during the stance phase of gait. The patient lies prone. Lines are then drawn on the distal one-third of the lower leg and a line is drawn bisecting the heel. The examiner's hand grasps the foot at the base of the fourth and fifth metatarsals, applying a downward distracting force to remove any resting ankle dorsiflexion. The foot is then passively inverted and everted as talar protrusion is palpated; the talus protrudes laterally with inversion and medially with eversion. The neutral position is that point at which protrusion is felt

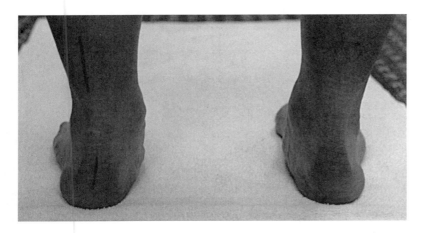

Figure 23–11. Rearfoot valgus (compensated).

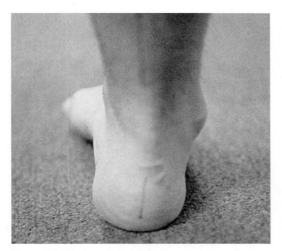

Figure 23–12. Standing rearfoot varus, neutral.

equally on the lateral and medial sides. Using the bisection line, this position is measured with a goniometer and recorded in degrees varus or valgus (Fig. 23–12). This position of the calcaneus then is compared with the calcaneus during standing to ascertain the amount of compensation in the subtalar joint.

The forefoot to rearfoot measurement can be taken as follows: The hand grasps the base of the fifth metatarsal. The subtalar joint is held in its predetermined neutral position. One arm of the goniometer rests against the metatarsal heads, while the other arm is perpendicular to the calcaneal bisection line. The axis of the goniometer is

placed laterally. The varus angle described by the metatarsal heads and the imaginary line perpendicular to the heel is recorded (Fig. 23–13). To measure forefoot valgus, the axis of the goniometer is held medially. Finally, as described earlier, the mobility of the midfoot should be assessed to determine the stability of the midtarsal joint area (see Fig. 23–7).

Assessment of leg length is performed clinically by either the direct or the indirect method. This is performed with the patient standing. Symmetrical landmarks, including the posterior superior iliac spine, ischial tuberosities, greater trochanters, and popliteal creases, are palpated and compared for height distances. If a consistent difference is found, the examiner places lifts of known heights under the foot of the lower leg to equalize leg length. The lifts are added and recorded to the half-centimeter. The indirect method is depicted in Figure 23–14*A*. The direct method is depicted in Figure 23–14*B* and is performed by measuring from the patient's anterior iliac spine to the lateral malleolus. Side-to-side differences are recorded to the half centimeter.

Assessment for soft tissue changes and potential muscle imbalances of the lower extremity should be performed in the presence of suspected malalignment. These tests include flexibility tests of the hamstrings, iliopsoas and rectus femoris, piriformis muscle, tensor fasciae latae/iliotibial band, and the gastrocnemius/soleus muscles. Manual

Figure 23–13. Forefoot varus measurement.

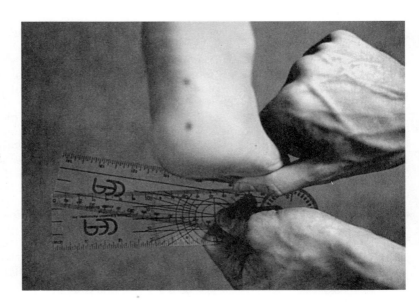

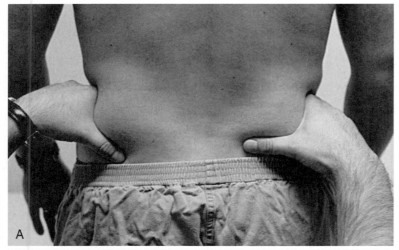

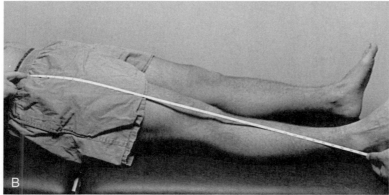

Figure 23–14. *A*, Indirect method to measure leg length asymmetry (iliac crest height). *B*, Direct method to measure leg length asymmetry, anterosuperior iliac spine to lateral malleolus.

muscle tests and isokinetic testing are performed to quantitate muscle parameters.

Principles of Treatment

In the presence of any orthopedic problem, identification of the pathologic condition is usually not sufficient to fully address and correct the condition. The rehabilitation specialist should perform a comprehensive clinical evaluation of the knee and the entire lower extremity to identify the relevant impairments (intrinsic factors) and, in the context of the history, the extrinsic factors of injury. Identification of these impairments constitutes the movement dysfunctions or pathomechanics of injury. Formalization of these impairments into short-term goals in conjunction with identifying the long-term functional goals provides the basis of treatment planning in rehabilitation. The rehabilitation specialist also considers the stage of

healing, clinical reactivity, and biomechanical constraint to exercise to complete overall treatment planning.

CORRECTION OF FOOT AND ANKLE MECHANICS

The most effective method of correcting malalignment of the foot is through the use of a biomechanical orthotic device. Foot orthotics can be flexible, semirigid, or rigid. The role of a biomechanical orthotic is to control abnormal movement of the subtalar joint during walking or running. Several studies have demonstrated the beneficial effects of foot orthoses in controlling pronation during the stance phase of gait.[28, 29] The studies indicated that use of a post or wedge placed in the forefoot or rearfoot will help to reduce overpronation of the rearfoot. Johanson et al.[29] demonstrated that a forefoot and rearfoot varus post produced the most significant reduction in abnormal pronation during the stance phase of gait (Fig. 23–15).

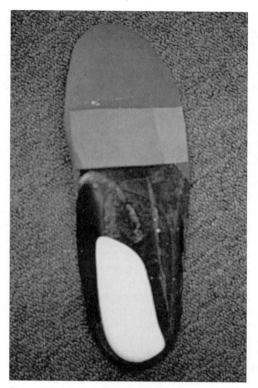

Figure 23–15. Forefoot and rearfoot varus post.

Brown et al.[28] demonstrated that the use of a device that controlled midtarsal joint (medial arch) motion was beneficial in controlling abnormal pronation during the stance phase of gait. Conversely, if the calcaneus is excessively inverted at heel strike, a lateral or valgus post helps control supination movements. The maximum amount of rearfoot posting is usually 5 to 6 degrees.

The forefoot post supports the forefoot deformity by bringing the ground closer to the metatarsal heads. The effect is to reduce the need for rearfoot compensation. The forefoot post is indicated when the forefoot deformity is creating problems during midstance to terminal stance. Generally, the maximum forefoot post that fits comfortably in a shoe is 6 to 8 degrees.

CORRECTION OF LEG LENGTH
DIFFERENCE

In the presence of a measured leg length difference, the clinician should determine whether the leg length is anatomic or functional. An anatomic leg length difference is due to a real difference in the bony anatomy in the lower extremity. In some cases as little as 0.5-cm correction in leg length discrepancies can help alter abnormal postures of the lower extremity kinetic chain. Clinical measure of anatomic leg length was described previously. A functional leg length difference is due to soft tissue changes in the lower extremity or a sacroiliac change that produces an apparent difference in leg length. A comprehensive evaluation will usually assess for a functional leg length that includes a closer analysis and correction of soft tissue dysfunction of joint positional faults.

CASE 1

The following cases illustrate clinical decision making in patients with knee conditions with associated foot and ankle malalignment.

Identifying the Patient's Problem

Ron is a 39-year-old computer programmer. Five months ago he suffered an isolated ACL tear in his left knee while playing basketball. He chose to undergo a comprehensive rehabilitation program rather than surgical reconstruction. After 3 months of aggressive physical therapy, Ron was fitted with an ACL functional brace and gradually returned to playing recreational basketball and tennis. Approximately 3 weeks ago he began to notice a sensation of slipping and "giving way" in his left knee. A revisit to his orthopedic surgeon indicated some increased lateral laxity and a mild "pivot shift" sign. He was re-referred to physical therapy for an additional 3 weeks of rehabilitation for strengthening and functional training.

Identifying the Characteristics of the Problem

1. Giving way of the knee with weight-bearing activities.

Identifying the Factors Affecting the Problem

Extrinsic Factors

1. Return to high-ballistic sports, including basketball and tennis.

Intrinsic Factors

1. Knee extension (concentric) isokinetic average torque across five repetitions at 90, 200, and 300 degrees per second indicated 25 percent bilateral deficits

(injured extremity weaker than uninjured).
2. Standing single-leg balance test (Stork test) indicated 30 seconds on right lower extremity and 15 seconds on left.
3. Standing calcaneal varus angle of 5 degrees bilaterally.
4. Forefoot valgus deformities of 10 degrees bilaterally.
5. Standing genu varum.
6. Lachman's test 3+ left (greater than 10-mm opening compared to contralateral side); varus test at 30 degrees 1+ left (less than 5-mm opening with firm end point); and pivot shift test 1+ left.

Determine a Method to Resolve the Problem

Program of Treatment
1. The patient was placed on an aggressive quadriceps strengthening program using both isotonic and closed kinetic chain applications. The exercises were to correct residual knee extension strength deficit to within 10 percent of bilateral comparisons, with application of closed kinetic chain rehabilitation to facilitate strength, balance, and proprioception as potential causes of functional instability.[30, 31]
2. Fabrication of foot orthoses with a 5-mm forefoot valgus post and 4-mm rearfoot valgus posts bilaterally. Compensatory abnormal external rotation and functional genu varum that result from abnormal subtalar joint supination may be increasing lateral tibiofemoral joint opening and stress along the lateral structures.

Evaluating the Effectiveness of the Treatment
The patient was instructed to perform his exercises three or four times weekly and slowly adjust to his orthotics. Some initial heel pain and aching in the subtalar joint were resolved with mobilization techniques applied to the calcaneus to improve eversion range of motion and to allow the calcaneus free movement toward the neutral position. Reassessment after the 3-week period included isokinetic retests (demonstrating bilateral deficits within 15 percent), and functional tests including the standing stork test, crossover test, and hop tests.[32] All the functional tests were performed with the orthotic inserted in the patient's shoes. In addition, reassessment of lower extremity alignment during static standing while the patient was wearing the orthotics indicated restoration close to the normal physiologic valgus angles.

CASE 2

Identifying the Patient's Problem
Ann is a 16-year-old high school volleyball player who developed gradual onset of bilateral anterior knee pain 2 weeks after the start of practice. She describes the pain as a constant dull ache, rated 3 out of 10 at rest, that increases to a sharp pain (5/10) with ascending or descending stairs, jumping, or prolonged sitting with her knee bent. She describes intermittent "popping" along the outside of her knee when squatting. The condition was diagnosed by her orthopedist as patellofemoral syndrome characterized by peripatellar soft tissue inflammation. She was referred to physical therapy for evaluation and treatment.

Identifying the Characteristics of the Problem
1. Pain increases with weight-bearing activities.
2. Pain increases with prolonged knee flexion.
3. Popping along the outside of the knee.

Identifying Factors Affecting the Problem

Extrinsic Factors
1. High ballistic activity (volleyball).

Intrinsic Factors
1. Q angle of 25 degrees bilaterally.
2. Lateral patellar tilt in a transverse plane (the medial facet of the patella is more prominent than the lateral facet)
3. Restricted medial patellar glide and tilt due to tight lateral retinaculum and distal iliotibial band.
4. Palpation of vastus medialis oblique muscle indicates fair contractions bilaterally (reduced bulk and moderately soft to palpation).
5. Isokinetic testing at 90 degrees indicated concentric peak torque to body weight ratios were 60 percent bilaterally. Isokinetic testing also reproduced anterior knee pain.

6. Standing calcaneal valgus angle of 10 degrees bilaterally.
7. Forefoot varus deformities of 15 degrees bilaterally.

Determine Method to Resolve the Problem

1. Fabrication of foot orthoses with 5-mm forefoot varus posting bilaterally. Rearfoot varus posting of 4 mm bilaterally. Compensatory abnormal tibial and femoral rotation that result from abnormal pronation may result in lateral patellofemoral tracking along the femoral trochlear groove, increasing lateral compression joint forces.[11]
2. Stretching tight lateral retinaculum and distal iliotibial band by applying a medial patellar glide or taping the patella medially. Increasing extensibility of the lateral patellar tissues potentially improves the ability of the vastus medialis oblique muscle to generate muscle tension to stabilize the patella in a medial direction.[33]
3. Resisted knee extension exercises performed at terminal knee extension (30 degrees to full extension) at least initially to minimize retropatellar forces, slowly increasing range of motion and incorporating closed kinetic chain partial squats as strength improves and reactivity reduces. The goals are to improve overall vastus medialis oblique muscle tone and knee extension strength.
4. The patient was instructed to temporarily defer volleyball until her anterior knee pain was resolved and the impairments were corrected. She was instructed to maintain her aerobic conditioning by performing stationary cycling with the seat positioned high to minimize the amount of knee flexion during pedaling. In the presence of overuse injuries, modification of extrinsic factors of injury are an important component in the overall treatment planning. Since athletes need at least to maintain cardiovascular conditioning, the clinician must come up with alternate exercises that are biomechanically appropriate for the patient's orthopedic condition.

Case Summaries

These two cases illustrate the intrinsic problems (impairments) and extrinsic problems associated with orthopedic conditions at the knee. The clinician must address all factors contributing to injury, including impairments, extrinsic factors, and tissue pathology, if possible, to successfully correct the problem.

SUMMARY

The diagnosis of movement dysfunction for rehabilitation specialists requires a thorough and profound background in anatomy, biomechanics, kinesiology, and neurology. That is because dysfunction that results in abnormal movement and pathologic conditions in the human body can encompass all systems. This chapter examined one aspect of dysfunction, the effect of musculoskeletal alignment and specifically the mechanics of the foot and ankle on the function and health of the knee. This chapter is not meant to be exhaustive in this area but rather to provide some insight for the reader into the relationship between structure and function and to encourage the reader to continue to assess this problem in both the clinic and research.

References

1. Herring SA, Nilson KL: Introduction to overuse injuries. Clin Sports Med 6:225, 1987.
2. Engles M: Tissue response. In Donatelli R, Wooden MJ (eds): Orthopaedic Physical Therapy. New York, Churchill Livingstone, 1994.
3. Cavanagh P: The biomechanics of the lower extremity action in distance running. Foot Ankle 7:127, 1987.
4. Renstrom P, Johnson RJ: Overuse injuries in sports: A review. Sports Med 6:40, 1978.
5. Greenfield B, Johanson M: Evaluation of overuse syndromes. In Donatelli R (ed): Biomechanics of the Foot and Ankle, 2nd ed. Philadelphia, F.A. Davis, 1996, pp. 191–272.
6. Andrews JR: Overuse injuries to lower extremities. Clin Sports Med 2:139, 1983.
7. Smith WB: Environmental factors in running. Am J Sports Med 8:138, 1980.
8. Clana WG: Runner's injuries. Am J Sports Med 8:137, 1980.
9. James SL: Chondromalacia of the patella in adolescent. In Kennedy JC (ed): The Injured Adolescent Knee. Baltimore, Williams & Wilkins, 1979, pp. 214–218.
10. Steindler A: Kinesiology of the Human Body Under Normal and Pathological Conditions. Springfield, IL, Charles C Thomas, 1973, p. 63.
11. Tiberio D: The effect of excessive subtalar joint pronation on patellofemoral mechanics: A theoretical model. J Orthop Sports Phy Ther 9:160, 1987.

12. Lutter LD: Foot-related problems in the long distance runner. Foot Ankle 1:112, 1980.
13. Taunton JE, Clement DB, Smart GW, et al.: A triplanar electrogonimeter investigation of running mechanics in runners with compensatory overpronation. Can J Sports Sci 10:104, 1985.
14. Norkin CC, Levangie PK: Joint Structure and Function: A Comprehensive Analysis, 2nd ed. Philadelphia, F.A. Davis, 1992, pp. 341–344.
15. Root ML, Orien WP, Weed JH: Normal and Abnormal Function of the Foot: Clinical Biomechanics, Vol 2. Los Angeles, Clinical Biomechanics Corporation, 1977.
16. Tiberio D, Larson RL, Cauband HE, et al.: The patellar compression syndrome: Surgical treatment by lateral retinacular release. Clin Orthop 134:158, 1978.
17. Fulkerson JP: Disorders of the Patellofemoral Joint, 3rd ed. Baltimore, Williams & Wilkins, 1997.
18. Fulkerson J, Tennant R, Javin J, et al.: Histological evidence of retinacular nerve injury associated with patellofemoral malalignment. Clin Orthop 197:196, 1985.
19. Taunton JE, Clement DB: Iliotibial tract friction syndrome in athletes. Can J Sports Sci 6:76, 1981.
20. Donatelli R: Normal anatomy and biomechanics. *In* Donatelli R (ed): The Biomechanics of the Foot and Ankle, 2nd ed. Philadelphia, F.A. Davis, 1996.
21. Garbalosa J, McClure M, Catlin PC, Wooden MJ: The frontal plane relationship of the forefoot to the rearfoot in asymptomatic population. J Orthop Sports Phy Ther 20:220, 1994.
22. Butler DL, Noyes FR, Grood ES: Ligamentous restraints of anterior-posterior drawer in human knee. J Bone Joint Surg 62A:259, 1980.
23. Smith J, Szczerba J, Arnold BL, et al.: Role of hyperpronation as a possible risk factor of anterior cruciate ligament injuries. Athletic Training 32:25, 1997.
24. Eng JJ, Pierrynowski MR: The effect of soft foot orthotics in three-dimensional lower-limb kinematics during walking and running. Phys Ther 74:836, 1994.
25. Eng JJ, Pierrynowski MR: Evaluation of soft foot orthotics in the treatment of patellofemoral pain syndrome. J Orthop Sports Phy Ther 73:62, 1993.
26. James SL: Chondromalacia of the patella in the adolescent. In Kennedy JC (ed): The Injured Adolescent Knee. Baltimore, Williams & Wilkins, 1979, pp. 214–218.
27. Noyes FR, Schipplein OD, Abdriacchi TP, et al.: The anterior cruciate-ligament deficient knee with varus alignment. An analysis of gait adaptations and dynamic loading. Am J Sports Med 20:707, 1992.
28. Brown GP, Donatelli R, Catlin PA, Wooden MJ: The effects of foot orthoses on rearfoot mechanics. J Orthop Sports Phys Ther 21:258, 1995.
29. Johanson MA, Donatelli R, Wooden MJ, et al.: Effects of three different posting methods on controlling abnormal subtalar pronation. Phys Ther 74:149, 1994.
30. Barrck RL, Skinner HB, Buckley SL: Proprioception in the anterior deficient knee. Am J Sports Med 17:1, 1989.
31. Laskowski ER, Newcomer-Aney K, Smith J: Refining rehabilitation with proprioception training. Physician Sports Med 25:89, 1997.
32. Juris PM, Edward PM, Dalpe C, et al.: A dynamic test of lower extremity function following anterior cruciate ligament reconstruction and rehabilitation. J Orthop Sports Rehab 26:184, 1997.
33. Kramer PG: Patella malalignment syndrome: Rationale to reduce excessive lateral patella pressure. J Orthop Sports Phys Ther 8:301, 1986.

24 Plyometrics in Rehabilitation

Donald A. Chu, PhD, PT, ATC, CSCS, and
Douglas J. Cordier, MS, PT, ATC, CSCS

HISTORY

Plyometrics is the term applied to exercises that have their roots in Europe, where they were first known as jump training.[1] In the early 1970s, East European athletes emerged as powers on the world track and field, gymnastics, and weightlifting scenes.[1] For a few years prior to this, coaches were using eccentric forms of exercise to train these athletes. Yuri Verhoshanki, then national track coach for the jumping events, wrote about the system being employed by the Soviet Union and simply called it "jump training."[2] Soon the rest of the world was interested in the European plyometric training methods. In 1975, the term *plyometrics* was first coined by an American track and field coach named Fred Wilt. Based on Latin origins, *plyo + metrics* is interpreted to mean "measurable increases."[3] Meanwhile, researchers in Europe were attempting to discern the physiologic basis and rationale for the exercise system. Komi, Bosco, and Cavagha were researchers who came up with information leading to the theory of the "stretch shortening" cycle as an aid to performance enhancement.[4-8]

During the 1980s, an original work was published by Chu[1] that was the first categorization of plyometric training in the United States. This article and others that followed attempted to encompass European literature to match the needs of the American athlete. Plyometrics soon became known as the link between strength and speed to produce increased power. Later coaches realized the potential plyometrics could have on increasing the power of athletes in other sports. Volleyball, football, basketball and weightlifting athletes began to use plyometrics to improve power. Today plyometrics have become essential for any athlete who jumps, throws, or lifts to compete at the elite level.

Plyometrics have also been incorporated into the rehabilitation setting. In the later stages of rehabilitation, patients and athletes begin exercises that employ the myotactic stretch reflex first described by researchers. The exercise system known as plyometrics was developed from the use of maximal voluntary muscle contractions in an effort to project the body vertically or linearly at the highest velocities possible. Rehabilitation patients often begin with exercises that are not maximal contractions and may not be performed with the full weight of the body; therefore, these types of exercises are termed "plyometric in nature."

When performed within the proper training regimen, and organized over time, plyometric training can lead to enhanced performance. Patients and athletes in their preparation to return to activity must employ specific functional exercises like plyometrics.

MUSCULAR AND NEUROPHYSIOLOGIC PRINCIPLES

Muscle Structure

Skeletal muscle is attached to bones of the skeleton to provide support and mobility. The cells of skeletal muscle are long and cylindrical. Running longitudinally throughout the muscle cells are regularly ordered thread-like arrays of proteins called myofibrils.[9] These myofibril bands have units called sarcomeres between them. The sarcomere is the functional unit of the muscle cell.[10] Sarcomeres contain myofilaments made up of proteins called actin, myosin, and tropomyosin. The thick filaments of myosin have small projections known as crossbridges extending from them (Fig. 24–1). Two types of muscle fiber make up mus-

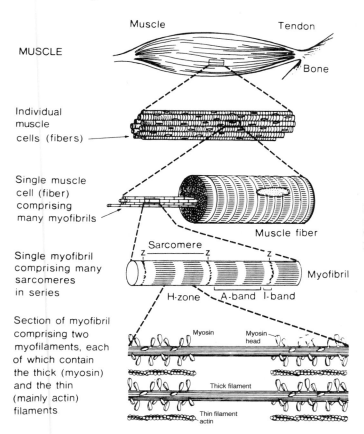

MUSCLE

Muscle   Tendon

Bone

Individual
muscle
cells (fibers)

Single muscle
cell (fiber)
comprising
many myofibrils

Muscle fiber

Single myofibril
comprising many
sarcomeres
in series

Sarcomere

Z   Z   Z

Myofibril

H-zone   A-band   I-band

Section of myofibril
comprising two
myofilaments, each
of which contain
the thick (myosin)
and the thin
(mainly actin)
filaments

Myosin   Myosin
head

Thick filament

Thin filament
actin

Figure 24–1. The architecture of the muscle. (From Nokes T: Lore of Running, 3rd ed. Champaign, IL, Leisure Press, 1991, reprinted with permission.)

cles: extrafusal and intrafusal. Extrafusal fibers receive nerve impulses from the brain, which causes a chemical reaction. This reaction allows the cross-bridges in myosin to collapse and actin and myosin to slide over, resulting in a muscle contraction. This is known as the sliding filament theory. The sliding filament theory proposes that a muscle shortens or lengthens because the thick and thin myofilaments slide past each other without the filaments themselves changing length.[10] Intrafusal fibers are also known as muscle spindles. Muscle spindles provide sensory information concerning changes in the length and tension of muscle fibers. Their main function is to respond to stretch on a muscle and, through reflex action, to initiate a stronger contraction to reduce this stretch.[10]

There are two classifications of muscle fiber. Fast-twitch (type II) is a fast-contracting fiber with its energy generated from anaerobic metabolism. These fibers are activated during change-of-pace and stop-and-go activities that require all-out powerful movements. Slow-twitch (type I) fibers are primar-

ily aerobic in nature. The primary role of type I fibers is to sustain continuous endurance-type activities that require a steady rate of aerobic energy transfer.[10]

Neurophysiology

When a muscle contracts, it tends to shorten toward the center of the muscle, pulling on its bony attachments.[11] Three modes of muscle activity associated with plyometrics are the concentric, eccentric, and isometric contractions. A concentric contraction occurs when the muscle shortens. Concentric contractions are also known as positive work and are associated with acceleration of the body or limb. Eccentric contractions occur when a muscle lengthens under tension. This contraction is commonly used to decelerate the body or limb. Eccentric contractions are also known as negatives or negative work. The isometric contraction is a static contraction. The muscle contracts with the associated body part not moving. There is no muscle shortening or lengthening visible. In sporting activities, the isometric contraction occurs during the brief instant between the eccentric and concentric contraction.

Eccentric (lengthening) muscle contractions are rapidly followed by concentric (shortening) contractions in many sport skills. This conversion from negative (eccentric) to positive (concentric) work is known as the amortization phase.[1] This split-second phase begins at the onset of the eccentric contraction and continues to the initiation of the concentric contraction. It is important to emphasize that the amortization phase of the plyometric activity be as brief as possible. This type of training is often utilized in sports that require speed and strength. This familiar speed-strength component is known as power. The primary goal when trying to improve power is to decrease time in the amortization phase. This will allow the stored energy of the eccentric phase to be better utilized during the concentric contraction and increase power.

The stretch-shortening cycle and stretch reflex are important factors in understanding the effectiveness of plyometrics. The stretch, or myotactic, reflex responds to the rate at which a muscle is stretched and is among the fastest in the human body.[1] It is linked from muscle fibers directly to the spinal cord through sensory receptors. The importance of this minimal delay in the stretch reflex is that muscle undergoes a contraction faster during a stretch-shortening cycle than in any other method of contraction.[1] The stretch-shortening cycle is characterized by rapid deceleration of a mass followed almost immediately by rapid acceleration of the mass in the opposite direction.[12] The stretch-shortening cycle is the eccentric-to-concentric component of plyometrics and is more powerful than a simple concentric muscle contraction. A National Strength and Conditioning Statement[12] states that the stretch-shortening cycle is essential in the performance of most competitive sports, particularly those involving running, jumping, and rapid changes in direction.

TRAINING CONSIDERATIONS

There are many factors to consider before beginning a plyometric training program. It is important to establish the patient's training level and consider his or her age. The clinician should pay attention to safety issues including exercise surface, equipment, and proper depth jump height. It is recommended that most individuals establish a reasonable amount of flexibility and have a basic strength training background prior to initiating plyometrics. Testing and assessment are essential to ascertain strength ratios and identify potential contraindications or precautions. All of these parameters will help the clinician establish a safe and injury-free plyometric program. The following sections discuss these parameters in greater detail.

Safety Concerns

The risk of injury from plyometrics is low.[13] To keep this risk low, the physical therapist must have a basic understanding of plyometrics and should always follow proper volume, intensity, and progression guidelines. Not adhering to pretraining requirements and proper progression will increase the risk of injury.[14] A qualified physical therapist, athletic trainer, or exercise professional, with education and training in plyometrics, should be present at all times to monitor and correct the exercise technique. Additionally, the therapist must be alert to signs of overtraining or injury. Areas of potential injuries associated with lower body plyometrics include feet, ankles, shins, knees, hips, and low back.[15] Injuries often happen when the patient is fatigued, during the end of the exercise session. Sprained ankles and twisted knees are among the common traumas associated with a lack of control due to excessive fatigue.[1] Insufficient strength and conditioning base, inadequate warm-up, poor shoes or surface, or simple lack of skill are also potential reasons for injury.[16] Although injuries can and do occur, it must be noted that in no epidemiologic studies have relative injury rates been addressed.[17] Borkowski[13] found that a pre-season plyometric program did not produce injuries but significantly reduced in-season muscle soreness in a group of collegiate volleyball players. Finally, previous injuries must be evaluated in relation to the potential risks of initiating a plyometric program.[15]

Depth jumps are probably the most "advertised" of all plyometric exercises and were originally designed for the athletic population with specific need to develop vertical velocity at take-off. Depth jumps are only necessary for a small percentage of athletes engaged in plyometric training.[17] As a rule, for athletes weighing over 220 lbs, depth jumping from platforms higher than 18 inches is not recommended.[17] Alternative drills to depth jumping for the heavy athlete (220 lbs and over) should be provided.[18] Information on proper depth jump height selection is provided in another section.

Flexibility

It is common sense that normal range-of-motion is necessary prior to performing plyometrics. Stretching and warm-up are a fundamental part of the plyometric training session. The individual should perform a thorough set of warm-up exercises before beginning a plyometric training session.[17] Static and ballistic stretching are two of the common stretching techniques used in the clinical setting. Static stretching increases flexibility by a prolonged hold, usually 15 seconds or longer and repeated three to four times. Ballistic stretching involves stretching the muscle to its normal length and gently bouncing at the end range for 10 to 15 repetitions. Static and ballistic stretching appear to be equally effective in increasing flexibility, and there is no significant difference between the two.[19] Physical therapists should keep in mind the principles of eliciting the stretch reflex and the serial elastic components of muscle to perform jumping activities. It might behoove the patient to "prime" the mechanism by doing controlled ballistic stretching.[1] Chu[20] recommends that the individual attain at least 90 percent of complete range-of-motion prior to initiating functional exercises.

Training Level and Age Considerations

Plyometric exercises, like all exercises, are geared toward the individual. A flexibility and strength base is an essential component when determining the training level. Maturity and age of the athlete are also important considerations. Allerheiligen and Rogers rec-

ommend that because of the potential risk of injury to growth plates, athletes under the age of 16 years should not perform shock-intensity level plyometrics like depth jumps.[15] They do not state what kind of injuries or which growth plates may be injured. Classifying an individual as beginner, intermediate, or advanced will help make program design more beneficial. A patient who has reached puberty and is relatively unskilled is considered a beginner. The age at which puberty occurs is often construed legally as 14 in boys and 12 in girls,[21] but we feel that some patients with an athletic background may begin low-intensity plyometrics at an earlier age. Post-injury or rehabilitation patients also fall into the beginner category. These beginners are placed in a complementary resistance training program and progress slowly into a program of low-intensity plyometrics such as skipping drills, 8-inch cone hops, and box drills of 6 to 12 inches.[1] Lateral bounding drills are also beneficial to the beginner who has sustained a valgus or varus stress injury to the ankle or knee. Certain injuries may preclude a patient from performing plyometrics that are more than low intensity. **If shock activities are a contraindication after surgery or rehabilitation, plyometrics of any intensity should not be performed**.

During the sport-specific stage of rehabilitation, when strength gains are normalized and a beginning plyometric program has been successfully completed, moderately intense plyometrics can begin. Patients who are high school competitors with some exposure to weight-training programs can benefit from moderately intense plyometrics.[1]

College and elite athletes often have strong strength-training backgrounds. Depending on the type of injury, and after complete rehabilitation, these athletes should be able to perform high-intensity plyometrics without problems.[1] It is not likely that high-intensity plyometrics will be performed in the clinical setting. More often, a high-intensity plyometric program will be under the supervision of a strength and conditioning professional. Furthermore, this program usually takes place after complete rehabilitation and discharge from the clinical setting.

Proper Depth-Jump Height

Depth jumps are performed by stepping out from a box and dropping to the ground,

From Chu DA: Jumping into Plyometrics. Champaign, IL, Human Kinetics, 1992.

○■ Table 24–1. **Determining Proper Depth-Jump Height**

1. The athlete is measured as accurately as possible for a standing jump-and-reach.
2. The athlete performs a depth jump from an 18-inch box height, trying to attain the same standing jump-and-reach score.
3. If the athlete successfully executes this task, he or she may move to a higher box. The box height should be increased in 6-inch increments. Step 2 is repeated until the athlete fails to reach the standing jump-and-reach height. This then becomes the athlete's maximum height for depth jumps.
4. If the athlete cannot reach the standing jump-and-reach height from an 18-inch box, either the height of the box should be lowered or depth jumping abandoned for a time in favor of strength development. If the athlete cannot rebound from a basic height of 18 inches, he or she probably does not have the musculoskeletal readiness for depth jumping.

then attempting to jump back up to the height of the box.[1] Depth-jumping presents a safety concern when performed in the clinical setting. Depth jumps should be used only by a small percentage of athletes engaged in plyometric training.[17] Therefore, we urge the clinician to be careful when determining whether an individual is going to perform the depth jump.

The key to this exercise is decreasing time in the amortization phase and stressing the "touch and go" action off the ground.[1] It is recommended to discontinue depth jumps 10 to 14 days prior to athletic competition.[18] Do not overuse depth-jump training in season.[18]

Past research on the proper depth-jump height varies. In practical terms, the task of determining a proper depth-jump height centers on the ability to achieve maximal elevation of the body's center of gravity after performing a depth jump.[1] If the depth-jump height is too great, the amortization phase will be extended because the athlete spends too much time absorbing the load on impact. Table 24–1 outlines one method of determining maximum depth-jump height.

EQUIPMENT

Plyometric training requires very little expensive equipment. Prefabricated equipment can be purchased at a local sporting goods store or through the various strength and conditioning periodicals. Items found in the clinic can be modified and used as plyometric equipment for little or no cost. The following is a list of equipment that will be useful for plyometric training.

Footwear and landing surfaces used in plyometric drills must have good shock-absorbing qualities.[17] The recommended shoe is forgiving yet still offers good support. A good cross-training shoe will do well for most circumstances. A soft or springy floor such as a "spring-loaded" floor may decrease injury prevalence and enhance the jump. Grass is also a good plyometric surface. Use of an area cleared of other equipment is important so that the patient does not injure himself or herself.

Solid boxes (Fig. 24–2) range from 6 to 24 inches. It is unlikely that boxes greater than 24 inches will be needed in the clinical setting. Plywood 3/4 inch thick or similar flexible wood is needed.[1] A variety of boxes ranging from 6 to 12 and then 24 inches will help with proper progression.

Plastic cones (Fig. 24–3) ranging in height from 6 to 24 inches serve as barriers over which to jump. The flexibility of cones makes them less likely to cause injuries if the patient lands directly on them.[1]

Hurdles and barriers (Fig. 24–4) are safe to use as plyometric equipment. This type of equipment is often found in physical therapy clinics. Barriers are constructed by balancing a pole across two cones. If the patient hits the pole, it will fall, which decreases the chance of injury.

Stairways or clinic steps (Fig. 24–5) are suitable for plyometric training, although they must be inspected carefully to make sure they are safe for jumping. Concrete steps are undesirable for jumping because they have unyielding surfaces.[1]

The Shuttle 2000-1 (Fig. 24–6) was first designed to stress an astronaut's cardiovascular system in a zero gravity environment. Today, the Shuttle 2000-1 is found in most orthopedic rehabilitation centers. The shuttle provides a controlled environment in which closed-kinetic chain and plyometric activities are performed. This is a rebound system with elasticords that are fixed to a horizontal platform. The platform glides back and forth on a rail. The patient lies on the platform with his or her feet on the kickplate. The kickplate is adjustable for the patient's height, desired range of motion,

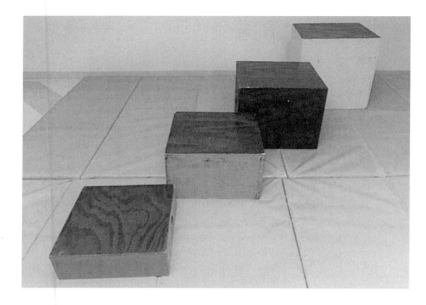

Figure 24-2. Solid boxes for plyometric training. (Courtesy of Baptist Health Systems Media Services Department, Miami, FL.)

and intensity of the workout. When the patient extends his or her legs, the elastic cords are stretched, creating the resistance. Sometimes the Shuttle has a tendency to migrate back and forth along the floor, especially when used for plyometrics. Therefore, it needs to be bolted to the floor or braced by the therapist to prevent movement.

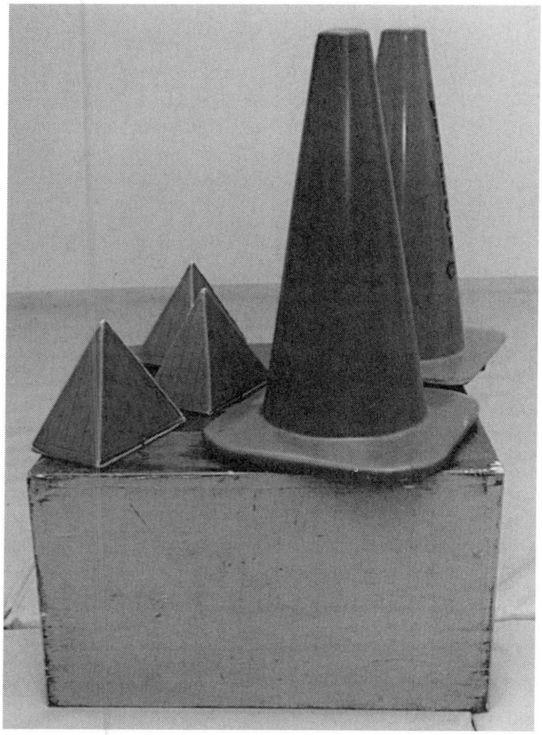

Calculating force is performed by measuring the distance the shuttle travels on the rail from the resting point and by using a chart provided by the manufacturer that is based on the number of elasticords utilized. For example, 20 inches of travel with one elasticord is equal to 24 pounds of force. Twenty inches of travel with two elasticords is equal to 48 lbs. It should be noted that over time the elasticords may stretch out, resulting in a deviation of the actual force produced. Force calculation is verified by placing a bathroom scale on the platform with the patient pushing on the scale.

The KYTEC Sidekick Box (Fig. 24-7) is a device that comes with a steel platform and two rugged end blocks that adjust to shorter and longer widths. The end blocks are positioned at 45-degree angles. The KYTEC is used for lateral plyometric type activities, to improve lateral speed and quickness, to improve balance, and for agility drills.

DESIGNING A TRAINING PROGRAM

Training Guidelines and Variables

Plyometric program design is similar to other strength and conditioning programs. Variables can be manipulated and the patient progressed by alterations in frequency,

Figure 24-3. Plastic cones for plyometric training. (Courtesy of Baptist Health Systems Media Services Department, Miami, FL.)

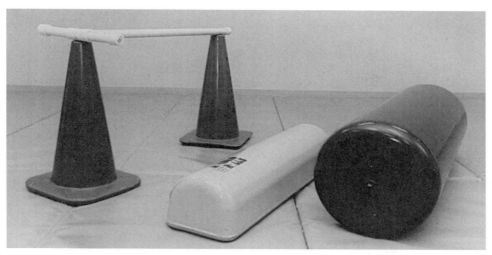

Figure 24–4. Hurdles and barriers for plyometric training. (Courtesy of Baptist Health Systems Media Services Department, Miami, FL.)

intensity, volume, and recovery. Use progression throughout the plyometric program to alter volume and intensity so that there is adaptation according to the SAID (specific adaptation to imposed demands) principle.

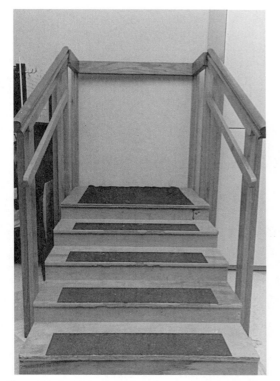

Figure 24–5. Clinic steps for plyometric training. (Courtesy of Baptist Health Systems Media Services Department, Miami, FL.)

It is important for the physical therapist to follow training guidelines. This will decrease the chance of injury or over-training. Basic plyometric knowledge is essential, as is proper progression and exercise technique. Allerheiligen and Rogers[22] recommend five steps to a good plyometric workout.

1. Warm-up, light 5-minute jog
2. Pre-workout stretching
3. Low-intensity strides, 30 to 50 yards or other dynamic warm-up
4. Plyometric training: simple to complex movements, low- to high-intensity drills
5. Post-workout stretching

Whereas this is a simple outline, further information will help the clinician have a greater understanding of plyometric program design.

Frequency

Frequency is the number of times an exercise is performed (repetitions), as well as the number of times exercise sessions take place during a training cycle.[1] It is recommended that 48 to 72 hours of rest is necessary for full recovery before the next plyometric session.[1] This will allow approximately two workouts per week. Either Monday and Thursday or Tuesday and Friday workouts will allow maximum recovery when doing plyometrics twice a week.[15] The

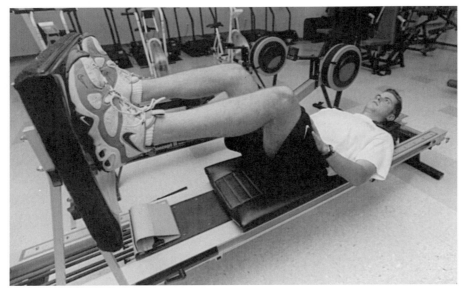

Figure 24–6. Shuttle 2000-1. (Courtesy of Baptist Health Systems Media Services Department, Miami, FL.)

individual should not perform plyometric drills affecting a particular muscle and joint complex on consecutive days.[17] The intensity of exercise must also be considered into the frequency equation. Skipping as a plyometric exercise is not as stressful as bounding and will not require the same amount of recovery time.[1] Three days (a week) of low-intensity drills may be lower in overall weekly intensity and physical fatigue than 2 days of high-intensity drills.[15]

Intensity

Intensity is the effort involved in performing a given task.[1] With plyometrics, *intensity* describes the complexity and amount of work necessary to complete the exercise. Plyometric exercise is classified as low-intensity, medium-intensity, and high-intensity. Stone and O'Bryant[18] recommend that the individual perform each plyometric exercise maximally to stimulate the neuromuscular

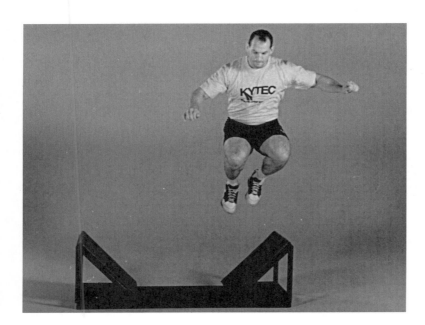

Figure 24–7. KYTEC Sidekick Box. (Reprinted from Perform Better Catalog, Cranston, RI, MF Corporation, 1998.)

system. Double-leg jumping is less stressful than single-leg jumping.[23] Raising the height of the box, step, or hurdle, will increase intensity. In the clinical setting, most plyometric exercises are low or medium intensity. Often some simple, low-intensity jumping drills are used as a precursor or warm-up to more intense plyometric drills. The six classifications of lower extremity plyometric exercises described by Chu[1] are listed below in increasing order of intensity.

1. Jumps in place
2. Standing jumps
3. Bounding
4. Multiple hops and jumps
5. Box jumps
6. Depth jumps

Some of these plyometrics are too intense for most outpatient orthopedic rehabilitation or sports medicine patients. The most common plyometrics utilized in this setting are jumps in place, standing jumps, low-intensity bounding, multiple hops (two or three), and box jumps. As previously stated, depth jumps and high-intensity plyometrics are used only with advanced athletes. In the clinical setting, a low-intensity form of depth jumping known as "jump from box," or "jump down" is used to improve eccentric strength and prepare the individual for possible depth jumping. To perform this exercise, the patient steps off a box and drops to the floor attempting to "freeze" as soon as contact is made with the ground, without jumping again.

Volume

Volume is the amount of work, or number of repetitions and sets, for an exercise session. With lower extremity plyometrics, volume of total work is measured in number of foot contacts. Orthopedic rehabilitation patients will fall into the beginner category and should start with 30 foot contacts of low-intensity exercises. The number of sets and repetitions varies with the patient's status. For bounding activities, a starting distance of 10 to 15 yards per repetition, and five to 10 repetitions is recommended. Two to three sets of eight to 10 repetitions of low-intensity exercise is a good starting point for jumping drills. If the patient tolerates these exercises without adverse joint or muscle

conditions (pain, swelling), intensity is gradually increased. If increased sets (3 to 5) are tolerated, the patient can advance to higher intensity plyometrics. Stone and O'Bryant[18] recommend using two to 10 sets of five to 12 repetitions per exercise, depending on the volume and intensity level of the drill.

Recovery

Wathen[17] recommends that time be allowed for complete recovery between plyometric exercise sets. A work-to-rest ratio of 1:5 to 1:10 is required to ensure proper execution and intensity of the exercise.[1] For example, if an exercise takes 10 seconds to complete, 50 to 100 seconds is allowed for recovery. Stone and O'Bryant[18] recommend 1 to 5 minutes of rest between plyometric exercises, depending on the volume and intensity level of the drill. Plyometrics in the purest sense is an anaerobic activity; therefore, shorter recovery periods (10 to 15 seconds) will not develop this energy system.

In the clinical setting, activities that are plyometric in nature are used to stress the anaerobic or aerobic system. When attempting to stress the aerobic endurance system a shorter work-to-rest ratio is required. This type of activity is often called *circuit training, conditioning drills,* or *functional training.* Voight and Tippett[23] recommend a shorter work-to-rest ratio of 1:1 or 1:2 for endurance training. Additionally, they state that for power training, a work-to-rest ratio of 1:3 or 1:4 should be used.

Ideally, if the individual is trying to improve power, then maximal effort should be performed. Improving power is an anaerobic activity that requires longer rest periods. Plyometrics in the clinical setting are of low intensity and the primary goal of each exercise may not be to improve power. Other goals for low-intensity plyometrics can include the following: improve eccentric strength and endurance, simulate sporting activities, perform close-kinetic chain strengthening, improve coordination or agility, promote normal myotactic and myoarthrokinetic reflexes, promote normal motor control and skill, and restore functional ability.

Progression

Progression is manipulated by adjusting volume and intensity. Rehabilitation patients will begin a plyometric program with low-intensity drills and progress to higher intensity as they master the easier drills. Twelve to 18 weeks of a basic plyometric program is advised to ensure that individuals can properly execute the mechanics of plyometric activities before they attempt higher volumes and intensities.[1] Not often does the physical therapist have a patient at end-stage rehabilitation for 12 to 18 more weeks. This is why most patients will only perform low- or moderate-intensity plyometrics prior to discharge from most physical therapy rehabilitation programs. Patients should begin with double-leg drills and progress to single-leg drills. Volume and number of foot contacts are increased as the patient progresses.

Complex Training

Patients who are experienced in weight training and have also been through basic plyometric training may choose a complex training method. Complex training occurs when the individual alternates weight training and plyometrics within the same workout session.[1] This training method is an effective way to stimulate the neuromuscular system and provides variety to the training session. Volume of plyometric exercises should be reduced to a number that is easily workable between strength training sets. This will also reduce the possibility of fatigue and overtraining. It is recommended that complex training be used with the major weight lifts, including squats, leg presses, split squats, bench press, power cleans, snatches, and push presses.[1] An example for the lower extremity may have the athlete perform one set of 10 squats followed by 10 to 15 box jumps, and repeated for three total sets of each exercise. As a rule of thumb, integrating two major lifts with plyometrics during a workout should yield maximum results.

Complex Training Example for Lower Extremity

- Individual performs one set of 10 leg presses or squats,
- Followed by 10 to 15, 6-inch box jumps;
- This is repeated for three total sets of each exercise.

TESTING AND ASSESSMENT

Dynamic Movement Testing

There are many ways the clinician can assess if an individual is ready to initiate a plyometric program. Testing is used to assess the patients' progress in their plyometric program and for data collection. Assessment is used to compare the gathered data and establish performance standards that can be compared with other patients in the same activity or sport. Dynamic movement testing assesses the individual's ability to produce explosive, coordinated movement.[23] This type of testing seems most appropriate to evaluate function prior to a plyometric program. Dynamic testing is performed before and after training periods and is important for measuring improvement and providing feedback, direction, and motivation. The description following describes two simple tests that will measure vertical and horizontal distance.

A. Standing Vertical Jump: (measures vertical jump height)
   1. Patient stands against a wall with his or her dominate arm extended vertically as high as possible.
   2. The point to which the tips of the fingers extend is marked.
   3. Patient jumps off both feet as high as possible and the highest point reached is marked.
   4. Three trials are taken and the greatest distance between the two points is the vertical jump height.
B. Standing Long Jump: (measures horizontal jump distance)
   1. Patient stands on a line with feet parallel and jumps forward as far as possible.
   2. Three trials are taken and the greatest distance is the horizontal jump distance.

Static Stability Testing

Voight and Tippett[23] recommend static stability testing in addition to dynamic testing prior to initiation of plyometrics. They state that an individual should be able to perform one-leg standing for 30 seconds with eyes open and closed before the initiation of plyometric training. There should be no notice-able shaking or wobbling of the support leg and a comparison to the contralateral leg should be made. They also recommend that for dynamic jump exercises to be initiated, there should be no wobbling of the support leg during quarter knee squats. Voight and Draovitch[24] recommend testing static balance, stabilization, and control by using the stork balance (30 seconds) (Fig. 24–8) and single-leg half-squat (Fig. 24–9). If the individual can perform these tests, then he or she is considered ready for basic jumping exercises.

Functional Testing

Functional tests are used in conjunction with more traditional objective tests to assess the patient's ability to perform dynamic activities. This type of testing can be useful to assist the clinician, who must determine when an individual should begin a plyometric program. Additionally, testing is helpful in determining the patient's readiness to

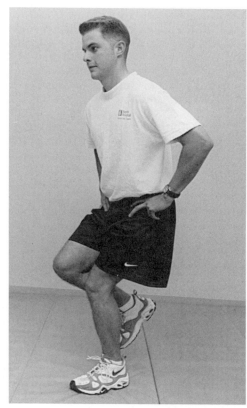

Figure 24–9. Single-leg half-squat. (Courtesy of Baptist Health Systems Media Services Department, Miami, FL.)

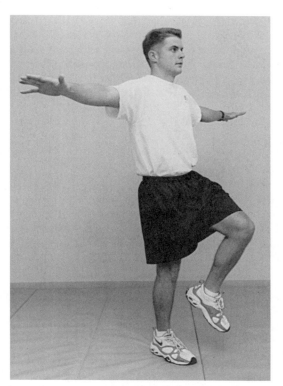

Figure 24–8. Stork balance. (Courtesy of Baptist Health Systems Media Services Department, Miami, FL.)

advance to more difficult functional activities or sport-specific training. A functional test is designed to incorporate movements that are used during sports participation. The objective is to stress the limb while in a controlled environment, in the same way it is stressed during the activity. These tests can assess the individuals' ability to perform activities such as running, jumping, twisting, and directional changes. The testing may stress individual movements or a combination of movements. Testing typically begins with double leg hops and advances from a one hop test to multiple hops and finally to crossover-type hops. The testing subject or patient must execute the test with good coordination, and the clinician should pay close attention to the subject's performance. Functional testing is performed in the later stages of the rehabilitation program, or to restore previous or maximal functional status. Barber et al.[25] recommend that an isokinetic evaluation be performed prior to functional testing to ascertain strength ratios.

According to Barber et al.,[25] contraindications to functional testing include moderate to severe symptoms with activities of daily living, a greater than 15 percent deficit for either the quadriceps or hamstrings at either 60 degrees per second or 300 degrees per second, severe patellofemoral or tibiofemoral crepitus, or a persistent joint effusion. They additionally state that functional tests alone do not have a high sensitivity rating and therefore are not used as a screening test, but can be used only to confirm lower limb limitations. They also found that using two functional tests, as opposed to one, showed a higher percentage of abnormal limb symmetry. Earlier research by Noyes et al.[26] confirmed that when two tests are performed, the number of abnormal cases on at least one of the two tests increased from 49 percent to 52 to 62 percent.

Barber and Noyes and colleagues recommend using at least two functional test results with the isokinetic dynamometer results and detailed patient questionnaires to determine whether an athlete can safely return to sports after anterior cruciate ligament injury or repair.[25–27] Their data suggest that an abnormal hop test result is an indication that the patient may be at serious risk for the knee giving-way during actual sports activities. The knee "giving-way," as they state, is also known as buckling and indicates instability or muscle imbalance of the knee. They found an 85 percent symmetry index score in more than 90 percent of their normal population with the one-legged hop for distance and timed hop tests.[27] They also state that patients who score normally may still have giving-way episodes under uncontrolled sports situations.[27] The one-legged hop tests are described.

One leg hop for distance.[27, 28] The patient stands on one limb, hops as far as possible, and lands on the same limb. Measure the distance and record the results. Each limb is tested twice. Calculate the symmetry index by dividing the mean of the involved limb by the noninvolved and multiply the result by 100.

Timed one leg hop.[27] The patient hops forcefully over a distance of 6 meters. Each limb is tested twice. For this test, the mean of the noninvolved limb is divided by the mean of the involved and multiplied by 100 to calculate the symmetry index.

Triple hop for distance.[26] The patient stands on one leg and takes three consecutive hops as far as possible, and lands on the same foot. The total distance hopped is measured.

Crossover hop test.[26] The course consists of a 15 cm marking strip on the floor, which extends approximately 6 meters. The patient hops three consecutive times on one foot, crossing over the center strip on each hop. The total distance hopped is measured.

Strength Base Testing

Poor strength in the lower extremities results in loss of stability when landing, and high-impact forces are excessively absorbed by the soft tissues of the body.[1] Anderson and Hall[29] recommend beginning power training after the injured limb has regained at least 80 percent of the muscle strength in the unaffected limb. Without adequate leg strength, fatigue becomes a factor and overuse injuries can occur.

Chu[1] recommends the power squat test as a good exercise to determine whether the patient has an adequate strength base. The exercise is performed with a weight equal to 60 percent of the individual's body weight. The patient performs five squat repetitions in 5 seconds. At the down position, the top of the individual's thighs should be parallel to the floor. If the patient cannot perform the test, the therapist should continue to emphasize the strength training program and begin plyometrics at a later date.

ORTHOPEDIC REHABILITATION

Understanding the physiologic basis of plyometric training is imperative to success in implementing these exercises in a rehabilitation program. It affords a basis for the analysis of the rationale for various treatment techniques and modalities, including plyometrics.

Treatment goals and strategies should correlate with deficits identified by the clinician during the assessment phase of the initial examination. Dryek[30] summarizes "Generic Treatment Goals" in the following manner:

1. Promote healing by improving the nutritional status of tissue.
2. Restore or prevent the loss of soft tis-

sue flexibility and length for contractile and noncontractile tissue.
3. Restore or prevent the loss of normal joint alignment.
4. Restore or prevent the loss of normal joint mobility.
5. Promote normal myotactic and myoarthrokinetic reflexes.
6. Promote normal motor control.
7. Resolve pain and associated symptoms.
8. Prevent recurrence of the lesion.
9. Restore the functional ability of the patient.

Promotion of normal myotactic and myoarthrokinetic reflexes such as the stretch reflex and stretch-shortening cycle of muscle tissue is achieved by accomplishing goals 1 through 4. An example is the inhibitory effect on surrounding musculature caused by joint effusion. Another is that ligament laxity is reported to decrease the normal protective response muscle gives a joint when it is under physical stress. This loss is believed to be secondary to sensory loss for the ligament.

The recovery of normal muscle control involves multiple factors such as strength, mobility, stability, motor control, and skill. The role of plyometric training is important in the recovery of all these areas. If this assumption is accepted, then the question becomes the timing and progression of plyometric training in the overall rehabilitation scheme.

The physical therapist must know and understand the etiology, symptomatology, physical manifestations, and natural course of musculoskeletal conditions. He or she must understand how to conduct a thorough examination and assess the patient's progress.

Treatment strategies developed by Dryek[30] are based on dividing the nine treatment goals into three categories of musculoskeletal lesions. The three plans are designed as a strategy for treatment of various musculoskeletal and structural deficits and are applicable to knee ligament rehabilitation.

Since plyometric training in its purest form involves maximal voluntary contractions, it fits into end-stage rehabilitation or as a part of "Restore previous or maximal functional status." In its more modified forms, plyometric training of very low inten-sity, or activities that are plyometric in nature, may be used to restore normal motor control. In no way should plyometric training be attempted prior to the treatment strategy's early levels (1–4) being accomplished.

PRACTICAL APPLICATIONS

Strength Training and Strength Base

A strength base is considered an important prerequisite, and therefore should be a precedent to bounding as well as plyometric training phases.[18, 31] To develop a strength base, the patient is engaged in a strength rehabilitation program for a minimum of 2 to 4 weeks.[14] Exercises generally begin with a moderate volume and low-intensity format. The strength program consists of six to eight core exercises. Two to three sets of 10 to 20 repetitions, performed three times a week, will be adequate to develop the strength base. Use two to three sets of 30 to 50 repetitions with lighter loads if the goal is to improve muscular endurance. With this format, the patient performs fewer (three to six) core exercises. Incorporate the major muscle groups that will be used during the plyometric activities for exercise selection. Emphasis is placed on performing closed-kinetic chain, eccentric, and functional activities utilizing large muscle groups.

Eccentric Strength

Eccentric muscular contractions occur when the muscle lengthens with applied resistance. Eccentric training is popular in the rehabilitation setting because of the increased force production within the muscle. Through a gradually progressed eccentric loading program, healing of tendinous tissue is stressed, yielding an increase in ultimate tensile strength.[23] Eccentric strength is an important component of plyometric training and is considered a precursor to success in plyometrics.[1] Eccentric strength decelerates the limbs when the patient is landing from the air during plyometric training. The prestretch phase associated with plyometric

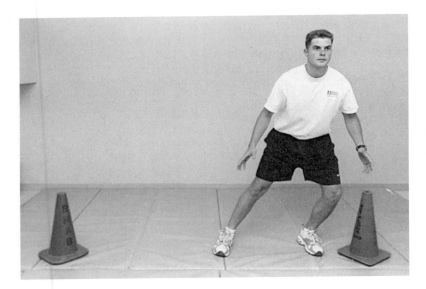

Figure 24–10. Shuffle agility drill. (Courtesy of Baptist Health Systems Media Services Department, Miami, FL.)

training is an eccentric contraction. Before an individual begins a plyometric regimen, a program of closed-chain stability training that focuses on eccentric lower quarter strength should be initiated.[23]

Footwork and Agility Drills

Once the patient passes previously described static and dynamic testing, introduction of footwork and agility drills is recommended. Footwork and agility drills are activities that have properties similar to ply-

ometrics and therefore are considered "plyometric in nature." In the rehabilitation, setting these drills are often not performed at full speed. Furthermore, they are less explosive than true plyometrics. They are similar in that they apply eccentric loads and the patient's lower extremity or extremities often leave the platform or ground.

The shuffle (Fig. 24–10), carioca (Fig. 24–11), and figure-of-eight (Fig. 24–12) are probably the three most common agility drills. Use of all three drills during each agility session stresses the hip, knee, and ankle in multiple planes. Initially the patient walks

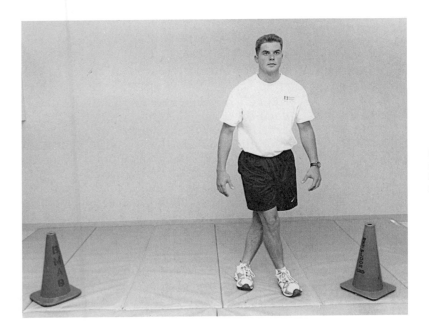

Figure 24–11. Carioca agility drill. (Courtesy of Baptist Health Systems Media Services Department, Miami, FL.)

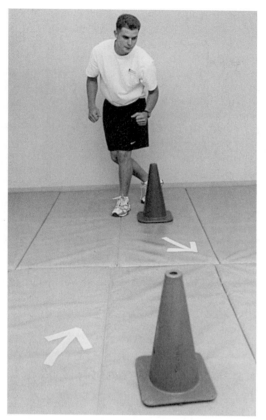

Figure 24–12. Figure-of-eight agility drill. (Courtesy of Baptist Health Systems Media Services Department, Miami, FL.)

through the drills, then gradually is progressed to jogging, and finally running. Markey[32] recommends an agility progression beginning with large figure-of-eights, advancing to 90-degree cuts or running in and out of pylons. Then he completes agility maneuvers with jumping (jumping rope with two legs then one leg) and finishes with stop-go-stop activities. He also states that the carioca drill is important in developing the kinesthetic sense of the lower extremity. After the patient is cleared to run, Antich and Brewster[33] begin straight plane activities such as running forward and backpedaling. They also emphasize the importance of assessing and training the individual to start and stop on command.

As stated, begin the agility program with the patient performing all three of the different drills. We recommend three to six repetitions of each drill, for approximately 20 yards (10 yards out, 10 back). Initially, the patient rests for 10 to 20 seconds between each repetition. To improve endurance, the

patient performs all repetitions (three to six) without rest, and is only allowed rest between each drill. After the patient is able to walk through the drills, he or she progresses to jogging and running at 50 percent, then 75 percent, and finally at 100 percent.

After the patient is able to perform basic agility drills, progress him or her to more advanced footwork activities. Increase the intensity of footwork and agility drills by increasing speed and complexity of the drill. Traditionally, a four-square jumping program has been used by clinicians to increase complexity and improve coordination to the lower extremity (specifically the ankle). This activity falls under the multiple hops category of plyometric training and is designed to be performed at full speed, although in the clinical setting this drill may be performed at 50 percent to 75 percent speed. The patient jumps from square to square in different variations (patterns) to stress the lower extremity in different planes.

The Acceleration Products company of Fargo, North Dakota has taken the basic four-square program and advanced the traditional technique and rationale. They include an eight-square program and other more advanced and complicated footwork drills. The rationale behind this type of training revolves around the "inverted funnel" principle. Based on the use of footwork patterns and the "inverted funnel" principle, these drills have been carefully protocolled to fit with a high-speed, intense-interval training program. This principle involves the body's center of gravity and its relationship to stability and movement. The person's center of gravity is the balance point about which all the particles of the body are evenly distributed. The "inverted funnel" concept is based on the fact that movements require the individual often to move the feet out from under the body's center of gravity, and then recover the position in a brief period of time, so as to regain balance and stability. The essence of the footwork drills is to teach the individual to maintain the center of gravity in a relatively constant position while the feet work out from under it in all directions. As the patient's feet move through the designated pattern, an attempt is made to keep the center of gravity in the middle of the pattern. This technique will help improve kinesthetic awareness. The description below is a sample program of the Acceleration eight-square plyometric formation.

Both legs

A. Box 1-2 Max. in 10 sec.   _____
B. Box 1-2-3 Max. in 10 sec.   _____
C. Box 1-3-2 Max. in 10 sec.   _____
D. Box 1-4-2 Max. in 10 sec.   _____
E. Box 1-2-4 Max. in 10 sec.   _____
F. Box 1-2-3-4 Max. in 10 sec.   _____
G. Box 1-4-3-2 Max. in 10 sec.   _____

Single leg

A. Box 1-2 (2 sets) Max. in 5 sec. R ____ ,
                                     L ____
B. Box 1-4 (2 sets) Max. in 5 sec. R ____ ,
                                     L ____

Clinical Lower Extremity

Lower extremity plyometrics are an effective functional closed-chain exercise that can be incorporated into the rehabilitation program.[23] It is important to apply the plyometric activities sensibly. Physical therapists should adhere to the previously described prerequisites to plyometric exercise. Plyometrics should not aggravate a patient's symptoms. Proper progression from strengthening to plyometrics is important to achieve increased functional strength and power, without reinjury. Plyometrics after injury are usually not started until the final stages of rehabilitation, or minimal protection phase, when flexibility and strength have returned to near pre-injury levels. However, activities that are plyometric in nature may be started sooner. Decreased body weight or low-impact plyometrics and agility drills are examples of activities that are "plyometric in nature." An individual recovering from a chronic overuse injury is closely monitored to prevent recurrence. After the patient has mastered decreased body weight plyometrics and agility drills, he or she will progress to low-intensity full-body weight plyometric activities. The individual must pass strength and functional testing prior to initiation of higher intensity plyometrics. Bilateral activities will always precede unilateral activities.

Have the patient practice initial plyometric activities on the leg press or shuttle 2000-1. The patient works on timing and muscle recruitment with less than full body weight impact forces. The Shuttle 2000-1 (see Fig. 24–6) is preferred because of its elastic qualities and low-impact forces. Start with 25 to 50 percent of the patient's body weight and have him or her perform two to three sets of 10 repetitions. If the patient does not experience pain or swelling from this activity, he or she can advance to increased repetitions and loads. Outlined below are two examples of shuttle protocols for knee ligament rehabilitation.[20]

Anterior Cruciate Ligament

Purpose: Increase range of motion to 90 + degrees (bilateral/single leg).

Volume: 30 to 50 repetitions; repetitions to fatigue; time intervals (30 - 90 seconds)

Intensity: four to eight cords

Frequency: Daily preferred

Medial Collateral Ligament

Purpose: Increase range of motion to 120 + degrees (bilateral/single leg).

Volume: 50 to 100 repetitions; repetitions to fatigue (three times); time intervals (60–120 seconds)

Intensity: six to eight cords

Frequency: Daily preferred

Bounding and Low-Intensity Full Body Weight Plyometrics

After the shuttle protocol and foot work drills are completed, the patient is ready to begin full weight-bearing plyometrics. At this time, the patient is ambulating with full weight and has achieved generic treatment goals 1 through 4 described by Dyrek.[30] At least 80 percent strength and 90 to 95 percent full range of motion is required before beginning functional exercises and power training.[20, 29] To make these plyometrics effective, the physical therapist emphasizes the "touch and go" principle to the patient. The ball of the foot touches first with the rest of the foot also making contact. The goal is to land and immediately take off, spending the least amount of time on the ground as possible. The double-arm swing, described by Chu,[1] will help develop force into the ground to "compress the spring." For this technique, the elbows are brought behind the midline of the body, so the arms can be brought rapidly forward and up, as the concentric contraction occurs for liftoff. These "true" plyometric techniques employ the stretch-shortening cycle and focus on decreasing amortization phase time, as plyometrics were originally intended.

Emphasize medial and lateral activities to accept greater valgus and varus loads with

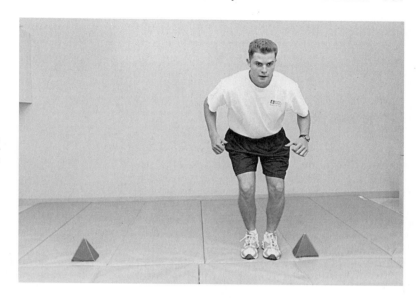

Figure 24–13. Lateral hops. (Courtesy of Baptist Health Systems Media Services Department, Miami, FL.)

lateral bounding drills. Emphasize these activities if the patient has sustained a valgus or varus injury to the knee. Also, have the patient perform the drills if the patient's goal is to return to activities that require him or her to perform cutting maneuvers. Lateral hops (Fig. 24–13) and lateral bounding (Fig. 24–14) are good drills to provide valgus and varus loads on the lower extremities.

Start the patient with two to three sets of 10 to 15 repetitions. Begin with one or two drills and progress the patient gradually if there is no pain or swelling. Through the imagination of the clinician, drills are administered and varied to stress different musculoskeletal areas. The program variation provides motivation and fun as the patient masters each drill. Progress from jumps in place to standing jumps. After these are easily performed, progress to bounding and multiple jumps. Finally, if applicable, introduce drop downs or depth jumps.

Figures 24–15 through 24–20 define different types of plyometric drills that are suitable for end-stage rehabilitation in the clinical setting. The plyometric exercises have been adapted from *Jumping into Plyometrics*.[1] This is a limited list, a complete list can be seen in *Jumping into Plyometrics*. Often the drill is performed to enhance the individu-

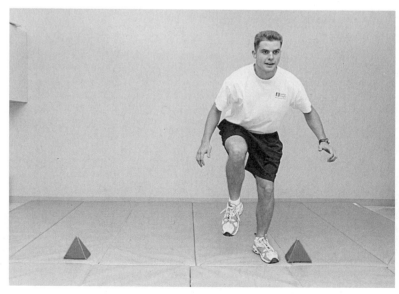

Figure 24–14. Lateral bounding. (Courtesy of Baptist Health Systems Media Services Department, Miami, FL.)

al's ability to perform the sporting activity. The equipment (if any), start position, and action of the drill are also described for the reader.

RETURNING TO SPORTS

There are many variables to consider when determining whether an athletic patient should return to his or her given activity or sport. Severity of injury, surgical technique, therapeutic intervention, and the individual's physiologic healing process are all factors affecting rehabilitation outcomes. Several rehabilitation protocols give time frames and criteria the individual must meet before returning to play.[34–42] Rehabilitation protocols vary greatly, even among the same surgical procedure. Anterior cruciate ligament reconstruction surgery is a good example and can vary from the longer traditional protocols to the faster accelerated programs. Literature review of ACL protocols reveals that an athlete is allowed to begin running anywhere from 5 weeks to 7.5 months after injury.[36, 41] Additionally, athletes are allowed to return to their sport from 4 months to 12 months.[41, 43] Regardless of the time frames, usually athletes must pass testing criteria before they are allowed to return to play. Functional, diagnostic, arthrometric, isokinetic, and clinical examination tests are just a few of the procedures often used to assess the athlete's status. Guidelines for return to competitive sports vary among the research and rehabilitation programs.[34–42]

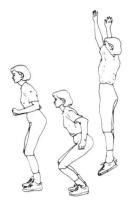

Figure 24–16. Standing jumps: standing jump and reach. *Equipment*: An object suspended overhead, or a wall with a target marked. *Start*: Stand with feet shoulder-width apart. *Action*: Squat slightly, and explode upward, reaching for a target or object. Do not step before jumping. (Reprinted with permission from Chu DA: Jumping into Plyometrics. Champaign, IL, Human Kinetics, 1992, p. 31.)

The application of a time table for return to activity is generally only utilized as a guide. Time tables are arbitrary, and objective testing criteria seem more appropriate. While rehabilitation time tables for return to sports vary among the research, the physical requirements to return are neighboring. Following is a theoretical model for criteria to return to sports or sport-specific training based on the previously reviewed literature.[34–43] We believe that this program can be adopted for any knee ligament injury, as criteria for returning to sport and or sport-specific training.

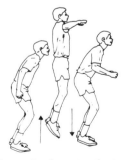

Figure 24–15. Jumps-in-place: two-foot ankle hop. *Equipment*: None. *Start*: Stand with feet shoulder-width apart and the body in a vertical position. *Action*: Using only the ankles for momentum, hop continuously in one place. Extend the ankles to their maximum range on each vertical hop. (Reprinted with permission from Chu DA: Jumping into Plyometrics. Champaign, IL, Human Kinetics, 1992, p. 27.)

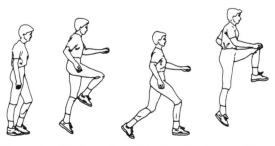

Figure 24–17. Bounding: skipping. *Equipment*: None. *Start*: Stand comfortably. *Action*: Lift the right leg with the knee bent 90 degrees while lifting the left arm, with the elbows also bent 90 degrees. As these two limbs come back down, lift the opposite limbs with the same motion. For added difficulty, push off the ground for more upward extension. (Reprinted with permission from Chu DA: Jumping into Plyometrics. Champaign, IL, Human Kinetics, 1992, p. 56.)

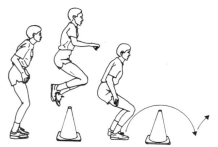

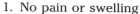

Figure 24–18. Multiple hops and jumps: front cone hops. *Equipment*: A row of 6 to 10 cones or small barriers (6 to 12 inches tall) set up approximately 3 to 6 feet apart. *Start*: Stand with feet shoulder-width apart at the end of the line of barriers (with their length spread out before you). *Action*: Keeping feet shoulder-width apart, jump over each barrier, landing on both feet at the same time. Use a double arm swing and work to decrease the time spent on the ground between each barrier. (Reprinted with permission from Chu DA: Jumping into Plyometrics. Champaign, IL, Human Kinetics, 1992, p. 37.)

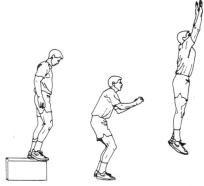

Figure 24–20. Depth jumps: depth jump. *Equipment*: A box 6 to 12 inches high. *Start*: Stand on the box, toes close to the front edge. *Action*: Step from the box and drop to land on both feet. Try to anticipate the landing and spring up as quickly as you can. Keep the body from "settling" on the landing, and make the ground contact as short as possible. (Reprinted with permission from Chu DA: Jumping into Plyometrics. Champaign, IL, Human Kinetics, 1992, p. 49.)

1. No pain or swelling
2. Flexion and extension range of motion equal to contralateral knee
3. Isokinetic test values: (when compared to contralateral knee) at 180, 240, 300 degrees per second, lower speeds can be used if there is no cruciate ligament involvement or patellofemoral symptoms.
   - Quadriceps: at least 80 to 85 percent
   - Hamstring: at least 85 to 90 percent
4. Joint laxity tests:
   - KT 1000 arthrometric test: (ACL or PCL injuries) unchanged from original test to a maximum of 2 mm bilateral difference[43]
   - Valgus-varus test: no laxity increase from original test

5. Proprioceptive test: (on a testing machine if available)
   - satisfactory result or injured limb 90 to 100 percent of uninjured
6. Complete jog-run program with satisfactory result
7. Complete functional training program with satisfactory result
8. Functional tests: satisfactory result (85 percent or greater) on two tests (tests to be determined by clinician)
9. Physician medical clearance

After the individual passes the criteria to return to sports, sport-specific plyometrics are begun. Soon, returning to sports participation will advance to returning to competition. The following list gives criteria for returning to athletic team competition or game situations.

1. Satisfactory performance in all tests for returning to sports
2. Execute sport-specific training drills with satisfactory skill
3. 1 to 2 weeks full participation in practice (depending on extent of injury)

Sport-Specific Training

Specificity of plyometric training is the key to improving an athlete's performance on the field. Stone and O'Bryant[18] state that specificity of movement is necessary for carry-over to athletic activities. The 1993

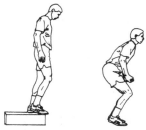

Figure 24–19. Box jumps: jump from box. *Equipment*: A box 6 to 8 inches high. *Start*: Stand on the box with feet shoulder-width apart. *Action*: Squat slightly and step from the box and drop to the floor. Attempt to quickly absorb the landing and "freeze" as soon as contact is made with the ground. (Reprinted with permission from Chu DA: Jumping into Plyometrics. Champaign, IL, Human Kinetics, 1992, p. 48.)

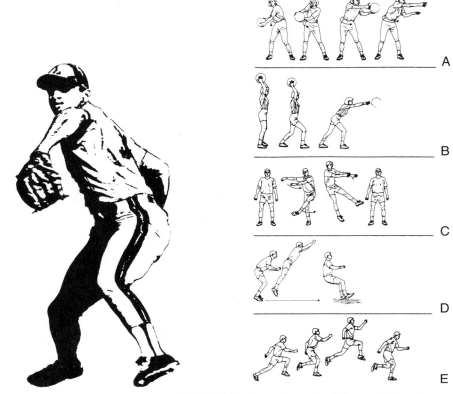

Figure 24–21. Plyometrics for baseball and softball. *A*, Side throw; *B*, overhead throw; *C*, lateral jump with two feet; *D*, standing long jump; *E*, alternate bounding with single arm action. (Reprinted with permission from Chu DA: Jumping into Plyometrics. Champaign, IL, Human Kinetics, 1992, p. 70.)

National Strength and Conditioning Association position paper[17] on plyometrics states that a plyometric exercise program can improve performance in most competitive sports, and a plyometric training program for athletes should include sport-specific exercises. Creating a sport-specific program requires understanding the mechanics of the sport by doing a needs analysis, and breaking down skill patterns into their most elementary parts.[1] The drills performed are similar to those used during actual sport practice and in game situations. The athlete is performing activities in a controlled environment without other athletes around. Previously practiced basic plyometric drills become sport specific.

At the end of this stage, the clinician can simulate other athletes and distract the patient. This increases the intensity and challenges the individual's balance, coordination, proprioception, and kinesthetic awareness in a more specific manner. This is an example of sports specificity at its highest level. Additionally, this approach allows the athlete to build confidence in his or her abilities before returning to an environment with other athletes. This is a good time to incorporate a medicine ball into the plyometric program. This will enhance the sport specificity for entire body utilization. The sport-specific drills are performed at 100 percent intensity. At this level, technique and execution of the drill are essential. Recovery periods should be sufficient to allow the athlete to perform the drill with proper technique and movement speed as applicable. Ultimately, the clinician should attempt to simulate actual recovery times used during the athlete's sport. If possible, have the athlete exercise on the actual or most similar sport playing surface. Suggested repetitions are adjusted according to the athlete's conditioning level. The individual should stretch and warm up with low-intensity plyometrics prior to the sport-specific plyometric session.

Illustrated in Figures 24–21 through 24–24 are four recommended sport-specific plyometric activities for five popular sports.

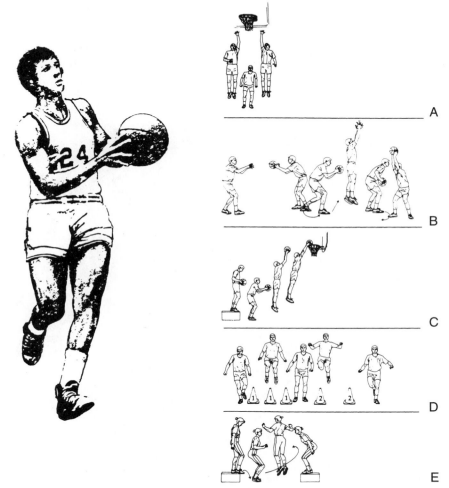

Figure 24–22. Plyometrics for basketball. *A,* Rim jump; *B,* low post drill; *C,* depth jump with stuff; *D,* lateral cone hops; *E,* depth jump with 180-degree turn. (Reprinted with permission from Chu DA: Jumping into Plyometrics. Champaign, IL, Human Kinetics, 1992, p. 70.)

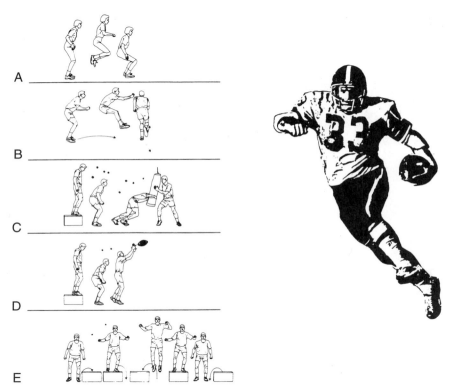

Figure 24–23. Plyometrics for football. *A*, Double leg hops; *B*, standing long jump with lateral sprint; *C*, depth jump with blocking bag; *D*, Depth jump with pass catching; *E*, 90-second box drill. (Reprinted with permission from Chu DA: Jumping into Plyometrics. Champaign, IL, Human Kinetics, 1992, p. 73.)

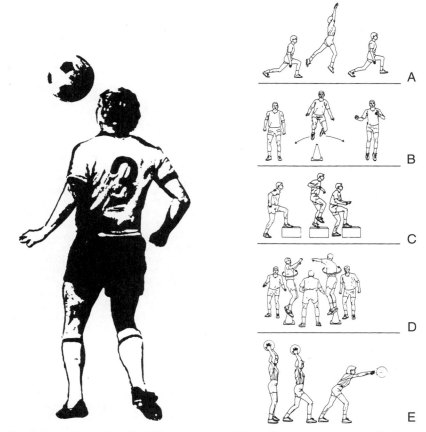

Figure 24–24. Plyometrics for soccer. *A*, Split squat jump; *B*, lateral jump over barrier; *C*, alternating push-off; *D*, cone hops with 180-degree turn; *E*, overhead throw. (Reprinted with permission from Chu DA: Jumping into Plyometrics. Champaign, IL, Human Kinetics, 1992, p. 74.)

Other sport-specific plyometric activities for various sports can be found in *Jumping into Plyometrics.*[1]

References

1. Chu DA: Jumping into Plyometrics. Champaign, IL, Human Kinetics, 1992.
2. Verhoshanski UV, Chernousov G: Jumps in the training of a sprinter. Track Field 9:16–17, 1974.
3. Wilt F. Plyometrics: What it is and How it Works. Athletic J 55(5):76–90, 1975.
4. Bosco C, Komi PV: Influence of aging on the mechanical behavior of leg extensor muscles. Eur J Appl Phys Neuromech Basis Kinesiol. 45:209–219, 1980.
5. Cavagna GA, Saibene FP, Margaria R: Mechanical work in running. J Appl Phys Neuromech Basis Kinesiol. 19:249–256, 1964.
6. Komi PV: Stretch-shortening cycle. *In* Komi PV (ed): Strength and Power in Sport: Neuromechanical Basis of Kinesiology. Champaign, IL, Human Kinetics; 1992, pp. 169–179.
7. Komi PV, Bosco C: Utilization of stored elastic energy in leg extensor muscles by men and women. Med Sci Sports Neuromech Basis Kinesiol 10:261–265, 1978.
8. Komi PV, Buskirk ER: Effects of eccentric and concentric muscle conditioning on tension and electrical activity of human muscle. Ergonomics Neuromech Basis Kinesiol. 15:417–434, 1972.
9. Spence AP: Basic Human Anatomy, 2nd ed. Menlo Park, CA, Benjamin/Cummings, 1986, pp. 66–67.
10. McArdle WD, Katch FI, Katch VL: Exercise Physiology: Energy, Nutrition, and Human Performance, 3rd ed. Malvern, PA, Lea & Febiger, 1991, pp. 367–383.
11. Howeley ET, Franks BD: Health/Fitness Instructor's Handbook. Champaign, IL, Human Kinetics, 1986, p. 41.
12. Wathen D: Literature Review: Explosive/Plyometric Exercises. Natl Strength Cond Assoc J 15(6):16–19, 1993.
13. Borkowski J: Prevention of preseason muscle soreness: Plyometric exercise. Athl Training 25(2):122, 1990.
14. Santos J: Jump training for speed and neuromuscular development. Track Field Q Rev 79(1):59, 1979.
15. Allerheiligen B, Rogers R: Plyometrics program design. NSCA J 17(4):26–31, 1995.
16. Allerheiligen WB: Speed development and plyo-

metric training. *In* Baechle TR (ed): Essentials of Strength Training and Conditioning. Champaign, IL, Human Kinetics; 1994, pp. 314–344.

17. Wathen D: Literature review: Explosive/plyometric exercises. NSCA J 15(6):16–19, 1993.

18. Stone MH, O'Bryant HS: Weight Training: A Scientific Approach. Minneapolis, MN, Bellwether Press, 1987, pp. 94–102.

19. Prentice WE: Maintaining and improving flexibility. *In* Prentice WE (ed): Rehabilitations Techniques in Sports Medicine, 2nd ed. St. Louis, Mosby, 1994, pp. 38–52.

20. Chu DA: Rehabilitation of the lower extremity. *In* Clinics in Sports Medicine, Racquet Sports. Philadelphia, W.B. Saunders, 1995, pp. 205–222.

21. Mish FC (ed): Webster's Ninth New Collegiate Dictionary. Springfield, MA, William A Llewellyn, Publisher, 1983, p. 952.

22. Allerheiligen B, Rogers R: Plyometrics program design, part 2. NSCA J 17(5):33–39, 1995.

23. Voight M, Tippett S: Plyometric exercise in rehabilitation. *In* Prentice WE (ed): Rehabilitation Techniques in Sports Medicine, 2nd ed. St. Louis, Mosby, 1994, pp. 88–97.

24. Voight ML, Draovitch P: Plyometrics. *In* Albert M (ed): Eccentric Muscle Training in Sports and Orthopaedics. New York,: Churchill Livingstone, 1991, p. 45.

25. Barber SD, Noyes FR, Mangine R, et al: Rehabilitation after ACL reconstuction: Functional testing. Orthopedics. 15:969–974, 1992.

26. Noyes FR, Barber SD, Mangine RE: Abnormal lower limb symmetry determined by functional hop tests after anterior cruciate ligament rupture. Am J Sports Med 19(5):513–518, 1991.

27. Barber SD, Noyes FR, Mangine RE, et al.: Quantitative assessment of functional limitations in normal and anterior cruciate ligament-deficient knees. Clin Orthop. 255:204–214, 1990.

28. Daniel D, Malcom L, Stone ML, et al.: Quantification of knee stability and function. Contemp Orthop 5(1):83–91, 1982.

29. Anderson MK, Hall SJ: Sports Injury Management. Media, PA, Williams & Wilkins, 1995, pp. 137–182.

30. Dyrek DA: Assessment and treatment planning strategies for musculoskeletal deficits. *In* O'Sullivan SB, Schmitz TJ, (eds): Physical Rehabilitation Assessment and Treatment, 3rd ed. Philadelphia, F.A. Davis, 1994, pp. 61–79.

31. Coaches Round Table, Improving Jumping Ability. NSCA J 6(2):10–20, 1984.

32. Markey KL: Functional rehabilitation of the cruciate-deficinet knee. Sports Med 12(6):407–417, 1991.

33. Antich TJ, Brewster CE: Rehabilitation of the nonreconstructed anterior cruciate ligamnet-deficient knee. Clin Sports Med 7(4):813–826, 1988.

34. Brotzman SB (ed): Clinical Orthopaedic Rehabilitation. St. Louis, Mosby Year Book, 1995.

35. DeMaio M, Mangine RE, Noyes FR et al.: Advanced muscle training after ACL reconstruction: Weeks 6 to 52. Orthopedics 15:757–767, 1992.

36. Frndak PA, Berasi CC: Rehabilitation concerns following anterior cruciate ligament reconstruction. Sports Med 12(5):338–346, 1991.

37. Mangine RE, Noyes FR: Rehabilitation of the allograft reconstruction. J Orthop Sports Phys Ther 15(6):294–302, 1992.

38. Markey KL: Functional rehabilitation of the cruciate-deficient knee. Sports Med 12(6):407–417, 1991.

39. Paulos LE, Stern J: Rehabilitation after anterior cruciate ligament surgery. *In* Jackson DW (ed): The Anterior Cruciate Ligament. New York, Raven Press, 1993.

40. Paulos LE, Wnorowski DC, Beck CL: Rehabilitation following knee surgery. Sports Med 11(4):257–275, 1991.

41. Shelbourne DK, Nitz P: Accelerated rehabilitation after anterior cruciate ligament reconstruction. Am J Sports Med 18(3):292–299, 1990.

42. Wilk KE, Andrews JR: Current concepts in the treatment of anterior cruciate ligament disruption. J Orthop Sports Phys Ther 15:279–293, 1992.

43. Bach BR, Warren RF, Flynn WM, et al.: Arthrometric evaluation of knees that have a torn ACL ligament. J Bone Joint Surg 72A(9):1299–1306, 1990.

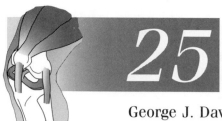

Functional Progression of Exercise During Rehabilitation

George J. Davies, MEd, PT, SCS, ATC, CSCS,
and Debra A. Zillmer, MD, PT

*T*here is consensus in the literature that there needs to be an evaluation and a systematic progression of any patient through a rehabilitation program.[1–6] How to perform this systematic progression is elusive, however, and there are as many methods and techniques as there are clinicians. Furthermore, there are few articles in the literature that describe specific methods or provide precise guidelines with objective documentation for functional progression of exercise during rehabilitation. Numerous descriptions of techniques exist to assess patients' performance,[7–22] but few articles have integrated all techniques into a systematic process. The purpose of this chapter is to provide a systematic, objective functional testing algorithm that is based on published research, empiric guidelines, and over 25 years of clinical experience using a similar format.

FUNCTIONAL TESTING ALGORITHM

We[23–26] have developed a functional testing algorithm (FTA) as one method to assess a patient in a systematic manner and to base the functional progression of exercise during a rehabilitation program. The FTA is discussed in a whole-part-whole system. We discuss the specific details of how the FTA is used in the evaluation and progression of a patient from postinjury or postsurgery through the rehabilitation program and back to functional activities and sports. An overview (whole) of the FTA is illustrated in Figure 25–1.

The FTA testing strategies are based on the principles of progression and "control." Each test in the progressive testing sequence increases different types of stresses to the patient with less clinical control. Early in the rehabilitation process and subsequent

testing, the FTA is based on maintaining careful clinical control of the stresses imposed on the patient, and as time goes on, to gradually introduce controlled progressive stresses. Each test in the FTA increases stress to the patient with less clinical control. Progression to the next higher level of testing difficulty is predicated on passing each test in the FTA sequence. The patient must pass a minimum level of performance on one level to progress to the next higher level in the FTA sequence.

The criteria for the progression through the FTA are currently based on limited research published in the literature, many years of clinical experience, and our empirically based clinical guidelines. Correlation research by other authors is in progress. In addition, a paper was submitted for publication that contains statistical correlations between many of the tests used in the FTA.[27] Table 25–1 provides the current empiric guidelines for clinical decision-making regarding the functional progression of exercise during rehabilitation.

The following information describes each stage of the FTA with emphasis on the empiric guidelines and rationales for their inclusion.

BASIC AND FUNDAMENTAL MEASUREMENTS

The basic and fundamental measurements consist of the various findings in the history, the subjective examination, and the objective physical examination of the patient. The various parts of the basic and fundamental measurements are listed in Table 25–2. Examples of how the basic and fundamental measurements can be used in the functional progression of exercise during rehabilitation is presented in the following sections.

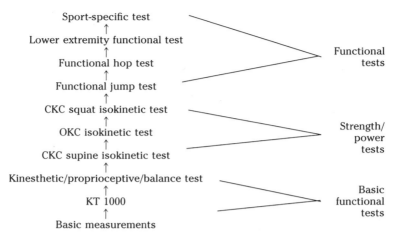

Figure 25–1. Functional testing algorithm (FTA), lower extremity. CKC = closed kinetic chain; OKC = open kinetic chain.

Subjective Examination

The patient's subjective symptoms are evaluated at rest, with activities of daily living, with vocational activities, and with avocational activities. A visual analog scale is used to assess the patient's response to different types of stress loading. The visual analog scale we use ranges from 0 (no pain) to 10 (worst pain). The clinician's experience and familiarity with the patient now become invaluable when trying to cause progression of a patient through a functional rehabilitation program. (What is one patient's pain may be another patient's pleasure.) Our present standard is for the patient to have no pain at rest and pain with activity at less than 1 or 2 on the visual analog scale before progressing to more exercises.

One of the reasons for this constraint is that pain produces a reflex inhibition resulting in muscle "weakness." In addition, the location of the symptoms and the specific anatomic structures involved often dictate the progression in the rehabilitation program. If pain is significant, discussion with the patient's physician or surgeon is recommended and progression is placed on

● Table 25–1. Empiric Guidelines for Patient Progression in the Functional Testing Algorithm

Tests	Empiric Guidelines
Sport-specific testing (SST)	
Lower extremity functional test (LEFT)	Female <2:00 min; Male <1:30 min
Functional hop test (FHT)	<15% bilateral comparison and norms
Functional jump test (FJT)	<20% compared with body height and norms
Closed kinetic chain (CKC) (standing)	<20% bilateral comparison
Open kinetic chain (OKC)	<25% bilateral comparison
Closed kinetic chain (CKC) (supine)	<30% bilateral comparison
Balance test	<30% bilateral comparison
KT 1000	<3 mm bilateral comparison
Basic measurements	<10% bilateral comparison
Subjective	Pain < 3 (analog pain scale: 0–10)

● Table 25–2. Functional Testing Algorithm (FTA): Basic/Fundamental Measurements

History and subjective examination
Objective examination
  Observation/posture
  Vital signs
  Gait evaluation
  Anthropometric measurements
  Leg length measurements
  Referral/related joints
  Palpation
  Neurologic examination
    Sensation
    Reflexes
  Balance/proprioception/kinesthesia
  Manual muscle testing
  Active range of motion
  Passive range of motion
  Flexibility tests
  Special tests
  Medical tests

hold. As a general clinical guideline, criteria for the progression of a patient to the next level of testing in the FTA include parameters within 10 percent in a bilateral comparison or relative to normative data and clinical experience and judgment.

KT 1000 Testing

If the patient has had an anterior or posterior cruciate ligament injury, evaluation of knee stability is performed with the KT 1000.[28] If surgery has been performed, ideally the difference between the uninvolved and the involved knee would be 3 mm or less. If a greater than 3 mm difference exists between the sides, medical discretion is used to determine whether the patient is ready to progress and be tested at the next stage of the FTA. If a patient has a KT 1000 reading that is greater than 3 mm early in the postoperative course, we try to protect the graft by protected weight-bearing, bracing, and modification of the rehabilitation program.

Balance, Kinesthesia, and Proprioception Testing

Measurement of balance, kinesthesia, and proprioception should be included as part of the FTA.[29–32] Both static and dynamic balance are measured. For many years, we used a digital balance evaluator, which was a single-plane balance board that had microswitches and counted the number of touches and time out of balance in a 30-second test protocol. During the last several years, however, we have used a FASTEX computerized neuromuscular assessment system. This allows us to measure both static and dynamic balance simultaneously. The current test protocols are described in Figures 25–2 and 25–3.

Limited information has been published on normative values for balance, kinesthesia, and proprioception. We therefore have our own internally generated testing data as empiric guidelines for the evaluation and progression of the patient in the FTA. Johnson-Stuhr (unpublished research, 1997) completed a test-retest reliability study on the FASTEX and found that it was a reliable device for measuring balance within the limita-

tions of the study. If, during testing, a patient's score is higher than the established norm, kinesthetic exercise for neuromuscular control is emphasized in his or her rehabilitation program. Variables are based on the specific pathologic condition and test scores. Retesting for progression takes place at a later date.

MUSCULAR STRENGTH AND POWER TESTING

Closed Kinetic Chain Isokinetic Testing Semisitting or Supine Position

With the increased emphasis on closed kinetic chain (CKC) exercises in many rehabilitation protocols, the need to test for CKC functional performance becomes an important part of the FTA. A concern is how to test safely with CKC exercises early in rehabilitation without iatrogenically creating more problems. It is often contraindicated to test using 1 repetition maximum or 10 repetition maximums too soon following injury or surgery because it may cause inappropriate stresses to the injured area or healing tissue structures.[33]

Historically, the reasons quoted for incorporating CKC exercises into the rehabilitation program are that (1) CKC exercises are functional,[34, 35] (2) CKC exercises are more effective in improving function, (3) the CKC position increases the joint compressive forces, increasing knee stability,[36–42] (4) CKC exercises promote co-contractions of the quadriceps and hamstrings to provide dynamic stability to the knee joint,[43–54] and (5) CKC exercises minimize translatory stresses to the ligaments, particularly the anterior cruciate ligament (ACL).[55] Interestingly, many of these reasons have been questioned.

As an example, one study using a prospective randomized controlled clinical trial series demonstrated that using only aggressive CKC exercises as the primary mode of rehabilitation for patients following ACL reconstruction did not normalize their quadricep function with gait.[56] Yet another study[57] demonstrated that in an unloaded bilateral squat, there was minimal electromyographic hamstring activity and minimal electromyographic gastrocnemius activity. This causes

Name _____ DOB _____ Gender M/F
GC # _____ PT _____ MD _____
Injury/Surgery _____ DOS/DOI _____

Procedure
1. Patient stands on uninvolved leg facing away from the computer, with head and eyes looking straight forward focusing on an object.
2. Non–weight-bearing knee is flexed to approximately a 90-degree angle, and the shin is held parallel to the floor.
3. NWB knee is abducted and not touching opposite leg.
4. Hands are clasped behind the back.
5. Allow one practice test for 20 seconds.
6. Each test is 20 seconds.
7. Repeat the test 3 times with a 20-second rest period in between each test.
8. Record the total stability index for each trial.
9. Repeat 1 to 8 on involved leg.

DATE	UNINVOLVED L/R	INVOLVED L/R	% DEFICIT
Trial 1			
Trial 2			
Trial 3			
Average			
DATE	UNINVOLVED L/R	INVOLVED L/R	% DEFICIT
Trial 1			
Trial 2			
Trial 3			
Average			
DATE	UNINVOLVED L/R	INVOLVED L/R	% DEFICIT
Trial 1			
Trial 2			
Trial 3			
Average			

Figure 25–2. Static balance test protocol and data collection sheet.

a question about the co-contraction loading to provide dynamic stability theory.

Nevertheless, accepting all the indications to do CKC testing and exercises as well as many of the limitations, we incorporate CKC testing at this point in the FTA. We use a Linea (Loredan Biomedical), which is a lower extremity computerized isokinetic/isotonic testing and rehabilitation system. We test the patient in a semisitting to supine position with CKC isokinetics. Davies and Heiderscheit[58] have published the results on the reliability of the Linea that demonstrates the intraclass correlation coefficients to be from .85 to .94, which demonstrates good to excellent test-retest reliability.

We begin the CKC testing in the semisitting or supine position for control of weight-bearing and range of motion. This testing position controls the stresses delivered to the knee and prevents varus-valgus and rotational forces. It is considered safe for operative and nonoperative patients early in rehabilitation.

Although the Linea provides numerous modes of testing (isometrics, isotonics, isokinetics), different muscle actions, including isometric, concentric, and eccentric, different patterns of testing, such as reciprocal lower extremity patterns or coupled or tandem symmetric leg press patterns, and a variety of speeds (0–30 inches per second), we primarily employ the following test protocol. The testing protocol has a CKC isokinetic reciprocal because it simulates the functional movements of gait or running. We use the isokinetic mode because of the safety afforded by the accommodating resistance and the ability to sample the muscle's performance through the velocity spectrum.

Name _____ DOB _____ Gender M/F
MH # _____ PT _____ MD _____
Injury/Surgery _____ DOS/DOI _____

Procedure
1. Patient stands on both legs.
2. Patient jumps side to side between two platforms, with the arms left free.
3. Allow one set of submax (easy side to side) warm-ups.
4. Each set consists of 20 jumps, with a 20-second rest period in between each set.
5. The objective is for the patient to complete the 20 jumps as quickly as possible.
6. The patient completes 3 sets of 20 jumps for the test. For each set the total elapsed time is recorded.

DATE	TOTAL ELAPSED TIME		DATE	TOTAL ELAPSED TIME
Trial 1			Trial 1	
Trial 2			Trial 2	
Trial 3			Trial 3	
Average			Average	

DATE	TOTAL ELAPSED TIME		DATE	TOTAL ELAPSED TIME
Trial 1			Trial 1	
Trial 2			Trial 2	
Trial 3			Trial 3	
Average			Average	

DATE	TOTAL ELAPSED TIME		DATE	TOTAL ELAPSED TIME
Trial 1			Trial 1	
Trial 2			Trial 2	
Trial 3			Trial 3	
Average			Average	

Figure 25–3. Dynamic balance test protocol and data collection sheet.

Many times, patients have normal function at one speed (such as slower speed) but then have a significant deficit at a faster speed. In these cases, it indicates that patients have a power deficit and the inability to produce the forces quickly that are necessary for functional activities. Research by Wojtys et al. has also illustrated the functional importance of the quadricep and hamstring and the power deficits or muscle reaction times.[59–62]

At the present time, the empirically based guidelines that we use to produce patient progression to the next stage of the FTA and to a higher level of functioning (increased stresses with less clinical control) are a bilateral comparison of less than 30 percent in peak force, total work, total work/body weight, average power, and average power/ body weight. If the patient has greater than a 30 percent deficit in bilateral comparison, we incorporate open kinetic chain (OKC) exercises along with the CKC program. The reason for the integrated OKC is to obtain isolated strengthening of the involved area without allowing other muscle groups to compensate and mask potential deficits. The emphasis is on motor re-education and power and endurance training before we re-test the patient's status.

Open Kinetic Chain Testing

As mentioned, OKC exercises are part of the total rehabilitation program so that no isolated muscle strength deficits are allowed to exist.[63] Although many practitioners believe that certain knee pathologies are contraindications to OKC testing, they also believe that it has an important place in evaluating recovering patients. Examples of conditions that would contraindicate OKC testing include limited joint range of motion, significant effusion, patellofemoral chondrosis and pain, tendinitis leading to pain with exertion, and insufficient soft tissue healing time since the surgery or injury. These conditions may change over time and the contraindication may be lifted.

Clinical controls that are inherent in OKC testing to improve its safety include the following:

1. No varus, valgus, or rotation applied during testing if the unit is properly applied.[50, 51]
2. A proximally placed tibial pad that helps reduce anterior translation of the tibia. (An important consideration for patients with ACL-deficient knees to prevent stretching the secondary restraints as well as with ACL reconstructions to prevent placing extra stresses on the healing or maturing ligament.)[64, 65]
3. Controlled speeds. (Faster speeds decrease the amount of anterior tibial translation.)[65, 66]
4. No applied compressive force during testing for joints with chondral abnormalities. (An exception exists across the patellofemoral joint.)
5. Precise control of range of motion. (By limiting range of motion, anterior tibial translation can be controlled.)[64, 65]
6. Isolation of the muscle to be tested so that results are "pure" for that muscle. (Also assesses the neural system's ability to "drive" the isolated muscle group and assess the muscle's power.)[67, 68]

Several authors[69, 70] have described and demonstrated the need for isolated joint testing. Furthermore, Nicholas et al.[71] and Gleim et al.[72] have demonstrated the need for creating a composite score of total leg strength. Davies[73] has documented the importance of performing isolated joint testing (OKC) in conjunction with CKC testing for patients with various knee pathologies. Rosenthal et al.[74] also compared OKC with CKC testing.

When performing the OKC testing, velocity spectrum testing is used[75] so that the muscle's performance can be sampled at different speeds.[76–78] Often, muscle deficits show up only at particular velocities.[79–82]

Research by Wojtys and colleagues reinforces the importance of evaluating isolated muscle function to identify the "weak link" in the kinetic chain.[59–62] Most studies employ isolated isokinetic testing to evaluate for deficits in peak torque production. Wojtys et al. and other investigators,[83–86] in contrast, demonstrated that the most important source of deficits is the neuromuscular timing and recruitment. Kannus et al. have extensively demonstrated the significance of measuring muscle power in an OKC test.[87–90]

The concept of muscle power or the ability to produce force or torque quickly is the basis of functional performance testing. It really does not matter how much force a muscle can produce in unlimited time.[91, 92] Real significance is placed on a muscle's ability to generate force quickly, which leads to functional dynamic stability of an adjacent joint. This ability can be measured as force development quickness, time rate of torque development, or torque acceleration energy.[83] Davies et al. have discussed the significance of this muscle contraction characteristic and its importance to functional performance since 1980.[75, 79, 80, 93–98] Furthermore, because more injuries occur in fatigued conditions, the status of muscle endurance is another parameter that should be assessed.[99]

The need certainly exists for more research in this area to determine the most significant muscle assessment parameters and how they correlate with functional performance. Admittedly, a patient and muscle group do not function in an isolated manner. There are numerous studies that demonstrate a correlation between OKC testing and functional performance,[100–107] and a few that dispute this association.[108, 109]

Data analysis involves many components, including bilateral comparison, unilateral ratios of agonist to antagonist, and peak torques to body weight, among others.[23, 81] The clinically based empiric guideline used for progression of the patient to the next level of the FTA is a bilateral comparison of less than 25 percent upon OKC testing. If the patient has a deficit in a particular isolated muscle, such as the quadriceps, greater than 25 percent (isolated weak link of the kinetic chain), then an integrated rehabilitation program utilizing both OKC and CKC exercises facilitates normal functional motor patterns (Table 25–3).

Closed Kinetic Chain Weight-Bearing Squat Position Isokinetic Testing

The next step is to move the patient from the OKC or partial CKC testing position to the actual weight-bearing position.[9, 27, 36, 110–113] In this test position, the Linea is placed in the upright position and the patient is tested in the CKC squat position using two legs. Then the patient can also progress to unilateral squat testing. With the single-leg squats, a bilateral comparison of the extremities is evaluated. We expect patients to have less than 20 percent bilateral deficit to go to the functional testing position. If the patient has greater than a 20 percent deficit, the rehabilitation program emphasizes single-leg concentrated training with integrated OKC and CKC techniques (Table 25–4).

FUNCTIONAL TESTING

At this time, there is a major change in the emphasis of the testing sequence. The focus of testing is now on functional activities. There is no longer clinical control superimposed on the patient. The patient's knee is now subjected to progressive varus-valgus and rotational stresses. Furthermore, speed, range of motion, and eccentric decelerative loading forces are no longer limited by the testing, as was done earlier in the sequence.

⊙━ Table 25–3. **Comparison of Open and Closed Kinetic Chain Isokinetic Testing with Body Weight**

The peak torque to body weight (BW) for the quadriceps with OKC was	
slow speed	60°/sec: ≈ 1 × BW
medium speed	180°/sec: ≈ ⅔ × BW
fast speed	300°/sec: ≈ ½ × BW
The peak force to body weight (BW) for the leg extensors with CKC was	
slow speed	25.4 cm/sec: ≈ 3 × BW
medium speed	50.8 cm/sec: ≈ 2½ × BW
fast speed	76.2 cm/sec: ≈ 2 × BW

BW = body weight; CKC = closed kinetic chain; OKC = open kinetic chain.

Functional Jump Test

We begin the functional testing sequence with a functional jump test (FJT), which is a simultaneous two-leg jump.[114] The purpose of the FJT is to measure simultaneous functional bilateral leg power. To prevent the segmental contributions of the arm, neck and trunk,[115, 116] we have the patient clasp the hands behind the back to minimize the neck and trunk movements. The patient performs four gradient submaximal to maximal warm-up jumps (25, 50, 75, and 100 percent effort). It is important to have the patient perform at least one maximal jump to create a positive transfer of learning from a warm-up activity to the actual test activity. If the patient performs only submaximal warm-ups and is then asked to perform a maximal effort in the testing, it creates a negative transfer of learning.

Moreover, this is an excellent test to assess the patient's readiness to perform "uncontrolled functional test activities." The patient then performs three maximal volitional effort jump tests. The distance the patient jumps is averaged and then normalized to the patient's height (distance is recorded as a percentage of patient height) to make it relative to the patient. We normalize the data to the patient's height because the absolute distance values provide limited usefulness in data analysis and interpretation, since patients vary in gender and body size. As an example, if a patient jumps 102 cm, 112 cm, and 107 cm in the three maximal test repetitions, is that excellent, good, fair, or poor performance? The normative data allow a standard for performance to be set and used for functional progression.

The descriptive normative data collected over the years at this center are listed in Table 25–5. Healthy recreational or competitive athletes under 40 years of age are expected to achieve the numbers listed in Table 25–5. The criterion for the patient to progress to the next level of the FTA is that the patient achieve scores with less than a 15 percent deficit compared with the descriptive normative data. If the patient has greater than a 15 percent deficit based on the normative data, then we continue the functional rehabilitation program with emphasis on bilateral lower extremity CKC exercises.

Table 25–4. Lido Linea Closed Kinetic Chain Computerized Isokinetic Testing Compared with Cybex Open Kinetic Chain Computerized Isokinetic Testing*

Cybex		Linea	
Test	% Deficit	Test	% Deficit
PT 60 degrees/sec quadriceps U - 142 ft-pounds I - 101 ft-pounds	29	PT 25.4 cm/sec U - 208 kg I - 189 kg	9
PT BW 60 degrees/sec quadriceps U - 95% I - 66%	31	PT % BW 25.4 cm/sec U - 134 kg I - 120 kg	11
PT 180 degrees/sec U - 99 ft-pounds I - 78 ft-pounds	21	PT 50.8 cm/sec U - 168 kg I - 149 kg	11
PT BW 180 degrees/sec U - 64% I - 48%	25	PT % BW 12.7 cm/sec U - 108 kg I - 97 kg	11
PT 300 degrees/sec U - 80 ft-pounds I - 64 ft-pounds	20	PT 76.2 cm/sec U - 137 kg I - 114 kg	16
PT BW 300 degrees/sec U - 51% I - 41%	20	PT % BW 76.2 cm/sec U - 87 kg I - 77 kg	11

*N = 250 patients (different knee injuries).
BW = body weight; I = involved side; PT = peak torque; U = uninvolved side.

Functional Hop Test

The functional hop test is a unilateral hop test that compares the normal with the involved extremity.[117] This test, which is recommended by the International Knee Documentation Committee, is a major progression in the FTA because uncontrolled stresses are placed exclusively on the involved extremity. This is also an important "psychologic readiness test" on the part of the patient. Often, even though the patient has passed all the tests prior to this stage of the FTA, the patient is not "psychologically" ready to take this test. The patient exhibits apprehension, hesitation, or unwillingness to perform the test. In some cases, the patient can concentrically hop off the involved leg but cannot land with the eccentric deceleration on the involved leg.[67, 118–120] Many times the patient hops off the involved leg but keeps landing on both feet. This demonstrates that the patient is not ready, whether psychologically or physiologically, to progress further in the FTA at this point, and the emphasis must be placed on a continued rehabilitation program to correct the patient's deficits. There are several reliability studies that demonstrate that this is an excellent test.[121–124]

We use guidelines for the functional hop test similar to those already described for the FJT. The techniques for testing are as follows: the patient's hands are clasped behind the back and the head and trunk movements are minimized for the reasons previously described relative to the FJT. Four gradient submaximal to maximal warm-ups are used prior to the three maximal volitional tests being performed. The data are analyzed as a bilateral comparison, as recommended by the International Knee Documentation Committee; however, these data are also normalized to the patient's height, similar to the FJT. This practice allows comparison with the general population of athletes and not simply side-to-side comparisons.[125, 126]

With the involved leg, the patient should hop within 10 percent bilateral comparison of the involved to the uninvolved side. Moreover, the patient should hop within 10 percent of the descriptive normative data de-

Table 25–5. Functional (Relative/Normalized) Jump and Hop Test Data for Males and Females

	Males (%/Ht)	Females (%/Ht)
Jump test (R + L)	90–100	80–90
Hop test (U)	80–90	70–80
Hop test (I)	80–90	70–80

Ht = patient's height.

scribed in Table 25–5. If the patient has greater than a 10 percent deficit in either data analysis or interpretation, functional rehabilitation exercises are continued. The emphasis of the rehabilitation is on single-leg CKC and OKC exercises as well as on the eccentric loading component of various activities. Once the patient performs and passes the test, then he or she progresses to the next level of the FTA.

Lower Extremity Functional Test

When the patient reaches the terminal phases of the rehabilitation program and is being considered for discharge from ongoing treatment, a lower extremity functional test (LEFT) is administered. The LEFT has evolved from several years of attempting to replicate numerous functional sporting activities into one practical test. It meets the criteria of being a test that can be performed within the constraints of the size of a clinical setting, requires minimal equipment to perform, takes a short time to administer, and is valid and reliable. A study by Negrete and Brophy[27] demonstrated the validity or correlation of the LEFT with other tests to measure performance.

The specific dimensions of the LEFT were designed based on in-clinic space constraints. The floor dimensions are in a diamond shape 30 feet in length and 10 feet in width (Fig. 25–4).

The test is designed to create progressively more demanding functional movement patterns to the lower extremity. The sequence of activities of the LEFT are described in Table 25–6.

When the patient performs the LEFT, the clinician evaluates the quantity of the performance (time required to complete the test) as well as the quality of the performance. Considerations regarding the quality of the performance come back to the "psychologic readiness" and willingness to put out during the test, any hesitation in performing the various maneuvers of the test, and any limping that may result during the test. The quality of the performance by the patient is an empiric assessment by the clinician. The tester's clinical judgment is important in determining whether the patient passes this stage of the FTA. On rare occasions, a patient may be able to complete the LEFT in a reasonable time but has poor quality of performance. Both components of the evaluation of this test are important in deciding whether the patient returns to limited practices, scrimmages, and so on. If the quality of the performance is poor, it may mean that the patient is still "favoring" the injured extremity and may be more vulnerable for reinjury, even though he or she has passed many of the prior objective tests.

The quality of the performance (time to complete the LEFT) for objective documentation is also recorded. The descriptive normative data collected at this center are described in Table 25–7.

There are certainly many considerations in evaluating a patient's performance during the LEFT. The analysis and interpretation of the results may take into consideration many factors, including age, sex, somatotype, physical fitness level, sport, and position within the sport. Each of these factors can certainly influence one's performance in this test. A need exists to develop patient-specific norms based on many of the aforementioned criteria. This massive undertaking is in its early stages.

An example of the need for these patient-specific norms is if we were testing a 15-year-old, 230-pound endomorphic wrestler who had injured his knee and was being assessed for possible return to practice. Most likely, this patient would score poorly on the test, not just because of the injury, but also because of age, size, condition, and so on. Consequently, the norms in Table 25–7 would have to altered. Furthermore, the interpretation of any patient's test performance relative to descriptive normative data is performed with caution. Good clinical judgment is not applied to poor research data (if the norms are not really inclusive of the particular patient's unique characteristics).

The LEFT is a very stressful test for the anaerobic cardiovascular system. Consequently, if the individual being tested has poor cardiovascular conditioning, it must also be considered in the interpretation. If cardiovascular limitations are noted, generalized training and specific cardiovascular training techniques through cross-training can help improve this component without causing further stress to the injured area.

If the patient does not pass the LEFT, both quantitatively and qualitatively, the focus of the rehabilitation is then on the areas of the

Patient Name: _____ GC # _____ DOB _____
MD _____ PT _____ DOS/DOI _____
Diagnosis _____ Gender   M/F
Dominant   L/R   Involved   L/R   Height _____ in   Weight _____ lb

Procedure
  1. Forward sprint (A-C-A)
  2. Retro sprint (A-C-A)
  3. Side shuffle right—face in (A-D-C-B-A)
  4. Side shuffle left—face in (A-B-C-D-A)
  5. Cariocas right—face in (A-D-C-B-A)
  6. Cariocas left—face in (A-B-C-D-A)
  7. Figure 8s right (A-D-C-B-A)
  8. Figure 8s left (A-B-C-D-A)
  9. 45° Cuts right—plant outside foot (A-D-C-B-A)
 10. 45° Cuts left—plant outside foot (A-B-C-D-A)
 11. 90° Cuts right—plant outside foot (A-D-B-A)
 12. 90° Cuts left—plant outside foot (A-B-D-A)
 13. Crossover 90° cuts right—plant inside foot (A-D-B-A)
 14. Crossover 90° cuts left—plant inside foot (A-B-D-A)
 15. Forward sprint (A-C-A)
 16. Retro sprint (A-C-A)

Data
Date _____   Date _____   Date _____
Time _____ sec   Time _____ sec   Time _____ sec

Date _____   Date _____   Date _____
Time _____ sec   Time _____ sec   Time _____ sec

NORMS	
Males	Females
90 sec–good	120 sec–good
100 sec–average	135 sec–average
125 sec–below average	150 sec–below average

Figure 25–4. Lower extremity functional test (LEFT) dimensions.

test where the patient did not perform well. As an example, if the patient had no problems with the straight-ahead running or gradual cutting maneuvers, but only had pain or disability during the sharper cutting motions, the emphasis in the rehabilitation program is on the sharper cutting motions. The problematic areas are analyzed and broken down into the component parts to try to determine as precisely as possible where the problematic areas were in the activity. The component parts are then addressed in the rehabilitation program. Slow submaximal activities may be performed initially, and the intensity of the effort, the speed of the activity, and the angle of the cut may all be gradually improved to obtain the adaptation response required to allow the patient to perform the activity with no limitations. Goals for the patient to achieve are to be within the range of the descriptive normative data in Table 25–7. If a surgical patient

Table 25–6. Sequence of the Lower Extremity Functional Test (LEFT)

  1. Sprint (frontward)
  2. Sprint (retro-run)
  3. Side shuffles (both ways)
  4. Cariocas (both ways)
  5. Figure-of-eights (both ways)
  6. 45-degree angle cuts (outside foot) (both ways)
  7. 90-degree angle cuts (outside foot) (both ways)
  8. Crossover step (both ways)
  9. Sprint (frontward)
 10. Sprint (retro-run)

Table 25–7. Lower Extremity Functional Test (LEFT) Descriptive Normative Data

	Norms (seconds)
Males	90–125
	100 average
Females	120–150
	135 average

is unable to achieve these goals and consistently has difficulty with this particular test, discussion of the deficit with the patient's surgeon is important. Once the patient performs in a satisfactory manner based on the established criteria, however, the patient progresses to the next level of the FTA.

Sport-Specific Testing

The final stage of the FTA is sport-specific testing. Often, because of the space limitations, equipment limitations, simulated environment, appropriate testing methodology, and so forth this cannot be performed in the clinical setting. Ideally, there is a health care

team approach in which the functional "field" testing can be performed by members at the respective competitive venues. These would include certified athletic trainers, certified strength and conditioning specialists, physical therapists, and so forth. Ideally, a consultation takes place between the "field" professional and the clinical therapist regarding the patient's status and the eventual disposition of the patient.

Figure 25–5 illustrates how the FTA (whole) provides the foundation for a precise (based on the test results from the FTA), progressive rehabilitation program that can be performed safely and efficiently to progress through the process to discharge and return to activities.

Most articles on ACL outcome studies are

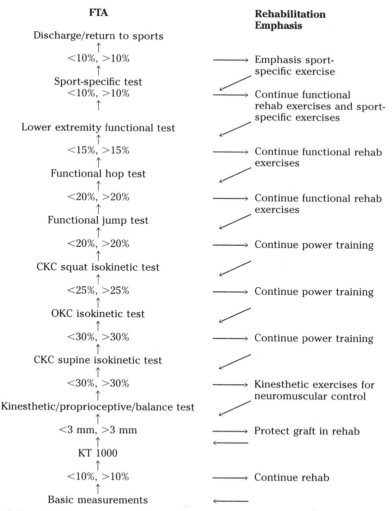

Figure 25–5. Functional testing algorithm as the foundation for a progressive rehabilitation program.

based on retrospective descriptive chart reviews.[127] Perhaps a comprehensive systematic FTA as described will facilitate more prospective randomized controlled clinical trial studies.

To those unaccustomed to this approach, the FTA may correctly seem long and impractical. In practice, it actually helps a patient to progress more quickly through a rehabilitation program. The primary reason is that patients are always being tested and monitored to know exactly where they are and what their status is. Instead of following the protocol or having patients continue with the generic home program, they are placed on specific in-clinic rehabilitation activities based on their test results and their deficits. Furthermore, their home program is also designed to specifically address the problematic area to complement the clinical program.

The functional progression can be explained to coaches and even to parents in the field by certified athletic trainers so that they develop a better understanding of where in the recovery phase their athlete is. Visual demonstration of progression can also be provided by using the algorithm (see Fig. 25–1).

Another important point about this treatment approach is how it works with managed care and limited numbers of physical therapy visits. The physical therapists' first goals after injury or surgery are to decrease pain and swelling, increase range of motion, and achieve muscle control. The treatments and home programs are thereafter based on test results. The patient's progression can then be more goal oriented, more efficient, and less time consuming.

SUMMARY

The FTA is a systematic, objective, progressive sequence that forms the scientific and clinical foundation for testing a patient to determine his or her status and then uses the results to guide the appropriate rehabilitation program. This approach has been effective in highly motivated individuals. It may prove less useful to focus on deficits in less goal-oriented individuals. However, in less goal-oriented patients, continuing to emphasize the positive progression and improvement through the FTA can still serve

as a motivational tool to help them return to their desired activity levels.

References

1. Bunton EE, Pitnez WA, Kane AW, et al.: The role of limb torque, muscle action and proprioception during closed kinetic chain rehabilitation of the lower extremity. J Athletic Train 28:10–20, 1993.
2. Harter RA, Osterning LR, Singer KM, et al.: Long term evaluation of knee stability and function following surgical reconstruction for anterior cruciate ligament insufficiency. Am J Sports Med 16:434–443, 1988.
3. Kegerreis S: The construction and implementation of functional progressions as a component of athletic rehabilitation. J Orthop Sports Phys Ther 5:14–19, 1983.
4. Kegerreis S, Malone T, McCarroll J: Functional progression: An aid to athletic rehabilitation. Physician Sports Med 12:67–71, 1984.
5. Snyder-Mackler L: Scientific rationale and physiologic basis for the use of closed kinetic chain exercise in the lower extremity. J Sports Rehab 5:2–13, 1996.
6. Timm KE: Post-surgical knee rehabilitation: A five year study of four methods and 5,381 patients. Am J Sports Med 16:463–468, 1988.
7. Ciccotti MG, Kerlan RK, Perry J, et al.: An EMG analysis of the knee during functional activities. I: The normal profile. Am J Sports Med 22:645–650, 1994.
8. Cicotti MG, Kerlan RK, Perry J, et al.: An EMG analysis of the knee during functional activities. II: The anterior cruciate ligament-deficient and reconstructed profiles. Am J Sports Med 22:651–658, 1994.
9. Decarlo M, Porter DA, Gehlsen G, et al.: Electromyographic and cinematrographic analysis of the lower extremity during closed and open kinetic chain exercise. Isokin Exerc Sci 2:24–29, 1992.
10. Graham VL, Gehlsen GM, Edwards JA: Electromyographic evaluation of closed and open kinetic chain rehabilitation exercises. J Athletic Train 28:23–30, 1993.
11. Lephart SM, et al.: Functional assessment of the anterior cruciate insufficient knee [abstract]. Med Sci Sports Exerc 20:2, 1988.
12. Lephart SM, Perrin DH, Fu FH, et al.: Functional performance tests for the anterior cruciate insufficient athlete. J Athletic Train 26:44–50, 1991.
13. Lephart SM, Perrin DH, Fu FH, et al.: Relationship between selected physical characteristics and functional capacity in the anterior cruciate ligament insufficient athlete. J Orthop Sports Phys Ther 16:174–181, 1992.
14. Reynolds NL, Worrell TW, Perrin DH: Effects of a lateral step-up exercise protocol on quadriceps isokinetic peak torque values and thigh girth. J Orthop Sports Phys Ther 15:151–155, 1992.
15. Rivera JE: Open versus closed kinetic chain rehabilitation of the lower extremity: A functional and biomechanical analysis. J Sports Rehab 3:154–167, 1994.
16. Seto JL, Orofino AS, Morrissey MC, et al.: Assessment of quadriceps/hamstring strength, knee ligament

stability, functional and sports activity levels five years after anterior cruciate ligament reconstruction. Am J Sports Med 16:170–180, 1988.

17. Smith MJ, Melton P: Isokinetic versus isotonic variable resistance training. Am J Sports Med 9:275–279, 1981.

18. Snyder-Mackler L, Fitzgerald GK, Bartolozzi AR, et al.: The relationship between passive joint laxity and functional outcome after anterior cruciate ligament injury. Am J Sports Med 25:191–195, 1997.

19. Tibone JE, Antich TJ, Fanton GS, et al.: Functional analysis of anterior cruciate instability. Am J Sports Med 14:276–284, 1986.

20. Wilk KE, Simoneau G, McGraw J: The EMG activity of the quadriceps femoris vastus medialis/lateralis ratio during squats, leg press, and knee extensions exercises. [abstract]. Phys Ther 73:580, 1993.

21. Wilk KE, Escamilla RF, Fleisig GS, et al.: Open and closed kinetic chain exercise for the lower extremity: Theory and clinical application. Athl Train Sports Health Care Perspect 1:336–346, 1995.

22. Yack HJ, Collins CE, Whieldon TJ: Comparison of closed and open kinetic chain exercise in the anterior cruciate ligament-deficient knee. Am J Sports Med 17:154–160, 1993.

23. Davies GJ, Malone T: Proprioception, open kinetic chain and closed kinetic chain exercises and their application to rehabilitation and assessment. AOSSM Proceedings, 1992.

24. Davies GJ: The need for critical thinking in rehabilitation. J Sports Rehab 4:1–22, 1995.

25. Davies GJ: Functional testing algorithm for patients with knee injuries [abstract]. Proceedings of the 12th International Congress of the World Confederation for Physical Therapy, Washington, DC, June, 1995, p. 912.

26. Davies GJ, Wilk K, Ellenbeck TS: Assessment of strength. In Malone TR, McPoil T, Nitz AJ (eds): Orthopaedic and Sports Physical Therapy, 3rd ed. St. Louis, Mosby, 1997, pp. 225–227.

27. Negrete R, Brophy J: Predicting performance of single leg hop, single leg vertical jump and a speed and agility test using isokinetic devices. J Sport Rehab (in press).

28. Daniel DL, Malcolm ML, Stone H, et al.: Quantification of knee stability and function. Contemp Orthop 5:83–91, 1982.

29. Anderson SB, Terwilliger DM, Denegar CR: Comparison of open versus closed kinetic chain test positions for measuring joint position sense. J Sport Rehab 4:165–171, 1995.

30. Davies GJ, Shenton D, Romeyn R: Objective quantification of kinesthesia (balance) in 116 patients with knee ligament injuries while wearing or not wearing a functional knee brace [abstract]. J Orthop Sports Phys Ther 15:54, 1992.

31. Lephart SM, Pincivero DM, Giraldo JL, et al.: The role of proprioception in the management and rehabilitation of athletic injuries. Am J Sports Med 25:130–137, 1997.

32. MacDonald PB, Hedden D, Pacin O, et al.: Proprioception in anterior cruciate ligament-deficient and reconstructed knee. Am J Sports Med 24:774–778, 1996.

33. LaFree J, Mozingo A, Worrell T: Comparison of open kinetic chain knee and hip extension to closed kinetic chain leg press performance. J Sports Rehab 4:99–107, 1995.

34. Lutz GE, Palmitier RA, An KN, et al.: Closed kinetic

chain exercises for athletes after reconstruction of the anterior cruciate ligament [abstract]. Med Sci Sports Exerc 23:413, 1991.

35. Lutz GE, Palmitier KN, An KN, et al.: Comparison of tibiofemoral joint forces during open-kinetic chain and closed-kinetic chain exercises. J Bone Joint Surg 75A:732–739, 1993.

36. Chandler TJ, Wilson GD, Stone MH: The effects of the squat exercise on knee stability. Med Sci Sports Exerc 21:229–303, 1989.

37. Hsieh H, Walker PS: Stabilizing mechanisms of the loaded and unloaded knee joint. J Bone Joint Surg 58A:87–93, 1976.

38. Markolf KL, Bargar WL, Shoemaker SC, et al.: Role of joint load in knee stability. J Bone Joint Surg 63A:579–585, 1981.

39. Shoemaker SC, Markolf KL: Effects of joint load on the stiffness and laxity of ligament-deficient knees. J Bone Joint Surg 67A:136–146, 1985.

40. Torzilli PA, Deng X, Warren RF: The effect of joint-compression load and quadriceps muscle force on knee motion in the intact and anterior cruciate ligament-sectioned knee. Am J Sports Med 2:105–112, 1994.

41. Wilk KE, Escamilla RF, Fleisig GS, et al.: A comparison of tibiofemoral joint forces and EMG activity during open and closed kinetic chain exercises. Am J Sports Med 24:518–527, 1996.

42. Yasuda K, Sasaki T: Exercise after anterior cruciate ligament reconstruction. The force exerted on the tibia by the separate isometric contractions of the quadriceps or the hamstrings. Clin Orthop 220:275–283, 1987.

43. Baratta R, Solomonow M, Zhou BH, et al.: Muscular coactivation: The role of the antagonist musculature in maintaining knee stability. Am J Sport Med 16:113–122, 1988.

44. Aune AK, Cawley PW, Ekeland A: Quadriceps muscle contraction protects the anterior cruciate ligament during anterior tibial translation. Am J Sports Med 25:187–190, 1997.

45. Draganich LF, Jaeger R, Kralj A: EMG activity of the quadriceps and hamstrings during monoarticular knee extension and flexion. Trans Orthop Res Soc 12:283, 1987.

46. Draganich LF, Vahey JW: An in-vivo study of anterior cruciate ligament strain induced by quadriceps and hamstring forces. J Orthop Res 8:57–63, 1990.

47. Fleming BC, Beynnon BD, Peura GD, et al.: Anterior cruciate ligament strain during an open and closed kinetic chain exercise: An in vivo study. Trans Orthop Res Soc 20:631, 1995.

48. Goldfuss AJ, Morehouse CA, LeVeau BF: Effect of muscular tension on knee stability. Med Sci Sports 5:267–271, 1973.

49. Hagood S, Solomonow M, Baratta R, et al.: The effect of joint velocity on the contribution of the antagonist musculature to knee stiffness and laxity. Am J Sports Med 18:182–187, 1990.

50. Hirokawa S, Solomonow M, Lu Y, et al.: Anterior-posterior and rotational displacement of the tibia elicited by quadriceps contraction. Am J Sports Med 20:299–306, 1992.

51. Howell SM: Anterior tibial translation during a maximum quadriceps contraction: Is it clinically significant? Am J Sports Med 18:573–578, 1990.

52. More RC, Karras BT, Neiman F, et al.: Hamstrings—an anterior cruciate ligament protagonist: An in-vivo study. Am J Sports Med 21:231–237, 1993.

53. Renstrom PS, Arms SW, Stanwyck TS, et al.: Strain within the anterior cruciate ligament during hamstring and quadriceps activity. Am J Sports Med 14:83–87, 1986.

54. Solomonow M, Barata R, Zhou BH, et al.: The synergistic action of the anterior cruciate ligament and thigh muscles in maintaining joint stability. Am J Sports Med 15:207–213, 1987.

55. Beynnon BD, Fleming BC, Johnson RJ, et al.: Anterior cruciate ligament strain behavior during rehabilitation exercises in vivo. Am J Sports Med 23:24–34, 1995.

56. Snyder-Mackler L, Delitto A, Bailey SL, et al.: Strength of the quadriceps femoris muscle and functional recovery after reconstruction of the anterior cruciate ligament. J Bone Joint Surg 77A:1166–1173, 1995.

57. Isear JA, Erickson JC, Worrell TW: EMG analysis of lower extremity muscle recruitment patterns during an unloaded squat. Med Sci Sports Exer 28:532–539, 1997.

58. Davies GJ, Heiderscheit BC: Reliability of the Lido Linea closed kinetic chain isokinetic dynamometer. J Orthop Sports Phys Ther 25:133–136, 1997.

59. Wojtys EM, Huston LJ: Neuromuscular performance in normal and anterior cruciate ligament-deficient lower extremities. Am J Sports Med 22:89–104, 1994.

60. Wojtys EM, Huston LJ, Taylor PD, et al.: Neuromuscular adaptations in isokinetic, isotonic, and agility training programs. Am J Sports Med 4:187–192, 1996.

61. Wojtys EM, Wylie BB, Huston LJ: The effects of muscle fatigue on neuromuscular function and anterior tibial translation in healthy knees. Am J Sports Med 24:615–621, 1996.

62. Wojtys EM, Huston LJ: Longitudinal effects of ACL injury and patellar tendon autograft reconstruction on neuromuscular performance [abstract]. AOSSM Proceedings, Sun Valley, ID, June, 1997, p. 812.

63. Davies GJ, Heiderscheit B, Clark M: Open kinetic chain assessment and rehabilitation. Athl Training Sports Hlth Care Perspect 1:347–370, 1995.

64. Jurist KA, Otis JC: Anteroposterior tibiofemoral displacements during isometric extension efforts. Am J Sports Med 13:254–258, 1985.

65. Wilk KE, Andrews JR: The effects of pad placement and angular velocity on tibial displacement during isokinetic exercise. J Orthop Sports Phys Ther 7:223–230, 1993.

66. Kaufman KR, An KN, Litchy WJ, et al.: Dynamic joint forces during knee isokinetic exercises. Am J Sports Med 19:305–316, 1991.

67. Davies GJ, Ellenbecker TS: Eccentric isokinetics. Orthop Phys Ther Clin North Am 1:297–336, 1992.

68. Storm KL, Waller TR, Davies GJ: Specificity of isokinetic exercise: Comparison of eccentric and concentric training of the quadriceps femoris muscle [abstract]. 72:S100, 1992.

69. Goslin BR, Chateris J: Isokinetic dynamometry: Normative data for clinical use in lower extremity (knee) cases. Scand J Rehabil Med 11:105–109, 1979.

70. Grace TG, Sweetser ER, Nelson MA, et al.: Isokinetic muscle imbalance and knee joint injuries. J Bone Joint Surg 66A:734–740, 1984.

71. Nicholas JA, Strizak AM, Veras G: A study of thigh muscle weakness in different pathological states of the lower extremity. Am J Sports Med 4:241–248, 1976.

72. Gleim GW, Nicholas JA, Webb JN: Isokinetic evaluation following leg injuries. Phys Sports Med 6:74–82, 1978.

73. Davies GJ: Descriptive study comparing open kinetic chain and closed kinetic chain isokinetic testing of the lower extremity in 200 patients with selected knee pathologies [abstract]. Proceedings of the 12th International Congress of the World Confederation for Physical Therapy, Washington, DC, June, 1995, p. 906.

74. Rosenthal MD, Baer LL, Griffith PP, et al.: Comparability of work output measures as determined by isokinetic dynamometry and a closed kinetic chain exercise. J Sports Rehab 3:218–227, 1994.

75. Davies GJ: A Compendium of Isokinetics in Clinical Usage. La Crosse, WI, S & S Publishers, 1984.

76. Davies GJ, Legler JC, Metropulos GG: A comparison of the effects of high velocity and lower velocity training of the quadriceps on closed kinetic chain functional performance [abstract]. Phys Ther 71:S119, 1991.

77. Davies GJ: A descriptive study of isokinetic knee flexion/extension testing from 300-600 degrees/second [abstract]. Phys Ther 72:S72, 1992.

78. Timm KE: Investigation of the physiological overflow effect from speed specific isokinetic activity. J Orthop Sports Phys 9:106, 1987.

79. Davies GJ, Halbach J, Gould J: Torque acceleration energy and average power changes in quadriceps and hamstring through the selected velocity spectrum as determined by computerized Cybex testing [abstract]. Med Sci Sports Exer 15:144, 1983.

80. Davies GJ, Gould JA, Ross D, et al.: Computerized Cybex testing of ACL reconstructions assessing quadriceps peak torque, torque acceleration energy, total work and average power [abstract]. Med Sci Sports Exerc 16:204, 1984.

81. Davies GJ: A Compendium of Isokinetics in Clinical Usage and Rehabilitation Techniques, 4th ed. Onalaska, WI, S & S Publishers, 1992.

82. Stafford MG, Grana WA: Hamstrings/quadriceps ratios in college football players: A high velocity evaluation. Am J Sports Med 12:209–211, 1984.

83. Bell DG, Jacobs I: Electro-mechanical response times and rate of force development in males and females. Med Sci Sports Exerc 18:31–36, 1986.

84. Huston LM, Wojtys, EM: Neuromuscular performance in elite women athletes. Am J Sports Med 24:427–436, 1996.

85. Kalund S, Sinkjaer T, Arendt-Nielsen L, et al.: Altered timing of hamstring muscle action in anterior cruciate deficient patients. Am J Sports Med 18:245–248, 1990.

86. Madsen OR: Torque, total work, power, torque acceleration energy and acceleration time assessed on a dynamometer: Reliability of knee and elbow extensor and flexor strength measurements. Eur J Appl Physiol 74:206–210, 1996.

87. Kannus P, Jarvinen M: Prediction of torque acceleration energy and power of thigh muscles from peak torque. Med Sci Sports Exerc 21:304–307, 1989.

88. Kannus P, Latvala K: Torque acceleration energy, power and peak torque in thigh muscles after pre-

vious knee sprain. Can J Sports Sci 14:103–106, 1989.

89. Kannus P: Normality, variability and predictability of work, power and torque acceleration energy with respect to peak torque in isokinetic muscle testing. Int J Sports Med 13:249–256, 1992.

90. Kannus P: Isokinetic evaluation of muscular performance: Implications for muscle testing and rehabilitation. Int J Sports Med 15(Suppl):s11–s18, 1994.

91. Knapik JJ, Bauman CL, Jones BH, et al.: Preseason strength and flexibility imbalances associated with athletic injuries in female collegiate athletes. Am J Sports Med 19:76–81, 1991.

92. Knight KL: Strength imbalance and knee injury. Physician Sports Med 8:140, 1980.

93. Davies GJ, Halbach J, Wilson PK, et al.: A descriptive muscular power analysis of the U.S. cross country ski team [abstract]. Med Sci Sports Exerc 12:141, 1980.

94. Davies GH, Kirkendall DT: Isokinetic characteristics of professional football players: I. Normative relationships between quadriceps and hamstring muscle groups and relative to body weight [abstract]. Med Sci Sports Exerc 13:76–77, 1981.

95. Davies GH, Bendle S: The optimum repetitions to increase average power in the quadriceps and hamstrings [abstract]. Phys Ther 65:666–744, 1985.

96. Gould J, Davies GJ, Ross D, et al.: Computerized Cybex testing of ACL reconstructions assessing hamstrings peak torque, torque acceleration energy, total work, and average power [abstract]. Med Sci Sports Exerc 16:204, 1984.

97. Kirkendall DT, Davies GJ: Isokinetic characteristics of professional football players: II. Absolute and relative power relationships [abstract]. Med Sci Sports Exerc 13:77, 1981.

98. Siewart MW, Davies GJ, Ariki P: The effects of short arc terminal extension isokinetic exercise on the torque acceleration energy of the quadriceps [abstract]. Phys Ther 65:732, 1985.

99. DeNuccio DK, Davies GJ, Rowinski MJ: Comparison of quadriceps isokinetic eccentric and isokinetic concentric data using a standard fatigue protocol. Isok Exerc 2:81–86, 1991.

100. Barber SD, Noyes FR, Mangine RE, et al.: Rehabilitation after ACL reconstruction: Functional testing. Orthopedics 15:969–974, 1992.

101. Barber SD, Noyes FR, Mangine RE, et al.: Quantitative assessment of functional limitations in normal and anterior cruciate ligament-deficient knees. Clin Orthop Rel Res 255:204–214, 1990.

102. Noyes FR, Barber SD, Mangine RE: Abnormal lower limb symmetry determined by functional hop tests after anterior cruciate ligament rupture. Am J Sports Med 19:513–518, 1991.

103. Sachs RA, Daniel DM, Stone ML, et al.: Patellofemoral problems after anterior cruciate ligament reconstruction. Am J Sports Med 17:760–764, 1989.

104. Shaffer SW, Payne ED, Gabbard MB, et al.: Relationship between isokinetic and functional tests of the quadriceps [abstract]. J Orthop Sports Phys Ther 19:55, 1994.

105. Tegner Y, Lysholm J, Lysholm M, et al.: Performance test to monitor rehabilitation and evaluate anterior cruciate ligament injuries. Am J Sports Med 14:156–159, 1986.

106. Wiklander J, Lysholm J: Simple tests for surveying

107. Wilk KE, Rominello BR, Soscia S, et al.: The correlation between subjective knee assessments, isokinetic muscle testing and functional hop testing in ACL reconstructed knees. J Orthop Sports Phys Ther 20:60, 1994.

108. Anderson MA, Geick JH, Perrin D, et al.: The relationship among isometric, isotonic and isokinetic concentric and eccentric quadriceps and hamstring force and three components of athletic performance. J Orthop Sports Phys Ther 14:114–120, 1991.

109. Greenberger HB, Paterno MV: Comparison of an isokinetic strength test and a functional performance test in the assessment of lower extremity function [abstract]. J Orthop Sports Phys Ther 19:61, 1994.

110. Oshkoshi Y, Yasuda K: Biomechanical analysis of shear force exerted to anterior cruciate ligament during half squat exercises. Orthop Trans 13:310, 1989.

111. Oshkoshi Y, Yasuda K, Kaneda K, et al.: Biomechanical analysis of rehabilation in the standing position. Am J Sports Med 19:605–510, 1991.

112. Palmitier RA, An KN, Scott SG, et al.: Kinetic chain exercise in knee rehabilitation. Sports Med 11:402–413, 1991.

113. Stuart MJ, Meglan DA, Lutz GE, et al.: Comparison of intersegmental tibiofemoral joint forces and muscle activity during various closed kinetic chain exercises. Am J Sports Med 4:792–799, 1996.

114. Robertson DG, Fleming D: Kinetics of standing broad and vertical jumping. Can J Sports Sci 12:19–23, 1987.

115. Hubley CS, Wells RP: A work energy approach to determine individual joint contribution to vertical jump performance. Eur J Appl Physiol 50:247–254, 1983.

116. Luhtanen P, Komi PV: Segmental contributions to forces in vertical jump. Eur J Appl Physiol 38:181–188, 1978.

117. Gauffin H, Tropp H: Altered movement and muscular activation patterns during the one-legged jump in patients with an old anterior cruciate ligament rupture. Am J Sports Med 20:182–192, 1992.

118. DeVita P, Skelly WA: Effect of landing stiffness on knee joint kinetics and energetics in the lower extremity. Med Sci Sports Exerc 24:108–115, 1992.

119. Dufek JS, Bates BT: Biomechanical factors associated with injury during landing in jump sports. Sports Med 12:326–337, 1991.

120. Hewett TE, Stroupe AL, Nance TA, et al.: Plyometric training in female athletes: Decreased impact forces and increased hamstring torques. Am J Sports Med 24:765–773, 1996.

121. Booher LD, Hench KM, Worrell TW, et al.: Reliability of three single leg hop tests. J Sports Rehab 2:165–170, 1993.

122. Greenberger HB, Paterno MV: The test-retest reliability of a one-legged hop for distance in healthy young adults [abstract]. J Orthop Sports Phys Ther 19:62, 1994.

123. Hu HS, Whitney SL, Irrgang J, et al.: Test-retest reliability of the one-legged vertical jump test and one-legged standing hop test [abstract]. J Orthop Sports Phys Ther 15:51, 1992.

124. Kramer JF, Nusca D, Fowler P, et al.: Test-retest

reliability of the one-leg hop test following ACL reconstruction. Clin J Sports Med 2:240–243, 1992.

125. Decarlo M, Sell KE: Range of motion and single leg hop values for normals and patients following anterior cruciate ligament reconstruction [abstract]. J Orthop Sports Phys Ther 19:73, 1994.

126. Decarlo MS, Sell KE: Normative data for range of motion and single-leg hop in high school athletes. J Sport Rehab 6:246–255, 1997.

127. Crandall D, Richmond J, Lau J, et al.: A meta-analysis of the treatment of the anterior cruciate ligament. Presented at American Orthopedic Society for Sports Medicine, Palm Desert, CA, June 1994.

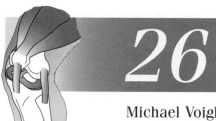

26 Proprioception and Balance Training and Testing Following Injury

Michael Voight, DPT, OCS, SCS, ATC, and
Turner Blackburn, MEd, PT, ATC

*T*he basic goal in rehabilitation is to enhance one's ability to function within the environment and to perform the specific activities of daily living. The entire rehabilitation process should be focused on improving the functional status of the patient. A functional progression for return to activity can be defined as breaking specific activities down into a hierarchy and then performing them in a sequence that allows for the acquisition or reacquisition of that skill. From a historical perspective, the rehabilitation process following injury has focused on the restoration of muscular strength, endurance, and joint flexibility without any consideration of the role of the neuromuscular mechanism. A common error in the rehabilitation process is in assuming that clinical programs alone using traditional methods will lead to a safe return to function. Limiting the rehabilitation program to these traditional programs often results in an incomplete restoration of ability and quite possibly an increased risk of re-injury.

The objective of the functional exercise program is to return the patient to the pre-injury level as quickly and as safely as possible. Specific training activities are designed to restore both dynamic stability about the joint and specific activities of daily living (ADL) skills. To accomplish this objective, a basic tenet of exercise physiology is employed. The SAID principle (*specific adaptions to imposed demands*) states that the body will adapt to the stress and strain placed upon it.[1] Athletes as well as patients cannot succeed if they have not been prepared to meet all of the demands of their specific activity.[1] Reactive neuromuscular training serves to help bridge the gap from traditional rehabilitation via proprioceptive and balance training to promote a more functional return to activity.[1]

In the normal healthy knee, both static and dynamic stabilizers provide support. Static stabilizers include ligaments, meniscus, and the joint capsule. Although the primary role of these structures is mechanical, by providing stabilization to the joint, the capsuloligamentous tissues also play an important sensory role by detecting joint position and motion.[2–4] The role of the capsuloligamentous tissues in the dynamic restraint of the knee has been well established in the literature.[3, 5–14] Sensory afferent feedback from the receptors in the capsuloligamentous structures projects directly to the reflex and cortical pathways, thereby mediating reactive muscle activity for dynamic restraint.[2, 3, 5, 6, 15]

PROPRIOCEPTION

Although there has been no definitive definition of proprioception, Beard et al.[16] described proprioception as consisting of three similar components: (1) a static awareness of joint position, (2) kinesthetic awareness, and (3) a closed-loop efferent reflex response required for the regulation of muscle tone and activity. From a physiologic perspective, proprioception is a specialized variation of the sensory modality of touch. Specifically defined, proprioception is the cumulative neural input to the central nervous system from mechanoreceptors in the joint capsules, ligaments, muscles, tendons, and skin.

Sherrington[4] first described the term *proprioception* in the early 1900s when he noted the presence of receptors in the joint capsular structures that were primarily reflexive in nature. Mechanoreceptors are specialized end organs that function as biologic transducers, which can convert the mechanical energy of physical deformation (elongation, compression, and pressure) into action nerve potentials yielding proprioceptive information.[8] Receptor discharge varies according to the intensity of the distortion. This neural signal is a repetitive discharge of action potentials whose rate directly relates to the intensity of the stimulus.

Once stimulated, mechanoreceptors are able to adapt. With constant stimulation, the frequency of the neural impulses decreases. The functional implication here is that mechanoreceptors detect change and rates of change, as opposed to steady state conditions.[17] This input is then analyzed in the central nervous system (CNS) for joint position and movement.[18] The status of the articular structures is sent to the CNS so that information regarding static versus dynamic conditions, equilibrium versus disequilibrium, or biomechanical stress and strain relations can be evaluated.[1, 19] Once processed and evaluated, this proprioceptive information becomes capable of influencing muscle tone, motor execution programs, and cognitive somatic perceptions or kinesthetic awareness.[20] Proprioceptive information also protects the joint from damage caused by movement exceeding the normal physiologic range of motion and helps determine the appropriate balance of synergistic and antagonistic forces. All of this information helps to generate a somatosensory image within the CNS. Therefore, the soft tissues surrounding a joint serve a double purpose: they provide biomechanical support to the bony partners making up the joint, keeping them in relative anatomic alignment, and, through an extensive afferent neurologic network, they provide valuable proprioceptive information.

Before the 1970s, articular receptors in the joint capsule were held primarily responsible for joint proprioception.[17] Since then, there has been considerable debate as to whether muscular and articular mechanoreceptors interact. Some studies have shown that capsular receptors only respond at the extremes of the range of motion or during other situations in which a strong stimulus is imparted onto the structures such as distraction or compression.[9, 10, 21, 22] Muscle receptors are thought to play a more important role in signaling joint position.[23, 24] Recent thought has focused on the muscle and joint receptors working complementary to one another in this complex afferent system, with each one modifying the function of the other.[11, 25] Both the articular and muscle

receptors have well-described cortical connections to substantiate a central role in proprioception.[4] Therefore, the sensory mechanoreceptors may represent a continuum rather than separate distinct classes of receptor.[4] This concept is further illustrated by research that demonstrated a relationship between the muscle spindle sensory afferent and joint mechanoreceptors.[26] McCloskey[27] has also demonstrated a relationship between the cutaneous afferent and joint mechanoreceptors. These studies suggest a complex role for the joint mechanoreceptors in smooth, coordinated, and controlled movement.

Information generated and encoded by the mechanoreceptors in the muscle tendon units are projected upward in the CNS to the cortex.[28] Articular joint mechanoreceptors project upward in the CNS to the cerebellum by three separate spinal pathways.[29] The ascending pathways to the cerebral cortex provide a conscious appreciate of motion and position sense. A rehabilitation program that addresses the need for restoring normal joint stability and proprioception cannot be constructed until one has a total appreciation of both the mechanical and sensory functions of the articular structures.[30] Knowledge of the basic physiology of how these muscular and joint mechanoreceptors work together in the production of smooth controlled coordinated motion is critical in developing a rehabilitation-training program. The role of the joint musculature extends beyond absolute strength and the capacity to resist fatigue. Simply restoring mechanical restraints or strengthening the associated muscles neglects the smooth coordinated neuromuscular controlling mechanisms required for joint stability.[30] The complexity of joint motion necessitates synergy and synchrony of muscle firing patterns, thereby permitting proper joint stabilization, especially during sudden changes in joint position, which is common in functional activities. Understanding these relationships and functional implications will allow the clinician greater variability and success in returning athletes safely to their playing environment.

Although the concept and value of proprioceptive mechanoreceptors have been documented in the literature, treatment techniques directed at improving their function generally have not been incorporated into the overall rehabilitation program. The neurosensory function of the capsuloligamentous structures has taken a back seat to the mechanical structural role. This is mainly due to the lack of information about how mechanoreceptors contribute to the specific functional activities and how they can be specifically activated.[24, 31] Following injury to the capsuloligamentous structures, a partial deafferentation of the joint occurs as the mechanoreceptors become disrupted. This partial deafferentation secondary to injury may be related to either direct or indirect injury. Direct trauma effects would include disruption of the joint capsule or ligaments, whereas post-traumatic joint effusion or hemarthrosis[15] can illustrate indirect effects. Whether by a direct or an indirect cause, the resultant partial deafferentation alters the reflex pathways to the dynamic stabilizing structures. There is considerable evidence in the literature that demonstrates a disruption in reflex muscle activity following injury to the capsuloligamentous structures.[7, 16, 32–34] This can inhibit normal neuromuscular joint stabilization and can contribute to repetitive injuries. Therefore, injury to the capsuloligamentous structures not only reduces the joint's mechanical stability but also diminishes the capability of the dynamic neuromuscular restraint system.

POSTURAL CONTROL

Both balance and proprioception training have been advocated to restore motor control to the lower extremity. In the clinic, the term *balance* is often used without a clear definition. It is important to remember that *proprioception* and *balance* are not synonymous. Proprioception is a precursor of good balance and adequate function. Balance is the process by which we control the body's center of mass with respect to the base of support, whether it is stationary or moving. Berg has attempted to define balance in three ways: the ability to maintain a position, the ability to voluntarily move, and the ability to react to a perturbation.[35] All three of these components of balance are important in the maintenance of upright posture. Static balance refers to an individual's ability to maintain a stable antigravity position while at rest by maintaining the center of mass within the available base of support.

Dynamic balance involves automatic postural responses to the disruption of the center of mass position. Reactive postural responses are activated to recapture stability when an unexpected force displaces the center of mass.[36]

Postural sway is a commonly used indicator of the integrity of the postural control system. Horak defined postural control as the ability to maintain equilibrium and orientation in the presence of gravity.[37] Researchers measure postural sway as either the maximum or the total excursion of center of pressure while standing on a force plate. Whereas little change is noted in healthy adults in quiet standing, the frequency, amplitude, and total area of sway increase with advancing age or when vision or proprioceptive inputs are altered.[38–41]

To maintain balance, the body must make continual adjustments. Most of what is currently known about postural control is based on stereotypical postural strategies activated in response to anteroposterior perturbation.[36, 37, 42] Horak and Nashner described several different strategies used to maintain balance.[42] These strategies include the ankle, the hip, and stepping strategies. These strategies adjust the body's center of gravity so that the body is maintained within the base of support to prevent the loss of balance or falling. Several factors determine which strategy would be the most effective response to postural challenge: speed and intensity of the displacing forces, characteristics of the support surface, and magnitude of the displacement of the center of mass. The automatic postural responses can be categorized as a class of functionally organized long-loop responses that produce muscle activation that brings the body's center of mass into a state of equilibrium.[36] Each of the strategies has reflex, automatic, and volitional components that interact to match the response to the challenge.

Small disturbances in the center of gravity can be compensated for by motion at the ankle. The ankle strategy repositions the center of mass after small displacements caused by slow-speed perturbations, which usually occur on a large, firm, supporting surface. The oscillations around the ankle joint with normal postural sway are an example of the ankle strategy. Anterior sway of the body is counteracted by gastrocnemius activity, which pulls the body posterior. Conversely, posterior sway of the body is counteracted by contraction of the anterior tibial muscles. If the disturbance in the center of gravity is too great to be counteracted by motion at the ankle, the patient will use a hip or stepping strategy to maintain the center of gravity within the base of support. The hip strategy utilizes a rapid compensatory hip flexion or extension to redistribute the body weight within the available base of support when the center of mass is near the edge of the sway envelope. The hip strategy is usually in response to a moderate or large postural disturbance, especially on an uneven, narrow, or moving surface. The hip strategy is often employed while standing on a bus that is rapidly accelerating. When sudden, large-amplitude forces displace the center of mass beyond the limits of control, a step is used to enlarge the base of support and redefine a new sway envelope. New postural control can then be re-established. An example of the stepping strategy is the uncoordinated step that often follows a stumble on an unexpected or uneven sidewalk.

Vision, vestibular, and proprioceptive information are all key ingredients for postural control. Most research suggests that people rely mostly on visual and proprioceptive inputs when maintaining balance under normal conditions.

Vestibular

The vestibular system is an important aspect of balance control. Information supplied by the vestibular apparatus assists in maintaining the body upright against the force of gravity and in determining linear and angular acceleration.[43] The otoliths provide information about gravitational forces and are composed of the utricle and saccule. The otoliths are also responsible for the detection of vertical and horizontal motion, and the saccule detects vertical information.

The semicircular canals are composed of three ducts, which are oriented at right angles to each other. These three canals are referred to as the posterior, lateral, and superior canals. Endolymph moving through the canals helps the nervous system detect angular acceleration. This information is integrated with information that is provided by the somatosensory and visual systems to maintain upright posture. When sudden perturbations are induced, causing a change

in head position, the automatic control provided by vestibular input becomes critical for stabilizing the direction of gaze. Therefore, vision becomes very important for maintaining control of balance, especially under conditions of postural perturbations. When both the support surface and visual surroundings are tilted, the vestibular input automatically takes precedence.

Vision

The visual system provides input to assist in balance control. Through vestibulo-ocular input, the patient gets information about his or her position in space and is able to keep a visual image centered on the fovea. When the head is suddenly tilted, signals from the semicircular canals cause the eyes to rotate in an equal and opposite direction to the rotation of the head. Eye movement counteracts the effects of head movement, with the eyes moving in a direction opposite to that of head movement.

Saccades are critical elements of most visual tracking tasks in ADL. Saccades are fast, jerking eye movements stimulated by retinal slips of the image on the fovea. Saccades are used to track or follow a slowly moving target.[44, 45] Schulmann et al.[45] feel that saccadic and visual fixation eye movements strengthen dynamic equilibrium whereas smooth-pursuit eye movements weaken dynamic equilibrium in healthy subjects. Visual acuity does not appear to be highly related to postural sway.[46]

Proprioception

Proprioception is important for adequate postural control. As previously described, proprioception is the ability to receive and process inputs from the soft tissue structures. Information received from the mechanoreceptors assists the patient in knowing where his or her limbs are in space. For most healthy adults, the preferred sense for balance control comes from proprioceptive information.

Balance is really a constellation of systems working together. In patients, these units must function optimally or performance in ADL will be affected. Probably the most important thing to consider during rehabilitation of patients is that they should be performing functional activities that stimulate their ADL requirements. Practice does appear to be task-specific in both athletes and people who have motor control deficits.[47] As retraining of balance continues, it is best to practice complex skills in their entirety rather than in isolation, because the skills will then transfer more effectively.[48]

ASSESSMENT OF JOINT PROPRIOCEPTION

Assessment of proprioception is valuable for identifying proprioceptive deficits. If deficiencies in proprioception can be clinically diagnosed in a reliable manner, a clinician would know when and if a problem exists and when the problem has been corrected.[1] There are several ways to measure or assess proprioception about a joint. From an anatomic perspective, histologic studies can be conducted to identify mechanoreceptors within the specific joint structures. Neurophysiologic testing can assess sensory thresholds and nerve conduction velocities. From a clinical perspective, proprioception can be assessed by measuring the components that make up the proprioceptive mechanism: kinesthesia (perception of motion) and joint position sensibility (perception of joint position).

Measuring either the angle or time threshold to detection of passive motion can as-sess kinesthetic sensibility. With the subject seated, the patient's limb is mechanically rotated at a slow constant angular velocity (2 degrees per second). With passive motion, the capsuloligamentous structures come under tension and deform the mechanoreceptors located within. The mechanoreceptor deformation is converted into an electrical impulse, which is then processed within the CNS. The patient is instructed to stop the lever arm movement as soon as he or she perceives motion. Depending on which measurement is used, either the time to detection or the degree of angular displacement is recorded.

Joint position sense is assessed through the reproduction of both active and passive joint repositioning. The examiner places the limb at a preset target angle and holds it there for a minimum of 10 seconds to allow the patient to mentally process the target angle. Following this, the limb is returned to the starting position. The patient is asked to either actively reproduce or stop the device when passive repositioning of the angle has been achieved (Fig. 26–1). The examiner measures the ability of an individual to accurately reproduce the preset target angle position. The angular displacement is recorded as the error in degrees from the preset target angle. Active angle reproduction measures the ability of both the muscle and the capsular receptors, whereas passive repositioning primarily measures the capsular receptors.

With both tests of proprioception, the patient is blindfolded during testing to elimi-

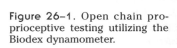

Figure 26–1. Open chain proprioceptive testing utilizing the Biodex dynamometer.

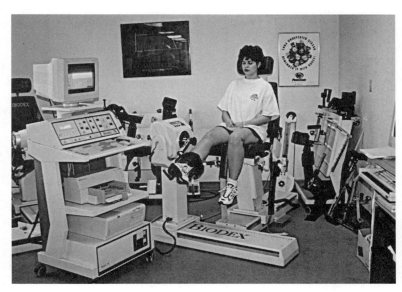

nate all visual cueing. In patients with unilateral involvement, the contralateral uninjured limb can serve as an external control for comparison.

The main limitation to current proprioceptive testing is that neither time nor angle threshold to detection of passive motion provides an assessment of the unconscious reflex arc believed to provide dynamic joint stability. The assessment of reflex capabilities is usually performed by measuring the latency of muscular activation to involuntary perturbation through electromyographic interpretation of firing patterns of those muscles crossing the respective joint (Fig. 26–2).[49] The ability to quantify the sequence of muscle firing can provide a valuable tool for the assessment of asynchronous neuromuscular activation patterns following injury.[34, 50] A delay or lag in the firing time of the dynamic stabilizers about the joint can result in recurrent joint subluxation and joint deterioration.

The functional assessment of the combined peripheral, visual, and vestibular contributions to neuromuscular control can be measured with computerized balance measures of postural stability. The sensory orga-

nization test protocol is used to evaluate the relative contribution of vision, vestibular, and proprioceptive input to the control of postural stability when conflicting sensory input occurs.[36] Postural sway is assessed (NeuroCom Smart System) under six increasingly challenging conditions. Baseline sway is recorded in quiet standing position with the eyes open. The reliance on vision is evaluated by asking the patient to close his or her eyes. A significant increase in sway or loss of balance suggests an over-reliance on visual input.[36, 51, 52] Sensory integration is evaluated when the visual surround moves in concert with sway (sway-referenced vision), creating inaccurate visual input. The patient is then re-tested on a support surface that moves with sway (sway-referenced support), thereby reducing the quality and availability of proprioceptive input for sensory integration. With the eyes open, vision and vestibular input contribute to the postural responses. With the eyes closed, vestibular input is the primary source of information, since proprioceptive input is altered. The most challenging condition combines sway-referenced vision and sway-referenced support surface.[36, 37, 51]

Knee Proprioception

Numerous studies have been performed examining the role of proprioception about the knee joint. Most studies suggest that following injury to the knee, there is some level of partial deafferentation to the capsuloligamentous structures.[14, 53, 54] A disruption in the proprioceptive pathway will result in an alteration of position sense and kinesthesia.[55, 56] Barrack showed an increase in the threshold to detection of passive motion in a majority of patients with anterior cruciate ligament (ACL) rupture and functional instability.[55] Corrigan,[54] who also found diminished proprioception after ACL rupture, confirmed this finding. Diminished proprioceptive sensitivity has also been shown to cause giving-way or episodes of instability in the ACL-deficient knee.[53]

Deficits in the neuromuscular reflex pathway may have a detrimental effect on the motor controls system as a protective mechanism. Diminished sensory feedback can alter the reflex stabilization pathway, thereby

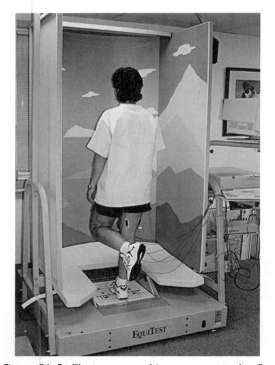

Figure 26–2. Electromyographic assessment of reflex muscle firing as a result of perturbation on the Neurocom Equitest.

causing a latent motor response when faced with unexpected forces or trauma. Beard demonstrated disruption of the protective reflex arc in subjects with ACL deficiency.[16] A significant deficit in reflex activation of the hamstring muscles after a 100 N anterior shear force in a single-leg closed chain position was identified, as compared with the contralateral uninjured limb.[16] Beard demonstrated that the latency was directly related to the degree of knee instability: the greater the instability, the greater the latency. Other researchers found similar alterations in the muscle firing patterns in the ACL-deficient patient.[34, 57, 58] Solomonow et al.[58] found that a direct stress applied to the ACL resulted in reflex hamstring activity, thereby contributing to the maintenance of joint stability. This response was also present in ACL-deficient knees, but the reflex was significantly slower.

It has been demonstrated that a proprioceptive deficit occurs following knee injury, but both kinesthetic awareness and reposition sense can be at least partially restored with surgery and rehabilitation. A number of studies have examined proprioception following ACL reconstruction. Barrett[59] measured proprioception after autogenous graft repair and found that the proprioception was better than that of the average ACL-deficient patient but still significantly worse than the proprioception in the normal knee. Barrett further noted that the patients' satisfaction was more closely correlated with their proprioception than with their clinical score. Harter et al.[60] could not demonstrate a significant difference in the reproduction of passive positioning between the operative and nonoperative knee at an average of 3 years after ACL reconstruction. Kinesthesia has been reported to be restored after surgery as detected by the threshold to the detection of passive motion in the midrange of motion.[55] A longer threshold to the detection of passive motion was observed in the ACL-reconstructed knee compared with the contralateral uninvolved knee when tested at the end range of motion (Barrack et al.[55]). Lephart et al.[50] found similar results in patients after either arthroscopically assisted patellar-tendon autograft or allograft ACL reconstruction.

The importance of incorporating a proprioceptive element in any comprehensive rehabilitation program is justified based on the results of these studies. The effects of how surgical and nonsurgical interventions may facilitate the restoration of the neurosensory roles is unclear; however, it has been shown that ligamentous re-tensioning coupled with rehabilitation can restore proprioceptive sensitivity.[61] Since afferent input is altered after joint injury, proprioceptive rehabilitation must focus on restoring proprioceptive sensitivity to retrain these altered afferent pathways and enhance the sensation of joint movement. Restoration may be facilitated by (1) enhancing mechanoreceptor sensitivity, (2) increasing the number of mechanoreceptors stimulated, and (3) enhancing the compensatory sensations from the secondary receptor sites. Research should be directed toward developing new techniques to improve proprioceptive sensitivity.

Methods to improve proprioception after injury or surgery could improve function and decrease the risk for re-injury. Ihara and Nakayama[57] demonstrated a reduction in the neuromuscular lag time with dynamic joint control on an unstable board. The maintenance of equilibrium and improvement in reaction to sudden perturbations on the unstable board served to improve the neuromuscular coordination. This phenomenon was first reported by Freeman and Wyke[3] in 1967 when they found that proprioceptive deficits could be reduced with training on an unstable surface. They found that proprioceptive training through stabilometry, or training on an unstable surface, significantly reduced the episodes of giving way following ankle sprains. Tropp et al.[62] confirmed the work of Freeman by demonstrating that the results of stabilometry could be improved with coordination training on an unstable board. Hocherman et al.[63] also showed an improvement in the movement amplitude of an unstable board and the weight distribution on the feet found in hemiplegic patients who received training on an unstable board.

Barrett[59] has demonstrated the relationship between proprioception and function. Barrett's study suggests that limb function relies more on proprioceptive input than on strength during activity. Borsa et al.[30] also found a high correlation between diminished kinesthesia with the single-leg hop test. The single-leg hop test was chosen for its integrative measure of neuromuscular control, since a high degree of proprioceptive sensibility and functional ability is required to successfully propel the body forward and land safely on the limb. Giove et al.[64] reported a higher success rate in returning athletes to competitive sports through adequate hamstring rehabilitation. Tibone et al.[65] and Ihara and Nakayama[57] found that simple hamstring strengthening alone was not adequate, it was necessary to obtain voluntary or reflex-level control of knee instability to return to functional activities. Walla et al.[33] found that 95 percent of patients were able to successfully avoid surgery after ACL injury when they were able to achieve "reflex-level" hamstring control. Ihara and Nakayama[57] found that the reflex arc between stressing the ACL and hamstring contraction can be shortened with training. With the use of unstable boards, the researchers were able to successfully decrease the reaction time. Since afferent input is altered after joint injury, proprioceptive sensitivity to retrain these altered afferent pathways are critical to shorten the time lag of muscular reaction to counteract the excessive strain on the passive structures and guard against injury.

Equally important in the area of rehabilitation is the effect of muscle fatigue on joint proprioception. There is evidence that exercise to the point of clinical fatigue does have an effect on proprioception.[19, 56] Skinner et al.[56] showed that the reproduction of passive positioning was significantly diminished following a fatigue protocol. Voight et al.[19] also demonstrated a significant proprioceptive deficit following a fatigue protocol. This suggests that patients who are fatigued may have a change in their proprioceptive abilities and be more prone to injury. Even if proprioceptive loss is not present with fatigue, the ability of the muscle to respond to mechanoreceptor signals is certainly diminished.[5]

EFFECTS OF INJURY ON BALANCE

The maintenance of balance requires the integration of sensory information from a number of different systems: vision, vestibular, and proprioception. Therefore, if proprioception is altered or diminished, balance will also be altered. Several studies have assessed the effect of ACL rupture on standing balance. Usually the balance characteristics of the injured extremity are compared to those of the uninjured extremity.

Mizuta et al.[66] measured postural sway in two groups: a functionally stable group and a functionally unstable group, both of which had unilateral ACL-deficient knees. An additional group of individuals were also studied to serve as a control group. When compared with the control group, an impaired standing balance was found in the functionally unstable group but not in the functionally stable group. These results suggest that stabilometry was a useful tool in the assessment of functional knee stability. Both Friden et al.[67] and Gauffin et al.[68] demonstrated impaired standing balance during unilateral stance in individuals with chronic ACL-deficient knees.

It is unknown at this time exactly how injuries to the knee affect performance on static and dynamic tests of balance control. It is known that the mechanoreceptors in and around the knee offer information about the change of position, motion, and loading of the joint to the CNS, which stimulates the muscles around the knee to function.[57] If a time lag exists in the neuromuscular reaction, injury may occur. The shorter the time lag, the less stress to the ligament and other soft tissue structures about the knee. Therefore, when faced with postural dysfunction, one-leg standing balance is maintained by a coordinated activation of the postural muscles of the trunk and lower limbs.[62] Tropp et al.[62] reported that this coordinated activation at the ankle joint was demonstrated by the activation of the peroneal muscles in patients with functional instability following lateral ligament injury to the ankle joint. An inadequate correction at the ankle joint might cause an impaired standing balance in patients with functional instability of the ankle joint. Therefore, neuromuscular coordination plays an important role in the maintenance of standing balance. Following injury to the knee, impaired standing balance may be due to the loss of muscular coordination, which could have resulted from the loss of normal proprioceptive feedback.[15, 55]

REACTIVE NEUROMUSCULAR TRAINING

The design and implementation of a reactive neuromuscular training (RNT) program is critical for restoring the synergy and synchrony of muscle firing patterns required for dynamic stability and fine motor control. The main objective of reactive neuromuscular training is to return the patient to his or her pre-injury activity level as quickly and as safely as possible. This is accomplished by enhancing the dynamic muscular stabilization of the joint and by increasing the cognitive appreciation of the respective joint in regard to both position and motion. Reactive neuromuscular training activities are designed both to restore functional stability about the joint and to enhance motor control skills. Program design manipulates the environment to facilitate an appropriate response. Clinical control is provided over the joints that dominate the task and in which plane that the activity is taking place.

The first objective that should be addressed in the RNT program is the restoration of dynamic stability. Dynamic stability allows for the control of abnormal joint translation during functional activities. The re-establishment of dynamic stability is dependent on the type of injury and whether or not surgical intervention was necessary. In either case, the RNT program will be similar because of the ultimate goal of returning the athlete back to his or her pre-injury level. Following the restoration of range of motion and strength, dynamic stability can be enhanced with reflex stabilization and basic motor learning exercises.

Once dynamic stability has been achieved, the focus of the RNT program is to restore ADL and sport-specific skills. Exercise and training drills should be incorporated into the program that will refine the physiologic parameters that are required for the return to pre-injury levels of function. Emphasis in the RNT program must be placed on a progression from simple to complex neuromotor patterns that are specific to the demands placed on the patient during function. The training program should begin with simple activities, such as walking/running, and then progress to highly complex motor skills requiring refined neuromuscular mechanisms, including proprioceptive and kinesthetic awareness that provides reflex joint stabilization.

Central Nervous System Motor Control Integration

It is important that the clinician have a good understanding of the central nervous system's influence on motor control to develop an appropriate rehabilitation program. The CNS input provided by the peripheral mechanoreceptors as well as the visual and vestibular receptors are all integrated by the CNS to generate a motor response. In general, the CNS response falls under three categories or levels of motor control: spinal reflexes, brain stem processing, and cognitive program planning. The goal of the rehabilitation process is to retrain the altered afferent pathways to enhance the neuromuscular control system. To accomplish this goal, the objective of the rehabilitation program should be to hyperstimulate the joint and muscle receptors to encourage maximal afferent discharge to the respective CNS levels.[34, 69–72]

In the simplest mechanism, the afferent fibers of the mechanoreceptors synapse with the spinal interneurons and produce a reflexive facilitation or inhibition of the motor neurons.[70, 72, 73] This mechanism is responsible for regulating motor control of the antagonistic and synergistic patterns of muscle contraction.[28] This serves to provide for reflex muscle splinting during conditions of abnormal stress about the joint.[30, 69, 70] At this level of motor control, activities to encourage reflex joint stabilization should dominate.[14, 30, 69, 72] These activities are characterized by sudden alterations in joint position that require reflex muscle stabilization. With sudden alterations or perturbations, both the articular and muscular mechanoreceptors will be stimulated for reflex stabilization. Rhythmic stabilization exercises encourage co-contraction of the musculature, thereby producing a dynamic neuromuscular stabilization.[74] These exercises serve to build a foundation for dynamic stability.

The second level of motor control interaction is at the level of the brain stem.[1, 70, 75] At this level, afferent mechanoreceptors interact with the vestibular system and visual input from the eyes to control or facilitate postural stability and equilibrium of the body.[1, 30, 69–71] Afferent mechanoreceptor input also works in concert with the muscle spindle complex by inhibiting antagonistic muscle activity under conditions of rapid lengthening and periarticular distortion, both of which accompany postural disruption.[20, 72] In conditions of disequilibrium in which simultaneous neural input exists, a neural pattern is generated that affects the muscular stabilizers, thereby returning equilibrium to the body's center of gravity.[70] Therefore, balance is influenced by the same peripheral afferent mechanism that mediates joint proprioception and is at least partially dependent on the individual's inherent ability to integrate joint position sense with neuromuscular control.[76]

Balance activities, both with and without visual input, will enhance motor function at the brain stem level.[70, 75] It is important that these activities remain specific to the types of activities or skills that will be required of the athlete upon return to his or her sport.[77] Static balance activities should be used as a precursor to more dynamic skill activity.[77] Static balance skills can be initiated once the individual is able to bear weight on the lower extremity. The general progression of static balance activities is from bilateral to unilateral and from eyes open to eyes closed.[69, 70, 77–79] With balance training, it is important to remember that sensory systems respond to environmental manipulation. To stimulate or facilitate the proprioceptive system, vision must be disadvantaged. This can be accomplished in several ways: remove vision with either the eyes closed or blindfolded, destabilize vision by demanding hand and eye movements (ball toss) or moving the visual surround, or confuse vision with unstable visual cues that disagree with the proprioceptive and vestibular inputs (sway referencing).

To stimulate vision, proprioception must be either destabilized or confused. The logical progression to destabilize proprioception is to start the balance training on a stable surface and then move to an unstable surface such as a mini-tramp, balance board, or dynamic stabilization trainer.[1, 69, 70] As joint position changes, dynamic stabilization must occur for the patient to control the unstable surface (Fig. 26–3). Vision can be confused during balance training by having the patient stand on a compliant surface such as a foam mat or utilizing a sway-referenced moving forceplate.

The vestibular system can be stimulated by disadvantaging both vision and proprioceptive information. This can be accomplished by several different methods. Absent vision with an unstable or compliant surface is achieved with eyes closed, training on an unstable surface. Demanding hand and eye movements while the patient is on a floor mat or foam pad will destabilize both vision and proprioception. A moving surround with

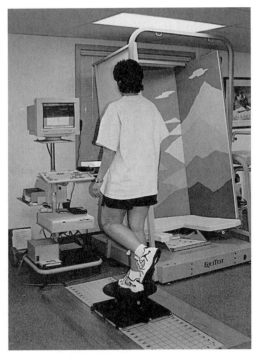

Figure 26–3. Unstable surface training on the Dynamic Stabilization Trainer and Neurocom BalanceMaster.

a moving forceplate will confuse both vision and proprioceptive input.

The patients should initially perform the static balance activities while concentrating on the specific task (position sense and neuromuscular control) to facilitate and maximize sensory output. As the task becomes easier, activities to distract the athlete's concentration (catching a ball or performing mental exercises) should be incorporated into the training program. This will help to facilitate the conversion of conscious to unconscious motor programming.[1, 70] Balance training exercises should induce joint perturbations to facilitate reflex muscle activation.

At the highest level of contribution to the CNS is the ability of the mechanoreceptors to interact and influence cognitive awareness of body position and movement in which motor commands are initiated for voluntary movements.[20, 28, 34, 70] Appreciation of joint position at the highest or cognitive level needs to be included in the RNT program. These types of activities are initiated on the cognitive level and include programming motor commands for voluntary movement. The repetitions of these movements will maximally stimulate the conversion of conscious programming to unconscious programming.[1, 30, 69–72] This information can then be stored as a central command and ultimately performed without continuous reference to the conscious.[30, 69–72] Both active and passive joint re-positioning should be utilized to enhance cognitive appreciation of joint position.

EXERCISE PROGRAM AND PROGRESSION

Dynamic reactive neuromuscular control activities should be integrated into the overall rehabilitation program once adequate healing has occurred. The progression to these activities is predicated on the athlete's having satisfactorily completed the activities that are considered prerequisites for the activity being considered. Keeping this in mind, the progression of activities must be goal-oriented and specific to the tasks, which will be expected of the athlete.

The general progression for activities to develop dynamic reactive neuromuscular control is from slow-speed to fast-speed activities, from low-force to high-force activities, and from controlled to uncontrolled activities. Initially these exercises should evoke a balance reaction or weight shift in the lower extremities and ultimately progress to a movement pattern. These reactions can be as simple as a static control with little or no visible movement or as complex as a dynamic plyometric response requiring explosive acceleration, deceleration, or change in direction. The exercises will allow the clinician to challenge the patient using visual and/or proprioceptive input via tubing and other devices (e.g., medicine balls, foam rolls, visual obstacles). Although these exercises will improve physiologic parameters, they are specifically designed to facilitate neuromuscular reactions. Therefore, the clinician must be concerned with the kinesthetic input and quality of the movement patterns rather than the particular number of sets and repetitions. Once fatigue occurs, motor control becomes poor and all training effects lost. During the exercise progression, all aspects of normal should be observed. These should include isometric, concentric, and eccentric muscle control; articular loading and unloading; balance control during weight shifting and direction changes; controlled acceleration and deceleration; and demonstration of both conscious and unconscious control.

Phase I: Static Stabilization (Closed Chain Loading and Unloading)

Phase I involves minimal joint motion and should always follow a complete open chain exercise program that restores near full active range of motion. The patient should stand bearing full weight with equal distribution on the affected and unaffected lower extremities. The feet should be positioned approximately shoulder-width apart. Greater emphasis can be placed on the affected lower extremity by having the patient put the unaffected lower extremity on a 6 to 8-inch stool or step bench. This flexes the hip and knee and forces a greater weight shift to the affected side, yet still allows the unaffected extremity to assist with balance reactions (Fig. 26–4). The weight-bearing status then progresses to having the unaffected extremity suspended in front or behind the

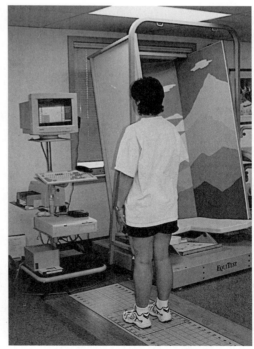

Figure 26–4. Static stabilization weight-shifting technique.

body, forcing a single-leg stance on the affected side. The patient is then asked to continue the single-leg stance while shifting weight to the forefoot and toes by lifting the heel and plantarflexing the ankle. This places the complete responsibility of weight-bearing and balance reactions on the affected lower extremity. This position will also require slight flexion of the hip and knee. Support devices are often helpful and can minimize confusion. When the patient is first asked to progress weight-bearing to the forefoot and toes, a heel lift device can be used. A support device can also be used to place the ankle in dorsiflexion, inversion, or eversion to increase kinesthetic input or decrease biomechanical stresses on the hip, knee, and ankle.

At each progression, the clinician may ask that the patient train with eyes closed to decrease the visual input and increase kinesthetic awareness. The clinician may also use an unstable surface with training in this phase, which will also increase the demands on the mechanoreceptor system. Single or multidirectional rocker devices will assist the progression to the next phase (Fig. 26–5).

The physiologic rationale for this phase of

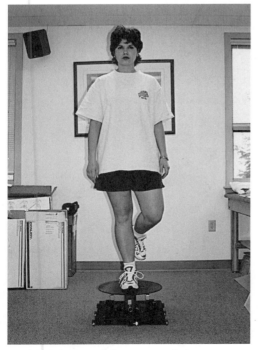

Figure 26–5. Static stabilization: single-leg stance on an unstable surface (DST).

reactive neuromuscular training is the utilization of static compression of the articular structures to facilitate isometric contractions of the musculature, thereby providing a dynamic reflex stabilization. The self-generated oscillations will help increase the interplay between visual, mechanoreceptor, and equilibrium reaction. Changes in the isometric muscle tension will assist in the sensitization of the muscle spindle (gamma bias).

The exercise tubing technique used in this phase is called oscillating technique for isometric stabilization (OTIS). This is accomplished by pulling two pieces of tubing toward the body and returning the tubing to a start position in a smooth rhythmical fashion with increasing speeds. Resistance builds as the tubing is stretched. This forces a transfer of weight in the direction of the tubing. Isometric contraction in the lower extremity must offset the change by producing a stabilizing force in the opposite direction. Four uniplanar exercises can be derived from this technique. Each technique is given a name, which is related to the weight shift produced by the applied tension. The body will then react with an equal and opposite stabilization response. Therefore, the exercise is named for the cause and not the effect.

The goal during this phase is static stabilization. Numerous successful repetitions demonstrating stability are required to achieve motor learning and control.

UNIPLANAR EXERCISE
  1. Anterior weight shift (AWS): The patient faces the tubing and pulls the tubing toward the body using a smooth comfortable motion. This causes forward weight shift, which is stabilized with an isometric counterforce consisting of hip extension, knee extension, and ankle plantar flexion. There should be little or no movement noted in the lower extremity. If movement is noted, resistance should be decreased to achieve the desired stability (Fig. 26–6).
  2. Lateral weight shift (LWS): The patient stands with the affected side facing the tubing. The tubing is pulled by one hand in front of the body and the other hand behind the body to equalize the force and minimize the rotation. This

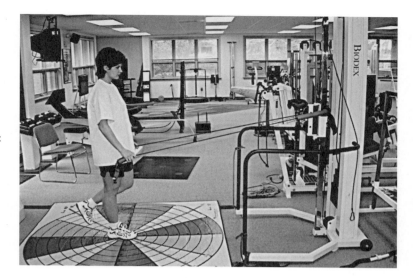

Figure 26–6. Static stabilization: uniplanar anterior weight shift.

causes a lateral weight shift, which is stabilized with an isometric counterforce consisting of hip abduction, knee co-contraction, and ankle eversion (Fig. 26–7).

3. Medial weight shift (MWS): The patient stands with the unaffected side facing the tubing. The tubing is pulled in the same fashion as for LWS. This causes a medial weight shift, which is stabilized with an isometric counterforce consisting of hip adduction, knee co-contraction, and ankle inversion (Fig. 26–8).

4. Posterior weight shift (PWS): The patient stands with his or her back to the tubing in the frontal plane. The tubing

is pulled to the body from behind, causing a posterior weight shift, which is stabilized by an isometric counterforce consisting of hip flexion, knee flexion, and ankle dorsiflexion (Fig. 26–9).

MULTIPLANAR EXERCISE

The exercise can be progressed to multiplanar activity by combining the proprioceptive neuromuscular facilitation (PNF) chop and lift patterns with the upper extremities. The chop patterns from the affected and unaffected side will cause a multiplanar stress requiring isometric stabilization. The patient will now be forced to

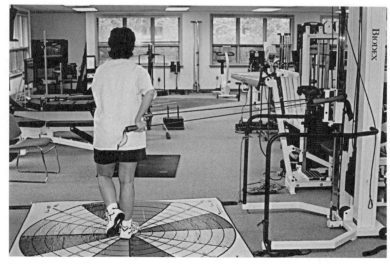

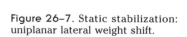

Figure 26–7. Static stabilization: uniplanar lateral weight shift.

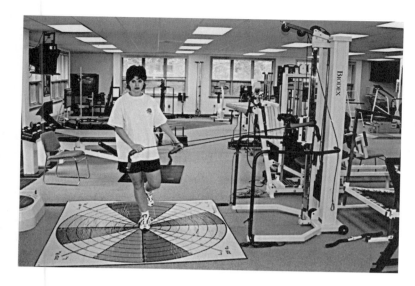

Figure 26–8. Static stabilization: uniplanar medial weight shift.

automatically integrate the isometric responses that were developed in the previous uniplanar exercises. The force will be representative of the PNF diagonals of the lower extremities (Fig. 26–10). The lift patterns from the affected to the unaffected side will add multiplanar stress in the opposite direction (Fig. 26–11). Modifications can be made by changing the resistance, the speed of movement, or spacial orientation relative to the resistance. If resistance is increased, the movement speed should be decreased to allow for a strong stabilizing counterforce. If the speed of movement is increased, then resistance should be decreased to allow for a quick counterforce response. By altering the angle of the body in relation to the resis-

tance, the quality of the movement is changed. A greater emphasis can be planned on one component while reducing the emphasis on another component.

Technique Modification

These techniques can also be used with medicine ball exercises. The posture and position are nearly the same, but the medicine ball does not allow for the oscillations provided by the tubing. The medicine ball provides impulse activity and a more complex gradient of loading and unloading. This is referred to as impulse technique for isometric stabilization (ITIS). As described earlier, the patient is positioned to achieve the de-

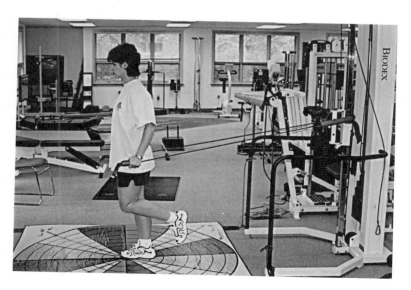

Figure 26–9. Static stabilization: uniplanar posterior weight shift.

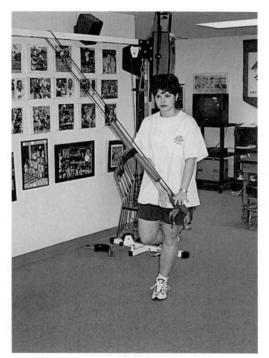

Figure 26–10. Static stabilization: multiplanar proprioceptive neuromuscular facilitation chop technique.

sired stress. The medicine ball is then used with a rebounding device or thrown by the clinician. The ball can also be used without a throw, just by having the patient move the ball in the desired plane at varying speeds. The elastic tubing and medicine ball techniques are similar in position but differ somewhat in physiologic demands. Therefore, they should be used to complement each other and not replace or substitute one another at random. When performing an ITIS activity with a medicine ball, the force exerted by the exercise device names the weight shift. The tubing will exert a pull and the ball will exert a push; therefore, they will be performed from the opposite sides to achieve the same weight shift.

Phase II: Transitional Stabilization (Conscious Controlled Motion Without Impact)

This phase replaces isometric activity with controlled concentric and eccentric activity progressing through a full range of functional motion. The forces of gravity are coupled with tubing to simulate stress in both the vertical and horizontal planes. In phase 1, gravitational forces statically load the neuromuscular system. Varying degrees of imposed lateral stress via the tubing are used to stimulate isometric stabilization. Phase II requires that the movement occur in the presence of varying degrees of imposed lateral stress. The movement stimulates the mechanoreceptors in two ways: (1) articular movement causes capsular stretch in a given direction at a given speed, and (2) the changes in the body position cause loading and unloading of the articular structures and pressure changes in the intracapsular fluid. The exercises in this phase use simple movements such as the squat and lunge. The addition of tubing adds a horizontal stress. Other simple movements such as walking, side-stepping, and the lateral slide board can also be emphasized to stimulate a more efficient and controlled movement.

The physiologic rationale for activities in this phase are the stimulation of dynamic postural responses and facilitation of concentric and eccentric contractions via the compression and translation of the articular structures. The self-generated movements require dynamic control in the mid-range

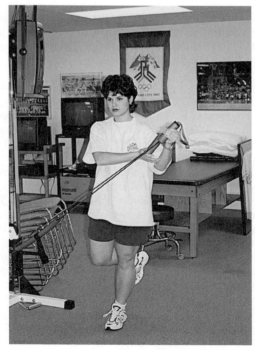

Figure 26–11. Static stabilization: multiplanar proprioceptive neuromuscular facilitation lift technique.

and static control at the end range of motion. Since a change in direction is required at the end ranges of motion, the interplay between visual, mechanoreceptor, and equilibrium reactions continues to increase. The "gamma bias" now responds to changes in both length and tension of the involved musculature.

Assisted techniques can also be used in this phase to progress patients who may find phase II exercise fatiguing or difficult. Assisted exercise is used to reduce the effect of gravity on the body or an extremity to allow for an increase in the quality or quantity of a desired movement. The assisted technique will offset the weight of the body or extremity by a percentage of the total weight. This will allow improved range of motion, a reduction in substitution, minimal eccentric stress, and a reduction in fatigue. The closed chain tubing program can also benefit from assisted techniques, which allow for a reduction in vertical forces by decreasing relative body weight on one or both lower extremities.

The need for assisted exercise is only transitional in nature. The goal is to progress from unweighted to weighted with overloading. The tubing, if utilized effectively, can also provide an overloading effect by causing exaggerated weight shifting. This overloading will be referred to as resisted techniques for all closed chain applications. The two basic exercises used are the squat and the lunge.

SQUAT

The squat is used first because it employs symmetrical movement of the lower extremities. This allows the affected lower extremity to benefit from the visual and proprioceptive feedback from the unaffected lower extremity. The clinician should observe the patient's posture and for weight shifting, which almost always occurs away from the affected limb. Each joint can be compared with its unaffected counterpart. The tubing is used to assist, resist, and modify movement patterns. The bench can be used as a range of motion block (range-limiting device) when necessary. This minimizes fear and increases safety.

1. Assisted technique: The patient faces the tubing, which is placed at a descending angle and is attached to a belt. The belt is placed under the but-

tocks to simulate a swing. The bench is used to allow a proper stopping point. The elastic tension of the tubing is at its greatest when the patient is in the seated position and decreases as the mechanical advantage increases. Therefore, the tension curve of the tubing complements the needs of the patient. The next four exercises follow the assisted squat in difficulty. The tubing is now used to cause weight shifting and demands a small amount of dynamic stability.

2. Anterior weight shift (AWS): The patient faces the tubing, which comes from a level halfway between the hips and the knees and attaches to a belt. The belt is worn around the waist and causes an anterior weight shift. During the squat movement, the ankles plantarflex as the knees extend.

3. Posterior weight shift (PWS): The patient faces away from the tubing at the same level as for the AWS and attaches to a belt. The belt is worn around the waist and causes a posterior weight shift. This places a greater emphasis on the hip extensors and less emphasis on the knee extensors and plantar flexors.

4. Medial weight shift (MWS): The patient stands with the unaffected side toward the tubing at the same level as for the AWS. The belt is around the waist and causes a medial weight shift. This places less stress on the affected lower extremity and allows the patient to lean onto the affected lower extremity without incurring excessive stress or loading.

5. Lateral weight shift (LWS): The patient stands with the affected side toward the tubing at the same level as for the AWS. The belt is worn around the waist, which causes a weight shift onto the affected lower extremity. This exercise will place a greater stress on the affected lower extremity, thereby demanding increased balance and control. The exercise simulates a single leg squat but adds balance and safety by allowing the unaffected extremity to remain on the ground.

LUNGE

The lunge is more specific in that it simulates sports and normal activity. The exercise decreases the base of support and increases the stress to one extremity at a given moment. The range of motion can be stressed to a slightly higher degree. If the patient is asked to alternate the lunge from the right to the left leg, the clinician can easily compare the quality of the movement between the limbs. When performing the lunge, the patient may often use exaggerated extension movements of the lumbar region to assist weak or uncoordinated hip extension. This substitution is not produced during the squat exercise. Therefore, the lunge must be utilized not only as an exercise but as a part of the functional assessment. The substitution must be addressed by asking the patient to maintain a vertical torso (note that the assisted technique will assist the clinician in minimizing this substitution).

1. Assisted technique—forward lunge: The patient faces away from the tubing, which descends at a sharp angle (approximately 60 degrees). This angle parallels the patient's center of gravity, which moves forward and down (Fig. 26–12). This places a stretch on the tubing and assists the patient up from the low point of the lunge position. The assistance also minimizes eccentric demands for deceleration when lowering and provides balance assistance by helping the patient focus on the center of gravity (anatomically located within the hip and pelvic region). The patient is asked to first alternate the activity to provide kinesthetic feedback. The clinician can then use variations of full and partial motion to stimulate the appropriate control before moving on the next exercise.

2. Resisted technique—forward lunge: The patient faces the tubing, which is at an ascending angle from the floor to the level of waist (Fig. 26–13). The tubing will now increase the eccentric loading on the quadriceps with the deceleration on the downward movement. For the upward movement, the patient is asked to focus on hip extension and not knee extension. The patient must learn to initiate movement from the hip and not from lumbar hyperextension or excessive knee extension. Initiation of hip extension should automatically stimulate isometric lumbar stabilization along with the appropriate amounts of knee extension and ankle plantarflexion. A foam block is often used to protect the rear knee from flexing beyond 90 degrees and touching the floor. The block can also be made larger to limit range of motion at any point in the lunge.

3. Resisted technique—lateral (LWS) and medial weight shift (MWS): Forward lunges can be performed to stimulate static lateral and medial stabilization during dynamic flexion and extension movements of the lower extremities. The LWS lunge is performed by positioning the patient with the affected lower extremity toward the direction of resistance. The tubing is placed at a level halfway between the waist and

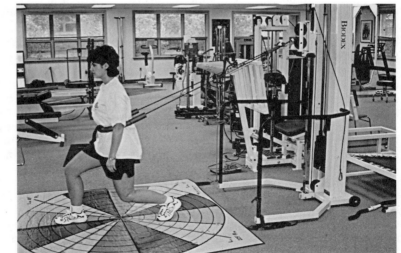

Figure 26–12. Transitional stabilization: assisted lunge technique.

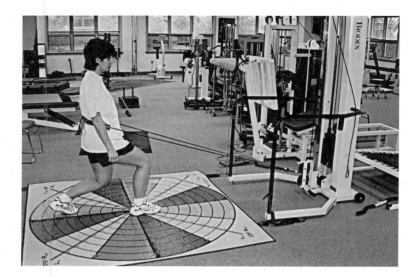

Figure 26–13. Transitional stabilization: resisted forward lunge.

the ankle. The patient is then asked to perform a lunge with minimal lateral movement. This movement stimulates static lateral stabilization of the hip, knee, ankle, and foot during dynamic flexion (unloading) and extension (loading). The MWS lunge is performed by positioning the patient with the affected extremity opposite to the resistance. The tubing is attached as described for the LWS. The movement stimulates static medial stabilization of the affected lower extremity in the presence of dynamic flexion and extension.

The lunge techniques teach weight shifting onto the affected lower extremity during lateral body movements. The assisted technique lateral lunge will complement the assisted technique forward lunge, since it also reduces relative body weight while allowing closed chain function. The prime mover is the unaffected lower extremity that moves the center of gravity over the affected lower extremity for the sole purpose of visual and proprioceptive input prior to excessive loading. The resisted technique lateral lunge will complement the resisted technique forward lunge, since it also provides an overloading effect on the affected lower extremity. In this exercise, the affected lower extremity is the prime mover as well as the primary weight-bearing extremity. The affected lower extremity must not only produce the weight shift but also react, respond, and repeat the movement. Sets, repetitions, and resistance for all of the above exercises are selected by the clinician to produce the appropriate reaction without pain or fatigue.

Technique Modification

As in phase I, the medicine ball can be used to add variety and increase stimulation. However, it is used to stimulate control in the beginning, middle, and end ranges of the squat and lunges. The tubing can also be used to create ITIS and OTIS applications to reinforce stability throughout the range of motion.

Functional Testing

Functional testing provides objective criteria and can help the clinician justify a progression to phase III or an indication that the patient should continue working in phase II. A single-leg body-weight squat or lunge can be performed. The quality and quantity of the repetitions are compared to the unaffected lower extremity and a deficit can be calculated. An isotonic leg press machine can also be used in this manner by setting the weight at the patient's body weight and comparing the repetitions. Open chain isotonic and isokinetic testing can also be helpful in identifying problem areas when specificity is needed. Regardless of the mode of testing, it is recommended that the affected lower extremity display 70 to 80 percent of the capacity demonstrated by the unaffected lower extremity, or no more than a 20 to 30 percent strength deficit. When the patient has met these criteria, he or she can move safely into phase III.

Phase III: Dynamic Stabilization (Unconscious Control and Loading)

Phase III exercises introduce impact and ballistic exercise to the patient. This movement will produce a stretch-shortening cycle that has been described in plyometric exercises. Plyometric function is not a result of the magnitude of the pre-stretch, but rather relies on the rate of stretch to produce a more forceful contraction. This is done in two ways: (1) The stretch reflex is a neuromuscular response to tension produced in the muscle passively. The muscle responds with an immediate contraction to re-orient itself to the new position, protect itself, and maintain posture. If a voluntary contraction is added in conjunction with this reflex, a more forceful contraction can be produced. (2) The elastic properties of the tendon allow it to temporarily store energy and release it. When a quick pre-stretch is followed by a voluntary contraction, the tendon will add to the strength of the contraction by providing force in the direction opposite to the pre-stretch.

A PNF technique called *timing for emphasis* is based upon Beevor's axiom that the brain knows not of individual muscle action but knows only of motion. The urge of the subject to accomplish a motion brings into action the muscle necessary for the performance of that motion.[80] Figure 26–14 shows a patient performing the mountain climber exercise with resistance applied to the left and right hip. The resistance is in opposition of hip flexion. The patient, however, has a problem with left knee flexion and not left hip flexion. By stimulating the hip to flex more forcefully, the entire pattern of flexion is facilitated, thus facilitating knee flexion. In timing for emphasis, maximal resistance is superimposed on patterns of facilitation with due regard for normal timing so that overflow or irradiation may occur from stronger to weaker major muscle components.[80] Mass movements in most sports can be replicated in the clinic setting with minimal space and equipment. The clinician must, however, use sport-specific or movement-specific knowledge in conjunction with techniques borrowed from the science of PNF, plyometrics, and closed chain exercise. Throughout the exercise progression, the patient will move from a conscious to an unconscious or automatic system of control. Following an injury, the patient's attention is drawn to the injured area. At some time during the rehabilitation program, the patient's attention should be drawn away from the injury. This is the final goal in Phase III.

Before the patient is asked to learn any new techniques, he or she is instructed to demonstrate unconscious control by performing various phase II activities while throwing and catching the medicine ball. The squat and lunge exercises are performed with various applications of tubing at the waist level. This activity removes the attention from the lower extremity exercise,

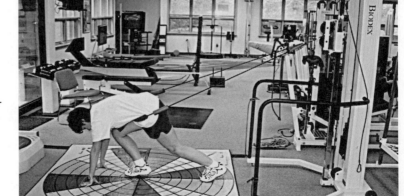

Figure 26–14. Dynamic stabilization: mountain climber drill.

thereby stimulating unconscious control. The forces added by throwing and catching the medicine ball stimulate balance reactions needed for the progression to plyometric activities. Simple rope jumping is another transitional exercise that can be used to provide early plyometric information. Double leg rope jumping is done first. The patient is then asked to perform alternating leg jumping. Rope jumping is effective in building confidence and restoring a plyometric rhythm to movement. Four-way resisted stationary running is an exercise technique used to orient the patient to light plyometric activity.

STATIONARY RUNNING

This technique simply involves jogging or running in place with tubing attached to a belt around the waist. The clinician can analyze the jogging or running activity since it is a stationary drill. The tubing resistance is applied in four different directions, providing simulation of the different forces that the patient will experience as he or she returns to full activity.

1. The posterior weight shift (PWS) run causes a balance reaction that results in an anterior weight shift (opposite direction) and simulates the acceleration phase of jogging or running (Fig. 26–15). The patient faces opposite the direction of the tubing resistance and should be encouraged to stay on the toes (for all running exercises). The

initial light stepping activity can be progressed to jogging and then running. The most advanced form of the PWS run involves the exaggeration of the hip flexion called "high knees." Exaggeration of hip flexion helps stimulate a plyometric action in the hip extensors, thus facilitating acceleration. This form of exercise lends itself to slow controlled endurance conditioning (greater than 3 minutes) or interval training, which depends greatly on the intensity of the resistance, cadence, and rest periods. The interval-training program is most effective and shows the greatest short-term gains. Intervals can be 10 seconds to 1 minute; however, the most common drills are 15 to 30 seconds in length. The patient is usually allowed a 1- to 2-minute rest and is required to perform three to five sets. To make sure that maximum intensity is being delivered by the patient, the clinician should count the amount of foot touches (repetitions) that occur during the interval. The clinician needs to count only the touches of the affected lower extremity. The patient is then asked to equal or exceed the amount of foot-touches on the next interval (set). This is also extremely effective as a functional test for acceleration. The interval time and number of repetitions can be recorded and compared with those of future tests. The clinician should note that the PWS

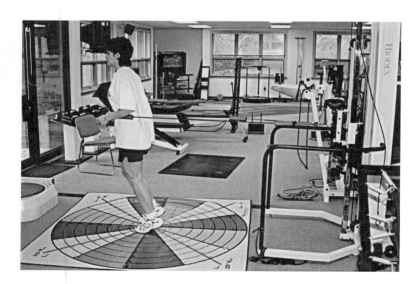

Figure 26–15. Dynamic stabilization: stationary run, posterior weight shift.

places particular emphasis on the hip flexors and extensors, as well as the plantar flexors of the ankle.

2. The medial weight shift (MWS) run follows the same progression as the PWS run (from light jogging to high knees) with the resistance now applied medial to the affected lower extremity (which causes an automatic weight shift laterally). Endurance training, interval training, and testing should also be performed for this technique. This technique simulates the forces that the patient will experience when cutting or turning quickly away from the affected side. This drill is the same as in phase I MWS. Although the phase I MWS is static, the same muscles are responsible for dynamic stability. This exercise represents the forces that the patient will encounter when sprinting into a turn on the affected side.

3. The lateral weight shift (LWS) run should follow the same progression as described for MWS with the exception that the resistance is now lateral to the affected lower extremity (which causes an automatic medial weight shift). This technique simulates the forces that the patient will experience when cutting or turning quickly toward the affected side. When performing the MWS and LWS runs, high knees should be used when working on acceleration. Instructing the patient to perform exaggerated knee flexion or "butt kicks" can emphasize deceleration. The exaggeration of knee flexion places greater plyometric stress on the knee, which has a large amount of eccentric responsibility during deceleration. This exercise represents the forces that the patient will encounter when sprinting into a turn on the unaffected side.

4. The anterior weight shift (AWS) run is probably the most difficult technique to perform correctly and is therefore taught last. The tubing that is set to pull the patient forward stimulates a posterior weight shift. This technique simulates deceleration and eccentric loading of the knee extensors. The patient should start with light jogging on the toes and progress to "butt kicks." This is a plyometric exercise that incorporates exaggerated knee flexion and extension. This exercise will then serve to assist the patient in developing eccentric and concentric reactions that are required in function. The clinician should note that injuries occur more frequently during deceleration and direction changes than on acceleration or straight forward running. Therefore, AWS training is extremely important to the athlete returning to the court or field.

The mountain-climber drill will complement the PWS run, since it exaggerates the need for hip flexion. The drill also places a greater responsibility for stabilization on the torso. If the torso is made rigid by a co-contraction of the spinal extensors, obliques, and abdominals, it will form a more efficient anchor for the hip flexors and extensors. The patient is instructed to get into a push-up position and maintain a near straight line from the shoulder to the ankle of the extended leg. The patient must bend at the hip and not the waist. Flexion at the waist will render the trunk less effective. Note that the desired angle of resistance can be changed from a high angle to a low angle to achieve the desired effect. A high angle will support the body weight somewhat and help to stimulate a need to flatten the back. The low angle will exert a force that pulls backward. This is more advanced and the patient will automatically have to increase his or her cadence to maintain the body's position on the floor. This drill also works well as a functional test; however, the clinician must be able to reproduce the tubing resistance, the angle of pull, the body position, and standardize the test time. To add greater difficulty to the drill, a partially deflated ball or compressible medicine ball can be added. This creates a greater demand for a rigid trunk, since the upper body is now on an unstable surface.

This exercise is a good building tool for sprinting. In sprinting, it is the gluteals that propel the body forward, but the ability to quickly flex the hip determines the stride length. A quick flexion of the hip will also render a more forceful firing of the hip extensors through the plyometric pre-stretch.

LATERAL BOUNDING

Bounding is an exercise technique that will place greater emphasis on the lateral movements. The progression of the bounding exercises will follow the same weight shifting sequence as the previous running exercise. It is suggested that the patient be taught how to perform the bounding exercise without the tubing first. A foam roll, cone, or other obstacle can be used to stimulate jump height and distance. The tubing can then be added to provide the secondary forces to cause anterior, lateral, medial, or posterior weight shifting. Bounding should be taught as a jump from one foot to another. A single lateral bound can be used as a supplementary functional test. Measurements can be taken for a left and right lateral bound. Bounding is considered valid only if the patient can maintain his or her balance when landing. To standardize the bounding exercise, the body height is used for the bound stride and markers can be placed for the left and right foot landings.

1. The anterior weight shift (AWS) bound combines lateral motion with an automatic posterior weight shift or deceleration reaction (Fig. 26–16). It is slightly more demanding than the stationary running exercises, since the body weight is driven a greater distance.
2. The lateral weight shift (LWS) bound causes an excessive lateral plyometric force and will help to develop lateral acceleration and deceleration in the affected lower extremity. This is the most strenuous of the lateral bounding activities, since it actually accelerates the body weight onto the affected lower extremity. This is, however, necessary so that the clinician can ob-

serve the ability of the affected limb to perform a quick direction change and controlled acceleration and deceleration.

3. The medial weight shift (MWS) bound is used as an assisted plyometric exercise. The patient works with his or her total body weight but impact is greatly lowered by reducing both acceleration and deceleration forces. This exercise is an excellent transitional exercise at the end of phase II as well as at the beginning of phase III. It also serves as a warm-up drill providing submaximal stimulation of the proprioceptive system prior to a phase III exercise session.
4. The posterior weight shift (PWS) bound facilitates an anterior lateral push-off of each leg and will stimulate an anterior weight shift. This exercise will assist in teaching acceleration and lateral cutting movements.

MULTIDIRECTIONAL DRILLS

Multidirectional drills include jumping (two-foot take-off followed by a two-foot landing), hopping (one-foot take-off followed by a landing on the same foot), and bounding (one foot take-off followed by an opposite foot landing). A series of floor markers can be placed in various patterns to simulate functional movements. A weight shift can be produced in any direction by the orientation of the tubing. Obstacles can

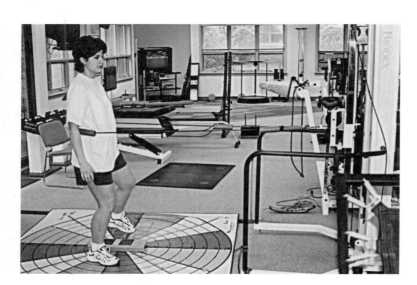

Figure 26–16. Dynamic stabilization: lateral bound, anterior weight shift.

also be used to make the exercise more complicated. The jumping exercise can be developed to simulate down-hill skiing, while the hopping exercise can be designed to stress single-leg push-off for vertical jumping sports such as basketball and volleyball.

SUMMARY

Increased attention has been given to the development of balance and proprioception in the rehabilitation and reconditioning of athletes following injury. It is believed that injury results in altered somatosensory input that influences neuromuscular control. If static and dynamic balance and neuromuscular control are not re-established following injury, then the patient will be susceptible to recurrent injury and his or her performance may decline. The rehabilitation program must focus on restoring the proprioceptive mechanism by enhancing cognitive appreciation of the respective joint and providing muscular stabilization of the joint in the absence of structural restraints. An organized progression is the key to success. Failing to plan is planning to fail.

References

1. Voight ML, Cook G, Blackburn TA: Functional lower quarter exercise through reactive neuromuscular training. *In* Bandy WD (ed): Current Trends for the Rehabilitation of the Athlete. Lacrosse, WI, SPTS Home Study Course, 1997.
2. Freeman MAR, Wyke B: Articular contributions to limb reflexes. Br J Surg 53:61–69, 1966.
3. Freeman MAR, Wyke B: Articular reflexes of the ankle joint. An electromyographic study of normal and abnormal influences of ankle-joint mechanoreceptors upon reflex activity in leg muscles. Br J Surg 54:990–1001, 1967.
4. Sherrington CS: The interactive action of the nervous system. New Haven, CT, Yale University Press. 1911.
5. Barrack RL, Lund PJ, Skinner HB: Knee joint proprioception revisited. J Sport Rehab 3:18–42, 1994.
6. Barrack RL, Skinner HB: The sensory function of knee ligaments. *In* Daniel D, Akeson W, O'Connor J, (eds): Knee Ligaments: Structure, Function, Injury, and Repair. New York, Raven Press, 1990.
7. Ciccotti MR, Kerlan R, Perry J, Pink M: An electromyographic analysis of the knee during functional activities: I. The normal profile. Am J Sports Med 22(5):645–650, 1994.
8. Grigg P: Peripheral neural mechanisms in proprioception. J Sport Rehab 3:1–17, 1994.
9. Grigg P, Hoffman AH: Ruffini mechanoreceptors in isolated joint capsule. Reflexes correlated with strain energy density. Somatosensory Res 2:149–162, 1984.
10. Grigg P, Hoffman AH: Properties of ruffini afferents revealed by stress analysis of isolated sections of cats knee capsule. J Neurophysol 47:41–54, 1982.
11. Grigg P: Response of joint afferent neurons in cat medial articular nerve to active and passive movements of the knee. Brain Res 118:482–485, 1976.
12. Grigg P, Finerman GA, Riley LH: Joint position sense after total hip replacement. J Bone Joint Surg 55:1016–1025, 1973.
13. Guyton AC: Textbook of Medical Physiology, 6th ed. Philadelphia: Saunders, 1991.
14. Skinner HB, Barrack RL, Cook SD, Haddad RJ: Joint position sense in total knee arthroplasty. J Orthop Res 1:276–283, 1984.
15. Kennedy JC, Alexander IJ, Hayes KC: Nerve supply to the human knee and its functional importance. Am J Sports Med 10:329–335, 1982.
16. Beard DJ, Kyberd PJ, Fergusson CM, Dodd CA: Proprioception after rupture of the ACL: An objective indication of the need for surgery? J Bone Joint Surg 75B:311, 1993.
17. Schulte MJ, Happel LT: Joint innervation in injury. Clin Sports Med 9:511–517, 1990.
18. Willis WD, Grossman RG: Medical Neurobiology, 3rd ed. St Louis, CV Mosby, 1981.
19. Voight ML, Blackburn TA, Hardin JA: Effects of muscle fatigue on shoulder proprioception. J Orthop Sports Phys Ther 21(5):348–352, 1996.
20. Phillips CG, Powell TS, Wiesendanger M: Protection from low threshold muscle afferents of hand and forearm area 3A of Babson's cortex. J Physiol 217:419–446, 1971.
21. Clark FJ, Burgess PR: Slowly adapting receptors in cat knee joint: Can they signal joint angle? J Neurophysiol 38:1448–1463, 1975.
22. Goodwin GM, McCloskey DI, Matthews PC: The contribution of muscle afferents to kinesthesia shown by vibration induced illusions of movement and by effects of paralyzing joint afferents. Brain 95:705–748, 1972.
23. Cross MJ, McCloskey DI: Position sense following surgical removal of joints in man. Brain Res 55:443–445, 1973.
24. Glenncross D, Thornton E: Position sense following joint injury. Am J Sports Med 21:23–27, 1981.
25. Braxendale RA, Ferrel WR, Wood L: Responses of quadriceps motor units to mechanical stimulation of knee joint receptors in decerebrate cat. Brain Res 453:150–156, 1988.
26. Cafarelli E, Bigland B: Sensation of static force in muscles of different length. Experimental Neurology 65:511–525, 1979.
27. McCloskey DI: Kinesthetic sensitivity. Physiol Rev 58:763–820, 1978.
28. Rowinski MJ: Afferent neurobiology of the joint. *In* ProClinics: The Role of Eccentric Exercise. Shirley, NY, Biodex, 1988.
29. Haddad B: Protection of afferent fibers from the knee joint to the cerebellum of the cat. Am J Physiol 172:511–514, 1953.
30. Borsa PA, Lephart SM, Kocher MS, Lephart SP: Functional assessment and rehabilitation of shoulder proprioception for glenohumeral instability. J Sports Rehab 3:84–104, 1994.
31. Gandevia SC, McCloskey DI: Joint sense, muscle sense and their contribution as position sense, measured at the distal interphalangeal joint of the middle finger. J Physiol 260:387–407, 1976.
32. Ciccotti MR, Kerlan R, Perry J, Pink M: An electro-

myographic analysis of the knee during functional activities: II. The anterior cruciate ligament–deficient knee and reconstructed profiles. Am J Sports Med 22(5):651–658, 1994.

33. Walla DJ, Albright JP, McAuley E, Martin V, Eldridge V, El-khoury G: Hamstring control and the unstable anterior cruciate ligament-deficient knee. Am J Sports Med 13:34–39, 1985.

34. Wojtys E, Huston L: Neuromuscular performance in normal and anterior cruciate ligament–deficient lower extremities. Am J Sports Med 22:89–104, 1994.

35. Berg K: Balance and its measure in the elderly: A review. Physiolother Can 41:240–246, 1989.

36. Nashner LM: Sensory, neuromuscular, and biomechanical contributions to human balance. *In* Duncan PW (ed): Balance: Proceedings of the APTA forum. Alexandria, VA, APTA, 1986.

37. Horak FB: Clinical measurement of postural control in adults. Phys Ther 67:1881–1885, 1989.

38. Era P, Heikkinen E: Postural sway during standing and unexpected disturbances of balance in random samples of men or different ages. J Gerontol 40:287–295, 1985.

39. Palta AE, Winter DA, Frank JS: Identification of age-related changes in the balance control system. In Duncan PW (ed): Balance: Proceedings of the APTA forum. Alexandria, VA, APTA, 1986.

40. Horak FB, Shupert CL, Mirka A: Components of postural dyscontrol in the elderly. Neurobiol Aging 10:727–738, 1989.

41. Peterka RJ, Black OF: Age related changes in human postural control: Sensory organizations tests. J Vestib Res 1:73–85, 1990.

42. Horak FB, Nashner LM: Central programming of postural movements. Adaption to altered support surface configurations. J Neurophysiol 55:1369–1381, 1986.

43. Crutchfield A, Barnes M: Motor Control and Motor Learning in Rehabilitation. Atlanta, GA: Stokesville, 1993.

44. Cohen H, Keshner E: Current concepts of the vestibular system reviewed: Visual/vestibular interaction and spacial orientation. Am J Occup Ther 43:331–338, 1989.

45. Schulmann D, Godfrey B, Fisher A: Effect of eye movements on dynamic equilibrium. Phys Ther 67:1054–1057, 1987.

46. Ekdhl C, Jarnlo G, Anderson S: Standing balance in healthy subjects. Scand J Rehab Med 21:187–195, 1989.

47. Tropp H, Odenrick P: Postural control in single limb stance. J Orthop Res 6:833–839, 1988.

48. Barnett M, Ross D, Schmidt R, Todd B: Motor skills learning and the specificity of training principle. Res Q 44:440–447, 1973.

49. Voight ML, Nashner LM, Blackburn TA: Neuromuscular function changes with ACL functional brace use: A measure of reflex latencies and lower quarter EMG responses. Abstract: American Orthopaedic Society of Sports Medicine Annual Conference 1998.

50. Lephart SM, Pincivero DM, Giraldo JL, Fu F: The role of proprioception in the management and rehabilitation of athletic injuries. Am J Sports Med 25:130–137, 1997.

51. Shumway-Cook A, Horak FB: Assessing the influence of sensory interaction on balance. Phys Ther 66:1548–1550, 1986.

52. Wollacott MH, Shumway-Cook A, Nashner LM: Aging and postural control: Changes in sensory organs

and muscular coordination. Int J Aging Hum Dev 23:97–114, 1986.

53. Borsa PA, Lephart SM, Irrgang JJ, Safran MR, Fu F: The effects of joint position and direction of joint motion on proprioceptive sensibility in anterior cruciate ligament deficient athletes. Am J Sports Med 25:336–340, 1997.

54. Corrigan JP, Cashman WF, Brady MP: Proprioception in the cruciate deficient knee. J Bone Joint Surg 74B:247–250, 1992.

55. Barrack RL, Skinner HB, Buckley SL: Proprioception in the anterior cruciate deficient knee. Am J Sports Med 17:1–6, 1989.

56. Skinner HB, Wyatt MP, Hodgdon JA, Conrad DW, Barrack RL: Effect of fatigue on joint position sense of the knee. J Orthop Res 4:112–118, 1986.

57. Ihara H, Nakayama A: Dynamic joint control training for knee ligament injuries. Am J Sports Med 14:309–315, 1986.

58. Solomonow M, Baratta R, Zhou BH, et al.: The synergistic action of the anterior cruciate ligament and thigh muscles in maintaining joint stability. Am J Sports Med 15:207–213, 1987.

59. Barrett DS: Proprioception and function after anterior cruciate reconstruction. J Bone Joint Surg 73B:833–837, 1991.

60. Harter RA, Osternig LR, Singer SL, Larsen RL, Jones DC: Long-term evaluation of knee stability and function following surgical reconstruction for anterior cruciate ligament insufficiency. Am J Sports Med 16:434–442, 1988.

61. Lephart SM, Henry TJ: Functional rehabilitation for the upper and lower extremity. Orthop Clin North Am 26:579–592, 1995.

62. Tropp H, Ekstrand J, Gillquist J: Factors affecting stabiliometry recordings of single leg stance. Am J Sports Med 12:185–188, 1984.

63. Hocherman S, Dickstein R, Pillar T: Platform training and postural stability in hemiplegia. Arch Phys Med Rehabil 65:588–592, 1984.

64. Giove TP, Miller SJ, Kent BE, Sanford TL, Garrick JG: Nonoperative treatment of the torn anterior cruciate ligament. J Bone Joint Surg 65A:184–192, 1983.

65. Tibone JE, Antich TJ, Funton GS, Moynes DR, Perry J: Functional analysis of anterior cruciate ligament instability. Am J Sports Med 14:276–284, 1986.

66. Mizuta H, Shiraishi M, Kubota K, Kai K, Takagi K: A stabiliometric technique for the evaluation of functional instability in the anterior cruciate ligament-deficient knee. Clin J Sports Med 2:235–239, 1992.

67. Friden T, Zatterstrom R, Lindstand A, Moritz U: Disability in anterior cruciate ligament insufficiency: An analysis of 19 untreated patients. Acta Orthop Scand 61:131–135, 1990.

68. Gauffin H, Pettersson G, Tegner Y, Tropp H: Function testing in patients with old rupture of the anterior cruciate ligament. Int J Sports Med 11:73–77, 1990.

69. Lephart S: Reestablishing proprioception, kinesthesia, joint position sense and neuromuscular control in rehab. *In* Prentice WE (ed): Rehabilitation Techniques in Sports Medicine, 2nd ed. St. Louis, Mosby, 1994.

70. Tippett S, Voight ML: Functional Progressions for Sports Rehabilitation. Champaign, IL, Human Kinetics, 1995.

71. Voight ML: Functional Exercise Training. Presented at the National Athletic Training Association Annual Conference, Indianapolis, IN, 1990.

72. Voight ML: Proprioceptive Concerns in Rehabilitation. *In* Proceedings of the XXVth FIMS World Congress of Sports Medicine, Athens, Greece, 1994.
73. Voight ML, Draovitch P: Plyometric training. *In* Albert M (ed): Muscle Training in Sports and Orthopaedics. New York, Churchill Livingstone, 1991.
74. Small C, Waters CL, Voight ML: Comparison of two methods for measuring hamstring reaction time using the Kin-Com Isokinetic Dynamometer. J Orthop Sports Phys Ther 19(6):335–340, 1994.
75. Blackburn TA, Voight ML: Single leg stance: Development of a reliable testing procedure. *In* Proceedings of the 12th International Congress of the World Confederation for Physical Therapy, 1995.
76. Swanik CB, Lephart SM, Giannantonio FP, Fu F: Reestablishing proprioception and neuromuscular control in the ACL-injured athlete. J Sport Rehab 6:183–206, 1997.
77. Rine RM, Voight ML, Laporta L, Mancini R: A paradigm to evaluate ankle instability using postural sway measures [abstract]. Phys Ther 74(5):S72, 1994.
78. Voight ML, Rine RM, Apfel P, et al: The effects of leg dominance and AFO on static and dynamic balance abilities [abstract]. Phys Ther 73(6):S51, 1993.
79. Voight ML, Rine RM, Briese K, Powell C: Comparison of sway in double versus single leg stance in unimpaired adults [abstract]. Phys Ther 73(6):S51, 1993.
80. Voss DE, Ionta MK, Myers BJ: Proprioceptive Neuromuscular Facilitation: Patterns and Techniques. Philadelphia, Harper & Row, 1985.

Bibliography

Burgess PR: Signal of kinesthetic information by peripheral sensory receptors. Ann Rev Neurosci 5:171, 1982.

Clark FJ, Burgess RC, Chapin JW, Lipscomb WT: Role of intramuscular receptors in the awareness of limb position. J Neurophysiol 54(6):1529–1540, 1985.

Eklund J: Position sense and state of contraction: the effects of vibration. J Neurol Neurosurg Psych 35:606, 1972.

Hellenbrant FA: Motor learning reconsidered: A study of change. *In* Neurophysiologic Approaches to Therapeutic Exercise. Philadelphia, FA Davis, 1978.

Matthews PC: Where does Sherrington's "muscular sense" originate? Muscle, joints, corollary discharges? Annu Rev Neurosci 5:189, 1982.

Schmidt RA: Motor Control and Learning. Champaign, IL, Human Kinetics, 1988.

Skoglund CT: Joint receptors and kinesthesia. *In* Iggo A (ed): Verlin, Handbook of Sensory Physiology, Berlin, Springer-Verlag, 1973.

Woollacott MH: Postural control mechanisms in the young and the old. *In* Duncan PW (ed): Balance: Proceedings of the APTA Forum. Alexandria, VA, APTA, 1990.

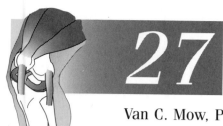

27 Effects of Instability on Articular Cartilage

Van C. Mow, PhD, Michael S. Roh, MD,
and David Joseph, MD

Both clinical and experimental observations of the unstable knee have supported a strong link between joint instability and accelerated degeneration of articular cartilage. The scientific exploration of this link has been pivotal in increasing our understanding of the etiology of osteoarthritis. From this work, insights have been made into the biochemical and biomechanical changes that occur with instability and, in turn, degenerative joint disease. Before initiating a meaningful discussion of this topic, however, one should begin by establishing a working definition of instability.

In its broadest sense, instability is the pathologic state caused by attenuation of the static or dynamic constraints that maintain normal, smooth, congruent joint motion. In the tibiofemoral joint of the knee, the ligaments, primarily the cruciate and the collateral ligaments, the menisci (to a lesser extent), and the anatomic form of the joint represent the static constraints (Fig. 27–1). The dynamic constraints are the muscles that cross the joint and contribute to stability with the force they generate around and through the joint. Any deficiency of these components will produce alterations in the loading of the articular surfaces[1] (Fig. 27–2) or their relative motion (Fig. 27–3).[2–4] In turn, these changes lead to altered contact areas and contact stresses on the articular cartilage. Though difficult to quantify in vivo, these alterations are believed to be responsible for initiating the process of cartilage degeneration seen with joint instability.

STRUCTURE OF ARTICULAR CARTILAGE

The building blocks of articular cartilage are water, collagen, proteoglycan, quantita-

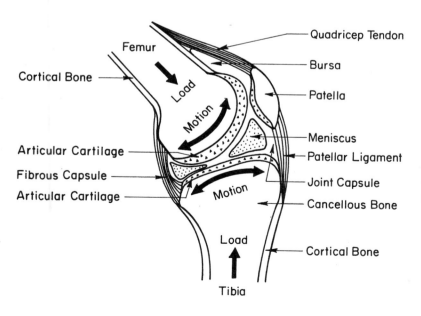

Figure 27–1. Lateral view of the knee showing the static and dynamic stabilizers.

Human Knee Joint

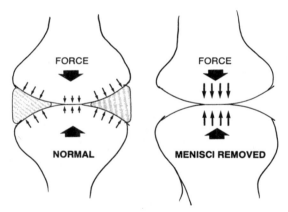

Figure 27–2. Schematic of load transfer with and without the menisci. Removal of the menisci increases the magnitude of stresses on the cartilage at the tibiofemoral articulation by changing its size and location. (From Nordin M, Frankel VH: Biomechanics of the Knee. *In* Nordin M, Frankel VH (eds): Basic Biomechanics of the Musculoskeletal System, 2nd ed. Williams & Wilkins, Baltimore, 1989, p. 128.)

tively minor glycoproteins, and living cells or chondrocytes. Between these elements arises a complex interplay of mechanical and molecular forces that gives cartilage its unique behavioral properties. Though a detailed description of all these interactions is beyond the scope of this chapter, a brief review of the basic structural considerations of cartilage is in order.

The composition of articular cartilage is well described. Water constitutes 60 to 80 percent of normal articular cartilage by weight. Next, 10 to 20 percent is made up of collagen, mainly type II collagen, and 4 to 7 percent of cartilage is composed of proteoglycan. Rife with negatively charged sulfate and carboxyl groups, these negative charges of the proteoglycans are countered by the free positively charged particles in the interstitial fluid, such as sodium ion.[5] Theoretically, with these components in mind, articular cartilage may be considered in three phases: liquid (water), solid (collagen, proteoglycan), and ionic (electrolytes, charged particles). This triphasic theory provides an elegant, albeit rigorous, method for bioengineers to model and study this complicated tissue.[6]

The major component of the solid phase, collagen makes up over 50 percent of the dry weight of articular cartilage. It is characterized by a triple helical structure composed of three alpha chains (Fig. 27–4). Although collagen type II is the primary form

in articular cartilage, collagen types V, VI, IX, X, and XI may also be found. Collagen fibers vary in diameter from 10 to 100 nm, $(1 \text{ nm} = 10^{-9} \text{ meter} = 10^{-3} \text{ } \mu\text{m})$ and this usually increases with age or disease. A protein, collagen is comprised mainly of three amino acids: hydroxyproline, hydroxylysine, and glycosylated hydroxylysine. The special nature of these helical chains of amino acids (like a rope) contributes to the tensile strength of the collagen fiber. These collagen fibers are cross-linked by hydroxypyridinium residues.[7] Type IX collagen is really a hybrid between collagen and proteoglycan, functioning to enhance proteoglycan retention within the fine collagen meshwork.[8]

Proteoglycans are macromolecules that consist of polysaccharide chains attached to a protein core. Aggrecan is a large aggregating proteoglycan that constitutes up to 90 percent of all cartilage proteoglycans. Nonaggregating proteoglycans do exist, although they make up only a small percentage of the total number of proteoglycans.[9] As many as 100 chondroitin sulfate and 50 keratan sulfate glycosaminoglycan chains can be

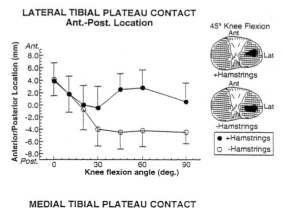

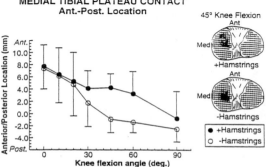

Figure 27–3. This diagram shows what happens to the tibiofemoral relationship with loss of hamstring contraction. Note the anterior tibial translation similar to that seen with anterior cruciate insufficiency.

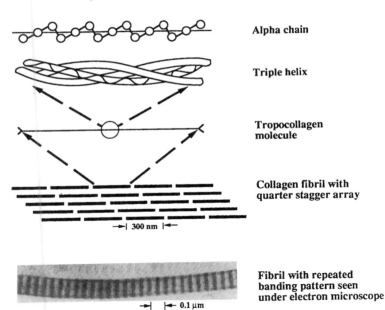

Alpha chain

Triple helix

Tropocollagen
molecule

Collagen fibril with
quarter stagger array

→| 300 nm |←

Fibril with repeated
banding pattern seen
under electron microscope

→| |← 0.1 μm

Figure 27–4. Schematic representation and photomicrograph of the collagen fibril structure. (Adapted from Eyre DR: Collagen: molecular diversity in the body's protein scaffold. Science 207:1315, 1980; copyright 1980 American Association for the Advancement of Science.)

attached to one protein core. Hence, proteoglycan assumes a "test-tube brush-like" appearance on electron microscopy (Fig. 27–5).

Collagen and proteoglycan molecules form a complex, the solid matrix, which is porous-permeable (Fig. 27–6). The size of the proteoglycans plays a major role in the structural properties of the articular cartilage. As there are no covalent bonds linking collagen to proteoglycan, the collagen fibers are free to move through the proteoglycans during compressive loading. As the cartilage deforms under compression, the fibers become taut as they resist the tensile forces that develop. Simultaneously, the interstitial water can be made to flow through the solid matrix. The drag that occurs as a result of interstitial fluid flow contributes to the compressive viscoelastic behavior of cartilage. Also, when the cartilage is subjected to a compressive load, it is the interstitial fluid pressure that resists the load, for the most part.[10, 11] In fact, for normal articular cartilage, the water supports 90 to 95 percent of the load. With time and under constant load, the solid matrix takes over this responsibility as the fluid pressure dissipates. Under normal loading conditions, however, not enough time passes for this load transfer to occur. Therefore, fluid pressure is the major load support mechanism of the knee during daily activity (Fig. 27–7).[5, 10–12]

Lastly, one must consider the living carti-

lage cells or chondrocytes that maintain the matrix and occupy only 5 percent of the total volume and weight. The histologic appearance of articular cartilage can be divided into four zones: superficial or tangential, middle, deep, and the zone of calcified cartilage (Fig. 27–8). Considerable variation exists among the different zones in terms of biochemical composition, metabolism, and chondrocyte shape. The superficial zone contains collagen fibers and chondrocytes aligned parallel to the articular surface and is a zone with very little proteoglycan, the highest collagen content, and the highest water content.[8] This structural organization suggests that the superficial zone experiences considerable tensile stress. Next, the middle zone contains collagen fibers with larger diameters than the superficial zone. The chondrocytes tend to have a round appearance, and the collagen fibers are obliquely arranged. This zone has the highest proteoglycan content. In contrast, the deep zone is characterized by columns of spherical chondrocytes with collagen fibers arranged vertically with respect to the surface. The proteoglycan content of this zone lies between most of the surface and the middle zones and the water content is lowest.[5] Farthest from the surface lies the zone of calcified cartilage, characterized by a wavy line, or tide mark, that separates the noncalcified zones of articular cartilage from the underlying calcified zone and subchon-

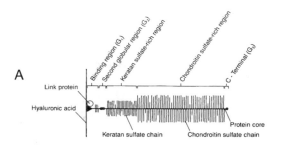

A

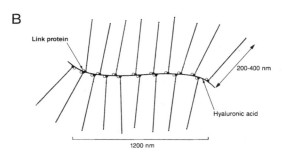

B

Figure 27–5. *A*, Schematic depiction of an aggregating proteoglycan molecule (aggrecan) composed of keratan sulfate and chondroitin sulfate chains bound covalently to a protein core molecule. *B*, A representation of a proteoglycan aggregate that is composed of aggrecans noncovalently attached to hyaluronan with stabilizing link proteins. *C*, Dark field electron micrograph of a proteoglycan aggregate from bovine humeral articular cartilage (×120,000). (Courtesy of Dr. Lawrence Rosenberg.) (From Mow VC, Ratcliffe A: Structure and function of articular cartilage and meniscus. *In* Mow VC, Hayes WC (eds): Basic Orthopaedic Biomechanics, 2nd ed. Philadelphia, Lippincott-Raven Publishers, 1997, p. 122.)

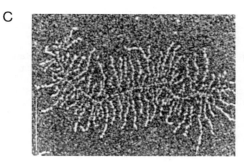

C

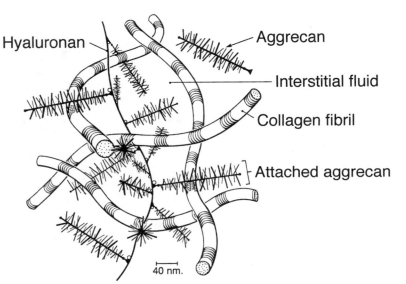

Figure 27–6. Schematic representation of the molecular organization of cartilage. The structural components of cartilage form a fiber-reinforced composite solid matrix. The swelling pressure exerted by the proteoglycan keeps the collagen network inflated. (Modified from Mow VC, Proctor CS, Kelly MA: Biomechanics of articular cartilage. *In* Nordin M, Frankel VH (eds): Basic Biomechanics of the Musculoskeletal System, 2nd ed. Baltimore, Williams & Wilkins, 1989, p. 38.)

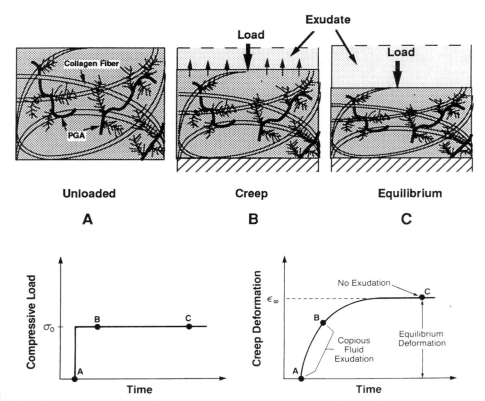

Figure 27–7. Biphasic creep behavior of a hydrated soft tissue such as articular cartilage during compression. Rate of creep is governed by the rate at which fluid can be forced out from the tissue, which in turn is governed by the permeability and stiffness of the porous-permeable, collagen-proteoglycan solid matrix. (Adapted from Mow VC, Proctor CS, Kelly MA: Biomechanics of articular cartilage. *In* Nordin M, Frankel VH (eds): Basic Biomechanics of the Musculoskeletal System, 2nd ed. Baltimore, Williams & Wilkins, 1989, p. 40.)

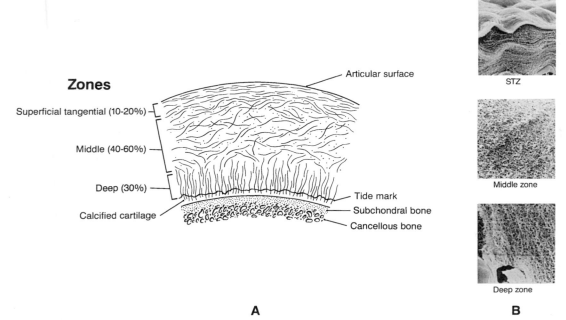

Figure 27–8. Layered structure of cartilage collagen network showing three distinct regions *(A)*, and corresponding scanning electron microscopic collagen fibrillar arrangement *(B)*. (Scanning electron microscope image courtesy of Dr. T. Takei.) (Modified from Mow VC, Proctor CS, Kelly MA: Biomechanics of articular cartilage. *In* Nordin M, Frankel VH (eds): Basic Biomechanics of the Musculoskeletal System, 2nd ed. Baltimore, Williams & Wilkins, 1989, p. 34.)

dral bone. The cells in this layer are smaller and the extracellular matrix is high in apatitic salts, heralding the proximity of bone tissue. Numerous studies over the years have shown that both the cellular and structural arrangements of articular cartilage are optimally suited for its physiologic role.[5, 12]

FUNCTION AND REPAIR OF ARTICULAR CARTILAGE

An extremely durable tissue, articular cartilage has two primary functions: (1) minimizing contact stresses through deformations that increase joint contact areas[10–13] (Fig. 27–9) and (2) contributing to lubrication of the joints by allowing fluid efflux and redistribution at the articular surface and within the tissue.[14] When an external load is applied to the knee joint, a complex distribution of compression (see Fig. 27–7), tension (Fig. 27–10), and shear (Fig. 27–11) stresses are generated within the articular cartilage. During compression, water within the extracellular matrix becomes pressurized, and a net efflux of interstitial fluid occurs from the cartilage. As discussed earlier, the hydrostatic pressure within the matrix supports the cartilaginous infrastructure and bears much of the load during weight-bearing activity. Simultaneously, the water that exudes

from the cartilage during loading aids in lubricating the articular surfaces (Fig. 27–12). When the load is removed, the cartilage resorbs the fluid exudate, allowing the tissue to recover its initial, unstressed shape. These fluid shifts give rise to the viscoelastic behaviors known as biphasic creep and stress-relaxation, which in turn enable articular cartilage to withstand the normally high and repetitive loading on the joint.[15] In addition, the flux of interstitial fluid is believed to be critical for the metabolic and nutritive maintenance of living chondrocytes.

During normal daily functioning, the cells and matrix of the articular cartilage are probably subjected to microtrauma. This trauma can directly injure chondrocytes, causing cell abnormalities and necrosis. Through poorly understood mechanisms, the chondrocytes detect such changes in mechanical stresses, and in the matrix environment. In response, they alter their synthetic, degradative, and possibly proliferative activities and, to a degree, are able to repair the surrounding extracellular matrix. However, following a destabilizing injury such as anterior cruciate ligament (ACL) or meniscal tear, the reparative capacity of the cells is often insufficient to keep up with the rate of microdamage production in the extracellular matrix, and hence maintain a normal, functioning cartilage.[15, 16] The point at which the accumulated microdamage be-

Figure 27–9. Comparison of hydrodynamic lubrication *(A)* and squeeze film lubrication *(B)* of rigid surfaces, and elastohydrodynamic lubrication of deformable bearing surfaces under a hydrodynamic (sliding) action *(C)* and a squeeze film action *(D)*. As is evident, surface deformation of elastohydrodynamically lubricated bearings increases the contact area, thus increasing the load-carrying capacity of these bearings. (From Mow VC, Proctor CS, Kelly MA: Biomechanics of articular cartilage. *In* Nordin M, Frankel VH (eds): Basic Biomechanics of the Musculoskeletal System, 2nd ed. Baltimore, Williams & Wilkins, 1989, p. 49.)

Rigid Bearings

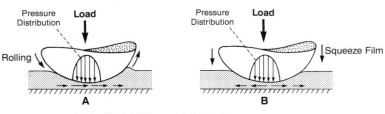

Thin Fluid Film and High Pressures

Deformable Bearings

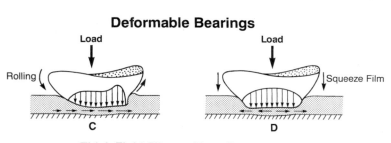

Thick Fluid Film and Low Pressures

Unloaded

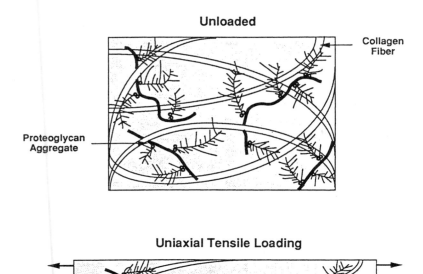

Collagen
Fiber

Proteoglycan
Aggregate

Uniaxial Tensile Loading

Figure 27–10. Schematic diagram of articular cartilage deformation in tension. When pulled in tension, collagen fibers stretch and align with the axis of loading. (From Mow VC, Setton LA, Ratcliffe A, Buckwalter JA, Howell DS: Structure-function relationships of articular cartilage and the effects of joint instability and trauma on cartilage function. *In* Brandt KD (ed): Cartilage Changes in Osteoarthritis. © 1990 Novartis, formerly CIBY-GEIGY Corporation.)

comes irreversible is unknown. But presumably, if the basic collagen meshwork remains intact and if enough chondrocytes remain viable, the chondrocytes can restore the matrix as long as the rate of loss of proteoglycan does not exceed the amount that can be rapidly produced by the cells. When these conditions are not met, the chondrocytes will be exposed to excessive loads, and the tissue will degenerate.[17]

Much of the experimental work on knee instability and cartilage has been done in animals. By transecting various stabilizing structures, scientists are able to reproduce clinical instability and subsequently record the changes that occur within the knee. Notable animal models include anterior cruciate ligament transection in dogs,[18] posterior cruciate ligament transection in rabbits,[19] and partial meniscectomy in dogs and rabbits.[20] Despite some minor variations between animal models, the existing body of research generally shows that the alterations of knee articular cartilage after destabilization are similar to those of degenerative joint disease. Some animal models utilize various combinations of destabilizing, surgical manipulations, leading to marked

joint laxity. Overall, more severe laxity led to more rapid and severe degenerative changes.[21, 22] These can be divided into biochemical, biomechanical, and pathologic changes.

BIOCHEMICAL EFFECTS OF INSTABILITY

The chondrocytes metabolically adapt to changes in stress and strain.[23, 24] Although the mechanisms by which chondrocytes are able to sense and respond to their environment are unclear, several theories exist. Chondrocytes may be able to sense deformations in its shape during stress loading or hydrostatic loading.[24] Alternatively, chondrocytes may detect alterations in the surrounding fluid flow and streaming electrochemical potentials.[25]

In the context of instability, it is hypothesized that a minimum level of abnormal joint load is required to induce chondrocyte necrosis and matrix abnormalities. Further characterization of this "minimum level" is an area of intense research. Nonetheless, the

Unloaded

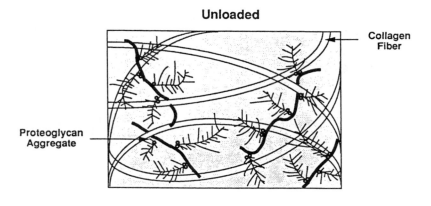

Pure Shear

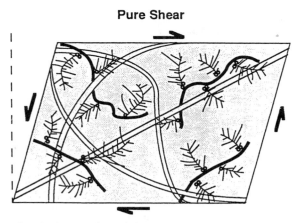

Figure 27–11. Schematic diagram of articular cartilage deformation in pure shear. As the tissue is deformed, collagen fibrils are stretched in the direction of shearing, as shown. Under small shear conditions, no pressure gradients or volume changes develop within the tissue. Thus, no interstitial fluid flow occurs. (From Mow VC, Setton LA, Ratcliffe A, Buckwalter JA, Howell DS: Structure-function relationships of articular cartilage and the effects of joint instability and trauma on cartilage function. *In* Brandt KD (ed): Cartilage Changes in Osteoarthritis. © 1990 Novartis, formerly CIBY-GEIGY Corporation.)

changes seen with instability in animal models are consistent with the early changes seen in osteoarthritis.[26] Within the first few weeks after surgery, chondrocyte swelling occurs, with a corresponding increase in hexuronic acid and water content. Associated with these changes are a higher collagen-to-proteoglycan ratio and greater permeability to interstitial flow.[5]

Instability also has both qualitative and quantitative deleterious effects on the solid phase of cartilage. Disruption of the collagen fibers is believed to be the initial cartilage injury that occurs with instability.[27] Similarly, production of smaller proteoglycan aggregates and a decrease in proteoglycan content have been observed.[28] These changes amount to a biochemical profile similar to that of immature cartilage, less suited to handling the demands of weight-bearing. Because the compressive stiffness of articular cartilage depends on the glycosaminoglycan content, the decrease in the proteoglycan or glycosaminoglycan contents may have a direct and injurious effect on cartilage.[29] Other biochemical changes include a higher galactosamine-to-glucosamine ratio and production of more easily extractable proteins. In response, an early repair reaction may be seen, consisting of increased cellular activity, production of collagen and proteoglycan, and cell proliferation. The response depends on the extent of the instability and articular cartilage dam-

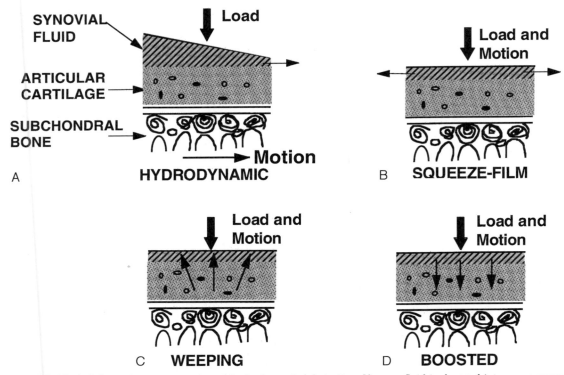

Figure 27–12. *A,* Schematic representation of hydrodynamic lubrication. Viscous fluid is dragged into a convergent channel, causing a pressure field to be generated in the lubricant. Fluid viscosity, gap geometry, and relative sliding speed determine the load-carrying capacity. *B,* As the bearing surfaces are squeezed together, the viscous fluid is forced from the gap in the transverse direction. This squeeze action generates a hydrodynamic pressure in the fluid for load support. The load-carrying capacity depends on the size of the surfaces, velocity of approach, and fluid viscosity. *C,* Weeping lubrication hypothesis for the uniform exudation of interstitial fluid from the cartilage. The driving mechanism is a self-pressurization of the interstitial fluid when the tissue is compressed. *D,* Direction of fluid flow under squeeze-film lubrication in the boosted mode for joint lubrication. (From Mow VC, Ateshian GA: Lubrication and wear of diarthrodial joints. *In* Mow VC, Hayes WC (eds): Basic Orthopaedic Biomechanics, 2nd ed. Philadelphia, Lippincott-Raven, 1997, p. 296.)

age.[30] Repair response may also vary with the depth of the lesion, as there is little functional repair of surface lesions.

BIOMECHANICAL EFFECTS OF INSTABILITY

The material properties of cartilage from animal models have elucidated the effects of instability on cartilage function. Using an ACL transection in a greyhound dog model, Setton and coworkers analyzed the mechanical properties of knee articular cartilage at 6 weeks and 12 weeks after surgery.[29, 30] At 6 weeks, significant decreases were noted in matrix stiffness of the cartilage when tested in compression, tension, and shear. Other studies that measured stiffness at serial intervals after surgery show these changes to

be progressive.[15, 31, 32] In other words, the abnormal pattern of loading associated with this altered kinematics of instability may have caused irreversible cumulative injury to the solid, collagen-proteoglycan matrix. This damaged matrix makes the cartilage softer and less capable of withstanding typical joint loads.

Significant increases occur in water content and permeability with joint instability. Basically, the surface zone of the articular cartilage becomes damaged, increasing the porosity and allowing the cartilage to swell.[33] Moreover, Setton and colleagues found that significant changes in water content and permeability occur after ACL transection, although somewhat later than the changes in the material properties.[29, 30] Given that the fluid pressurization in cartilage is the dominant mechanism essential to its load-bearing and self-lubricating characteristics, the loss

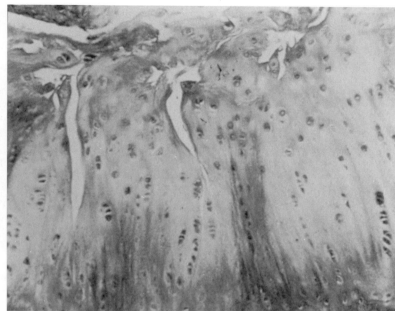

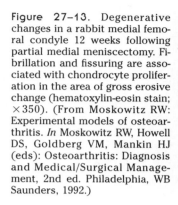

Figure 27–13. Degenerative changes in a rabbit medial femoral condyle 12 weeks following partial medial meniscectomy. Fibrillation and fissuring are associated with chondrocyte proliferation in the area of gross erosive change (hematoxylin-eosin stain; ×350). (From Moskowitz RW: Experimental models of osteoarthritis. *In* Moskowitz RW, Howell DS, Goldberg VM, Mankin HJ (eds): Osteoarthritis: Diagnosis and Medical/Surgical Management, 2nd ed. Philadelphia, WB Saunders, 1992.)

of its ability to regulate hydration severely impairs cartilage function in the joint.[8, 12] Other proposed effects of increased permeability include increased deformations of the solid matrix and elevated interstitial fluid velocities (with associated increased proteoglycan loss), both of which may have a deleterious impact on the long-term survival of articular cartilage.[29]

ANATOMIC EFFECTS OF INSTABILITY

The biochemical and material changes are accompanied by gross pathologic changes similar to those of osteoarthritis.[34] Progressive lesions of the articular cartilage include softening, fibrillation and fissuring, pitting and ulceration (Fig. 27–13), pitting, fissuring (Fig. 27–14), ulceration, and erosions. In the ACL model, gross degenerative changes are most severe at the medial aspect of the medial tibial plateau, with less involvement of the lateral tibial plateau and femur.[30, 35] Likewise, the knees of posterior cruciate ligament–deficient rabbits most frequently developed degenerative changes on the medial tibial plateau.[19] In contrast, in the partial medial meniscectomy model, fissuring and ulceration is seen primarily on the medial femoral condyle, as early as the first 3 weeks after surgery. These degenerative changes were limited when evidence of meniscal re-

generation was noted.[20] Given that studies have not shown any significant site-specific difference in the intrinsic material properties of tibial and femoral cartilage, the location of these changes probably have more to do with the loading characteristics of the medial compartment of the knee. With continued instability, however, the joint becomes severely afflicted with degenerative

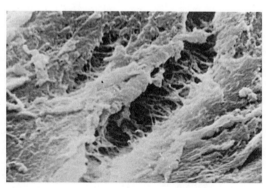

Figure 27–14. Scanning electron micrograph of a human cartilage specimen demonstrates fissure in the articular surface. This type of damage not only weakens the surface in tension but also allows large pores to be created in the surface, thus decreasing its effectiveness as a filter and its ability to provide a membrane to limit the rate of fluid exudation (original magnification ×3000). (Adapted from Armstrong CG, Mow VC: Friction, lubrication, and wear of synovial joints. *In* Owen R, Goodfellow J, Bullough P (eds): Scientific Foundations of Orthopaedics and Traumatology. London, William Heinemann Medical Books, 1980, p. 227.)

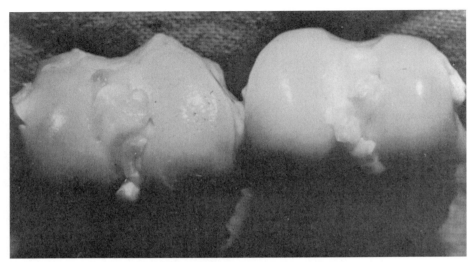

Figure 27–15. Right femur of rabbit (on the left) 12 weeks following partial meniscectomy is compared with an unoperated contralateral left knee (on the right). Pitting and ulceration are most marked in the medial femoral condyle *(left)*. (From Moskowitz RW: Osteoarthritis—studies with experimental models. Arthritis Rheum 20:S104, 1977.)

joint disease, indistinguishable from primary osteoarthritis.

Osteophytes are an early and common finding in all animal models of knee instability. In the ACL-deficient dog model, osteophyte formation on the femoral condyles occurred as early as 2 weeks after surgery, with progression to involve all surfaces with increasing size and number.[36] Similarly, in partial medial meniscectomy models, osteophytes are prominent on the medial femoral condyle (Fig. 27–15) and on the inner aspect of the medial tibial plateau (Fig. 27–16).[20] In the posterior cruciate ligament–deficient rabbit, osteophytes occurred frequently, primarily on the tibial plateaus.[19] Evidence of

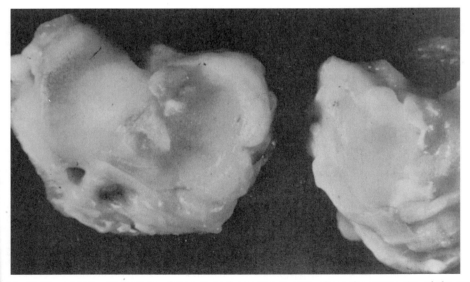

Figure 27–16. Right and left rabbit tibias. Osteophyte formation is seen along the entire rim of the medial tibial plateau of the right tibia 12 weeks after partial medial meniscectomy. The left knee shows normal soft synovial reflection. (From Moskowitz RW: Experimental models of osteoarthritis. *In* Moskowitz RW, Howell DS, Goldberg VM, Mankin HJ (eds): Osteoarthritis: Diagnosis and Medical/Surgical Management, 2nd ed. Philadelphia, WB Saunders, 1992, p. 226.)

increased synovial and periosteal cellular activity at the site of osteophyte formation suggests that instability may rapidly incite a hypertrophic response at the joint line. The prevalence of osteophytes may represent either a reparative effort of damaged cartilage, or perhaps a direct response to abnormal loading conditions. It remains unclear why osteophyte formation in animal models of knee instability is so prominent or so rapid compared to the human knee.

SUMMARY

Science has convincingly demonstrated that knee instability from injuries such as rupture of the ACL has deleterious effects on otherwise healthy articular cartilage. And although many questions remain unanswered, the study of instability has provided many valuable insights into the larger picture of degenerative joint disease. Of particular importance are the two recent comprehensive studies on this subject.[29, 30] Readers should familiarize themselves with these two studies. For now, current therapeutic modalities, both operative and nonoperative, may focus on minimizing knee instability in an attempt to repair normal knee motion and to delay the progression of osteoarthritis. With continued research into the properties and metabolism of articular cartilage, however, science may one day unlock the secrets of cartilage restoration and repair.[8]

References

1. Nordin M, Frankel VH: Biomechanics of the knee. *In* Nordin M, Frankel VH (eds): Basic Biomechanics of the Musculoskeletal System, 2nd ed., Philadelphia, Lea & Febiger, 1989, p. 115.
2. Markolf KL, Mensch JS, Amstutz HC: Stiffness and laxity of the knee: The contributions of the supporting structures. J Bone Joint Surg 50A:583–593, 1976.
3. Frankel VH, Burstein AH, Brooks DB: Biomechanics of internal derangement of the knee. Pathomechanics as determined by analysis of the instant centers of motion. J Bone Joint Surg 53A:945–962, 1971.
4. Grana WA: Physiologic and biomechanical considerations. In Larsen RL, Grana WA (eds): The Knee: Form, Function, Pathology, and Treatment. Philadelphia, W. B. Saunders, 1993, p. 51.
5. Mankin HJ, Mow VC, Buckwalter JA, et al.: Form and function of articular cartilage. *In* Simon SR (ed): Orthopaedic Basic Science. Rosemont, IL, AAOS Publishing, 1994, p. 1.
6. Lai WM, Hou JS, Mow VC: A triphasic theory for swelling and deformation behaviors of articular cartilage. J Biomech Eng 113:245–258, 1991.
7. Wu JJ, Eyre DR: Cartilage type IX collagen is cross linked by hydroxypyridinium residues. Biochem Biophys Res Commun 123:1033–1039, 1984.
8. Ratcliffe A, Mow VC: Articular cartilage. *In* Comper WD (ed): Extracellular Matrix. Amsterdam, Harwood Academic Publishers, 1996, p. 234.
9. Simunek Z, Muir H: Changes in the protein-polysaccharides of pig articular cartilage during prenatal life, development and old age. J Biochem 126:515–523, 1972.
10. Mow VC, Holmes MH, Lai WM: Fluid transport and mechanical properties of articular cartilage. J Biomech 17:377–394, 1984.
11. Mow VC, Kuei SC, Lai WM, Armstrong CG: Biphasic creep and stress relaxation of articular cartilage in compression: Theory and experiments. J Biomech Eng 102:73–84, 1980.
12. Ateshian GA, Lai WM, Zhu WB, Mow VC: An asymptotic solution for two contacting biphasic cartilage layers. J Biomech 27:1347–1360, 1994.
13. Askew MJ, Mow VC: The biomechanical function of the collagen ultrastructure of articular cartilage. J Biomech Eng 100:105–115, 1978.
14. Mow VC, Ateshian GA: Lubrication and wear of diarthrodial joints. *In* Mow VC, Hayes WC (eds): Basic Orthopaedic Biomechanics. Philadelphia, Lippincott-Raven, 1997, p. 275.
15. Mow VC, Setton LA, Ratcliffe A, et al.: Structure-function relationships of articular cartilage and the effects of joint instability and trauma on cartilage function. *In* Brandt KD (ed): Cartilage Changes in Osteoarthritis. Indianapolis, University of Indiana Press, 1990, p. 22.
16. Buckwalter JA, Mow VC, Ratcliffe A: Restoration of injured or degenerated articular cartilage. J Am Acad Orthop Surg 2(4):192–201, 1994.
17. Buckwalter JA, Mow VC: Sports injuries to articular cartilage. *In* Drez D Jr, DeLee JC (eds): Orthopaedic Sports Medicine: Principles and Practice. Philadelphia, WB Saunders, 1994, p. I:82.
18. Pond MJ, Nuki G: Experimentally-induced osteoarthritis in the dog. Ann Rheum Dis 32:387–388, 1973.
19. Davis W, Moskowitz RW: Degenerative joint changes following posterior cruciate ligament section in the rabbit. Clin Orthop 93:307–312, 1973.
20. Moskowitz RW, Davis W, Sammarco J, et al.: Experimentally induced degenerative joint lesions following partial meniscectomy in the rabbit. Arthritis Rheum 16:397–405, 1973.
21. Telhag H, Lindberg L: A method for inducing osteoarthritic changes in rabbits' knees. Clin Orthop 86:224–229, 1972.
22. Ehrlich MG, Mankin HJ, Jones H, et al.: Biochemical confirmation of an experimental osteoarthritis model. J Bone Joint Surg 57A:392–396, 1975.
23. Hall AC, Horwitz ER, Wilkins RJ: The cellular physiology of articular cartilage. Exp Physiol 81:535–545, 1996.
24. Bacharach NM, Valhmu WB, Stazzone E, et al.: Changes in articular cartilage are associated with time-dependent changes in their mechanical environment. J Biomech 28:1561–1569, 1995.
25. Urban JP, Hall AC: Physical modifiers of matrix metabolism. *In* Kuettner KE, Schleyerbach RP, Hascall VC (eds): Articular Cartilage and Osteoarthritis. New York, Raven Press, 1992, p. 393.

26. McDevitt CA, Muir H: Biochemical changes in the cartilage of the knee in experimental and natural osteoarthritis in the dog. J Bone Joint Surg 58B:94–101, 1976.

27. Bayliss MT: Proteoglycan structure in normal and osteoarthrotic human cartilage. *In* Kuettner KE, Schleyrbach R, Hascall VC (eds): Articular Cartilage Biochemistry. New York, Raven Press, 1986, p. 295.

28. Thonar EJ-MA, Bjornsson S, Kuettner KE: Age-related changes in cartilage proteoglycans. In Kuettner KE, Schleyrbach R, Hascall VC (eds): Articular Cartilage Biochemistry. New York, Raven Press, 1986, p. 273.

29. Setton LA, Mow VC, Müller FJ, et al.: Mechanical properties of canine articular cartilage are significantly altered following transection of the anterior cruciate ligament. J Orthop Res 12:451–463, 1994.

30. Setton LA, Mow VC, Howell DS: Mechanical behavior of articular cartilage in shear is altered by transection of the anterior cruciate ligament. J Orthop Res 13:473–482, 1995.

31. Sandy JD, Adams ME, Billingham ME, et al.: In vivo and in vitro stimulation of chondrocyte biosynthetic activity in early experimental osteoarthritis. Arthritis Rheum 27:388–397, 1984.

32. Myers ER, Hardingham TE, Billingham MEJ, Muir H: Changes in the tensile and compressive properties of articular cartilage in a canine model of osteoarthritis. Trans Orthop Res Soc 11:231, 1986.

33. Setton LA, Zhu W, Mow VC: The biphasic poroviscoelastic behavior of articular cartilage: Role of the surface zone in governing the compressive behavior. J Biomech 26:581–592, 1993.

34. Goldberg VM, Moskowitz RW, Malemud CJ, Mansour J: Response of articular cartilage to instability. *In* Finerman GAM, Noyes FR (eds): Biology and Biomechanics of the Traumatized Synovial Joint: The Knee as a Model. Rosemont, IL, AAOS Publishing, 1992, p. 97.

35. McDevitt C, Gilbertson E, Muir H: An experimental model of osteoarthritis: Early morphological and biochemical changes. J Bone Joint Surg 59B:24–35, 1977.

36. Moskowitz RW, Goldberg VM: Studies of osteophyte pathogenesis in experimentally induced osteoarthritis. J Rheumatol 14:311–320, 1987.

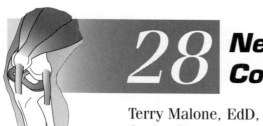

28 Neuromuscular Concepts

Terry Malone, EdD, PT, ATC, Arthur J. Nitz, PhD, PT, OCS, ECS,
Janice Kuperstein, PT, MSEd, Del-CHA, and
William Garrett, Jr., MD, PhD

*The autonomic nervous system is involved in any injury
no matter how slight.*
**—Fulkerson & Hungerford
Disorders of the Patellofemoral Joint**

*T*his brief chapter presents the classic factors of neuromuscular rehabilitation (structure and role of muscle, relationship of muscle and ligament, neural drive and inhibition, and effects of training on normal and involved muscular structure) and introduces the often underacknowledged role of the autonomic nervous system. We believe that the lack of appreciation for these arthrogenic and neurogenic responses impedes successful rehabilitation for many patients and leads to delay and frustration for many others. The opening quote is an excellent reminder for clinicians of the realities of our medical, surgical, and rehabilitative interventions.

SKELETAL MUSCLE AND KNEE

The typical initial focus of muscle function at the knee is the (appreciation of the) quadriceps femoris, serving to extend the joint. This is then followed by the flexors (hamstrings) for their role in moving the joint into flexion. However, an analysis of movement during function enables the clinician to quickly recognize that these roles are frequently reversed to control the body weight placed through the joint via dynamic actions. Secondary actions related to the kinetic chain require synchronous actions at multiple joints to allow normal function. This process is easily visualized but very difficult to analyze, particularly when the role of gravity is added to the equation. This is especially true in those muscles that are biarticulate, as they may be serving different roles at each joint simultaneously.

Researchers often differentiate muscle activation as being concentric, isometric, or eccentric. We believe it is probably better to indicate whether muscle is activated (tension developed) and provides shortening (resulting in joint approximation—concentric action); stabilization (no motion but joint control—isometric); or controlled lengthening (resulting in a controlled lengthening—eccentric action). This is a more functional sequence, particularly when agonists and antagonists are considered. During function, a strong concentric action is usually preceded by a "passive" eccentric loading, permitting a potentiation of the movement producer described as the stretch-shortening cycle by Komi in 1986[1] and serves as the cornerstone of plyometric training technique.[2] Further examination of this concept increases awareness of the role of muscle to absorb or dissipate shock (eccentric or stretch action) while also preparing the stretched but activated muscle for response. It is our opinion that these absorbing actions do not receive adequate focus in many rehabilitation protocols, particularly when actions are required at higher intensities as speed and load are increased. Eccentric loads are the highest demands placed on the muscle-tendon unit and are thus often the most difficult for the patient to tolerate.[3]

STRUCTURAL-FUNCTIONAL RELATIONSHIPS

The muscle-tendon unit is designed to generate tension and is controlled through

399

an intricate neural process of efferent (to the muscle) and afferent (feedback from tissues to the neural system) fibers. The afferents thus have the ability to impact directly and indirectly on the efferent signal to the muscle.[4] Janda[4] describes direct effects as those typically related to pain and swelling or effusion, which results in muscle inhibition and atrophy. Indirect effects (inhibition) are a result of impaired afferentiation influencing multiple muscles often remote to the specific site of involvement. He believes that indirect inhibition may include reprogramming of motor patterns, as they may be seen following significant insults to ligaments or articular structure (anterior cruciate ligament [ACL] rupture, patellar dislocation, articular cartilage injury, and so on).

The process of afferent information being transmitted from the knee has been outlined by numerous authors. The arrangement and distinct patterns of innervation were presented by Gardiner (1948)[5] and Kennedy et al. (1982),[6] and reflexive concepts were presented by Solomonow and D'Ambrosia[7] examining the linkage of ligaments to muscular activation. Nyland et al.[8] describe this overall system in detail. This information is outlined in Table 28–1 and is diagrammed in Figure 28–1.[9]

Each of the receptors provides specific information, with the complete picture only seen when all facets are normal. This is nicely demonstrated by the traditional classification scheme, which includes four distinct mechanoreceptors. Type I receptors are of a low threshold; are slow-adapting, which enables them to provide continuous information; and are more densely represented in proximal joint capsules. Type II receptors are quite sensitive to dynamic joint position changes (tension, acceleration, and deceleration) and are of low threshold. Type III receptors are primarily in structural ligaments, are slow-adapting, and have a high threshold. Type IV are free nerve endings, which provide information related to pain and inflammation. Quite appropriately, Nyland et al. state, "There appears to be an intricate relationship involving peripheral mechanoreceptors found in inert and contractile tissues of the knee. This relationship should not be ignored during treatment planning."[8]

Joint afferent information is added to afferent data from other tissues (eg, muscle, skin) and other systems (visual and vestibular), thus enabling the patients to have awareness of position and the ability to purposefully move or alter position in relation to the acquired data. These actions are often referred to as proprioception (joint position sense) and kinesthesia (awareness of joint motion).[9] These activities are vital to the normal function of the patient and are frequently altered following insult to the knee.

Kennedy et al.[6] theorized that the failure of mechanoreceptor feedback following ligamentous injury of the knee (laxity) led to reduced or absent reflex muscular splinting, rendering the joint more vulnerable to repetitive major and minor injuries, and ultimately to progressive joint instability. Animal studies conducted by O'Connor et al.[10, 11] have partially confirmed the close link between joint afference and the protective effects of proprioceptive information in the event of joint injury and instability. These studies established that some measure of adaptability in the presence of injury is built into the joint afferent-efferent system. Proprioceptive input from one source or another enables the animal with an unstable joint to organize movement strategies that lessen tissue stress and minimize otherwise undampened joint reactive forces. This fact may explain why proprioceptive and kinesthetic tasks often seem to be the most beneficial component of the rehabilitation protocol for patients who have sustained joint injury.

RELATIONSHIP OF LIGAMENT TO MUSCLE

The structural pattern of ligament is specific to function and location. Collagen fibers are typically aligned parallel to the length of the ligament, enabling it to efficiently resist the tensile loads of function. A key feature of these structures is their nonlinear mechanical responses to loading. Frisen et al.[12] described this in their early work in 1969 as a theoretical model of nonlinear elasticity as displayed by Figure 28–2. Frank and colleagues have advanced our knowledge of this process and apply the concept of viscoelasticity to describe ligament function.[13, 14] Their work has defined the traditional stress-strain curve often used in ligament applications as seen in Figure 28–3. We must appreciate the actual role of ligament as that

● Table 28–1. Joint Receptors

Receptor	Location	Description	Sensitivity	Distribution (of Receptor Type)	Functional Classification	Parent Axon (Fiber Diameter, Conduction Velocity)
Pacinian corpuscles	Fibrous layer of capsule, on capsule-synovium border, close to small blood vessels	Single terminal within lamellated encapsulation; appears in clusters of five or less (20–40 × 150–250 μm cylindrical)	Sensitive to high frequency vibration (>60 Hz), acceleration, and high velocity changes in joint position; possible sensitivity to hemohydraulic, transient events and rapid contractile events of adjacent muscles	Found in all joints examined; sole corpuscular receptor in laryngeal and middle ear joints; greater density in distal than in proximal joints	Very rapidly adapting (RA); very low mechanical threshold	Group II (8–12 μm, 49 ms; terminal branch at 3–5 μm diameter
Golgi-Mazzoni corpuscles	Inner surface of joint capsule between fibrous layer and subcapsular fibroadipose tissue	Multiple terminating endings within thin encapsulation (30 × 200 μm cylindrical)	Sensitive to compression of joint capsule in plane perpendicular to its inner surface; insensitive to stretching capsule	Knee joint and many others likely; may have specific distribution within joint capsule	Slowly adapting (SA); response is linear function of compressive stress on capsule; low mechanical threshold	Group II–III (5–8 μm; estimate ≈30 ms)
Ruffini endings	Fibrous layer of capsule; few present in extrinsic ligaments	Spray-type terminal endings within thin encapsulation, having investment of collagen fibers (330 × 300–800 μm, two to six endings per axon)	Sensitive to capsule stretching along either of its long axes within capsular plane, direction and speed of capsular stretch, intracapsular fluid pressure change, amplitude and velocity of joint position change	Few present in distal joints; greater density in proximal joints; concentrated in capsular regions of most stress	Slowly adapting (SA); low mechanical threshold; response is linear function of axial components of capsular plane stress	Group I–II (13–17 or 8–12 μm, 51 ms)
Golgi ligament endings (Golgi tendon organ-like)	Extrinsic and intrinsic ligaments; adjacent to bony attachments of ligaments	Thick encapsulation; profuse branching (100 × 600 μm total terminal spread)	Sensitive to tension or stretch on ligaments	Present in most joints except cervical vertebral, laryngeal, ossicular ligaments	Slowly adapting (SA); low-to-high mechanical threshold	Group I (13–17 μm; estimate ≈51 ms)
Free nerve endings (nociceptive and non-nociceptive)	Fibrous capsule, ligaments subsynovial capsule, synovium, fat pads	Thin, bare nerve endings of small myelinated or unmyelinated axons; profuse branching	One type sensitive to non-noxious mechanical stress; other type sensitive to noxious mechanical or biochemical stimuli	Present in all joints examined but density varies with joint component; most joints have relatively higher density in ligaments	Slowly adapting (SA); low-to-high mechanical threshold	Group III–IV (2–5 μm, <2 μm; 2.5–20 ms)

From Malone TR, McPoil T, Nitz AJ: Orthopaedic and Sports Physical Therapy, 3rd ed. St. Louis, CV Mosby, 1997, p. 52.

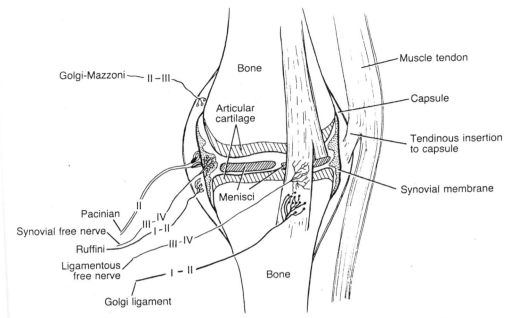

Figure 28–1. Composite diagram of total joint innervation pattern, showing interrelations of afferent receptors. (From Malone TR, McPoil T, Nitz AJ: Orthopaedic and Sports Physical Therapy, 3rd ed. St. Louis, CV Mosby, 1997, p. 51.)

of guiding and directing normal movements, while providing significant restraint at the extremes of the range of motion to further abnormal joint displacement.

Musculature is required to support the ligamentous system and functions synergistically to enable joint control. The stiffness of the joint to displacement is a combination of active elements (musculature if activated) and passive elements (ligamentous and soft tissue envelope of muscle). Ligament alone is incapable of total control under the loads seen in high demand situations, as its ultimate strength is greatly enhanced through active muscle.[15] This was further confirmed by Pope et al.,[16] who elegantly demonstrated

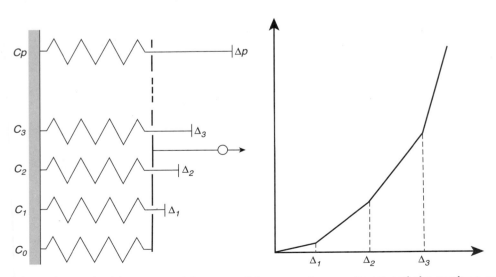

Figure 28–2. Nonlinear elasticity expressed by sequential, progressive recruitment and the resultant nonlinear stress-strain curve.

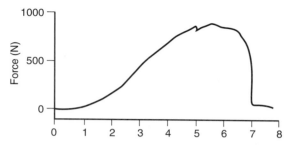

Figure 28–3. Traditional stress-strain curve. Significant joint displacement occurs prior to complete disruption.

that the time required for efferent response would preclude a protective role for muscle unless the muscle was activated prior to stress. It is our opinion that while ligamentous structures are most important at the extremes of motion, their presence is required to maintain optimal relationships throughout joint movement. This combination (ligament and musculature) can only function well when appropriate afferent data allow proper efferent drive to the active elements.

Factors that would thus create alterations in this process include loss or inappropriate afferent information, inhibitory influences to the efferents, altered muscle-tendon structure or capability (injury or fatigue), altered articular or biomechanical structure, neurologic damage or injury, and other modifiers of ligament and muscle. The ability of muscle or ligament to function in an isolated manner rather than in its interrelated pattern is quickly dispelled when the complexity of human motion is examined. As greater than two thirds of all nerve fibers in mixed nerve connecting the spinal cord with muscle are afferent, we must conclude that feedback is vital to normal function.[17] Although some afferents are directly connected to enable monosynaptic reflexive action (tendon jerk), many internuncial connections exist to allow inhibition of antagonists and facilitation of synergists enhancing function. The stretch reflex involves a sustained tension within the muscle-tendon unit, resulting in excitation to resist further stretch (thus protecting the muscle-tendon unit).[17] These actions have led investigators to consider the abilities of muscles to work as agonist or antagonist to specific ligaments. The most examined of these relationships is that of the cruciate ligaments and the quadriceps and hamstring muscles. Numerous authors

have discussed the antagonist actions of the quadriceps and the ACL. Arms et al.[18] and Draganich et al. were early presentations of the ACL induced forces with quadriceps action.[19] Renstrom et al.[20] examined ACL strain with quadriceps and hamstring action, better defining angle-to-effect relationships. Some authors speculate that this ACL-quadriceps relationship can be a part of the actual cause of injury to the ligament. Although hypothesized, other authors have demonstrated that activation of the quadriceps "stiffens" the joint and actually serves to require greater load to disrupt the ligament.[21, 22] The hamstrings are seen as agonists to the ACL, absorbing energy and thus decreasing injury. As outlined by Renstrom, the hamstrings, when activated, decrease ACL strain significantly, including when co-contraction with the quadriceps is present.[20] These results are supported by Yasuda and Sasaki[21] and therefore clinicians often attempt to use these activations to minimize early strain to the ACL graft. Markolf et al.[22] have further investigated the concepts of co-contraction and have demonstrated increased knee stiffness (by a factor of two to four times), resulting in decreased laxity. Numerous others have documented similar results, implying the hypothesis that these actions may be quite important in ligament injury and may possibly serve a role in prevention.[23–25]

The role of fatigue presents an interesting factor, particularly as we view the hamstrings. Since the hamstrings are more fast twitch–oriented, they may be more sensitive to fatigue development, thus permitting greater opportunity for quadriceps dominance to be present. McNair et al.[26] describe hamstring stiffness and function in ACL-deficient patients and hypothesize on the importance of these structures. Huston and Wojtys[27] present the neuromuscular characteristics of ACL-deficient females and believe that these patients may be more quadriceps dominant or oriented than their noninjured peers or male counterparts. We would like to add the hypothesis that hamstring flexibility and strength play a role in this process. Female basketball players have significantly more ACL injuries than their male counterparts[28] while demonstrating significantly greater flexibility (unpublished data, 1990–1992: in intercollegiate basketball participants, females averaged more than 100 degrees of flexibility while males averaged less than 80 degrees). Some of these athletes were able to hyperextend their knees 10 degrees and often stood in such a pattern at rest. Anecdotally, we refer to this as "living on your ligaments," since the ACL is under larger loads with minimal muscular support in this position.

Fatigue is also quite likely to alter the ability of the soft tissues to dissipate loads and therefore to require the other structures to be forced into a loaded state. This could play a role in articular problems or other functional alterations at the knee. One could see this analogous to decreased muscular control following strenuous exercise affecting bone, as presented in Figure 28–4.

Neural Drive and Inhibition

Following injury, a key question relates to initial response to and implications for function. Magnetic resonance imaging has provided a much better appreciation of injury and resultant underlying bony response but also the inherent limitations of MRI itself.[29] The loss of primary restraint, bony contusion, articular insult, hemarthrosis, and possible concomitant structural disrup-

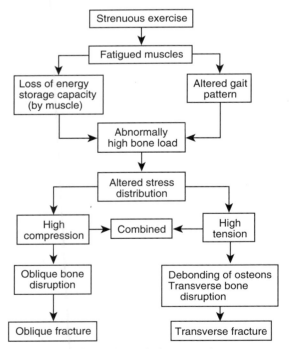

Figure 28–4. Effects of muscle fatigue on bone.

tion all present specific challenges to the rehabilitation specialist. Early inflammatory activities and significant inhibition through pain and pressure afferents often dramatically limit muscular recruitment (neural drive inhibition). The classic work related to this topic is by de Andrade et al. from 1965.[30] Their premise was that joint distension resulted in reflexive muscle inhibition. Spencer et al.[31] further elucidated these actions when they demonstrated a progressive loss of neural drive through progressive infusion (effusion) of the joint. Interestingly, they showed that the earliest detected alterations were to the vastus medialis with a relatively small level of effusion.

Numerous authors have investigated the effects of effusion on the proprioception "system." Barrack and associates have examined this in the loss of the ACL and also in relationship to laxity.[32, 33] Freeman et al.[34] demonstrated how changes at the ankle affect the function of the entire lower extremity and coined the term *functional instability*, a state ascribed to the loss of proprioceptive capabilities.[34] Guido et al.[35] examined the effects of chronic effusion of the knee joint on proprioception. They used a single-subject design and evaluated active and passive repositioning as a measure of proprioception in a subject with a chronic knee effusion. Measurements were taken prior to, 15 minutes after, and 24 hours after aspiration of 60 mL of aspirant. Interestingly, the passive repositioning reading improved after aspiration but the active one did not, whereas both readings were back to preaspiration levels at 24 hours as the effusion re-developed. The authors speculate that this aspiration enables a "resetting" of the capsular afferent system, resulting in the passive improvement, but that the active system relies on other inputs and is not solely dependent on capsule. However, factors other than the isolated loss of joint afference contribute to the observed muscle recruitment inhibition associated with joint inflammation and instability. One likely factor is muscle denervation, for which research and clinical observations are beginning to emerge.[36–38]

The selective effects of inhibition are difficult to explain. Quadriceps femoris maximal torque output is significantly decreased in the ACL-deficient patient.[39, 40] These changes are also reflected by atrophy resulting in loss of cross-sectional area.[41, 42] However, these changes do not correlate well, as the loss in area is much less than the loss in strength. A 5 percent loss in cross-sectional area led to approximately a 25 percent decrease in peak torque assessment.[39] Some authors believe that the cruciate ligament injury leads to diminished central neural drive as evidenced by alterations in the electromyogram.[43]

Muscle atrophy following knee joint injury or surgery is a ubiquitous observation that has historically been attributed to disuse. However, the rate at which the atrophy progresses following insult suggests a neurologic explanation rather than simple inhibition or disuse.[44] It has been our experience that some patients have significantly more difficulty than others in regaining normal motor and functional patterns of movement following surgery of the knee. During the late 1970s, electromyographic changes following extra-articular and intra-articular ACL surgical procedures were investigated (Malone, unpublished data). Nearly all (more than 90 percent) demonstrated considerable alterations in neural drive and denervation potentials in the surgical limb, but also approximately 50 percent presented with changes reflective of denervation on the nonsurgical limb, although of a lesser degree than seen in the surgical limb. These data have been confirmed by Nitz[36] and correspond to similar findings in patients following meniscectomy.[38] Electrophysiologic testing (electromyography) has documented evidence of motor denervation in lower extremity muscles following knee surgery accomplished with[38] and without[45] pneumatic tourniquet application and after ACL tear attended by significant capsular effusion (Nitz, unpublished data). The compressive and ischemic effects of tourniquet application are the likely explanation for muscle impairments observed after surgery accomplished with pneumatic cuff use.[45, 46] Pedowitz and co-workers review experimental and clinical data ascribed to tourniquet use and conclude that tourniquet ischemia or compression does have significant sequelae, which can often result in significant functional alterations.[47, 48] Somewhat unfortunately, we have collected data from patients post-surgery without tourniquet use that still display the aforementioned alterations, which leads us to recognize that multiple factors are involved with this complex process.

Although early functional changes can be explained through acute injury, surgical or surgically related trauma; the long-term effects are more difficult to identify. Cicotti et al.[49] elegantly evaluated and described the electromyograph profiles of normal subjects, ACL-deficient patients, and ACL-reconstructed patients. Their findings support ACL reconstruction, as those patients' profiles were very similar to the profiles of the normal subjects, whereas ACL-deficient patients had significant alterations. They also describe a coordinated response between the hamstrings and quadriceps that was present regardless of the ACL, thus indicating that receptors outside of the ligament exist to either provide or assist in conveyance of afferent information. Dvir et al.[50] reiterate these ideas in their evaluation of static position sense in ACL-reconstructed patients, as no significant differences existed 1 year postoperatively. It has been our experience that ACL-reconstructed patients begin to look and feel more normal approximately 4 to 6 months postoperatively. Our earlier discussed findings of denervation potentials in our postoperative patients, interestingly, typically dissipate during this time frame (Malone, Nitz, and Benz, unpublished data). Although the precise cause of muscle denervation observed after ACL injury (prior to surgery) and following ACL reconstruction accomplished without benefit of the pneumatic tourniquet is not known with certainty, there is evidence to indicate that the best explanation is *neurogenic inflammation*. This correlates well with the hypothesis offered by Levine et al.[51] in their description of reflex neurogenic inflammation. Levine et al. have shown in an animal model that soft tissue inflammation in peripheral tissues leads to spatially remote inflammatory responses, which affects the joints. This response has been linked experimentally to the development of arthritis and is mediated by biogenic amines (histamines) or a wide variety of other possible potent neurotransmitters such as substance P, vasoactive intestinal polypetide (VIP), and calcitonin gene related peptide (CGRP). In sufficiently strong concentrations following joint injury or surgery, these biochemical substances may have a denervating effect on the motor end-plate. It is reasonable to suggest that the profound muscle atrophy so often noted following knee joint injury or surgery and the electromyographically documented evidence of denervation in patients may be partially explained by *neurogenic inflammation*.

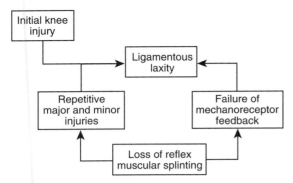

Figure 28–5. Hypothesized neurogenic contribution to progressive knee instability. (Modified from Kennedy JC, Alexander IJ, Hayes KC: Nerve supply of the human knee and its functional importance. Am J Sports Med 10:329, 1982.)

It is important to note that the observed signs and symptoms of muscle change do not appear to be of the classically described reflex sympathetic dystrophy or complex regional pain variety. Rather, evidence indicates that they are of an as-yet autonomic or neurotransmitter-mediated process.

Motor denervation may further affect the protective muscle responses (reflexive) and the voluntary muscle activations that normally dampen joint reactive forces during functional movement (Fig. 28–5). Levine et al. examined the humoral and neural factors related to injury and demonstrated the contralateral limb's response.[51] Their data support a reflex neurogenic inflammation that was neurally mediated through a spinal cord level. We would propose that some of the challenges seen during the first weeks and months following significant insult (injury or surgery) are related to this neurally mediated process. This helps explain the general pattern seen with so many of these patients and might also better enable us to tailor our rehabilitation to address these specific autonomic factors.

BRIEF CASE REPORT

The following brief clinical description is an example of a patient who experienced rehabilitation difficulty as a result of muscle denervation and impairment. Patient JD is a 44-year-old woman who underwent left knee arthroscopy for meniscal repair in February 1998. She began physical therapy approximately 2 weeks following surgery, at which point she exhibited severe muscle atrophy (thigh girth difference) and residual joint effusion (2+). Active range of motion was limited to 15 degrees of extension and 40 degrees of flexion and the patient could not accomplish a straight leg raise without significant effort and difficulty. The quality of quadriceps muscle contraction was considered to be far less than optimal. Because the patient was experiencing severe difficulty with motor recruitment 4 weeks after arthroscopy, electromyographic assessment was performed. The initial electromyographic findings of interest were severe (3/4+) fibrillations and positive sharp waves (evidence of denervation) in the quadriceps muscle and mild-to-moderate level denervation in the tibial and peroneal innervated leg muscles. Motor recruitment of the quadriceps muscle was severely affected, whereas the leg muscles below the knee showed moderate amounts of motor unit impairment. No abnormalities were identified in the hamstrings or paraspinals. The interpretation of these findings was that they best represented evidence of neurogenic inflammation, as a tourniquet was not used for the surgery and the patient had no clinical or other indicators of nerve root lesion. The presence of this level of muscle impairment radically altered the intensity and timing of early rehabilitative efforts so as not to give rise to secondary soft tissue breakdown (eg, patellar tendinitis, excessive quadriceps muscle fatigue).

Eight weeks after arthroscopy, the protracted course of rehabilitation led the patient to seek further confirmation of her muscle impairment. A second electromyogram was obtained at a different facility, which identified 1–2+ fibrillations and positive sharp waves primarily in the quadriceps muscles. The number of motor units recruited was reduced by 25–50 percent and the percentage of polyphasic motor units (evidence of re-innervation) was significantly elevated. The tibial and peroneal innervated muscle abnormalities noted with the initial study had essentially resolved by the 8-week mark. The improvement in the patient's electrophysiologic findings roughly corresponded to her clinical evidence of progression, which allowed the rehabilitative protocol to be intensified accordingly (without unnecessarily compromising further soft tissue healing). Four months following initial evaluation, a final electromyogram was obtained to track the patient's electrophysiologic progress. At this time, all denervation potentials (fibrillations, positive sharp waves) had resolved. Motor unit recruitment continued to be characterized by increased polyphasicity (30–40 percent) and reduced numbers of motor units during maximal interference (60–80 percent) of normal. At this point, the patient made the most obvious improvements in girth acquisition and indicators of muscle performance (open and closed chain, fatigue resistance). The patient was ultimately discharged with $4+/5$ quadriceps muscle strength and had returned to full functional activity level.

This case serves to indicate the unfortunate prolongation associated with impaired muscle recruitment, which often follows knee injury or surgery. Since denervated muscle is both weak and easily fatigable, the clinician should be alert for evidence of deleterious response to rehabilitative efforts (eg, inflammation, inordinate joint discomfort, deterioration in muscle performance).[52] We have found high amplitude neuromuscular electrical stimulation and electromyographic biofeedback to be two rehabilitative measures which promote physiologic motor unit recruitment capabilities when the patient has sustained denervation.[53–57]

EFFECTS OF TRAINING AND REHABILITATION

Rehabilitation following ACL surgery has seen enormous changes since the classic article of Paulos et al. in 1981.[58] During this era, the primary limiting factor in rehabilitation was the concern for the healing graft and fixation of this developing structure to the tibia and femur. Unfortunately, many of these patients developed secondary problems related to limited range of motion and soft tissue restraints. Shelbourne and Nitz published their recommendation for accelerated rehabilitation in 1990,[59] which was predicated on their noncompliant patients'

outcomes, which were retrospectively compared with those of their more compliant peers.[59] They have followed these patients and additional cohorts and have provided additional supporting publications.[60] They now espouse a process of surgical intervention only after the initial inflammatory state is minimized (essentially full range of motion), implementation of a rehabilitation sequence that prevents iatrogenic complications, restoration of full range of motion, and restoration of normal function through a progression of activities. Quite interesting are their data reflecting that the average time to return to full athletic competition is 6.2 months.

Although the acceptance of closed chain exercises as being most efficacious in ACL rehabilitation has been widespread, we question the overly broad interpretation of these activities. Since closed chain actions are typically multi-joint oriented, the body is provided additional opportunities for patterns of substitution. These patterns of recruitment are often impaired or altered, as discussed previously, following insult to the knee structures. Limbird and Shiavi demonstrated altered sequences of muscle recruitment (electromyographic-profile) in gait in ACL-deficient patients and further demonstrated functional alterations associated with pivoting.[61, 62] Functional outcome is correlated to muscular performance, but the chicken-or-the-egg question is always valid. Seto et al.[63] assessed ACL-reconstructed patients in a long-term study. Strength, stability, function, and muscle activity were assessed with significant correlation between quadriceps and hamstring strength and functional activities. In fact, muscle performance correlated better than did stability with function. Wexler et al.[64] indicated that a progression of alterations develops in ACL deficiency, which demonstrates the importance of intervention but also the alterations of muscle patterns (recruitment) used by these patients. The difficulty in designing a protocol for rehabilitation is the need to address the specific needs of the individual patient but also using a scientific rather than an anecdotal approach. Functional return requires the quadriceps to absorb and dissipate forces, thus avoiding the development of effusion or other joint reactions. Shelbourne and Gray[60] recommend that patients achieve a 65 percent level of quadriceps performance prior to initiation of demanding functional tasks. This is in agreement with our recommendation of 70 to 75 percent for general patients in the outpatient environment.[65] If patients attempt to run or perform pivoting tasks with lower levels of quadriceps outputs, the result is often effusion and pain. Snyder-Mackler et al.[66] speak to this issue, as their measurements of joint kinematics were correlated to quadriceps strength even in the early postoperative period. One of their key findings is that the strength of the quadriceps had a significant relation to functional recovery, and that closed chain exercise alone did not provide adequate stimulus for quadriceps development. This is likewise in agreement with our previous work, as an integrative approach of open chain (enabling isolation and determination of neural drive) and closed chain (enabling the integration of normalized muscle into proper recruitment sequences) exercise provides the best method for comprehensive rehabilitation. Other authors use the terminology of "neuromuscular control" as a guiding principle.[67] Some would describe this as a program that focuses on development or redevelopment of proprioceptive and kinesthetic awareness, dynamic stability, reactive control, and functional motor patterns, much as is seen in traditional functional progressions. Wojtys et al.[68] demonstrate the specificity of training, which points toward the need for variety yet focus in rehabilitation. We recommend an integrative approach cognizant of afferent feedback and neuromuscular demands to enable an expeditious and safe return to function following joint insult. The following case study illustrates these concepts in an applied fashion.

CASE REPORT

JJ was referred to our clinic 6 months after intra-articular ACL reconstruction (patellar tendon graft, right knee). He had full range of motion and approximately equal patellar mobility bilaterally. He was referred by a community physician because he continued to be unable to progress into running activities. During the previous 8 weeks, the patient had attempted to initiate a series of running and jogging maneuvers with no success. After each attempt, his knee would swell and would be painful for 2 to 3 days.

Review of the patient's rehabilitation protocol revealed that all activities had been of a closed kinetic chain design to minimize anterior tibial shear. In our experience, this patient's profile is representative of a lack of quadriceps "capacity" related to both maximal efforts and eccentric absorbency. We frequently see patients complaining of swelling and pain after exercise when they have allowed "joint abuse" to occur. This is our expression for situations in which patients expose their joint to abnormal loads when their quadriceps do not have adequate ability to absorb the loads or attempt to do things beyond the endurance of the muscle group. We recommend assessing the patient's quadriceps strength both concentrically and eccentrically. Concentric assessment is typically done at 60 degrees per second and at 300 degrees per second, whereas eccentric assessment is accomplished at 60 degrees per second. Assessment is performed in a seated position and is of an open kinetic chain pattern. The typical patient at 6 months post-ACL reconstruction should develop approximately 80 percent of the noninvolved quadriceps.

JJ was able to generate 48 percent of his normal quadriceps at 60 degrees per second and 55 percent at 300 degrees per second concentrically. His eccentric values were approximately 55 percent, but these values are not as reliable in a single test collection according to our data. Interestingly, he was able to do a single-leg hop approximately to 85 percent of his normal limb with some difficulty upon landing. These data (15 percent closed chain deficit versus a 50 percent deficit open chain) are fairly consistent with our normative data, reflecting approximately a factor of two to three times greater effect of open chain versus closed chain exercise. We believe that this is related to the ability of closed chain exercise to allow greater substitution, whereas open chain exercise provides much greater isolation. It has been our experience that 70 to 75 percent concentric performance is required for most patients prior to significant running activities being tolerated (Shelbourne and Gray[60] recommend 65 percent).

Our recommendation for JJ was to add open chain quadriceps strengthening exercises to his protocol. He began these in the lower portion of the range of motion (90 degrees to 30 degrees), which enabled him to use heavier loads (which we believe are helpful to provide adequate stimulus) while protecting his graft. We also had him add single-leg maximal eccentric exercises in a similar range of motion. This was accomplished by concentrically extending with both legs followed by a single leg return or lowering and is required to provide maximal stimulus to the eccentric elements, as they are otherwise limited to what is accomplished concentrically. The activity would thus always be submaximal for the eccentric elements if this exercise were not added. We also had him do leg presses in a similar fashion (bilateral extension, single leg return) to enable maximal eccentric loading. He was to perform three sets of 10 repetitions three or four days weekly at his high school for the next month.

After 1 month, JJ's concentric values were in the 70 percent level and his eccentric values were greater than 65 percent. He was provided a running progression but one that is somewhat different than typically perceived. He was to run on his high school track in a straight line. His sequence was to increase speed smoothly over 10 yards, run hard (on the ball of the foot, or "up on the toes like a true sprint") for 40 yards, followed by a gradual decrease of speed over 10 yards. This pattern has enabled us to introduce running more efficiently and safely for many patients. The pattern requires heavy muscular effort but is not as likely to cause joint irritation because staying on the ball of the foot helps keep the knee flexed and requires absorbency of the musculature, whereas landing flat-footed or on the heel (as in jogging) is more likely to provide inadequately dampened impact loads. He was to introduce five to eight repetitions of these "runs" and ice after exercise (running and weight lifting).

Fortunately, he progressed quite nicely and began an overall progression to enable his return to basketball. He gradually introduced his skill acquisition or reacquisition over the next 3 months. It has been our experience that most high-demand or high-skill activities require approximately 3 to 4 months of performance prior to the

individual's performing at what he or she perceives to be normal (similar to Shelbourne and Gray's[60] finding that the average return is accomplished at 6.2 months with activities begun at 6 weeks). JJ returned to his desired activities 4 months after introduction of the integrated activities, including open chain and maximal eccentric exercises. His concentric values were greater than 85 percent and his eccentric value was 80+ percent on his return to sport. This case illustrates the conclusion of Snyder-Mackler et al. that quadriceps strength is required and that closed chain exercise training alone may not provide adequate stimulus.[66] This has been our experience and the reason we recommend an integrated approach to rehabilitation. The functional progression model is presented as Table 28–2.

SUMMARY

In this chapter, we provided information to remind and alert clinicians of the extent of neurologic involvement following joint injury and surgery. Successful recovery following knee injury or surgery requires that the clinician design rehabilitation activities that meet the specific needs of the individual patient. Avoidance of pitfalls such as joint reactivity to impaired muscle dampening (eg, effusion, soft tissue inflammation, impingement) or deterioration in performance resulting from muscle fatigue is contingent upon careful patient evaluation prior to rehabilitation and constant monitoring of the patient's condition. The appropriate inclu-

Table 28–2. Functional Progression: The Knee

Range of motion
Strength
Progressive weight-bearing
Balance and proprioceptive activities
Functional strengthening
Straight running (meniscal or loading problems)
Straight jogging (non-meniscal or impact concerns)
Sprinting running
Agility drills (related to needs)
Cutting/pivoting actions
Specific activities (demanded by sport or task)
Progressive return to sport or task

sion of isolated or total extremity patterns of movement and the intensity and duration of individual bouts of rehabilitation activities are determined by the evidence-based clinical decision-maker on the basis of thorough initial examination and regular assessment of patient response.

The authors have provided case report examples of the value of careful electrophysiologic assessment (electromyography and nerve conduction study) and how such information serves to provide a tailored plan of rehabilitation for the patient following injury and surgical intervention for the knee.

References

1. Komi PV: The stretch-shortening cycle and human power output. *In* Jones NL, McCartney N, McComas AJ (eds): Human Muscle Power. Champlain, IL, Human Kinetics, 1986, p. 27.
2. Malone TR, Garrett WE Jr: Exercise and assessment equipment for the knee: appropriate use and function. *In* Griffin LY (ed): Rehabilitation of the Injured Knee, 2nd ed. St. Louis, CV Mosby, 1995, p. 72.
3. Henriksson J, Hickner RC: Adaptations in skeletal muscle in response to endurance training. *In* Harries M, Williams C, Stanish WD, Micheli LJ (eds.): Oxford Textbook of Sports Medicine, 2nd ed. Oxford, England, Oxford University Press, 1998, p. 1.1.3:45.
4. Janda V: Muscle strength in relation to muscle length, pain and muscle imbalance. *In* Harms-Ringdahl K (ed): Muscle Strength, Vol 8. New York, Churchill Livingstone, 1993, p. 83.
5. Gardiner E: The innervation of the knee joint. Anat Rec 101:109, 1948.
6. Kennedy JC, Alexander IJ, Hayes KC: Nerve supply of the human knee and its functional importance. Am J Sports Med 10:329, 1982.
7. Solomonow J, D'Ambrosia R: Neural reflex arcs and muscle control of knee stability and motion. *In* Scott WN (ed): Ligament and Extensor Mechanisms of the Knee: Diagnosis and Treatment. St. Louis, CV Mosby, 1991.
8. Nyland J, Brosky T, Currier D, et al.: Review of the afferent neural system of the knee and its contribution of motor learning. J Orthop Sports Phys Ther 19:2, 1994.
9. Grigg P: Peripheral neural mechanisms in proprioception. J Sports Rehab 3:2, 1994.
10. O'Connor B, Palmoski MJ, Brandt KD: Neurogenic acceleration of degenerative joint lesions. J Bone Joint Surg 67A:562, 1985.
11. O'Connor B, Visco D, Brandt K, et al: Neurogenic acceleration of osteoarthritis. J Bone Joint Surg 74A:367, 1992.
12. Frisen J, Magi M, Sonnerup L, et al.: Rheological analysis of soft collagenous tissue. Part I: Theoretical considerations. J Biomech 2:13, 1969.
13. Frank C, Amiel D, Woo SLY, et al.: Normal ligament properties and ligament healing. Clin Orthop Rel Res 196:15, 1985.
14. Frank C, Woo SL, Amiel D, et al: Medical collateral ligament healing. Am J Sports Med 11:379, 1983.
15. Wojtys EM, Wylie BB, Huston LJ: The effects of muscle fatigue on neuromuscular function and anterior tibial translation in healthy knees. Am J Sports 24:615, 1996.
16. Pope MH, Johnson RJ, Brown DW, et al: The role of the musculature in injuries to the medial collateral ligament. J Bone Joint Surg 61A:398, 1979.
17. Garrett WE Jr, Kuester DJ, Best TM: Skeletal muscle and the knee joint. *In* Gordon S (ed): Biology and Biomechanics of the Synovial Joint: The Knee. Chicago, American Academy of Orthopaedic Surgeons, 1991.
18. Arms SW, Pope MH, Johnson RJ, et al: The biomechanics of anterior cruciate ligament rehabilitation and reconstruction. Am J Sports Med 12:8, 1984.
19. Aune AK, Schaff P, Nordletten L: Contraction of knee flexors and extensors in alpine skiing related to the backward fall mechanism of injury to the anterior cruciate ligament. Scand J Med Sci Sports 5:165, 1995.
20. Renstrom P, Arms SW, Stanwyck TS, et al.: Strain within the anterior cruciate ligament during hamstring and quadriceps activity. Am J Sports Med 14:83, 1986.
21. Yasuda K, Sasaki T: Exercise after anterior cruciate ligament reconstruction: The force exerted on the tibia by the separate isometric contractions of the quadriceps or the hamstrings. Clin Orthop 220:275, 1987.
22. Markolf KL, Graff-Radford A, Amstutz HC: In vivo knee stability: A quantitative assessment using an instrumented clinical testing apparatus. J Bone Joint Surg 60A:664, 1978.
23. Draganich LF, Jaeger RJ, Kralj AR: Coactivation of the hamstring and quadriceps during extension of the knee. J Bone Joint Surg 71A:1075, 1989.
24. Baratta R, Solomonow M, Shou BH, et al: Muscular coactivation: The role of the antagonist musculature in maintaining knee stability. Am J Sports Med 16:113, 1988.
25. Giove TP, Miller SJ III, Kent B, et al.: Non-operative treatment of the torn anterior cruciate ligament. J Bone Joint Surg 65A:184, 1983.
26. McNair PJ, Wood GA, Marshall RN: Stiffness of the hamstring muscles and its relationship to function in anterior cruciate deficient individuals. Clin Biomech 7:131, 1992.
27. Huston LJ, Wojtys EM: Neuromuscular characteristics in the ACL-deficient female. Am J Sports Med 24:427, 1996.
28. Malone TR, Hardaker WT, Garrett WE, et al: Relationship of gender to anterior cruciate ligament injuries in intercollegiate basketball players. J So Orthop Assoc 2:36, 1993.
29. Adalberth T, Roos H, Lauren M, et al: Magnetic resonance imaging, scintigraphy, and arthroscopic evaluation of traumatic hemarthrosis of the knee. Am J Sports Med 25:231, 1997.
30. de Andrade JR, Grant C, Dixon A: Joint distension and reflex muscle inhibition. J Bone Joint Surg 2A:313, 1965.
31. Spencer JD, Hayes KC, Alexander IJ: Knee joint effusion and quadriceps reflex inhibition in man. Arch Phys Med Rehabil 65:171, 1984.
32. Barrack R, Bruckner J, Kneis J, et al: The outcome of nonoperatively treated complete tears of the anterior cruciate ligament in active young adults. Clin Orthop 259:192, 1990.

33. Barrack R, Skinner H, Buckley S: Proprioception in the anterior cruciate deficient knee. Am J Sports Med 17:1, 1989.
34. Freeman MAR, Dean MRE, Hanham IWF: The etiology and prevention of functional instability of the foot. J Bone Joint Surg 47B:687, 1965.
35. Guido J Jr, Voight ML, Blackburn TA, et al.: The effects of chronic effusion on knee joint proprioception. A cast study. J Orthop Sports Phy Ther 25:208, 1997.
36. Nitz AJ: Limb denervation following anterior cruciate (ACL) reconstruction without tourniquet application. Phys Ther 68:822, 1988.
37. Kleinrensink GJ, Stoekart R, Meulstee J, et al.: Lowered motor conduction velocity of the peroneal nerve after inversion trauma. Med Sci Sports Exerc 26:877, 1994.
38. Dobner JJ, Nitz AJ: Postmeniscectomy tourniquet palsy and functional sequelae. Am J Sports Med 10:211, 1982.
39. Lorentzon R, Elmqvist LG, Sjostrom J, et al.: Thigh musculature in relation to chronic anterior cruciate ligament tear: Muscle size, morphology, and mechanical output before reconstruction. Am J Sports Med 17:423, 1989.
40. Elmqvist LG, Lorentzon R, Johansson C, et al.: Knee extensor muscle function before and after reconstruction of anterior cruciate ligament tear. Scand J Rehab Med 21:131, 1989.
41. LoPresti C, Kirkendall DT, Streete GM, et al.: Quadriceps insufficiency following repair of the anterior cruciate ligament. J Orthop Sports Phys Ther 9:245, 1988.
42. Karlya Y, Itoh M, Nakamura T, et al.: Magnetic resonance imaging and spectroscopy of thigh muscles in cruciate ligament insufficiency. Acta Orthop Scand 60:322, 1989.
43. Emqvist LG, Lorentzon R, Langstrom M, et al.: Reconstruction of the anterior cruciate ligament: Long-term effects of different knee angles at primary immobilization and different modes of early training. Am J Sports Med 16:455, 1988.
44. Herbison GJ: Effect of electrical stimulation on denervated muscle of rat. Arch Phys Med Rehab 52:516, 1971.
45. Nitz AJ, Matulionis DH: Ultrastructural changes in peripheral nerve following pneumatic tourniquet compression. J Neurosurg 57:600, 1982.
46. Nitz AJ, Dobner JJ, Matulionis DH: Pneumatic tourniquet application and nerve integrity: Motor function and electrophysiology. Exp Neurol 94:264, 1986.
47. Pedowitz RA: Tourniquet induced neuromuscular injury: A recent review of rabbit and clinical experiments. Acta Orthop Scand 62(suppl. 245):1, 1991.
48. Jacobson MD, Pedowitz RA, Oyama BK, et al.: Muscle functional deficits after tourniquet ischemia. Am J Sports Med 22:372, 1994.
49. Cicotti MG, Kerlan RK, Perry J, Pink M: An electromyographic analysis of the knee during functional activities. Am J Sports Med 22:651, 1994.
50. Dvir Z, Koren E, Halperin N: Knee joint position sense following reconstruction of the anterior cruciate ligament. J Orthop Sports Phys Ther 10:117, 1988.
51. Levine JD, Dardick SJ, Basbaum AI, Scipio E: Reflex neurogenic inflammation. J Neuro 5:1380, 1985.
52. Bohannon RW, Gajdoski RL: Spinal nerve root compression: Some clinical implications. Phys Ther 67:367, 1987.
53. Delitto A, McKowen J, McCarthy J, et al.: Electrically elicited co-contraction of thigh musculature after anterior cruciate ligament surgery. Phys Ther 68:45, 1988.
54. Delitto A, Rose S, McKowen J, et al.: Electrical stimulation versus voluntary exercise in strengthening thigh musculature after anterior cruciate ligament surgery. Phys Ther 68:660, 1988.
55. Lopriesti C, Kirkendall D, Street G, et al.: Quadriceps insufficiency following repair of the anterior cruciate ligament. J Orthop Sports Phys Ther 9:245, 1988.
56. Sinacore D, Delitto A, Kind D, et al.: Type II fiber activation with electrical stimulation: A preliminary report. Phys Ther 70:416, 1990.
57. Draper V: Electromyographic biofeedback and recovery of quadriceps femoris muscle function following anterior cruciate ligament reconstruction. Phys Ther 70:11, 1990.
58. Pavlos LFR, Noyes E, Grood E, et al.: Knee rehabilitation after ACL reconstruction and repair. Am J Sports Med 9:140, 1981.
59. Shelbourne KD, Nitz P: Accelerated rehabilitation after anterior cruciate ligament reconstruction. Am J Sports Med 18:292, 1990.
60. Shelbourne KD, Gray T: Anterior cruciate ligament reconstruction with autogenous patellar tendon graft followed by accelerated rehabilitation. A two- to nine-year follow up. Am J Sports Med 25:786, 1997.
61. Limbird TJ, Shiavi R, Frazer M, et al.: EMG profiles of knee joint musculature during walking: Changes induced by anterior cruciate ligament deficiency. J Orthop Res 6:630, 1988.
62. Shiavi R, Limbird T, Borra H, et al.: Electromyography profiles of knee joint musculature during pivoting: Changes induced by anterior cruciate ligament deficiency. J Electromyograph Kinesiol 1:49, 1991.
63. Seto JL, Orofino AS, Morrissey MC, et al.: Assessment of quadriceps/hamstring strength, knee ligament stability, functional and sports activity levels five years after anterior cruciate ligament reconstruction. Am J Sports Med 16:170, 1988.
64. Wexler G, Hurwitz DE, Bush-Joseph CA, et al.: Functional gait adaptations in patients with anterior cruciate ligament deficiency over time. Clin Orthop Rel Res 348:166, 1998.
65. Malone TR: Muscle Injury and Rehabilitation, Vol 1. Baltimore, Williams & Wilkins, 1988.
66. Snyder-Mackler L, Delitto A, Bailey SL, et al.: Strength of the quadriceps femoris muscle and functional recovery after reconstruction of the anterior cruciate ligament. J Bone Joint Surg 77A:1166, 1995.
67. DeMont R, Lephart S: Repetition drives neuromuscular recovery after ACL injury. Biomechanics 5:31, 1998.
68. Wojtys EM, Huston LJ, Taylor PD, Bastian SD: Neuromuscular adaptations in isokinetic, isotonic and agility training programs. Am J Sports Med 24:187, 1996.

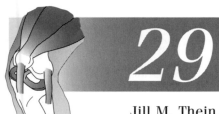

29 Aquatic Therapy

Jill M. Thein, MPT, ATC, and
Lori Thein Brody, MS, PT, SCS, ATC

*I*n the past few decades, ligamentous knee injuries have been studied with increasing interest. With medical advancements, including improved imaging techniques, an accurate diagnosis and an appropriate course of action for various knee injuries have been established. Owing to its high incidence of injury, the anterior cruciate ligament (ACL) has been studied and discussed most often in the literature. Because of medical advancements, the surgical technique to reconstruct the ACL has changed tremendously.[1–4] The reader is referred to Chapter 7 for further discussion of current surgical techniques. As surgical techniques became more refined, postoperative care and rehabilitation also underwent significant changes. Historically, early postoperative rehabilitation consisted of prolonged immobilization, often in slight flexion, non-weight-bearing, and avoidance of quadriceps setting to decrease stresses on the graft.[5–7]

In the early 1990s, with the intent of documenting the success of their postoperative rehabilitation protocol, Shelbourne and Wilckens compiled outcomes of patients undergoing ACL reconstruction using bone-patellar tendon-bone autografts.[8] Follow-up data revealed that compliance to rehabilitation was inversely related to success, and that patients with poor compliance to immobilization and weight-bearing guidelines in the early phase of rehabilitation did better without long-term complications.[8] Questions were raised regarding rehabilitation, and changes were made. The outcome was accelerated rehabilitation programs, which were actually modeled after noncompliant patients.[8] Rehabilitation programs have become more aggressive, encouraging early postoperative range of motion and strengthening, primarily focusing on closed kinetic chain exercises.[9–12] The reader is referred to Chapter 21 for further discussion of closed

kinetic chain concepts in knee ligament rehabilitation.

A variety of modalities have also been used in the course of ACL rehabilitation, including continuous passive motion (CPM),[5, 8, 9, 11, 13] electrical muscle stimulation,[5, 9, 14] electromyographic biofeedback,[14, 15] transcutaneous electrical nerve stimulation (TENS),[5, 9] and cryotherapy.[5, 8, 10, 13] One treatment tool that has been in existence for centuries but is often overlooked and underutilized in rehabilitation is the swimming pool. It was not until the past few decades that clinicians discovered utilization of a water-based program to be of great benefit to their patients. They can regain mobility and strength and maintain or improve cardiovascular endurance. The pool may also be used to increase flexibility, speed, balance, and coordination. Although a vast amount of research exists for land-based ACL rehabilitation,[5, 8–11, 13] little research exists regarding the utilization of aquatic-based therapy.[16, 17]

Prior to implementing the pool in any rehabilitation program, the clinician must have knowledge of the physical properties of water, the physiologic responses seen with immersion and exercise, and the effect water temperature may have on exercise. By utilizing water's unique properties, patients can receive the fullest benefit from aquatic-based rehabilitation programs.

PHYSICAL PROPERTIES OF WATER

Buoyancy

Archimedes' principle of buoyancy states that a body partially or completely immersed in a fluid will experience an upward thrust equal to the weight of the fluid that was displaced. Buoyancy is defined as the upward thrust acting in the opposite direction of gravity.[18] Buoyancy is related to the specific gravity of the immersed object. Specific gravity is the ratio of the mass of one substance to the mass of the same value of water.[18] Therefore, by definition, the specific gravity of water is 1.0 and any body with a specific gravity of less than 1.0 will float. The average values for the human body range from 0.97 to 0.95, so human bodies can float.[19] However, many individuals still have difficulty floating because of their body composition and body fat distribution. They may rest just below the surface of the water, or their legs may sink while their trunk remains at the surface. This is of particular importance in treating an athlete who may be very lean. Buoyant equipment may be necessary on the trunk or at various points along the limb to maintain equilibrium in the pool.

Buoyancy can be used in rehabilitation in three ways: as assistance, as support, and as resistance. Buoyancy used as assistance occurs when movements are toward the surface of the water, as when allowing the leg to float up in the front of the body. This would be an example of buoyancy-assisted exercise for the iliopsoas muscle. Buoyancy-assisted exercises are frequently used to increase range of motion. A long lever arm and the use of a floatation device will enhance buoyancy-assisted exercises. It is essential that the antagonist muscle groups remain relaxed during the movement to avoid eccentric contraction of these muscles.[20]

Buoyancy-supported exercises are movements that are perpendicular to the upward thrust of buoyancy and parallel to the bottom of the pool. Typically, the limb will float just below the surface of the water, but this is dependent on the density of the extremity and the use of floatation devices. The more fatty tissue present, the less dense the extremity and the better floatation will be. Examples of buoyancy-supported exercise include horizontal abduction and adduction of the hip with the patient in a standing position, and trunk flexion and extension with the patient floating in a side-lying position at the surface of the water (Fig. 29–1).

Buoyancy-resisted exercises are those movements that directly oppose the upward thrust of buoyancy. Buoyancy-resisted hip extension is performed while standing with the hip in 90 degrees of flexion and extending the hip to neutral. The most resistance is noted when the limb is at a right angle to the buoyant force and reaches zero as the limb reaches vertical (Fig. 29–2A).[20] In this example, the hip extensors would become buoyancy-assisted if the hip were to extend past neutral (Fig. 29–2B). Muscle work can be assisted by increasing the lever arm or by adding floatation devices, which cause the patient to push down against a greater resistance. If enough floatation is added, the return motion can become an eccentrically resisted activity.

Hydrostatic Pressure

Pascal's law states that at any given depth, the pressure from the liquid is exerted

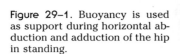

Figure 29–1. Buoyancy is used as support during horizontal abduction and adduction of the hip in standing.

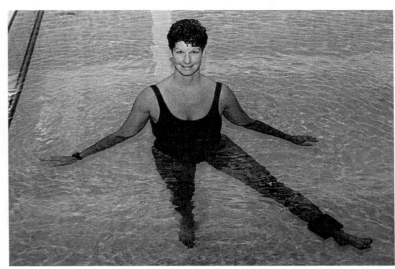

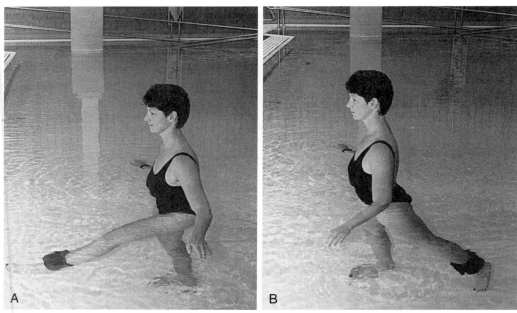

Figure 29–2. *A,* Buoyancy-resisted hip extension from 90 degrees flexion to neutral. *B,* Buoyancy-assisted hip extension beyond neutral.

equally on all surfaces of the immersed object.[21] As the density and depth of the liquid increases, so does the volume of liquid overhead and, therefore, the hydrostatic pressure. As such, hydrostatic pressure can be used in rehabilitation to reduce effusion or to allow the patient to exercise an injured extremity without an increase in effusion. This is especially important in the rehabilitation of lower extremity injuries; the patient may perform activities with the injured extremity in a dependent position without deleterious effects of increased effusion. Hydrostatic pressure is also responsible for the cardiovascular changes seen with immersion and has a significant impact on exercise training parameters.

Viscosity

Viscosity is defined as the friction occurring between individual molecules in a liquid, causing resistance to flow.[21] Viscosity is only noticeable when there is motion through the liquid and it acts as resistance to movement because the liquid molecules adhere to the surface of the body.[21] Because water is more viscous than air, there is resistance to most movement in the water regardless of buoyancy.

Fluid Dynamics

Two different types of water flow exist: laminar flow and turbulent flow. Laminar flow, defined as the smooth flow of water molecules, has the least amount of resistance because the water molecules are all traveling in the same direction and at the same speed. Turbulent flow is interrupted flow, as when laminar flow encounters an object causing water molecules to rebound in all directions. Turbulent flow can be visualized as the white water and air bubbles next to the skin when a body is moved through the water (Fig. 29–3).

The shape of the object moving the water also affects drag. A tapered, streamlined object will produce minimal disruption of flow, whereas an unstreamlined object will create rapid disruption of flow, causing turbulence.[18] For example, forward walking is more resistive than walking sideways, and shoulder internal and external rotation with the forearms pronated creates less drag than performing the same exercise in forearm neutral.

Muscle contraction type is a key consideration when designing an exercise program with increasing resistance based on viscosity. Exercises performed against the water's resistance almost always elicit concentric

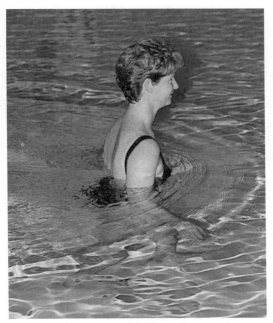

Figure 29–3. Eddy currents behind the walking individual create a negative pressure and drag posteriorly.

muscle contractions. Consider performance of the above example of shoulder internal and external rotation; the movements elicit reciprocal concentric contractions of the rotator cuff muscles. Alternately, eccentric muscle contractions can be elicited using buoyancy if enough floatation is used. For example, the upward abduction motion of the leg away from the side will elicit an eccentric contraction of the hip adductors if a large floatation device is placed on the ankle. Eccentric contractions in the lower extremity can also be achieved if the water is shallow enough to minimize buoyancy. For example, lunges in hip-deep water can elicit eccentric quadricep muscle contractions.

Effect of Depth of Immersion on Weight-Bearing

Weight-bearing is affected by the depth of water, owing to buoyancy. This becomes an important issue in rehabilitation, especially when rehabilitating patients with lower extremity injuries. In general, at the seventh cervical vertebral level, the xiphoid, and the anterior superior iliac spine, female athletes will bear 8 percent, 28 percent, and 47 percent of their body weight, respectively. Male

athletes are approximately 8 percent, 35 percent, and 54 percent weight-bearing at the same levels.[18] However, these numbers reflect static weight-bearing, and increasing to a fast walking speed can increase weight-bearing by as much as 76 percent.[22] Decreasing the depth of water is one way to progress lower extremity weight-bearing.

PHYSIOLOGIC RESPONSES TO AQUATIC EXERCISE

Physiologic Responses to Water Immersion

When humans are immersed in water, physiologic changes occur, both at rest and during exercise. Therefore, it is important that the clinician be aware of these differences so that training programs can be appropriately modified. Changes that occur at rest during water immersion are the result of hydrostatic pressure and include, most importantly, a cephalad redistribution of blood flow.[23] Included in these alterations is an increase in right atrial venous pressure, which results in a Frank-Starling reflex and a subsequent increase in stroke volume (SV).[23–28] Hormonal changes and diuresis have been observed with sustained periods of water immersion (Table 29–1).[29–33]

Immersion and Exercise Response

Several studies have been conducted to determine whether central blood volume

Table 29–1. **Cardiovascular Responses to Immersion at Rest**

Measure	Response
Right atrial venous pressure	Increase (8–12 mm Hg)
Heart blood volume	Increase (180–250 mL)
Cardiac output	Increase (25% +)
Stroke volume	Increase (25% +)
Central venous pressure	Increase
Heart rate	Remains the same or decreases slightly
Systemic blood pressure	Remains the same or increases slightly

Data from Skinner et al.[18]; Arborelius et al.[23]; Begin et al.[24]; Echt et al.[25]; Fahri and Linnarson[26]; Lange et al.[27]; Epstein et al.[30]; Lin[33]; Christie et al.[34]; and Sheldahl et al.[35]

continues to remain elevated during exercise in water. Christie et al.[34] studied 10 men performing upright bicycle ergometry both on land and immersed in water to the suprasternal notch. Subjects exercised at 40, 60, 80, and 100 percent VO_{2max} while numerous cardiac responses were observed. Although VO_{2max} did not differ between groups, other cardiac responses were significantly greater during water exercise than on land. Cardiac preload was elevated both at rest and during water exercise, suggesting that the centralization of peripheral blood flow exists despite the redistribution of blood known to occur during exercise. Sheldahl et al.[35] studied two groups of nine males performing supervised bicycle ergometry, three times a week for 12 weeks, one group on land, the other immersed to the suprasternal notch. Results showed a similar increase in stroke volume and decrease in heart rate (HR) and blood pressure, as well as a similar increase in VO_{2max} in both groups. The authors concluded that exercise training is not affected by the cephalad shift in blood volume during water exercise.

These two studies highlight the issue of immersion and exercise. As cardiovascular changes are immersion-related, exercise prescription in deep water becomes difficult. Deep water running is commonly used in the rehabilitation of athletic injuries and has been extensively studied. A study of 20 trained males running at four submaximal loads and maximal intensity in both deep water and on land showed that submaximal workload heart rates and VO_{2max} were lower during water running.[36] The authors believed that the lower submaximal HR relative to VO_2 may be due to increased SV, which is an effect of increased central blood volume or increased preload.

A similar study of 12 female cross-country runners compared VO_{2max} on a treadmill with deep water immersion.[37] Results found VO_{2max} values to be 17 percent lower in water when compared with land, a finding similar to that of previous studies. Peak HR responses during water running were 17 beats/minute (bpm) lower than those during a treadmill run. The authors suggested the lower HR response was due to increased SV and the cooling effects of the water.

An important factor in deep water running is the skill of the patient. Studies found the HR-VO_2 relationship and the rate of perceived exertion in deep water running to be skill-dependent.[36, 38] Those individuals who were less skilled used greater arm movement to maintain position in the water, thereby increasing their heart rate and rate of perceived exertion. A period of technique training should precede any testing or establishing of a training HR.

Training HR should be established in the pool, rather than attempting to apply land-based HRs to pool exercises.[39] In general, HRs during deep water exercise will be approximately 17 bpm lower than comparable exercise on land.[40]

Effects of Water Temperature

Water temperature can have a profound effect on the cardiovascular response to exercise. Avellini et al.[41] studied three groups of five males; group I exercised on land, and groups II and III exercised in 32°C and 20°C water, respectively. Maximal oxygen consumption was tested before and after the training period on land via treadmill and cycle ergometer. Subjects trained on a cycle ergometer 5 days/week for 1 hour at 75 percent VO_{2max}, which was adjusted throughout the study. Results showed that the water groups exercised at a lower HR for a prescribed VO_{2max} level than the land group. Maximal oxygen consumption increased for all three groups, but no significant difference was found between groups. The authors hypothesized that the lower water temperature caused vasoconstriction in the periphery to decrease heat loss, forcing blood centrally, enhancing venous return, and increasing SV. Since cardiac output at the same VO_2 is similar when exercising on land or in water, the exercise could be achieved at a lower HR. Since group III demonstrated similar improvements in maximal aerobic power while exercising at an HR 20 bpm lower than groups I and II, the authors concluded that training in cold water enhanced SV and decreased HR, increasing exercise efficiency.

In contrast, exercising in warm water can cause increased cardiovascular demands above those of exercise alone. Choukroun and Varene[42] studied the effects of water temperature on the cardiovascular system on subjects at rest. Subjects were immersed to the neck in 25°C, 34°C, and 40°C water and cardiovascular demands were measured. Cardiac output increased significantly at 40°C. Gleim and Nicholas[43] studied the effects of water temperature on individuals exercising in waist-deep water. The authors found that the centralization of peripheral blood flow was overcome by the thermal stimulus to increase HR at 36°C.

Owing to the potential for heat illness, temperature recommendations for intense training of the patient should be between 26°C and 28°C to prevent any heat-related complications.

REHABILITATION

The pool can be used throughout rehabilitation, barring any contraindications, which include incontinence (unless catheterized), discharging wounds, upper respiratory infection, uncontrolled blood pressure, febrile conditions, cardiac or pulmonary disorders, or a great fear of water.[44] In the early postoperative phase, it can be used to work on range of motion, gait, stretching, strengthening, balance, and proprioception. Because of the buoyancy water provides, many activities can be initiated sooner in water than on land. Later in the rehabilitation process, the pool can be used for continued strength training, cardiovascular conditioning, and to initiate and progress impact activities.

Knee ligament rehabilitation is often broken up into phases, with progression based on criteria, rather than based exclusively on time. Pool progression will differ from progression on land, and may not necessarily coincide. The concepts discussed in the following section may or may not be used in conjunction with land-based rehabilitation. Patients may find the variety in their exercise program enjoyable, overcoming the boredom and burnout sometimes seen in rehabilitation. Rehabilitation of patients with ACL reconstructions with or without meniscectomy will be discussed first, followed by reconstructions with meniscal repair. Rehabilitation of the ACL with injury or repair of other ligaments will be discussed, and lastly, rehabilitation of patients with posterior cruciate ligament (PCL) injuries and reconstruction will be presented.

Anterior Cruciate Ligament Rehabilitation with or without Meniscectomy

The ACL may be injured alone or in conjunction with the meniscus. Depending on the size and location of the meniscal tear, the patient may undergo either a meniscectomy or a meniscal repair. The surgical indications for each procedure are beyond the scope of this chapter. Isolated ACL reconstructions and ACL reconstructions with meniscectomies are typically rehabilitated in the same manner, unless otherwise indicated. The location and size of the meniscectomy, as well as any degenerative changes present, are salient points the physical therapist should be cognizant of. Good communication with the orthopedic surgeon proves to be extremely important.

EARLY PHASE

The goals of the early phase of rehabilitation include controlling edema, obtaining full knee extension, achieving a good quadriceps set, initiating knee flexion range of motion exercises, restoring flexibility of the lower extremity, beginning light cardiovascular conditioning, and ambulating without an assistive device. Bearing no contraindications, the patient may begin pool rehabilitation within the first week postoperatively. It is imperative that the incision is well covered to avoid any complications or infection. Products such as Bioclusive or Tagaderm can be used to keep the incision dry.

Range of Motion and Flexibility

The athlete may perform any or all of the stretching and range of motion routine in the water. A warm water pool (32°C to 35°C) provides a relaxing environment, which may allow for increased soft tissue extensibility. Additionally, the buoyancy of the water may make stretching easier to perform and optimal positions easier to maintain. The duration of the stretch can vary; however, a low-intensity, long-duration (20–30 seconds) stretch has proved to be most beneficial in promoting lasting changes.[45] To work on knee flexion activities, patients can sit on a step or chair and actively flex their knee, as they would on land. They may utilize their uninvolved lower extremity to passively flex the knee farther. Another way to increase knee flexion while concurrently stretching the quadriceps is in standing. While maintaining the femur in a vertical position, the patient can allow buoyancy to lift the lower leg posteriorly. A floatation device on the affected ankle will increase the intensity of

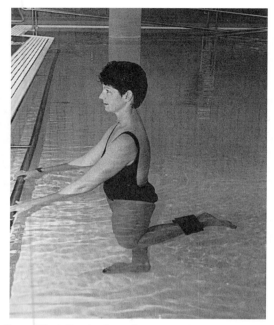

Figure 29–4. Passive knee flexion may be increased with the use of a floatation device.

the stretch (Fig. 29–4). To obtain knee extension, the patient may use a floatation device and allow buoyancy to passively bring the leg toward the surface of the water in the sagittal plane. If an anterior pelvic tilt is maintained, this also becomes an optimal hamstring stretch (Fig. 29–5). Other lower extremity musculature, such as the gastroc-

soleus complex, iliotibial band, and iliopsoas may be stretched in water (Fig. 29–6).

Strength Training

Strength training for the postoperative patient is critical and should be initiated early in rehabilitation. By utilizing equipment and implementing the basic principles of water, the athletic trainer or physical therapist can create a complete aquatic strengthening program for the patient, which can be performed while minimizing the risk of re-injury to the ACL.

A variety of open and closed chain exercises can be performed in the pool and all exercises can be performed completely non-weight-bearing if necessary. One goal in early rehabilitation is achieving a good quadriceps muscle contraction. Standing leg lifts with the knee in full extension, which are buoyancy-assisted, may be beneficial for the patient who has difficulty eliciting a quadriceps contraction. A similar exercise, while the patient is seated and actively extends the knee from a flexed position, is another example of buoyancy-assisted strength training for the quadriceps. Although this activity involves full extension in the open kinetic chain, excess anterior shear is avoided if the exercise is performed slowly. Another exercise that may facilitate a quadriceps muscle contraction is "soldier walking," in which the patient walks in the water with the knees in full extension.

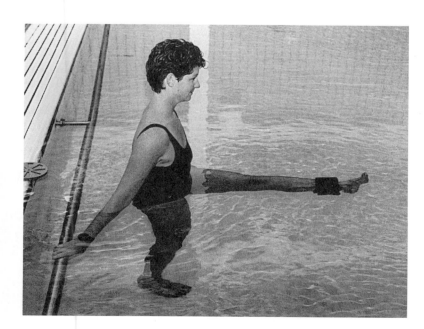

Figure 29–5. Hamstring stretching and passive knee extension can be accomplished in the pool.

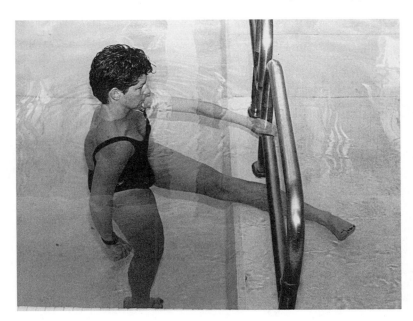

Figure 29–6. Stretching of the iliotibial band with hip flexion, adduction, and internal rotation using a ramp.

Active knee extension when starting from a flexed position with the femur in vertical is an example of buoyancy-resisted strength training. Patients must actively fire their quadriceps muscle to obtain extension. To make the exercise more difficult, a floatation device can be added to the ankle. This exercise can be combined with passive knee flexion as previously described.

Hamstring strengthening can be performed in standing with the femur vertical, or with the hip in 90 degrees of flexion, adding floatation as necessary (Fig. 29–7). Other lower extremity musculature should be included in any comprehensive strength-training program. Hip abduction-adduction and flexion-extension with or without floatation devices are useful exercises in the early phases of rehabilitation. Calf raises for gastrocnemius and soleus strengthening may also be included, bearing in mind they are buoyancy-assisted and will be much less challenging in the pool than on land.

Closed chain exercises can be initiated in this phase of rehabilitation. The closed kinetic chain causes increased compressive forces between the femur and tibia, encouraging vascularization and healing, all while minimizing the amount of anterior shear in the knee.[46–49] To strengthen the quadriceps and gluteals, exercises such as mini-lunges, step-downs, and squats should be incorporated. Lunges may be performed either in a stationary position or on alternating legs.

Tethered walking—forward, backward and sideways—may also be added to the patient's program. Owing to buoyancy, the quadriceps eccentric work with most aquatic exercise is decreased relative to comparable land-based exercise. Buoyancy will allow the patient to work only a small range of knee flexion and extension, unless the depth of water is decreased.

Cardiovascular Training

Cardiovascular conditioning is a large component of any rehabilitation program, especially if the patient is athletic. Research has shown that 3 weeks of inactivity can lead to a significant loss of cardiovascular fitness, and 6 weeks of rest can lead to a decrease of as much as 14 to 16 percent of maximal oxygen consumption.[50–52] With utilization of a pool for rehabilitation, the loss in cardiovascular conditioning typically seen immediately after surgery can be minimized, and the patient's goal of restoring cardiovascular function can be achieved without risk of injury to the newly reconstructed knee. This is particularly useful for the patient with weight-bearing or impact restrictions. Because of the physiologic changes incurred while immersed, it is recommended that the patient train at a heart rate 17 to 20 bpm lower than he or she does on land. The rate of perceived exertion is often unreliable

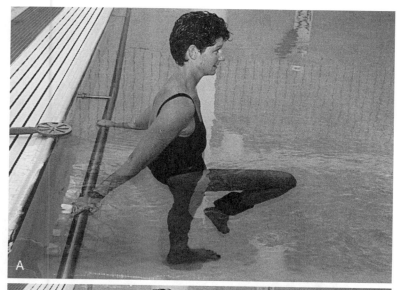

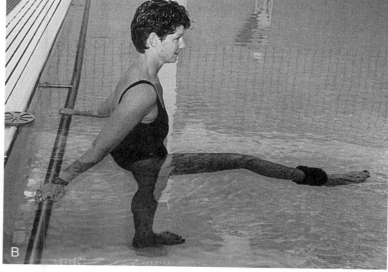

Figure 29–7. Buoyancy-assisted (A) and buoyancy-resisted (B) hamstring strengthening.

because of the effects of skill and comfort on perceived exertion.

The patient can be introduced to aquatic-based cardiovascular conditioning early in the postoperative phase. As with any exercise session, an appropriate warm-up and cool-down are essential. These should be performed in the pool and may consist of forward and backward walking, soldier-walking and high knees, followed by stretching. The patient will want to avoid rapid, repetitive knee flexion and extension movements, as this may stress the graft. Rather, cardiovascular conditioning should focus primarily on activities requiring minimal knee motion. An excellent but often overlooked activity is

swimming. It provides cardiovascular benefits, neuromuscular coordination, and stretching and elongation through the legs, trunk, and upper extremities, yet requires minimal movement at the knee. Initially, the patient may feel more comfortable using a floatation device between the thighs to minimize leg motion, focusing exclusively on the upper extremity. As the patient's confidence increases, the floatation device can be removed. If breathing is a concern for the patient, a snorkel can be used during freestyle swimming. Backstroke swimming eliminates the issue of breathing and incorporates increased hip extension and hamstring activity. The patient should be instructed to avoid a whip kick, as with breaststroke, as this causes increased rotation at the knee, potentially stressing the graft. Remember that the patient does not necessarily have to be able to swim for 25 minutes for the training session; the swimming may be just one component of an interval program.

Another example of cardiovascular conditioning is cross-country skiing, which emphasizes leg and trunk extension. Both the shoulders and hips move through a large range of motion, although the knees stay relatively straight. The patient may perform this activity in deep water either free-floating or tethered to the side of the pool (Fig. 29–8). Floatation vests may be used when teaching the patient a deep-water technique or if safety is a concern. When possible, the vest should be discontinued to increase the difficulty of the work-out. This activity proves to be good quadriceps, hamstring, and hip strengthening. Initially, the patient may be required to perform intervals of cross-country skiing, complementing it with swimming, because of lower extremity fatigue. Both cross-country skiing and swimming utilize upper extremity movement to assist with increasing the work on the heart.

A third example, focusing solely on the lower extremity, is straight knee kicking, either with a kickboard or stationary at the side of the pool. Fins may be used if the patient demonstrates good quadriceps control (Fig. 29–9). Again, minimal motion is re-quired at the knee. Because of quadriceps and hamstring fatigue, the patient may tire quickly, and it should be introduced in rehabilitation only after the patient is comfortable with kicking while swimming.

Balance and Proprioception

Balance and proprioception are important to any patient and should be part of any thorough rehabilitation program. Balance is controlled by sensory input, central processing, and neuromuscular responses.[53] Proprioception is defined as position sense that orients the body or specific body parts to space or other objects.[54] Balance and proprioception can be trained in a water-based program and can start early in rehabilitation. Often, patients feel more comfortable performing single leg balance activities in the pool than on land because of the increased support of the water. The fear of falling is eliminated and patients with decreased quadriceps control may feel more stable. Examples of balance exercises include single-leg toe raises without upper extremity support, hip flexion-extension, and circumduction in waist-deep water while standing on the injured leg, progressing to shallower water. Other non-impact balance activities include single-leg balance on the injured leg while altering the center of gravity by moving the upper extremity, as in a push-pull motion with a kickboard, or with

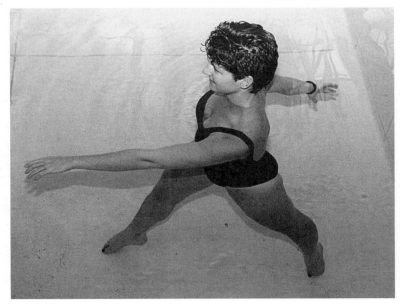

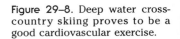
Figure 29–8. Deep water cross-country skiing proves to be a good cardiovascular exercise.

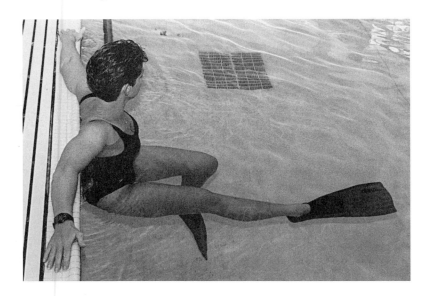

Figure 29–9. Kicking at the side of the pool with fins is a very fatiguing exercise for the quadriceps muscle. The athlete should keep the knees extended acutely to avoid stressing the graft.

horizontal adduction and abduction of the upper extremity while using water paddles as resistance, causing increased postural sway in the sagittal plane. Increasing knee flexion on the weight-bearing leg will increase the challenge to these muscles (Fig. 29–10). Additionally, the patient may close his or her eyes, relying more heavily on neuromuscular rather than visual input.

INTERMEDIATE PHASE

The intermediate phase of rehabilitation is started when the patient demonstrates good quadriceps control, full knee extension, flexion greater than 100 degrees, controlled effusion, and a normal gait on land without a brace or assistive device. This typically occurs approximately 3 to 4 weeks postoperatively but may take longer depending on a multitude of factors. The patient may continue to utilize the pool throughout this phase of rehabilitation, either exclusively or complementing a land-based program.

Range of Motion and Flexibility

Range of motion at the knee will require continued work, and flexibility should also continue to be addressed. The patient may find standing in a posterior pelvic tilt with

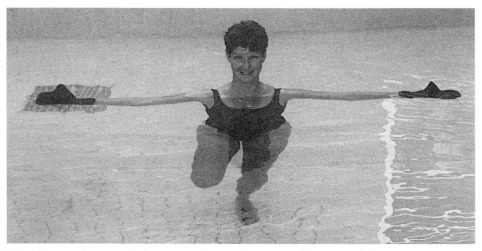

Figure 29–10. Balance activities include resisted shoulder horizontal adduction and abduction to increase neuromuscular input via postural sway.

the knee flexed with a floatation device on the ankle a comfortable way to elicit a prolonged quadriceps muscle stretch. Other lower extremity musculature, such as the hamstrings, iliotibial band, and gastrocnemius-soleus complex should continue to be stretched to achieve normal flexibility. Any or all of these activities can be incorporated into the patient's routine and performed prior to any strength training, cardiovascular conditioning, or balance and proprioception activities.

Strength Training

A comprehensive lower extremity strength training program is important for every patient. Consequently, the muscles of the lower extremity must continually be challenged and loaded. As the patient achieves good quadriceps control, exercises in the pool may be advanced. Step downs, lunges, and squats may all be progressed by decreasing the depth of the water, subsequently increasing the weight-bearing through the knee. These exercises can be done while the patient is tethered to the side of the pool to make them more challenging. To progress hamstring strengthening, the patient may perform standing hamstring curls with the hip flexed to 90 degrees with ankle floats. If enough resistance is added, the exercise becomes eccentric for the hamstrings as the knee is extended. Other lower extremity strength training should also be advanced. Standing hip extension with ankle floatation starting at 90 degrees of hip flexion is a good gluteal strengthening exercise.

Although impact on land may not be appropriate at this time, the physical therapist or athletic trainer may start the patient with some light impact in the pool during this phase. Activities should be started in shoulder- or neck-deep water, thereby decreasing weight-bearing forces. Bear in mind, however, that impact activities will increase weight-bearing by as much as 76 percent.[22] Even so, some light, double-leg impact activities may be introduced without stressing the graft. Double-leg hopping in place will strengthen the gastrocnemius yet decrease the amount of quadriceps eccentric control required when compared with the same activity on land. The patient can add side-to-side or forward-backward hopping when he or she feels ready. Easy pike or tuck jumping

can be started, as they assist in strengthening the hip flexors. Side shuffling, skipping, and jumping jacks also prove to be beneficial activities, as they address neuromuscular coordination, impact, and strength.

Cardiovascular Training

As the patient's range of motion and flexibility improves, other cardiovascular activities may be added to the program, giving the patient some variety. This will allow variety in lower extremity strengthening and endurance training, which will minimize joint and muscle soreness. Deep water running may be introduced at this time (Fig. 29–11). When teaching deep water running, have the patient "run off the bottom" of the shallow end into the deep end, trying to maintain form. Once the feet leave the bottom, some forward progress will be made owing to slight forward lean, but excessive lean, which begins to mimic a swimming stroke, should be avoided. Deep water running requires minimal range of motion at the shoulders and a large range of hip and knee motion when performed optimally. Of course, the technique may be modified as needed. For example, the patient may have to start deep water running with floatation devices and moving the lower extremities through a small range, progressing to a full range of motion without floatation.

The patient can also begin cardiovascular exercise in shoulder-deep water. Shallow water running and cross-country skiing are both effective training techniques. Bear in mind that running requires increased knee range of motion, whereas cross-country skiing requires little knee motion. The therapist must be aware that the patient is experiencing a small amount of impact; appropriate footwear should be suggested.

The fundamental guidelines for cardiovascular training should be at the core of program design. Twenty-five minutes, five times per week or more, is recommended as a minimum, whereas a high level athlete may need a longer training period, depending upon the season and sport. Like land-based exercise, the pool can also be used for interval training. A number of stations, or a variety of exercises performed within a single session, can alleviate boredom and ensure a well-rounded workout. The cardiovascular program does not have to be limited to the pool and can complement land-based cardio-

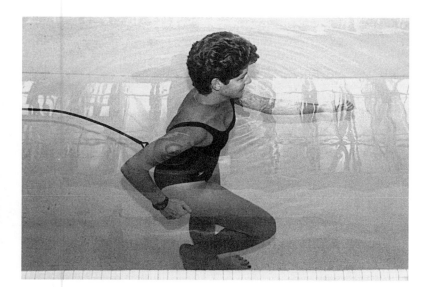

Figure 29–11. Deep water running tethered to the side of the pool.

vascular activities, such as bicycling and stairclimbing.

Balance and Proprioception

The concepts of balance and proprioception should continue to be addressed throughout rehabilitation. Activities previously mentioned—hip flexion-extension and abduction-adduction while standing on the rehabilitation leg—can be progressed by adding floatation devices to the ankle of the moving leg or by having the patient increase the speed of movement. The clinician can play catch with the patient from the side of the pool while performing this activity to make it more challenging for the patient. Another option to increase the level of difficulty is to have the patient perform the balance exercises with his or her eyes closed or by decreasing the depth of the water.

Impact activities also challenge balance. Athletes who require explosive push-offs, such as in track and baseball, as well as athletes in jumping sports will benefit from the jumping and hopping drills previously mentioned. These drills can be done while playing catch with a therapist, or mimicking a basketball shot or volleyball block to make the activity more sport-specific. The patient can also be tethered to the side of the pool and perform stationary or side-to-side jumping, adding challenge to core body strength as well as balance (Fig. 29–12). Shock-absorptive shoes may be necessary for these activities.

ADVANCED PHASE

As stated previously, the phases of aquatic rehabilitation do not necessarily coincide with the advancement of phases on land. The advanced phase of aquatic rehabilitation may be started at approximately 6 weeks. Again, a multitude of factors dictate time of progression into the advanced phase, including quadriceps strength, pain, motivation, results of land-based functional testing, and increased laxity as determined by arthrokinematic testing. Good communication between the patient, physical therapist, and physician proves beneficial when determining when to advance a patient's program.

Strength Training

Vertical kicking can be performed with or without fins and should be initiated with a small flutter kick. Once mastered, a dolphin kick can be added, keeping in mind that it requires a high level of dynamic lumbar control. Kicking should be performed without arm assistance, with the arms held behind the back or hands out of the water. This training technique is particularly effective for those athletes who perform rapid movements in a small range of motion (Fig. 29–13).

Floating squats, in which the athlete stands on a floatation board and pushes down, requires coordination and eccentric control. This activity also challenges balance and can be made sport-specific by play-

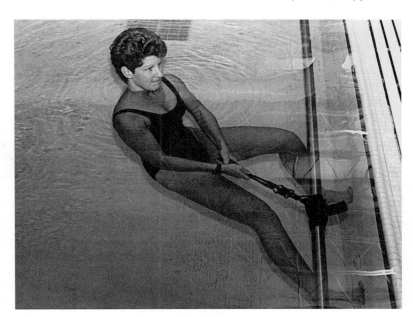

Figure 29–12. Tethered side-to-side jumping trains balance, proprioception, and strength.

ing catch with the patient or by having the patient mimic a basketball shot or a volleyball block.

Sitting on a floatation device while performing repetitive knee flexion and extension with or without fins is a very fatiguing quadriceps and hamstring exercise and

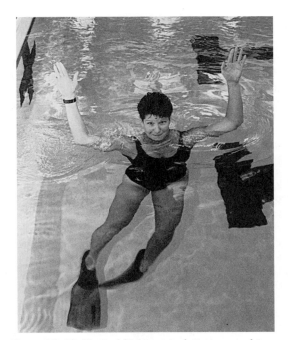

Figure 29–13. Vertical kicking is a fatiguing quadriceps exercise, and it challenges balance when the hands are out of the water.

proves beneficial for those involved in kicking sports such as football and soccer. Resistive boots can increase the resistance in the open kinetic chain as much as fourfold and may be useful in sports requiring power, such as figure skating and gymnastics.[55, 56] Bear in mind, however, that increased anterior shear may occur, and large amounts of resistance at the ankle may be contraindicated at this time.

Cardiovascular Conditioning

Many of the previously described cardiovascular techniques can be incorporated in the patient's training program, making the program as sport-specific as possible. For example, the sprinter can perform interval sprinting, working at peak oxygen consumption, with intermittent jogging for recovery. In contrast, the marathon runner might perform low-intensity, long-duration cardiovascular exercise, maintaining the workload at 70 to 80 percent maximal oxygen consumption. Likewise, a football lineman may perform shallow water sprinting with a plow for 6- to 10-second intervals, with light jogging during recovery, to replicate the demands of his sport.

Balance and Proprioception

Proprioception can continue to be addressed via impact drills. Two-foot jumping is progressed to single-leg jumping and jumping with 90-degree turns. A step can also be used to train the athlete to jump and hop to and from different levels. These jumping drills are especially useful with figure skaters, gymnasts, and volleyball, soccer, and basketball players for whom jumping and turning skills are essential. Side-to-side bounding and leaping are also useful jumping drills. All balance and proprioception drills can be made more challenging by having the patient close his or her eyes or by decreasing the depth of the water.

Anterior Cruciate Ligament Reconstruction with Meniscal Repair

As stated previously, meniscal tears can be surgically excised or repaired, depending on the size, depth, location, and experience of the surgeon. The cause of the tear—degenerative versus instability—may also dictate the surgical preference.[57–59]

Rehabilitation after meniscal repair with and without concurrent ACL reconstruction has been studied. Results have shown that accelerated rehabilitation—early weight-bearing, range of motion, and closed kinetic chain strengthening—can be prescribed without deleterious effects.[59, 60] Consequently, the suggested protocol for ACL reconstructions with meniscectomy may be appropriate for the patient undergoing a concurrent meniscal repair. Bear in mind, however, that the physician may restrict weight-bearing in the flexed position, especially if the repair site is considerably large, in the early phases of rehabilitation. Even with such restrictions, the pool may be of great benefit, as the patient can work on closed chain activities in chest- or neck-deep water and maintain a minimal amount of weight-bearing. The patient can be progressed through rehabilitation as previously described after weight-bearing restrictions in a closed chain are discontinued, usually by the recommendation of the surgeon. Again, establishing good oral and written communication skills with the surgeon proves to be important.

Collateral Ligament Injury and Repair

Isolated injuries to the medial collateral ligament or lateral collateral ligament may occur via valgus or varus stress to the knee, respectively. The ACL may be injured in combination with the medial collateral ligament; however, the lateral collateral ligament is rarely injured with the ACL.[58, 61] Partial disruption of the collateral ligaments warrants conservative treatment consisting of rest, range of motion, icing, elevation, and avoidance of valgus or varus stressing.[58] Complete disruption may require surgical repair, although outcomes show similar results for nonoperative and operative treatment.[58] Rehabilitation would once again consist of avoiding stressing these ligaments. The patient may progress through ACL rehabilitation as outlined previously, with the exception of avoiding activities that cause valgus or varus stress to the knee. Activities in the frontal plane—side stepping, side-to-side hopping, and rapid hip abduction and adduction—may need to be avoided early in rehabilitation. Activities in the sagittal plane such as squats, forward and backward walking, deep water running, and cross-country skiing may be continued and progressed according to the patient's tolerance.

Posterior Cruciate Ligament Injury and Repair

Injuries to the PCL occur less often than those of the ACL and the collateral ligaments. The PCL is injured from a posteriorly directed force to the anterior and superior aspect of the tibia, often with the knee in flexion.[58] A common mechanism of injury is the "dashboard injury," in which a patient is forced into the dashboard of the car during a collision. Often PCL injuries occur in conjunction with damage to other ligamentous structures.[62, 63] Treatment of PCL tears remains a controversial issue and the reader is referred to Chapters 12 and 13 for surgical indications and techniques. For the nonsurgical patient, early rehabilitation should focus on ROM, effusion, gait, and pain control strategies, all of which can be addressed in the pool, using similar techniques discussed in the early phase of ACL rehabilitation. As studies have shown that closed kinetic chain exercises reduce tibiofemoral compression forces, this approach is often incorporated into the rehabilitation program.[49] As such, activities mentioned previously such as squats, mini-lunges, and step downs, prove to be beneficial. Progression for the nonsurgical patient will depend on a multitude of factors including pain, effusion, range of motion, episodes of instability, and weakness in the quadriceps and hamstrings. Patients may be progressed through the phases of ACL rehabilitation on a "symptom-limited" or an "as tolerated" basis.

Although occurring less frequently than the reconstruction of the ACL, the PCL may be reconstructed or repaired, usually arthroscopically.[62, 63] Postoperative rehabilitation may consist of bracing, weight-bearing ambulation, range of motion exercises, and quadricep strengthening. The pool can be used throughout the PCL rehabilitation process as for ACL rehabilitation. As rapid knee flexion causes an increased posterior shear, activities such as rapid hamstring curls with ankle resistance need to be avoided until later stages in the rehabilitation process. Once again, the patient can be progressed through the previously outlined protocol, progressing as tolerated and avoiding posterior shear activities.

SUMMARY

Rehabilitation of the knee following ligamentous repair or reconstruction in a water-based program was discussed. The physiologic changes incurred by the body while immersed, both at rest and during exercise, were reviewed. Recommendations regarding both weight-bearing and non-weight-bearing cardiovascular conditioning were made, as well as suggestions regarding aerobic and anaerobic sport-specific conditioning. Stretching frequency and duration, and concentric and eccentric strength training were discussed. Balance and proprioception activities were suggested and progression to impact was reviewed. Suggestions regarding rehabilitation of various knee ligament injuries with and without meniscal pathology were discussed. The pool is an effective medium for many aspects of knee ligament rehabilitation. An understanding of the difference between land-based and water-based exercise allows the clinician to establish a comprehensive and effective training program for the patient.

References

1. Clancy WG, Nelson DA, Reider B, Narechania RG: Anterior cruciate ligament reconstruction using one-third of the patellar ligament, augmented by extra-articular tendon transfers. J Bone Joint Surg 64A:352–359, 1982.
2. Noyes FR, Butler DL, Paulos LE, et al.: Intra-articular cruciate reconstruction I: perspectives on graft strength, vascularization, and immediate motion after replacement. Clin Orthop 172:71–77, 1983.
3. Kurosaka M, Yoshiya S, Andrish JT: A biomechanical comparison of different surgical techniques of graft fixation in anterior cruciate ligament reconstruction. Am J Sports Med 15:225–229, 1987.
4. Swenson TM, Fu FH: Anterior cruciate ligament reconstruction: Long-term results using autograft tissue. Clin Sports Med 12:709–722, 1993.
5. Stanish WD, Lai L: New concepts of rehabilitation following anterior cruciate ligament reconstruction. Clin Sports Med 12:25–58, 1993.
6. Huegel M, Indelicato PA: Trends in rehabilitation following anterior cruciate ligament reconstruction. Clin Sports Med 7:801–811, 1988.
7. Paulos L, Noyes FR, Grood E, Butler DL: Knee rehabilitation after anterior cruciate ligament reconstruction and repair. Am J Sports Med 9:140–149, 1981.
8. Shelbourne KD, Wilckens JH: Current concepts in anterior cruciate ligament rehabilitation. Orthop Rev 19:957–964, 1990.
9. Silfverskoid JP, Steadman JR, Higgins RW, et al.: Rehabilitation of the anterior cruciate ligament in the athlete. Sports Med 6:308–319, 1988.
10. Shelbourne KD, Rowdon GA: Anterior cruciate ligament injury: The competitive athlete. Sports Med 17:132–140, 1994.
11. O'Meara PM: Rehabilitation following reconstruction of the anterior cruciate ligament. Orthopedics 16:301–306, 1993.
12. Palmitier RA, An KN, Scott SG, Chao EYS: Kinetic chain exercise in knee rehabilitation. Sports Med 11:402–413, 1991.
13. Lutz GE, Stuart MJ, Sim FH: Rehabilitative techniques for athletes after reconstruction of the anterior cruciate ligament. Mayo Clin Proc 65:1322–1329, 1990.
14. Draper V, Ballard L: Electrical stimulation versus electromyographic biofeedback in the recovery of quadriceps femoris muscle function following anterior cruciate ligament surgery. Phys Ther 71:455–461, 1991.
15. Draper V: Electromyographic biofeedback and recovery of quadriceps femoris muscle function following anterior cruciate ligament reconstruction. Phys Ther 70:11–17, 1990.
16. Tovin BJ, Wolf SL, Greenfield BH, et al.: Comparison of the effects of exercise in water and on land on the rehabilitation of patients with intra-articular anterior cruciate ligament reconstructions. Phys Ther 74:710–719, 1994.
17. Curl WW, Markey KL, Mitchell WA: Agility training following anterior cruciate ligament reconstruction. Clin Orthop Rel Res 172:133–136, 1983.
18. Skinner AT, Thompson AM: Duffield's Exercise in Water. London, Bailliere-Tindall, 1983.
19. Davis BC, Harrison RA: Hydrotherapy in Practice. New York, Churchill Livingstone, 1988.
20. Golland A: Basic hydrotherapy. Physiotherapy 67:258–262, 1981.
21. Beiser A: Physics, 2nd ed. Menlo Park, CA, Benjamin/Cummings Publishing, 1978.
22. Harrison RA, Bulstrode S: Percentage weightbearing

during partial immersion in the hydrotherapy pool. Physiother Pract 3:60–63, 1987.
23. Arborelius M Jr, Balldin UI, Lilja B, Lundgren CEG: Hemodynamic changes in man during immersion with the head above water. Aerospace Med 43:592–598, 1972.
24. Begin R, Epstein M, Sackner MA, et al.: Effects of water immersion to the neck on pulmonary circulation and tissue volume in man. J Appl Physiol 40:293–299, 1976.
25. Echt M, Lange L, Gauer OH: Changes of peripheral venous tone and central transmural venous pressure during immersion in a thermo-neutral bath. Pfluegers Arch 352:211–217, 1974.
26. Farhi LE, Linnarsson D: Cardiopulmonary readjustments during graded immersion in water at 35° C. Respir Physiol 30:35–50, 1977.
27. Lange L, Lange S, Echt M, Gauer OH: Heart volume in relation to body posture and immersion in a thermoneutral bath: A roentgenometric study. Pfluegers Arch 352:219–226, 1974.
28. Risch WD, Koubenec HJ, Beckmann U, et al.: The effect of graded immersion on heart volume, central venous pressure, pulmonary blood distribution, and heart rate in man. Pfluegers Arch 374:115–118, 1978.
29. Epstein M: Renal effects of head-out water immersion in man: Implications for an understanding of volume homeostasis. Physiol Rev 58:529–581, 1978.
30. Epstein M, Preston S, Weitzman RE: Isoosmotic central blood volume expansion suppresses plasma arginine vasopressin in normal man. J Clin Endocrinol Metab 52:256–262, 1981.
31. Gauer OH, Henry JP: Neurohormonal control of plasma volume. In Guyton AC, Cowley AW (eds): Cardiovascular Physiology II, Vol 9. Baltimore, University Park, 1976.
32. Greenleaf JE, Shvartz E, Keil LC: Hemodilution, vasopressin suppression, and diuresis during water immersion in man. Aviat Space Environ Med 52:329–336, 1981.
33. Lin YC: Circulatory functions during immersion and breath-hold dives in humans. Undersea Biomed Res 11:123–138, 1984.
34. Christie JL, Sheldahl LM, Tristani FE, et al.: Cardiovascular regulation during head-out water immersion exercise. J Appl Physiol 69:657–664, 1990.
35. Sheldahl LM, Tristani FE, Clifford PS, et al.: Effect of head-out water immersion on response to exercise training. J Appl Physiol 60:1878–1881, 1986.
36. Svedenhag J, Seger J: Running on land and in water: Comparative exercise physiology. Med Sci Sport Exerc 24:1155–1160, 1992.
37. Butts NK, Tucker M, Smith R: Maximal response to treadmill and deep water running in high school female cross country runners. Res Qt Exerc Sport 62:236–239, 1991.
38. Bishop PA, Frazier S, Smith J, Jacobs D: Physiologic responses to treadmill and water running. Phys Sports Med 17:87–94, 1989.
39. Wilder RP, Brennan D, Schotte DE: A standard measure for exercise prescription for aqua running. Am J Sports Med 21:45–48, 1993.
40. McArdle WD, Katch FI, Datch VL: Exercise Physiology: Energy, Nutrition, and Human Performance, 3rd ed. Philadelphia, Lea & Febiger, 1991.
41. Avellini BA, Shapiro Y, Pandolf KB: Cardio-respiratory physical training in water and on land. Eur J Appl Physiol 50:255–263, 1983.

42. Choukroun ML, Varene P: Adjustments in oxygen transport during head-out immersion in water at different temperatures. J Appl Physiol 68:1475–1480, 1990.
43. Gleim GW, Nicholas JA: Metabolic costs and heart rate responses to treadmill walking in water at different depths and temperatures. Am J Sports Med 17:248–252, 1989.
44. Walsh MT: Hydrotherapy: The use of water as a therapeutic agent. In Michlovitz SL (ed): Thermal Agents in Rehabilitation, 2nd ed. Philadelphia, F.A. Davis, 1990.
45. Malone TR, Garrett WE, Zachazewski JE: Muscle: Deformation, injury, repair. In Zachazewski JE, Magee DJ, Quillen WS (eds): Athletic Injuries and Rehabilitation. Philadelphia, W.B. Saunders, 1996.
46. Jenkins WL, Munns SW, Jayaraman G, et al.: A measurement of anterior tibial displacement in the closed and open kinetic chain. J Orthop Sports Phys Ther 25:49–56, 1997.
47. Yack HJ, Riley LM, Whieldon TR: Anterior tibial translation during progressive loading of the ACL-deficient knee during weight-bearing and non-weight-bearing isometric exercise. J Orthop Sports Phys Ther 20:247–253, 1994.
48. Stuart MJ, Meglan DA, Lutz GA, et al.: Comparison of intersegmental tibiofemoral joint forces and muscle activity during various closed kinetic chain exercises. Am J Sports Med 24:792–799, 1996.
49. Lutz GE, Palmitier RA, An KA, Chao EYS: Comparison of tibiofemoral joint forces during open-kinetic-chain and closed-kinetic-chain exercises. J Bone Joint Surg 75A:732–739, 1993.
50. Coyle EF, Hemmert MK, Coggan AR: Effects of detraining on cardiovascular responses to exercise: Role of blood volume. J Appl Physiol 60:95–99, 1986.
51. Coyle EF, Martin WH, Sinacore DR, et al.: Time course of loss of adaptations after stopping prolonged intense endurance training. J Appl Physiol 57:1857–1864, 1984.
52. Pedersen PK, Jorgensen K: Maximal oxygen uptake in young women with training, inactivity, and retraining. Med Sci Sport Exerc 10:223–227, 1978.
53. Wegener L, Kisner C, Nichols D: Static and dynamic balance responses in persons with bilateral knee osteoarthritis. J Orthop Sports Phys Ther 25:13–18, 1997.
54. Anderson MA, Foreman TL: Return to competition: Functional rehabilitation. In Zachazewski JE, Magee DJ, Quillen WS (eds): Athletic Injuries and Rehabilitation, Philadelphia, W.B. Saunders, 1996.
55. Law LA, Smidt GL: Underwater forces produced by the Hydro-Tone Bell. J Orthop Sports Phys Ther 23:267–271, 1996.
56. Visnic MA: Aquatic physical therapy comes of age. Aquatic Phys Ther Reports 1:6–8, 1994.
57. Barber FA: Accelerated rehabilitation for meniscus repairs. Arthroscopy 10:206–210, 1994.
58. Paletta GA, Warren RF: Knee injuries and alpine skiing, treatment and rehabilitation. Sports Med 17:411–423, 1994.
59. Shelbourne KD, Patel DV, Adsit WS, Porter DA: Rehabilitation after meniscal repair. Clin Sports Med 15:595–612, 1996.
60. Mariani PP, Santori N, Adriani E, Mastantuono M: Accelerated rehabilitation after arthroscopic meniscal repair: A clinical and magnetic resonance imaging evaluation. Arthroscopy 12:680–686, 1996.

61. Shelbourne KD, Nitz PA: The O'Donoghue triad revisited. Combined knee injuries involving anterior cruciate and medial collateral ligament tears. Am J Sports Med 19:474–497, 1991.
62. Littlejohn SG, Geissler WB: Arthroscopic repair of a posterior cruciate ligament avulsion. Arthroscopy 11:235–238, 1995.
63. Fanelli GC, Giannotti BF, Edson CJ: The posterior cruciate ligament arthroscopic evaluation and treatment. Arthroscopy 10:673–688, 1994.

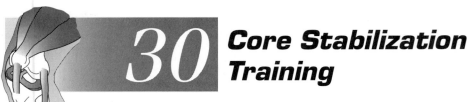

30 Core Stabilization Training

Micheal A. Clark, MS, PT, CSCS, and P. Dean Cummings, MD

*T*o stay on the cutting edge of research, science, and practical application, the sports medicine professional needs to follow a comprehensive, systematic, and integrated functional approach when rehabilitating an athlete with a knee ligament injury. To develop a comprehensive functional rehabilitation program, the sports medicine professional must fully understand what function is. Function is integrated, multidimensional movement.[1-3] Functional rehabilitation is a comprehensive approach that strives to improve all components necessary to allow an athlete to return to high levels of participation. Functional rehabilitation strives to develop functional strength. Functional strength is the ability of the neuromuscular system to perform dynamic eccentric, concentric, and isometric stabilization contractions upon demand in a smooth, coordinated fashion.[4]

Traditionally, sports medicine rehabilitation has focused on isolated absolute strength gains, in isolated muscles, utilizing one plane of motion. However, all functional activities require acceleration, deceleration, and dynamic stabilization.[2, 3, 5] Although a movement may appear to be one-plane dominant, the other planes need to be dynamically stabilized to allow for optimal neuromuscular efficiency.[4] Understanding that functional movements require a highly complex, integrated system allows the sports medicine professional to make a paradigm shift. The paradigm shift focuses on training the entire kinetic chain in all planes of movement instead of isolating one muscle.[6-11] Also, the paradigm shift dictates that we train force reduction, and dynamic stabilization as much as we train force production.[1, 12]

A dynamic, core stabilization training program is an important component of all comprehensive functional rehabilitation programs.[1-3, 13-16] A core stabilization program will improve dynamic postural control, ensure appropriate muscular balance around the lumbar-pelvic-hip complex, allow for dynamic three-dimensional flexibility, allow for the expression of dynamic functional strength, and improve neuromuscular efficiency.[1, 2, 4, 6, 7, 9, 11, 12, 17-22]

WHAT IS THE CORE?

The core is defined as the lumbar-pelvic-hip complex.[1, 4] The core is where our center of gravity is located and where all movement begins.[10, 23-25] There are 29 muscles that take their attachment to the pelvic complex.[1, 26-28] An efficient core allows for maintenance of the normal length-tension relationship of functional agonists and antagonists. This allows for the maintenance of the normal force-couple relationships in the lumbar-pelvic-hip complex. Maintaining the normal length-tension relationships and force-couple relationships allows for the maintenance of the normal path of instantaneous center of rotation in the lumbar-pelvic-hip complex during normal functional movements.[11, 22, 29] This provides optimal neuromuscular efficiency in the entire kinetic chain, which allows for optimal acceleration, deceleration, and dynamic stabilization of the entire kinetic chain during functional movements. This provides proximal stability for efficient lower extremity movements.[1, 3, 4, 10, 11, 22-25, 30]

The core functions as an integrated functional unit, whereby the entire kinetic chain works synergistically to produce force, reduce force, and dynamically stabilize against abnormal force.[4] In an efficient state, each structural component distributes weight, absorbs force, and transfers ground reaction forces.[4]

TRAINING CONCEPTS

Many individuals have developed the functional strength, power, neuromuscular control, and muscular endurance in specific muscles that enable them to perform functional activities.[1, 3, 4, 31] However, few people have developed the muscles required for spinal stabilization.[30–32] The body's stabilization system has to be functioning optimally to effectively utilize the strength, power, neuromuscular control, and muscular endurance that they have developed in their prime movers. If the extremity muscles are strong and the core is weak, then there will not be enough force created to produce efficient movements. A weak core is a fundamental problem of inefficient movements, which leads to injury.[3, 30–32]

Muscles produce force (concentric contractions), reduce force (eccentric contractions), and provide dynamic stabilization (isometric contractions) during functional movements.[17] The core musculature is an integral component of the protective mechanism that relieves the spine of the deleterious forces that are inherent during functional activities.[6] A core stabilization training program is designed to help an individual gain strength, neuromuscular control, power, and muscle endurance of the lumbar-pelvic-hip complex. This approach facilitates a balanced muscular functioning of the entire kinetic chain.[4] Greater neuromuscular control and stabilization strength will offer a more biomechanically efficient position for optimal neuromuscular efficiency.

Neuromuscular efficiency is established by the appropriate combination of postural alignment (static/dynamic) and stability strength, which allows the body to decelerate gravity, ground reaction forces, and momentum at the right joint, in the right plane, and at the right time.[2, 7, 12] If the neuromuscular system is not efficient, it will be unable to respond to the demands placed on it during functional activities.[4] As the efficiency of the neuromuscular system decreases, the ability of the kinetic chain to maintain appropriate forces and dynamic stabilization decreases significantly. This decreased neuromuscular efficiency leads to compensation and substitution patterns, as well as poor posture during functional activities.[11, 17, 22] This leads to increased mechanical stress on the contractile and noncontractile tissue, leading to repetitive microtrauma, abnormal biomechanics, and injury.[6, 8, 17, 33]

REVIEW OF FUNCTIONAL ANATOMY

To fully understand a functional core stabilization training program, the sports medicine professional must fully understand functional anatomy.[26–28, 34] A brief review of the key lumbar-pelvic-hip complex muscles will allow us to more fully understand integrated functional anatomy and therefore develop a comprehensive rehabilitation program based on function. The key lumbar spine muscles include the transversospinalis group, erector spinae, quadratus lumborum, and latissimus dorsi. The transversospinalis group includes the rotatores, interspinales, intertransversarii, semispinalis, and multifidus. The transversospinalis group is primarily responsible for intersegmental proprioception and segmental eccentric deceleration of flexion and rotation during functional movements.[28, 34] The transversospinalis is constantly put under a variety of compressive and tensile forces during functional movements and therefore needs to be trained adequately to allow dynamic postural stabilization and optimal neuromuscular efficiency of the entire kinetic chain.[28]

The abdominals are made up of four muscles, the rectus abdominus, external oblique, internal oblique, and transverse abdominus.[28] The abdominals function as an integrated functional unit, which helps maintain normal spinal kinematics.[26–28, 34] When working efficiently, the abdominals offer sagittal, frontal, and transverse plane stabilization by controlling forces that reach the lumbar-pelvic-hip complex.[28] The rectus abdominus eccentrically decelerates trunk extension and lateral flexion, as well as provides dynamic stabilization during functional movements. The external obliques work concentrically to produce contralateral rotation and ipsilateral lateral flexion, and work eccentrically to decelerate trunk extension, rotation, and lateral flexion during functional movements. The internal oblique works synergistically with the transverse abdominus to provide dynamic stabilization against rotational and translational forces during functional movements. The internal oblique and transverse abdominus contract in a feed-forward mechanism, contracting prior to the initiation of limb movement. This provides dynamic stabilization for the lumbar-pelvic-hip complex.

Key hip muscles include the psoas, gluteus medius, gluteus maximus, and hamstrings.[26–28] The psoas produces hip flexion and external rotation in the open chain position. The psoas produces hip flexion, lumbar extension, lateral flexion, and rotation in the closed chain position. The psoas eccentrically decelerates hip extension and internal rotation, as well as trunk extension, lateral flexion, and rotation. The psoas works synergistically with the superficial erector spinae and creates an anterior shear force at L4-L5.[28] The deep erector spinae, multifidus, and deep abdominal wall (transverse, internal oblique, and external oblique)[28] counteract this force. It is extremely common for athletes to develop tightness in their psoas. A tight psoas increases the anterior shear force and compressive force at the L4-L5 junction.[28] A tight psoas also causes reciprocal inhibition of the gluteus maximus, multifidus, deep erector spinae, internal oblique, and transverse abdominus. This leads to extensor mechanism dysfunction during functional movement patterns.[18–22, 28, 33] Lack of lumbar-pelvic-hip complex stabilization prevents appropriate movement sequencing and leads to synergistic dominance by the hamstrings and superficial erector spinae during hip extension. This complex movement dysfunction also decreases the ability of the gluteus maximus to decelerate femoral internal rotation during heel strike, which predisposes an individual with a knee ligament injury to abnormal forces and repetitive microtrauma.[6, 18, 20, 21, 35]

The gluteus medius functions as the primary frontal plane stabilizer during functional movement.[28] During closed chain movements, the gluteus medius decelerates femoral adduction and internal rotation. A weak gluteus medius increases frontal and transverse plane stress at the patellofemoral joint and the tibiofemoral joint.[28] A weak gluteus medius leads to synergistic dominance of the tensor fascia latae and the quadratus lumborum.[18, 35, 36] This leads to tightness in the iliotibial band and the lumbar spine. This will affect the normal biomechanics of the lumbar-pelvic-hip complex and the tibiofemoral joint as well as the patellofemoral

joint. Research by Beckman and Buchanan[37] has demonstrated decreased electromyographic (EMG) activity of the gluteus medius following an ankle sprain. Clinicians must address the altered hip muscle recruitment patterns or accept this recruitment pattern as an injury-adaptive strategy and thus accept the unknown long-term consequences of premature muscle activation and synergistic dominance.[17, 37]

The gluteus maximus functions concentrically in the open chain to accelerate hip extension and external rotation. It functions eccentrically to decelerate hip flexion and femoral internal rotation. It also functions through the iliotibial band to decelerate tibial internal rotation.[28] It has been demonstrated by Bullock-Saxton[38, 39] that the EMG activity of the gluteus maximus is decreased following an ankle sprain. Lack of proper gluteus maximus activity during functional activities leads to pelvic instability and decreased neuromuscular control. This can eventually lead to the development of muscle imbalances, poor movement patterns, and injury.

The hamstrings work concentrically to flex the knee, extend the hip, and rotate the tibia. They work eccentrically to decelerate knee extension, hip flexion, and tibial rotation. The hamstrings work synergistically with the anterior cruciate ligament.[28]

These are only some of the muscles of the lumbar-pelvic-hip complex. They have been reviewed so that the sports medicine professional realizes that muscles not only produce force (concentric contractions) in one plane of motion, but also reduce force (eccentric contractions) and provide dynamic stabilization in all planes of movement during functional activities. To effectively design a comprehensive rehabilitation program, we must understand functional anatomy and functional biomechanics.

POSTURAL CONSIDERATIONS

The core functions to maintain postural alignment and dynamic postural equilibrium during functional activities. Optimal alignment of each body part is a cornerstone to a functional training and rehabilitation program. Optimal posture and alignment will allow for maximal neuromuscular efficiency because the normal length-tension relationship, force-couple relationship, and path of instantaneous center of rotation will be maintained during functional movement patterns.[1, 3, 6, 8, 9, 11, 17, 18, 22, 36, 40, 41] If one segment in the kinetic chain is out of alignment, it will create predictable patterns of dysfunction throughout the entire kinetic chain. These predictable patterns of dysfunction are referred to as *serial distortion patterns*.[1] Serial distortion patterns represent the state in which the body's structural integrity is compromised because segments in the kinetic chain are out of alignment. This leads to abnormal distorting forces being placed on the segments in the kinetic chain that are above and below the dysfunctional segment.[1, 3, 6, 17] To avoid serial distortion patterns and the chain reaction that one misaligned segment creates, we must emphasize stable positions to maintain the structural integrity of the entire kinetic chain.[1, 3, 6, 20, 21] A comprehensive core stabilization program will prevent the development of serial distortion patterns and provide optimal dynamic postural control during functional movements.

MUSCULAR IMBALANCES

An optimally functioning core helps prevent the development of muscle imbalances and synergistic dominance. The human movement system is a well-orchestrated system of inter-related and interdependent components.[6, 19] The functional interaction of each component in the human movement system allows for optimal neuromuscular efficiency. Alterations in joint arthrokinematics, muscular balance, and neuromuscular control affect the optimal functioning of the entire kinetic chain.[6, 11, 22] Dysfunction of the kinetic chain is rarely an isolated event. Typically, any pathology of the kinetic chain is part of a chain reaction involving some key links in the kinetic chain with numerous compensations and adaptations developing.[19] The interplay of many muscles about a joint is responsible for the coordinated control of movement. If the core is weak, normal arthrokinematics are altered. This changes the normal length-tension relationship and the normal force-couple relationship, which in turn affects neuromuscular control. If one muscle becomes weak or tight or changes its degree of activation,

then synergists, stabilizers, and neutralizers have to compensate.[6, 9, 11, 17, 19–22]

Muscle tightness has a significant impact on the kinetic chain. Muscle tightness affects the normal length-tension relationship. This affects the normal force-couple relationship. When one muscle in a force-couple becomes tight, it changes the normal path of instantaneous center of rotation of two articular partners.[6, 11, 19] Altered arthrokinematics affect the synergistic function of the kinetic chain.[6, 11, 17, 19] This leads to abnormal pressure distribution over articular surfaces and soft tissues. Muscle tightness also leads to reciprocal inhibition.[6, 17–19, 29, 36, 40, 42, 43] If one develops muscle imbalances throughout the lumbar-pelvic-hip complex, it can affect the entire kinetic chain. For example, a tight psoas causes reciprocal inhibition of the gluteus maximus, transverse abdominus, internal oblique, and multifidus.[18, 28, 32, 36, 44] This muscle imbalance pattern may decrease normal lumbar-pelvic-hip stability. Specific substitution patterns develop to compensate for the lack of stabilization, including tightness in the iliotibial band.[17] This muscle imbalance pattern will lead to increased frontal and transverse plane stress at the knee. A strong core with optimal neuromuscular efficiency can help prevent the development of muscle imbalances. A comprehensive core stabilization training program should be an integral component of all rehabilitation programs.

NEUROMUSCULAR CONSIDERATIONS

A strong and stable core can improve optimal neuromuscular efficiency throughout the entire kinetic chain by helping to improve dynamic postural control.[11, 22, 30, 32, 45–47] Several authors have demonstrated kinetic chain imbalances in individuals with altered neuromuscular control.[6–9, 11, 18–21, 33–33, 36–39, 40, 42, 44, 47–49] Research has demonstrated that people with low back pain have an abnormal neuromotor response to the trunk stabilizers accompanying limb movement.[31, 32, 44] It has been demonstrated that individuals with low back pain had significantly greater postural sway and decreased limits of stability. Research has also been demonstrated that approximately 70 percent of athletes suffer from recurrent episodes of back pain. Furthermore, it has been demonstrated that individuals have decreased dynamic postural stability in the proximal stabilizers of the lumbar-pelvic-hip complex following lower extremity ligamentous injuries.[6, 37–39] It has also been demonstrated that joint and ligamentous injury can lead to decreased muscle activity.[17, 29, 43, 50] Joint and ligament injury can lead to joint effusion, which in turn leads to muscle inhibition.[50] Joint injury involving sensory afferents influences all of the muscles that function about that joint (Hilton's law). This leads to altered neuromuscular control in other segments of the kinetic chain secondary to altered proprioception and kinesthesia.[37, 38] Therefore, when an individual with a knee ligament injury has joint effusion, all of the muscles that cross the knee can be inhibited. Several muscles that cross the knee joint are attached to the lumbar-pelvic-hip complex.[28] Therefore, a comprehensive rehabilitation approach should focus on re-establishing optimal core function.

Research has also demonstrated that muscles can be inhibited from an arthrokinetic reflex.[6, 19, 29, 43] This is referred to as arthrogenic muscle inhibition. Arthrokinetic reflexes are reflexes that are mediated by joint receptor activity. If an individual has abnormal arthrokinematics, the muscles that move the joint will be inhibited. For example, if an individual has a sacral torsion, the multifidus and the gluteus medius can be inhibited.[51] This leads to abnormal movement in the kinetic chain. The tensor fascia latae will become synergistically dominant and become the primary frontal plane stabilizer.[28] This can lead to tightness in the iliotibial band. This can also decrease the frontal and transverse plane control at the knee. Furthermore, if the multifidus is inhibited,[51] the erector spinae and the psoas become facilitated. This will further inhibit the lower abdominals (internal oblique and transverse abdominus) and the gluteus maximus.[31, 32] This also decreases frontal and transverse plane stability at the knee. As previously mentioned, an efficient core will improve neuromuscular efficiency of the entire kinetic chain by providing dynamic stabilization of the lumbar-pelvic-hip complex and therefore improve pelvifemoral biomechanics. This is yet another reason that all rehabilitation programs should include a comprehensive core stabilization-training program.

ASSESSMENT

Before a comprehensive core stabilization program is implemented, an individual must undergo a comprehensive assessment to determine muscle imbalances, core strength, core neuromuscular control, core muscle endurance, core power, and overall function of the lower extremity kinetic chain.

It has been previously stated that muscle imbalances can cause abnormal movement patterns to develop throughout the entire kinetic chain. It is therefore extremely important to thoroughly assess each individual with a knee ligament injury for muscle imbalances. It is beyond the scope of this chapter to thoroughly explain a comprehensive muscle imbalance assessment procedure. It is therefore recommended that the interested reader use the reference list to more thoroughly review this important area.[1, 3, 4, 6, 7, 9, 11, 15, 16, 22, 29, 35, 42, 48]

Core strength can be assessed by utilizing the straight-leg lowering test (Fig. 30–1).[11, 22, 41, 48, 49, 52] The individual is placed supine. A blood pressure cuff is placed under the lumbar spine at approximately L4-L5. The cuff pressure is raised to 40 mm Hg. The individual's legs are maintained in full extension while flexing the hips to 90 degrees. The individual is instructed to perform a drawing-in maneuver (pull bellybutton to spine) (Fig. 30–2) and then flatten the back maximally into the table and pressure cuff. The individual is instructed to lower the legs toward the table while maintaining the back flat. The test is over when the pressure in the cuff decreases. The hip angle is then measured with a goniometer to determine the angle. Table 30–1 gives an approximation of an individual's lower abdominal strength.

Lower abdominal neuromuscular control is assessed in a similar fashion.[48, 52] The individual is supine with the knees and hips flexed to 90 degrees. The pressure cuff is placed under the lumbar spine at L4-L5 and

Table 30–1. Assessment of Core Strength

Range of Motion (Degrees)	Percent Strength
90	0
75	15
60	30
45	45
30	60
15	75
0	100

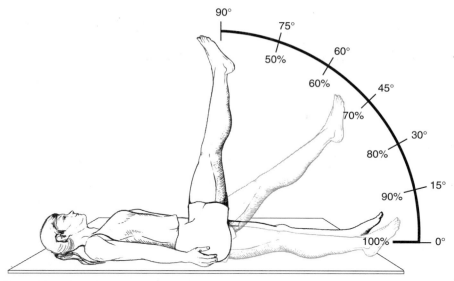

Figure 30–1. Straight-leg lowering test.

inflated to 40 mm Hg. The individual is instructed to perform a drawing-in maneuver to stabilize the lumbar spine. The individual is instructed to slowly lower the legs until the pressure in the cuff decreases. This indicates the ability of the lower abdominal wall to preferentially stabilize the lumbar-pelvic-hip complex. When the lumbar spine begins to move into extension, the hip flexors begin to work as stabilizers. This increases anterior shear forces and compressive forces at the L4-L5 lumbar segments and inhibits the transverse abdominus, internal oblique, and multifidus.

It has been demonstrated that approximately 80 to 85 percent of the general population suffers from low back pain.[52] It has also been demonstrated that individuals with low back pain have decreased muscle endurance in the erector spinae muscle group.[23, 24, 38, 52, 53] This leads to abnormal dynamic stabilization and movement during functional activities. This will lead to abnormal neuromuscular control. Therefore, all individuals should undergo an assessment of muscle endurance in the lumbar spine. Erector spinae performance can be assessed by having the individual lie prone on a treatment table, hands crossed behind the head. The axilla is used as a reference for the axis of a goniometer. The adjustable arm is aligned with the lateral side of the body and chin while the stationary arm is parallel to the table. The individual is instructed to extend at the lumbar spine to 30 degrees and hold the position for as long as he or she can while the clinician times the test.[52]

Power of the core musculature needs to

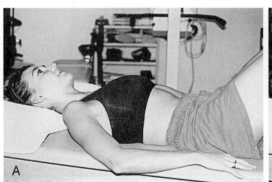
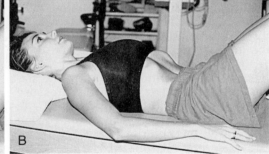

Figure 30–2. Drawing-in technique.

be assessed as well. Power production of the core musculature can be assessed by performing an overhead medicine ball throw.[54] The individual is instructed to hold a 4 kg medicine ball between the legs as he or she squats down. He or she is instructed to jump as high as possible while simultaneously throwing the medicine ball backward over the head. The distance is measured from a starting line to the point where the medicine ball stops. This is an assessment of total body power production with an emphasis on the core.

A lower extremity functional profile should also be carried out on all individuals with ligament injuries.[55] These tests should include isokinetic tests, balance tests, jump tests, power tests, and sports-specific functional tests.

A sports demand analysis profile (SDAP) should also be performed to determine the specific demands that each individual must return to. Please see Appendix I for an example of a sports demand analysis profile.

Scientific Rationale

Most individuals train their core stabilizers inadequately compared to other muscle groups.[4] Although adequate strength, power, muscle endurance, and neuromuscular control are important for lumbar-pelvic-hip stabilization, performing exercises incorrectly or performing ones that are too advanced is detrimental. Several authors have found decreased firing of the transverse abdominus, internal oblique, multifidus, and deep erector spinae in individuals with chronic low back pain.[30–32, 44, 48, 56] Performing core training with inhibition of these key stabilizers leads to the development of muscle imbalances and inefficient neuromuscular control in the kinetic chain. It has been demonstrated that abdominal training without proper pelvic stabilization increases intradiscal pressure and compressive forces in the lumbar spine.[13, 30–32, 48, 52, 57, 58] Furthermore, it has been demonstrated that hyperextension training without proper pelvic stabilization can increase intradiscal pressure to dangerous levels, cause buckling of the ligamentum flavum, and lead to narrowing of the intervertebral foramen.[13, 52, 58] Research has also demonstrated decreased stabilization endurance in individu-

als with chronic low back pain.[13, 23, 24, 59] The core stabilizers are primarily type I slow twitch muscle fibers.[10, 23–25] These muscles respond best to time under tension. Time under tension is a method of contraction that lasts for 6 to 20 seconds and emphasizes hypercontractions at end ranges of motion. This method improves intramuscular coordination, which improves static and dynamic stabilization. To get the appropriate training stimulus, you must prescribe the appropriate speed of movement for all aspects of exercises.[15, 16] Core strength endurance must be trained appropriately to allow an individual to maintain dynamic postural control for prolonged periods of time.[52]

Research has also demonstrated that the traditional curl up (Fig. 30–3) increases intradiscal pressure and increases compressive forces at L2-L3.[13, 52, 57, 58] It was also demonstrated that abnormally high levels of hip flexor EMG activity was elicited. This can lead to the development of inefficient stabilization and abnormal neuromuscular control in the entire kinetic chain.

Additional research has demonstrated increased EMG activity and increased pelvic stabilization when an abdominal drawing-in maneuver was performed prior to initiating core training.[13, 14, 16, 45, 47–49, 52, 61] Also, maintaining the cervical spine in a neutral position during core training will improve posture, muscle balance, and stabilization. If the head protracts during movement, then the sternocleidomastoid is preferentially recruited. This increases the compressive forces at the C0-C1 vertebral junction. This can also lead to pelvic instability and muscle imbalances secondary to the pelvo-occular reflex. This reflex is important to maintain

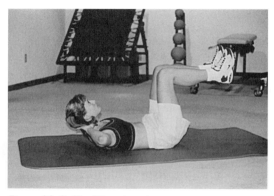

Figure 30–3. Traditional curl-up.

Table 30–2. Program Variation

1. Plane of motion	5. Speed of movement
2. Range of motion	6. Amount of control
3. Loading parameter	7. Duration
4. Body position	8. Frequency

Table 30–4. Exercise Selection

1. Safe
2. Challenging
3. Stress multiple planes
4. Proprioceptively enriched
5. Activity-specific

the eyes level. If the sternocleidomastoid muscle is hyperactive and extends the upper cervical spine, then the pelvis will rotate anteriorly to re-align the eyes. This can lead to muscle imbalances and decreased pelvic stabilization.[8, 19]

GUIDELINES

Prior to performing a comprehensive core stabilization program, each individual must undergo a comprehensive evaluation to determine the following: muscle imbalances, myokinematic deficits, arthrokinematic deficits, core strength/neuromuscular control/power, and overall kinetic chain function. All muscle imbalances, myokinetic deficits, and arthrokinematic deficits need to be corrected prior to initiating an aggressive core-training program.

A comprehensive core stabilization training program should be systematic, progressive, and functional. The rehabilitation program should emphasize the entire muscle contraction spectrum, focusing on force production (concentric contractions), force reduction (eccentric contractions), and dynamic stabilization (isometric contractions). The core stabilization program should begin in the most challenging environment the individual can control. A progressive continuum of function should be followed to systematically progress the individual (Table 30–2). The program should be manipulated regularly by changing any of the following variables; plane of motion, range of motion, loading parameters (eg, physioball, medi-

Table 30–3. Guidelines for Core Stabilization Training Program

1. Base program on science.
2. Program should be systematic, progressive, and functional.
3. Program should begin in the most challenging environment an athlete can control.
4. Program should be performed in a proprioceptively enriched environment.

cine ball, bodyblade, power sports trainer, weight vest, dumbbell, tubing), body position, amount of control, speed of execution, amount of feedback, duration (sets, repetitions, tempo, time under tension), and frequency.[1–4, 7, 9, 11–16, 39, 46–49, 54, 56, 58, 60–69]

SPECIFIC GUIDELINES

When designing a functional core stabilization training program, the clinician should create a proprioceptively enriched environment and select the appropriate exercises to elicit a maximal training response (Table 30–3). The exercises must be safe and challenging, stress multiple planes, incorporate a multisensory environment, be derived from fundamental movement skills, and be sports and position specific (Table 30–4).

The clinician should follow a progressive functional continuum to allow optimal adaptations.[1–3, 60] The following are key concepts for proper exercise progression: slow to fast, simple to complex, known to unknown, low-force to high-force, eyes open to eyes closed, static to dynamic, correct execution to increased repetitions, sets, and intensity (Table 30–5).[1–3, 15, 16, 60]

The goal of core stabilization should be to develop optimal levels of functional strength and dynamic stabilization.[4, 13] Neural adaptations become the focus of the program instead of striving for absolute strength gains.[1, 6, 7, 30, 49] Increasing proprioceptive demand by utilizing a multisensory, multimodal (eg, tubing, bodyblade, physioball, medicine ball, power sports trainer, weight vest, cobra belt, dumbbell) environ-

Table 30–5. Exercise Progression

1. Slow to fast
2. Simple to complex
3. Stable to unstable
4. Low force to high force
5. General to specific
6. Correct execution to increased intensity

ment becomes more important than increasing the external resistance (Fig. 30–4). The concept of quality before quantity is stressed. Core stabilization training is specifically designed to improve core stabilization and neuromuscular efficiency. You must be concerned with the sensory information that is stimulating your central nervous system. If you train with poor technique and poor neuromuscular control, then you develop poor motor patterns and poor stabilization.[1, 3] The focus of your program must be on function. To determine whether your program is functional, answer to following questions: Is it dynamic? Is it multiplanar? Is it multidimensional? Is it proprioceptively challenging? Is it systematic? Is it progressive? Is it based on functional anatomy and science? Is it sport-specific? (Table 30–6).[1–3]

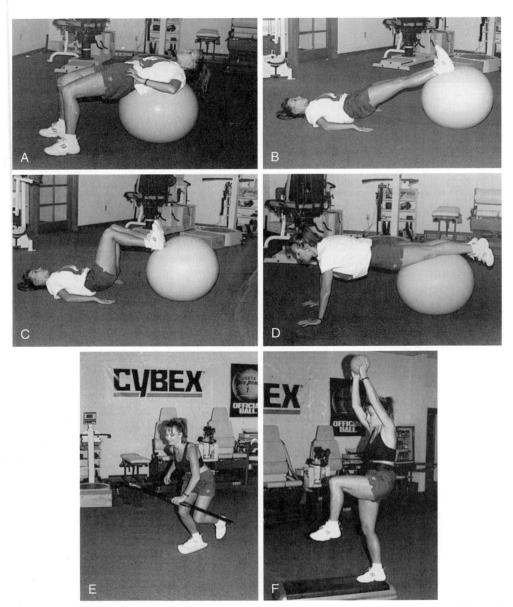

Figure 30–4. Multisensory, multimodal exercises. *A*, Ball bridging; *B*, ball hip extension; *C*, ball hamstring curl; *D*, ball push-ups; *E*, foam roll bodyblade deceleration; *F*, medicine ball step-ups.

○━ Table 30–6. **Guidelines for a Functional Core Stabilization Program**

1. Is it dynamic?
2. Is it multiplanar?
3. Is it proprioceptively enriched?
4. Is it systematic?
5. Is it progressive?
6. Is it activity-specific?

TRAINING PROGRAM

Please see appendices 2 and 3 for examples of comprehensive core stabilization-training programs. Individuals are started at the highest level at which they can maintain stability and optimal neuromuscular control. They are progressed through the program when they achieve mastery of the exercises in the previous level.[1–4, 6, 7, 9, 12–16, 23, 24, 30, 39, 46, 48, 49, 52, 54, 55, 58, 62, 63, 68, 69]

SUMMARY

A core stabilization program should be an integral component for all individuals rehabilitating from an injured knee ligament. A core stabilization training program will allow an individual to gain optimal neuromuscular control of the lumbar-pelvic-hip complex and allow the individual with a knee ligament injury to return to activity much faster and safer. Research has demonstrated that it is important to follow a systematic, progressive, and activity-specific core stabilization training program following injury.

References

1. Dominguez RH: Total Body Training. East Dundee, IL, Moving Force Systems, 1982.
2. Gambetta V: Building the complete athlete: Course Manual. Chicago, 1996.
3. Jesse J: Hidden causes of injury, prevention, and correction for running athletes. Pasadena, CA, The Athletic Press, 1977.
4. Aaron G: The use of stabilization training in the rehabilitation of the athlete. Sports Physical Therapy Home Study Course, 1996.
5. Crisco J, Panjabi MM: The intersegmental and multisegmental muscles of the lumbar spine. Spine 16:793–799, 1991.
6. Bullock-Saxton JE: Muscles and Joint: Inter-relationships with Pain and Movement Dysfunction. Course Manual, November, 1997.
7. Janda V, Vavrova M: Sensory Motor Stimulation video. Brisbane, Australia, Body Control Systems, 1990.
8. Lewit K: Manipulative Therapy in the Rehabilitation of the Locomotor System. London, Butterworths, 1985.
9. Liebenson CL: Rehabilitation of the Spine. Baltimore, Williams & Wilkins, 1996.
10. Panjabi MM: The stabilizing system of the spine. Part I: Function, dysfunction, adaptation, and enhancement. J Spinal Disord 5:383–389, 1992.
11. Sahrmann S: Diagnosis and Treatment of Muscle Imbalances and Musculoskeletal Pain Syndrome. Continuing Education Course. St. Louis, 1997.
12. Blievernicht J: Balance: Course Manual. Chicago, IL, 1996.
13. Beim G, Giraldo JL, Pincivero DM, et al.: Abdominal strengthening exercises: A comparative EMG study. J Sport Rehab 6:11–20, 1997.
14. Brittenham D, Brittenham G: Stronger Abs and Back. Champaign, IL, Human Kinetics, 1997.
15. Chek P: Scientific back training. Correspondence Course, Paul Chek Seminars, La Jolla, CA, 1994.
16. Chek P: Scientific abdominal training. Correspondence Course, Paul Chek Seminars, La Jolla, CA, 1992.
17. Edgerton VR, Wolf S, Roy RR: Theoreical basis for patterning EMG amplitudes to assess muscle dysfunction. Med Sci Sports Exerc 28(6):744–751, 1996.
18. Janda V: Muscle weakness and inhibition in back pain syndromes. In Grieve GP (ed.): Modern Manual Therapy of the Vertebral Column. New York, Churchill Livingstone, 1986.
19. Lewit K: Muscular and articular factors in movement restriction. Man Med (In print).
20. Liebenson CL: Active muscle relaxation techniques. Part I. Basic principles and methods. J Manipulative Physiol Ther 12(6):446–454, 1989.
21. Liebenson CL: Active muscle relaxation techniques. Part II. Clinical application. J Manipulative Physiol Ther 13(2):2–6, 1989.
22. Sahrmann S: Posture and muscle imbalance: Faulty lumbo-pelvic alignment and associated musculoskeletal pain syndromes. Orthop Div Rev Can Phys Ther 12:13–20, 1992.
23. Gracovetsky S, Farfan H: The optimum spine. Spine 11:543–573, 1986.
24. Gracovetsky S, Farfan H, Heuller C: The abdominal mechanism. Spine 10:317–324, 1985.
25. Panjabi MM, Tech D, White AA: Basic biomechanics of the spine. Neurosurgery 7:76–93, 1980.
26. Basmajian J: Muscles Alive. Baltimore, Williams & Wilkins, 1974.
27. Basmajian J: Muscles Alive: Their Functions Revealed by EMG, 5th ed. Baltimore, Williams & Wilkins, 1985.
28. Porterfield JA, DeRosa C: Mechanical low back pain; Perspectives in functional anatomy. Philadelphia, WB Saunders, 1991.
29. Warmerdam ALA: Arthrokinetic Therapy: Manual Therapy to Improve Muscle and Joint Functioning. Orthopaedic Physical Therapy Products, Continuing Education Course. Marshfield, WI, 1996.
30. Hodges PW, Richardson CA: Contraction of the abdominal muscles associated with movement of the lower limb. Phys Ther 77:132–114, 1997.
31. Hodges PW, Richardson CA: Inefficient muscular stabilization of the lumbar spine associated with low back pain. Spine 21(22):2640–2650, 1996.

32. Hodges PW, Richardson CA: Neuromotor dysfunction of the trunk musculature in low back pain patients. *In* Proceedings of the International Congress of the World Confederation of Physical Therapists, Washington, DC, 1995.
33. Lewit K: Myofascial Pain: Relief by Post-Isometric Relaxation. Arch Phys Med Rehabil 65:452, 1984.
34. Aspden RM: Review of the functional anatomy of the spinal ligaments and the erector spinae muscles. Clin Anat 5:372–387, 1992.
35. Chaitow L: Muscle Energy Techniques. New York, Churchill Livingstone, 1997.
36. Janda V: Muscles, central nervous system regulation and back problems. *In* Korr IM (ed): Neurobiologic Mechanisms in Manipulative Therapy. New York, Plenum Press, 1978.
37. Beckman SM, Buchanan TS: Ankle inversion and hypermobility: Effect on hip and ankle muscle electromyography onset latency. Arch Phys Med Rehabil 76(12):1138–1143, 1995.
38. Bullock-Saxton JE: Local sensation changes and altered hip muscle function following severe ankle sprain. Phys Ther 74(1):17–23, 1994.
39. Bullock-Saxton JE, Janda V, Bullock M: Reflex activation of gluteal muscles in walking: An approach to restoration of muscle function for patients with low back pain. Spine 18(6):704–708, 1993.
40. Janda V: Physical therapy of the Cervical and Thoracic Spine. *In* Grant R (ed). New York, Churchill Livingstone, 1988.
41. Jull G, Richardson CA, Hamilton C, et al.: Towards the validation of a clinical test for the deep abdominal muscles in back pain patients. Gold Coast, Queensland, Manipulative Physiotherapists Association of Australia, 1995.
42. Janda V: Muscle Function Testing. London, Butterworths, 1983.
43. Stokes M, Young A: The contribution of reflex inhibition to arthrogenous muscle weakness. Clin Sci 67:7–14, 1984.
44. O'Sullivan PE, Twomey L, Allison G, et al.: Altered patterns of abdominal muscle activation in patients with chronic low back pain. Austr J Physiother 43(2):91–98, 1997.
45. Hall T, David A, Geere J, Salvenson K: Relative Recruitment of the Abdominal Muscles During Three Levels of Exertion During Abdominal Hollowing. Gold Coast, Queensland, Manipulative Physiotherapists Association of Australia. 1995.
46. Jull G, Richardson CA, Comerford M: Strategies for the initial activation of dynamic lumbar stabilization. *In* Proceedings of Manipulative Physiotherapists Association of Australia. New South Wales, 1991.
47. Richardson CA, Jull G, Toppenberg R, Comerford M: Techniques for active lumbar stabilization for spinal protection. Austr J Physiother 38:105–112, 1992.
48. Hodges PW, Richardson CA, Jull G: Evaluation of the relationship between laboratory and clinical tests of transverse abdominus function. Physiother Res Int 1:30–40, 1996.
49. O'Sullivan PE, Twomey L, Allison G: Evaluation of Specific Stabilizing Exercises in the Treatment of Chronic Low Back Pain with Radiological Diagnosis of Spondylolisthesis. Gold Coast, Queensland, Manipulative Physiotherapists Association of Australia, 1995.
50. DeAndre JR, Grant C, Dixon ASJ: Joint distension and reflex muscle inhibition in the knee. J Bone Joint Surg (Am) 47:313–322, 1965.
51. Hides JA, Stokes MJ, Saide M, et al.: Evidence of lumbar multifidus wasting ipsilateral to symptoms in subjects with acute/subacute low back pain. Spine 19:165–177, 1994.
52. Ashmen KJ, Swanik CB, Lephart SM: Strength and flexibility characteristics of athletes with chronic low back pain. J Sports Rehab 5:275–286, 1996.
53. Boduk N, Twomey L: Clinical Anatomy of the Lumbar Spine. New York, Churchill Livingstone, 1987.
54. Gambetta V: The Complete Guide to Medicine Ball Training. Sarasota, FL, Optimum Sports Training, 1991.
55. Gray GW: Chain reaction festival. Course Manual, Wynn Marketing, Adrian, MI, 1996.
56. Richardson CA, Jull G: Muscle control—pain control. What exercises would you prescribe? Man Med 1:2–10, 195.
57. Nachemson A: The load on the lumbar discs in different positions of the body. Clin Orthop 45:107–122, 1966.
58. Norris CM: Abdominal muscle training in sports. Br J Sports Med 27(1):19–27, 1993.
59. Calliet R: Low back pain syndrome. Oxford, Blackwell, 1962.
60. Gustavsen R, Streeck R: Training Therapy: Prophylaxis and Rehabilitation. New York, Thieme Medical Publishers, 1993.
61. Miller MI, Medeiros JM: Recruitment of the internal oblique and transverse abdominus muscles on the eccentric phase of the curl-up. Phys Ther 67(8):1213–1217, 1987.
62. Chek P: Swiss Ball Training. Correspondence Course, Paul Chek Seminars, La Jolla, CA, 1996.
63. Creager C: Therapeutic Exercise Using Foam Rollers. Berthoud, CO, Executive Physical Therapy, 1996.
64. Kennedy B: An Australian program for management of back problems. Physiotherapy 66:108–111, 1980.
65. Mayer TG, Gatchel RJ: Functional restoration for spinal disorders. The sports medicine approach. Philadelphia, Lea & Febiger, 1988.
66. Mayer-Posner J: Swiss ball applications for orthopedic and sports medicine. Ball Dynamics International. Denver, CO, 1995.
67. Robinson R: The new back school prescription: Stabilization training. Part I. Occup Med 7:17–31, 1992.
68. Saal JA: The new back school prescription: Stabilization training. Part II. Occup Med 7:33–42, 1992.
69. Saal JA: Nonoperative treatment of herniated disc: An outcome study. Spine 14:431–437, 1989.
70. Aaron G: Clinical Guideline Manual for Spine. Healthsouth Corporation 1996.
71. Chek P: Dynamic Medicine Ball Training. Correspondence Course, Paul Chek Seminars, La Jolla, CA, 1996.
72. Freeman MAR: Coordination exercises in the treatment of functional instability of the foot. Phys Ther 44:393–395, 1964.
73. Gambetta V: Following a functional path. Train Condition 5(2):25–30, 1995.
74. Gambetta V: Everything in balance. Train Condition 1(2):15–21, 1996.
75. Chek P: Program Design. Correspondence Course, Paul Chek Seminars, La Jolla, CA, 1995.
76. Chek P: Strong and Stable. Three-Volume Video Series. Paul Chek Seminars, La Jolla, CA, 1995.
77. Cook G, Fields K: Functional Training for the Torso. Internet access: www.funct.html, 1998.

Bibliography

Aruin As, Latash ML: Directional specificity of postural muscles in feed-forward postural reactions during fast voluntary arm movements. Exp Brain Res 103:323–332, 1995.

Axler CT, McGill SM: Low back loads over a variety of abdominal exercises: Searching for the safest abdominal challenge. Med Sci Sports Exerc 29(6):804–810, 1997.

Beimborn DS, Morrissey MC: A review of the literature related to trunk muscle performance. Spine 13(6):655–670, 1988.

Bousiett S, Zattara M: A sequence of postural adjustments precedes voluntary movement. Neurosci Lett 22:263–270, 1981.

Chaitow L: Soft Tissue Manipulation. Rochester, VT, Healing Arts Press, 1988.

Cresswell AG, Grundstrom H, Thorstensson A: Observations on intra-abdominal pressure and patterns of abdominal intra-muscular activity in man. Acta Physiol Scand 144:409–418, 1992.

Cresswell AG, Oddson L, Thorstensson A: The influence of sudden perturbations on trunk muscle activity and intra-abdominal pressure while standing. Exp Brain Res 98:336–341, 1994.

Dvorak J, Dvorak V: Manual Medicine-Diagnostics. New York, Georg Theim Verlag, 1984.

Evjenth O: Muscle Stretching in Manual Therapy. Sweden, Alfta Rehab, 1984.

Fairbanks JCT, O'Brien JP: The abdominal cavity and the thoracolumbar fascia as stabilizers of the lumbar spine in patients with low back pain. Engineering Aspects of the Spine: Conference. London, 1980.

Freyette: Principles of Osteopathic Technique. Yearbook of the Academy of Applied Osteopathy, American Osteopathic Association, 1954.

Greenman PE: Principles of Manual Medicine. Baltimore, Williams & Wilkins, 1991.

Holt LE: Scientific Stretching for Sport. Halifax, Dalhouise University Press, 1976.

Lavender SA, Tsuang YH, Andersson GBJ: Trunk muscle activation and co-contraction while resisting movements in a twisted posture. Ergonomics 36:1145–1157, 1993.

Paquet N, Malouin F, Richards CL: Hip-spine movement interaction and muscle activation patterns during sagittal trunk movements in low back pain patients. Spine 19(5):596–603, 1994.

Peck D, Buxton DF, Nitz AJ: A comparison of spindle concentrations in large and small muscles acting in parallel combinations. J Morphology 180:243–252, 1984.

Pope M, Frymoyer J, Krag M: Diagnosing instability. Clin Orthop Rel Res 296:60–67, 1992.

Strohl K, Mead J, Banzett R, et al.: Regional differences in abdominal activity during various maneuvers in humans. J Appl Physiol 51:1471–1476, 1981.

Tesh KM, ShawDunn J, Evans JH: The abdominal muscles and vertebral stability. Spine 12:501–508, 1987.

Thorstensson A, Ardidson A: Trunk strength and low back pain. Scand J Rehabil Med 14:69–75, 1982.

Wilke HJ, Wolf S, Claes LE: Stability increase of the lumbar spine with different muscle groups: A biomechanical in vitro study. Spine 20:192–198, 1995.

I *Sport Demands Analysis Profile (SDAP)*

Sport analyzed: _____

Type of Sport

Endurance 1 2 3 4 5   Speed/power 1 2 3 4 5

Skill 1 2 3 4 5   Strength 1 2 3 4 5

☐ Aquatic   ☐ Combative   ☐ Artistic

1 = High Demand   5 = Low Demand

Characteristics of the Sport

☐ Team   ☐ Individual

☐ Collision   ☐ Contact

☐ Equipment dominant   ☐ Weight-bearing

☐ Non-weight-bearing

Length of Competition (Time/Motion Analysis)

Time of Actual Competition

Work time _____ Rest time _____

Distribution of intensity of effort

1   2   3   4   5   6   7   8   9   10

Infrequent maximal   Frequent maximal
effort   effort

Temporal classification

☐ Set time frame   ☐ Open time frame

Nature of Competitive Season

Length _____ Competition venue _____

Number of competitions _____ Travel _____

Competition frequency ____ Multiple season ____

From Gambetta V: Building the Complete Athlete. Course Manual. Chicago, 1996.

From Building and Rebuilding the Athlete, Seminar Workbook. Vern Gambetta, Gambetta Sports Training, 1999.

442

II Therapeutic Exercise Ball Training Program

A. WARM-UP

1. Pelvic rock forward/backward
2. Pelvic rock side-to-side
3. Pelvic rock figure-of-eight
4. Back/abdominal stretch
5. Quadratus lumborum/oblique stretch
6. Adductor stretch
7. Hamstring stretch
8. Hip flexor stretch
9. Rotational stretch
10. Latissimus dorsi stretch

B. FUNCTIONAL EXERCISE PROGRESSION

1. Beginner
   a. Pelvic tilt
   b. Prone jackknife stabilization
   c. Two-leg bridge stabilization
   d. Supine hip extension stabilization
   e. Supine leg extension stabilization
   f. Prone hip extension stabilization
   g. Prone hip/leg extension stabilization
   h. Seated posture trainer knee lift
   i. Alternating superman upper extremity/lower extremity flexed
   j. Back extension, arms at side
   k. Ball crunch, arms across chest
   l. Ball oblique crunch, arms across chest
   m. Torso side flexion, arms across chest
2. Intermediate
   a. Pelvic tilt with crunch
   b. Prone jackknife at knees
   c. Two-leg bridge
   d. Supine hip extension stabilization, two legs
   e. Supine leg extension, two legs
   f. Prone hip extension, one leg
   g. Prone hip/leg extension, stabilization neutral
   h. Seated posture trainer leg extension
   i. Alternating superman upper extremity/lower extremity extended
   j. Back extension, hands on head
   k. Ball crunch, arms behind head
   l. Ball oblique crunch, arms behind head
   m. Torso side flexion, arms behind head
3. Advanced
   a. Pelvic tilt with cross crunch
   b. Prone jackknife at feet
   c. One-leg bridging
   d. Supine hip extension, one leg
   e. Supine leg extension, one leg
   f. Prone hip extension, two legs
   g. Prone hip/leg extension, vertical
   h. Seated posture trainer opposite upper extremity/lower extremity
   i. Alternating superman upper extremity/lower extremity flexed
   j. Back extension, arms extended
   k. Ball crunch, arms overhead
   l. Ball oblique crunch, arms overhead
   m. Torso side flexion, arms overhead

C. FUNCTIONAL CORE STABILIZATION PROGRAM

1. Beginner
   a. Supine pelvic tilt
   b. Supine pelvic tilt, single leg
   c. Supine pelvic tilt, unsupported
   d. Supine pelvic tilt half knee-ups
   e. Oblique crunch 90/90 degrees
   f. Standard crunch
   g. Prone cobra
   h. Trunk and hip extension
   i. Alternating superman
   j. Quadruped vertical
   k. Wall squats with ball
2. Intermediate
   a. Supine pelvic tilt, single leg
   b. Supine pelvic tilt unsupported
   c. Supine pelvic tilt half knee-ups
   d. Supine pelvic tilt reverse crunch
   e. Oblique crunch, straight legs
   f. Jackknife crunch

g. Prone cobra with resistance
h. Trunk and hip extension with resistance
i. Quadruped horizontal
j. Chops and lifts
k. Static lunges
l. Tube walking

3. Advanced
   a. Supine pelvic tilt unsupported
   b. Supine pelvic tilt, double leg lowering
   c. Supine pelvic tilts half knee-ups incline
   d. Supine pelvic tilts reverse crunch incline
   e. Hanging reverse crunch
   f. Oblique crunch with counter-rotation
   g. Alternating oblique crunch
   h. Seated oblique torso rotation with cable
   i. Lower body rotation with cable
   j. Lower body rotation with ball
   k. Standard crunch on progressive incline
   l. Jackknife crunch with resistance
   m. Cable/machine-resisted crunch
   n. Prone cobra on ball
   o. Alternating superman on ball
   p. Quadruped horizontal
   q. Quadruped alphabet
   r. Quadruped dynamic

NOTE: PROGRESSIVE FUNCTIONAL CONTINUUM

1. Accumulation phase = increase training load by increasing volume.
2. Intensification phase = increase training load by increasing intensity.
3. Add functional implements (bodyblade, tubing, dumbbell, manual resistance) to increase neuromuscular recruitment.

III Core Stabilization Training Program

LEVEL I: NEUROMUSCULAR STABILIZATION

Exercise Selection

- Abdominal exercises
  Drawing-in
  Drawing-in one leg to chest
  Drawing-in one leg slide
  Drawing-in unsupported
  Drawing-in two knees to chest
  Drawing-in two leg slide
  Drawing-in long lever crunch
  Drawing-in alternate cross crunch
  Drawing-in with knee-up
- Back exercises
  Prone gluteal squeeze with drawing-in
    maneuver
  Prone cobra
  Prone arm raise
  Prone leg raise
  Prone alternate arm/leg raise
  Prone superman
  Quadruped drawing-in
  Quadruped arm raise
  Quadruped leg raise
  Quadruped opposite arm/leg raise
- Hip exercises
  Bridging with drawing-in
  Single leg raise with drawing-in
  Hip abduction
  Hip adduction
  Hip extension
  Tube walking
    Side-to-side
    Front-to-back
    Front-to-back at 45-degree diagonal
- Balance exercises
  Balance shoes
    In place balance with drawing-in
      maneuver
    Forward walking
    Backward walking
    Side walking
  Balance board
    Standing in alignment
    Squatting with proper alignment

Overhead press with proper alignment
Squat to calve raise with proper alignment
Sport beam
  Standing in balance
  One-leg standing
  Forward walking
  Backward walking
  Side walking
  Lunge in place
Mini-tramp
  Multi-angle stabilization squats
  Single-leg stabilization squats
  Calf raise
  Squat to calve raise
Floor drills
  One-leg standing with tubing resistance (three planes)
  Two-leg standing with proprioceptive neuromuscular facilitation movements
  One-leg standing with proprioceptive neuromuscular facilitation movements

LEVEL II: DYNAMIC STABILIZATION

Exercise Selection

- Active warm-up exercises (utilizing a physioball)
  Pelvic tilts
    Forward
    Backward
    Side
    Circles
    Figure-of-eights
  Abdominal wall stretch
  Side stretch
  Adductor stretch
  Supine Russian twist
  Trunk rotation
  Standing trunk rotation
  Foam roller active myofascial release
    Tibiofemoral ligament/iliotibial band

Piriformis
Gluteus medius
Latissimus dorsi
Teres major
Three-dimensional flexibility
Psoas
Adductors
Rectus femoris
Hamstrings
• Abdominal exercises
Reverse crunch on horizontal
Reverse crunch on physioball
Reverse crunch on incline
Knee-ups on horizontal
Knee-ups on physioball
Knee-ups on incline
Physioball crunch
Physioball rotational crunch
Physioball side sit-up
Physioball stabilization push-up
• Back exercises
Standing on one leg opposite arm/leg
Physioball exercises
Bridging
Back extension
Hamstring curls
Hip and leg extension
Alternating upper extremity/lower
extremity raise
• Hip exercises
Quadruped exercises
Dynamic upper extremity/lower
extremity movement
Alphabet
Fire hydrant clockwise/counter-
clockwise
Tube walking
Carioca
Low and long carioca
Step-ups
Hurdle walking
Dynamic mobility
• Balance exercises
Balance shoes
Squat
Squat and side walk
Carioca walk
Heel to toe walk forward and back-
ward
Balance board
Squat with weight on balls of feet
Squat to calf raise
Squat with extrinsic resistance
Sport beam
Dynamic lunge
Forward backward walking on toes
Squat on toes side walk

Squat on heels side walk
Lateral walk in squat position
Single leg squats
Single leg squat touchdowns
Hip closed kinetic chain internal/ex-
ternal rotation
Mini-tramp
Stabilization jumps
Single-leg squat
Single-leg touchdown
Single-leg calf raise
Hip closed kinetic chain internal/ex-
ternal rotation
Slide board
Lateral slides
Fitter
Side to side
Forward and backward
Floor
Tubing drills
Lunge with Dumbbell Press (three
planes)
Step-ups with Dumbbell Press
(three planes)
Dumbbell matrix

LEVEL III: REACTIVE FUNCTIONAL STABILIZATION

Exercise Selection

• Dynamic functional warm-up
Prisoner squats
Single-leg squats
Touchdowns
Three-position lunges
Knee-ups
Standing opposite upper extremity/
lower extremity raise
Squat push press
Standing torso twist
Good morning
Bent over row
Bend and reach
Dynamic side stretch
Walking lunge with opposite rotation
• Dynamic medicine ball exercises
Abdominal crunch on physioball with
medicine ball pass
Rotational crunch on physioball with
medicine ball pass
Side sit-up on physioball with medi-
cine ball pass
Wood chopper
Overhead toss (multiplane)

Standing oblique toss
Seated oblique toss
Chest pass
Soccer pass
Two medicine ball push-up
Medicine ball cross-over push-up
Lunge with medicine ball pass
  (three positions)
Step-up with medicine ball pass
  (three positions)
Overhead throw
Forward throw
Rotational throw
Squat jumps with medicine ball throw
Squat throw and chase
• Dynamic balance exercises
Balance shoes
  Single-leg squat
  Touchdown
  Lunge
  Upper extremity lifting while
    maintaining center of gravity
Balance board
  Squat to calf raise with external
    loading
  Stabilization jumps
  Squat while throwing and catching
    medicine ball
  Single-leg squat
  Touchdown
Sport beam
  Lunging while catching medicine
    ball
  Side shuffling while throwing medi-
    cine ball
  Carioca while throwing medicine
    ball
Mini-tramp
  Running in place
  Jump while throwing and catching
  Single leg stabilization hops
Slide board
  Lateral movement with external
    loading
  Interval training
  Complex training
Fitter
  Lateral movement with medicine
    ball
  Lateral movement with bodyblade
Floor drills
  Running in place with tubing
    (three planes)
  Lateral shuffle with tubing (three
    planes)
  Carioca with tubing (three planes)
  Lateral bounding with tubing

Multidirectional drills
Single-leg squat/touchdown with
  external loading using an un-
  stable surface
In-place reactive jumps
Dynamic lunging with medicine ball
  and tubing system
Agility ladder drills

LEVEL IV: EXPLOSIVE STABILIZATION

Exercise Selection

• Plyometric exercises
Reactive jumps
  Jump rope (two legs)
  Jump rope (one leg)
  Jump rope (alternating legs)
  Jump rope (crossover)
  Jump rope (jumps)
  Jump rope (hops)
  Jump rope (patterns)
  Proprioceptive jumps (90, 180, 270,
    360 degrees)
  Jump squats
  Tuck jumps
  Butt kickers
  Ice skaters
  Scissor jumps
  Pattern jumps
  Skipping
  Repetitive long jumps
  Repetitive vertical jumps
  Cone jumps
  Diagonal cord jumps/hops
  Bounding
  Hurdle hops
  Bound into a run
  Long jump into a run
  Vertical jump into a run
  Multiple box jumps
  Depth jumps
• Lateral speed and agility exercises
Speed ladder drills
  Forward 1 ins
  Forward 2 ins
  Lateral 2 ins
  Lateral cross-step
  Lateral step in/out
  Left/right shuffle
  Slalom jumps
  Cross-over steps
  Forward in/in/out
  Forward out/out/in/in

Shuffle bounds
Cross-step bounds
Be creative and sports specific
Use resistance (tubing, weight vests)
Hills and different surfaces
Utilize medicine balls and sports implements
Lateral speed and agility drills
Wheel drills
Short shuttle drills
Four cone drills
LEFT test
Cone drills
Bag drills
Sport-specific drills with cobra belt or power trainer
Straight ahead speed exercises (42)
Hips tall, fall, and catch
Drop and go
Lean, fall, run
Mechanics with cobra belt, core trainer
Exchange drill
Arm action drill
Push/push drill
Contrast drill

Push-up start
Roll over start
Track start
Jump into sprint
Bound into a sprint
Acceleration ladder
Low hurdle runs
Straight leg bounding
Dynamic butt kicks
Weight sled running
Parachute running
Cobra belt assisted/resisted running
Pulley resistance running
Super speed trainer running
Sport-specific technical drills
Resistance
Assistance
Game Speed

Data from Dominguez,[1] Gambetta,[2] Jesse,[3] Aaron,[4] Janda and Vavrova,[7] Liebenson,[9] Blievernicht,[12] Beim et al.,[13] Brittenham and Brittenham,[14] Chek,[15, 16] Bullock-Saxton et al.,[39] Jull et al.,[46] Richardson et al.,[47] O'Sullivan et al.,[49] Gambetta,[54] Norris,[58] Gustavsen,[60] Chek,[62] Creager,[63] Kennedy,[64] Mayer and Gatchel,[65] Robinson,[67] Saal,[68, 69] Chek,[71] Gambetta,[73, 74] Chek,[75, 76] and Cook and Fields.[77]

Index

Note: Page numbers in *italics* refer to illustrations; page numbers followed by t indicate tables.

Unloading, using braces, after lateral, posterolateral graft reconstruction, 178, *182*
with cartilage repair, 84–86
using tape, for soft tissue inflammation, 215–216, *216*
Upper body ergometer (UBE), for conditioning, after anterior cruciate ligament reconstruction, 142
after posterior cruciate ligament reconstruction, 175
Utricle, 364

Valgus angle, physiologic, 308, *308, 309*
Valgus deformity, of forefoot, 309, *310*
measurement of, 315
of great toe, indications of, in clinical examination, 25t
of knee, 308, *309*
functional, due to abnormal foot pronation, 312
indications of, in clinical examination, 25t
of rearfoot, measurement of, 314–315
Valgus stress, medial soft tissue restraints to, in extension, 92, *92*
in flexion, 92, *92*
Valgus stress test, 29, *29*, 95–96, *95*
in posterolateral instability detection, 162
Varus deformity, of forefoot, 309–311, *310, 311*
measurement of, 315, *315*
of knee, 308, *309*
functional, due to abnormal foot supination, 313–314
indications of, in clinical examination, 25t
tibial osteotomy for, before lateral and posterolateral reconstruction, 184
using resorbable wedge, 75, *75, 76*, 84
of rearfoot, 313–314, *313*
measurement of, 314–315, *315*
of tibia, 25t
Varus stress test, 29–30, *30*
in posterolateral instability detection, 162
Vastus intermedius, 10, *11*
in patellar stabilization, 203
Vastus lateralis, 10, *11*, 12, *12*, 202
activity of, patellofemoral pain and, 206–207

Vastus lateralis *(Continued)*
in patellar stabilization, 203
Vastus medialis, 7, 8, 10–12, *11, 12*
in patellar stabilization, 203
Vastus medialis longus, 10
in patellar stabilization, 203
Vastus medialis obliquus, 10–12
activity of, patellofemoral pain and, 206–207
in patellar stabilization, 203
selective training of, for patellofemoral pain, 217–219, *218, 219*
Velocity, angular, in isokinetic evaluation, 56, 56t
Velocity spectrum rehabilitation protocol (VSRP), 282
Velocity spectrum testing, 293
Verbal feedback, in isokinetic evaluation, 56
Vertical box hopping, after anterior cruciate ligament reconstruction, 141
after posterior cruciate ligament reconstruction, 174
Vertical jump test, *165*, 330
Vertical kicking, in water, 424, *425*
Vestibular system, in postural control, 364
stimulation of, in balance training, 370
Viscosity of water, 414
resistance and, 414–415
Vision, disadvantaging techniques for, in balance training, 370
in postural control, 364
stimulation of, in balance training, 370
Visual analog pain scale, 25, 37
Visual feedback, in isokinetic evaluation, 55–56
Vitamin C, connective tissue repair and, 245
Vitamin E, connective tissue repair and, 245
Voshell's (anserine) bursa, 9, *9*, 89
VSRP (velocity spectrum rehabilitation protocol), 282

Walking, soldier, 418
tethered, in water, 419
Wall sitting, after anterior cruciate ligament reconstruction, 139–140
after posterior cruciate ligament reconstruction, 172–173
Wall slides, after anterior cruciate ligament reconstruction, 125, *126*

Warm-ups, in isokinetic evaluation, 55
Water, depth of, weight-bearing and, 415
exercise in. See *Aquatic exercise.*
in articular cartilage, 71, 387, 388, *390*
physical properties of, 412–415, *413–415*
temperature of, cardiovascular response to exercise and, 416–417
Wedge, resorbable, opening wedge tibial osteotomy using, 75, *75, 76*, 84
Weight, body. See also *Weight bearing; Weight shifting.*
ratio of peak torque to, in isokinetic dynamometry, 57, 57t
Weight bearing, after anterior cruciate ligament reconstruction, 124, 126, *127*, 136
after posterior cruciate ligament reconstruction, 170–171
assessment of posture in, in clinical examination, 25, 25t
in water exercise, water depth and, 415
Weight machines, advantages of, 140
after anterior cruciate ligament reconstruction, 140
after posterior cruciate ligament reconstruction, 173
Weight shifting, for balance training, after anterior cruciate ligament reconstruction, 140
after posterior cruciate ligament reconstruction, 173
in reactive neuromuscular training, 372–373, *373, 374*
lateral bounding with, 382, *382*
lunge with, 377–378
squat with, 376
stationary running with, 380–381, *380*
Weight training. See also *Strength training.*
plyometric training alternating with, 330
Winslow's ligament, *8*, 9
Women. See *Female athlete.*
Work, in isokinetic dynamometry, 58–59
Work-to-rest ratio, in plyometric training, 329
Wrisberg's ligament, 5, 195. See also *Meniscofemoral ligaments.*
function of, 16, 186